Nephrology
In 30 Days

Notice

Nephrology

In 30 Days

ROBERT F. REILLY, JR., M.D.

Frederic L. Coe Professor of Nephrolithiasis Research in Mineral Metabolism
Chief, Section of Nephrology
Veterans Administration North Texas Health Care System
Professor of Medicine
Department of Medicine
The Charles and Jane Pak Center for Mineral Metabolism and Clinical Research
The University of Texas Southwestern Medical Center at Dallas
Dallas, Texas

MARK A. PERAZELLA, M.D., F.A.C.P.

Associate Professor of Medicine
Director, Renal Fellowship Program
Director, Acute Dialysis Services
Section of Nephrology
Department of Medicine
Yale University School of Medicine
New Haven, Connecticut

McGraw-Hill
Medical Publishing Division

New York   Chicago   San Francisco   Lisbon   London   Madrid   Mexico City   Milan
New Delhi   San Juan   Seoul   Singapore   Sydney   Toronto

Nephrology in 30 Days

Copyright © 2005 by The McGraw-Hill Companies, Inc. All rights reserved. Printed in the United States of America. Except as permitted under the United States Copyright Act of 1976, no part of this publication may be reproduced or distributed in any form or by any means, or stored in a database or retrieval system, without the prior written permission of the publisher.

3 4 5 6 7 8 9 0   DOC/DOC   0 9 8 7

ISBN 0-07-143701-0

This book was set in Garamond by International Typesetting and Composition.
The editors were James Shanahan and Robert Pancotti.
The production supervisor was Rick Ruzycka.
Project management was provided by International Typesetting and Composition.
The indexer was Roger Wall.
RR Donnelley was printer and binder.

This book is printed on acid-free paper.

Library of Congress Cataloging-in-Publication Data

Reilly, Robert F., M.D.
   Nephrology in 30 days / Robert F. Reilly Jr., Mark A. Perazella.
      p. ; cm.
   Includes bibliographical references and index.
   ISBN 0-07-143701-0 (alk. paper)
   1. Nephrology. 2. Kidneys—Diseases. I. Title: Nephrology in thirty days. II. Perazella, Mark A. III. Title.
   [DNLM: 1. Kidney Diseases. 2. Metabolic Diseases. WJ 300 R3626n 2005]
RC902.R363 2005
616.6′1—dc22

                                                                    2004055997

To my wife Sheli,
my parents Robert Sr. and Nancy,
my son Rob, and
my brothers Steven and Fred
whose help and support are invaluable
in both my life and career.

Robert F. Reilly, Jr.

To my parents Joe and Santina Perazella
who sacrificed much to educate me,
to my brothers Joe and Scott
for their encouragement,
to my wife Donna
who wholeheartedly supported
my efforts in this endeavor, and
to my boys Mark and Andrew
who gave up their time with me.

Mark A. Perazella

Contents

Contributors

Richard Formica, M.D.
Assistant Professor of Medicine and Surgery
Director, Transplant Nephrology
Co-Director, Outpatient Transplant Service
Section of Nephrology
Department of Medicine
Yale University School of Medicine
New Haven, Connecticut

Dinkar Kaw, M.D.
Assistant Professor of Medicine
Division of Nephrology
Department of Medicine
Medical College of Ohio
Toledo, Ohio

Aldo J. Peixoto, M.D.
Associate Professor of Medicine
Section of Nephrology
Department of Medicine
Yale University School of Medicine
Director, Hypertension Clinic
Veterans Affairs Connecticut Healthcare System
West Haven Campus
West Haven, Connecticut

Mark A. Perazella, M.D., F.A.C.P.
Associate Professor of Medicine
Director, Renal Fellowship Program
Director, Acute Dialysis Services
Section of Nephrology
Department of Medicine
Yale University School of Medicine
New Haven, Connecticut

Robert F. Reilly, Jr., M.D.
Frederic L. Coe Professor of Nephrolithiasis
  Research in Mineral Metabolism
Chief, Section of Nephrology
Veterans Administration North Texas Health
  Care System
Professor of Medicine
Department of Medicine
The Charles and Jane Pak Center for Mineral
  Metabolism and Clinical Research
The University of Texas Southwestern Medical
  Center at Dallas
Dallas, Texas

Sergio F. F. Santos, M.D., Ph.D.
Associate Professor of Medicine (Nephrology)
Nephrology Division
State University of Rio de Janeiro
Rio de Janeiro, Brazil

Joseph I. Shapiro, M.D.
Mercy Health Partners Education Professor
Chairman, Department of Medicine
Professor of Medicine and Pharmacology
Medical College of Ohio
Toledo, Ohio

Youngsook Yoon, M.D.
Assistant Professor of Medicine
Division of Pulmonary and Critical Care Medicine
Department of Medicine
Medical College of Ohio
Toledo, Ohio

Preface

Nephrology is a discipline that combines basic science and clinical disease. Recent times have seen a narrowing of the gap between basic and clinical science, bringing the "research bench to the patient's bedside." As a result, a better understanding of clinical disease states has been achieved. Perhaps more than any other subspecialty of medicine, kidney disease has no specialty boundaries. One such example includes the patient with diabetic nephropathy who manifests end-organ disease requiring expert care from the nephrologist, internist, cardiologist, endocrinologist, emergency medicine physician, vascular surgeon, intensivist, podiatrist, ophthalmologist, interventional radiologist, and renal transplantation surgeon. It is imperative, therefore, that physicians early in their training as medical students, physician assistants, house officers, and subspecialty fellows gain a solid understanding of basic aspects of nephrology. Kidney disease, disturbances of fluid and electrolyte balance, and disorders of acid-base and mineral metabolism homeostasis can be confusing to many trainees and non-nephrology physicians. This book was conceived to remove that confusion. *Nephrology in 30 Days* provides a comprehensive and concise text for physicians in training and practitioners.

This textbook is an ideal tool for health care providers to attain rapidly a complete understanding of the basics of nephrology, allowing an *educated approach* to diagnosis and management of kidney disease and its associated complications. As the title suggests, those who read the book will gain this knowledge within 30 days. Such a time frame is ideal for medical students, physician assistants, and medical residents rotating on the clinical nephrology service elective.

The book will be a foundation on which they can build by intelligently using other sources of information such as primary literature from journals and more detailed reference textbooks. It will also serve as an efficient resource for non-nephrology practitioners in internal medicine and other fields of medicine and surgery.

Nephrology in 30 Days is broken down into three major sections. The first section discusses electrolyte and acid-base disturbances. Experts in the field review disorders of sodium and potassium balance, use of intravenous fluids, pathogenesis and treatment of diuretic resistance, and respiratory and metabolic acidosis/alkalosis. The second section deals primarily with disturbances of mineral metabolism. Concise discussions on calcium, phosphate, and magnesium homeostasis are presented. Clinical disease states associated with these divalent disorders are reviewed, as are the pathogenesis and treatment of nephrolithiasis. The last section is dedicated to structural kidney disease. Acute renal failure and chronic kidney disease are explored separately. Aspects of urinalysis and examination of the urine sediment are reviewed. Diseases of various structures within the kidney are also examined. Included are the glomerulopathies, both primary and those due to systemic processes, tubulointerstitial diseases, and abnormalities of the urinary tract including infection and obstruction. Finally, essential hypertension and secondary causes of hypertension are reviewed. Importantly, renal imaging and genetic causes of kidney disease are covered within each of the chapters where they figure prominently.

Homer Smith in his book *From Fish to Philosopher* stated "What engineer, wishing to regulate the composition of the internal environment of the body on which the function of every bone, gland, muscle, and nerve depends, would devise a scheme that operated by throwing the whole thing out sixteen times a day—and rely on grabbing from it, as it fell to earth, only those precious elements which he wanted to keep?" Hopefully, after reading this book the reader will begin to comprehend the wonderful complexity and ingenuity of the engineer that is the kidney.

Acknowledgments

I wish to thank Drs. Peter Igarashi, Peter Aronson, David Ellison, Gary Desir, Asghar Rastegar, Norman Siegel, Herbert Chase, John Forrest, John Hayslett, Robert Schrier, Allen Alfrey, Laurence Chan, and Tomas Berl who served as mentors and teachers during my career. I would also like to thank Gregory Fitz, Clark Gregg, Charles Pak, Orson Moe, and Khashayar Sakhaee for their help in recruiting me to my current position. Dr. Perazella and I would also like to express our sincere appreciation and gratitude to our contributors for their prompt and outstanding contributions, as well as Dr. Michael Kashgarian (Pathology Department, Yale University School of Medicine) for kindly providing many of the images of renal biopsy specimens and Drs. Arthur Rosenfield and Leslie Scoutt (Diagnostic Radiology Department, Yale University School of Medicine) for the ultrasound and CT images. Thanks to Jim Shanahan of McGraw-Hill for his outstanding efforts on behalf of the book. I would also like to thank the patients, medical students, house officers, and nephrology fellows who I have cared for, trained, and learned from over the years.

Robert F. Reilly, Jr.

I wish to thank Dr. Robert Reilly who had the vision to conceive this book and encouraged my role as a coeditor. I would like to extend my gratitude to the too numerous to name former and current mentors and colleagues who shaped my career in medicine and nephrology—they know who they are and I thank them all. Many thanks to Jim Shanahan of McGraw-Hill as publication of this book would not have been possible without his support. Finally, I would like to extend my most sincere thanks to the medical students, house officers, and in particular clinical nephrology fellows (Dinna Cruz, Tony Cayco, Aldo Peixoto, Raj Alappan, James Wood, Chris Cosgrove, Kory Tray, Marc Ciampi, Ursula Brewster, and Brian Rifkin) who I have had the distinct honor to train and who in the process, have also taught me a great deal.

Mark A. Perazella

Nephrology
In 30 Days

Introduction

Recommended Time to Complete: 1 day

Guiding Questions

1. What are the essential functions of the kidney?
2. The nephron is the basic unit of the kidney. What are its major components?
3. How does the glomerular capillary loop prevent the filtration of macromolecules?
4. What factors are integral to the formation of glomerular ultrafiltrate?
5. How is glomerular filtration rate (GFR) regulated in normal subjects on a day-to-day basis?
6. What factors maintain renal perfusion and GFR during states of severe intravascular volume depletion?
7. How is GFR best measured in the clinical setting?
8. Are there accurate estimates of GFR that can substitute for a 24-hour urine collection?

Introduction

The kidney is designed to perform a number of essential functions. First, it contributes importantly to the maintenance of the extracellular environment that is essential for normal cellular function. The kidney achieves an optimal extracellular environment through excretion of waste products such as urea, creatinine, uric acid, and other substances. Balanced excretion of water and electrolytes is another important role of the kidney. Second, the kidney regulates systemic and renal hemodynamics through the production

1

of various hormones, as well as the regulation of salt and water balance. Hormones such as renin, angiotensin II (AII), prostaglandins (PGs), endothelin, nitric oxide, adenosine, and bradykinin regulate vascular reactivity and renal blood flow. Third, the kidney produces other hormones that influence various end organ functions. Red blood cell production is stimulated by renal erythropoietin synthesis, which is controlled by a highly regulated oxygen sensor in the proximal nephron. Hence the kidney can be viewed as a "critmeter." Bone metabolism is influenced by renal production of calcitriol, as well as proper balance of calcium and phosphorus. Finally, the kidney participates in gluconeogenesis during fasting to prevent hypoglycemia. It also contributes to the catabolism of various peptide hormones filtered by the glomerulus such as insulin.

In order to perform these functions, the kidney is uniquely constructed to filter, reabsorb, and secrete a variety of substances in a very precise manner through integrated regulation of renal hemodynamics and tubular handling of water and solutes. Secretion of hormones such as erythropoietin and calcitriol closely link kidney function with control of red cell mass and bone metabolism. Metabolism of peptide hormones and clearance of medications is another important kidney function to maintain health. Disturbances in these processes lead to several harmful and potentially life-threatening clinical syndromes.

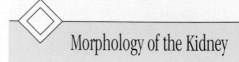

Morphology of the Kidney

Gross examination of the kidney reveals an outer portion, the cortex, and inner portion, the medulla (Figure 1.1). Blood is supplied to the kidney via the renal artery (or arteries) and is drained via the renal vein. As will be discussed next, the glomeruli, which are the filtering units of the nephron, are found within the cortex. Tubules are located in both cortex and medulla. The medulla consists of an inner and outer stripe. Collecting tubules form a large part of the inner medulla and papilla. Urine is formed by glomerular filtration and modified by the tubules, leaves the collecting ducts and drains sequentially into the calyces, renal pelvis, ureter, and finally into the bladder.

The nephron is the basic unit of the kidney. There are approximately 1.0–1.3 million nephrons in the normal adult kidney. The nephron consists of a glomerulus and a series of tubules (Figure 1.2). The glomerulus is composed of a tuft of capillaries with a unique vascular supply. Glomerular capillaries are interposed between an afferent and efferent arteriole. They reside in the cortex and corticomedullary junction. Within the tubular lumen, glomerular filtrate is modified by tubular cells. Tubules are lined by a continuous layer of epithelial cells, each of which possesses

KEY POINTS

Functions of the Kidney

1. The kidney maintains the extracellular environment through excretion of waste products and proper electrolyte and water balance.
2. Several hormones are produced in the kidney that act to control renal hemodynamics, stimulate red cell production, and maintain normal bone homeostasis.

Figure 1.1

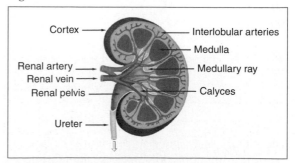

Anatomy of the kidney. Shown are the cortex, medulla, calyces, renal pelvis, and ureter.

Figure 1.2

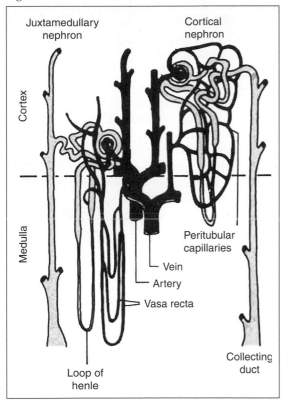

The nephron. The nephron consists of a glomerulus and series of tubules. Nephrons can be subdivided into those in the cortex and those in the juxtamedullary region. The glomerulus is composed of a capillary tuft interposed between the afferent and efferent arteriole. Tubules are supplied by a peritubular capillary network that includes the vasa recta, which runs parallel to the loop of Henle.

characteristic morphology and function depending on its location in the nephron.

An ultrafiltrate of plasma is formed by the glomerulus and passes into the tubules where it is modified by reabsorption (removal of a substance from the ultrafiltrate) and secretion (addition of a substance to the ultrafiltrate). Different tubular segments alter fluid contents by varying reabsorption and secretion. Division of the nephron is based on morphology, as well as permeability and transport characteristics of the segments. For example, the proximal tubule and loop of Henle reabsorb the bulk of filtered water and solutes. In the distal nephron, and particularly in collecting tubules, fine adjustments in urinary composition are undertaken. Also, there is heterogeneity of cell types within the cortical collecting tubule. In this segment, the principal cell reabsorbs sodium and secretes potassium while the intercalated cell secretes hydrogen ion and reabsorbs potassium.

The formation of urine occurs as glomerular filtrate is sequentially modified in tubular segments. Plasma is ultrafiltered by the glomerulus and passes from Bowman's space into the proximal tubule. This nephron segment consists anatomically of an initial convoluted segment, followed by a straight segment, the pars recta, that enters the outer medulla. The loop of Henle, which possesses a hairpin configuration, follows the pars recta and includes a thin descending limb, and thin and thick ascending limb. The loop of Henle is not uniform in its length. Approximately 40% are short loops that don't enter the medulla or enter only the outer medulla. These loops do not have a thin ascending limb and are located predominantly in the outer cortex. The remaining loops of Henle are long and extend into the medulla and may reach the inner medulla and papilla. Long loops are located in the juxtamedullary region. Both short and long loops are found in the midcortex.

The thick ascending limb of the loop of Henle has a cortical segment that returns to its own glomerulus. This tubule, which has specialized epithelial cells known as the macula densa, approximates the afferent arteriole, forming the juxtaglomerular (JG) apparatus. As will be discussed later, the JG apparatus participates importantly in regulation of GFR.

Four cortical tubular segments follow the macula densa. They are the distal convoluted tubule, the connecting tubule, the initial collecting tubule, and the cortical collecting tubule. The connecting tubule drains into a single cortical collecting tubule, which then connects to the medullary collecting tubule. In cortex, initial collecting tubules drain into collecting ducts, whereas deeper connecting tubules join to form an arcade that drains into a cortical collecting tubule. From this segment, urine drains into the calyces, renal pelvis, ureters, and bladder.

Morphology of the Kidney

1. On gross examination, the kidney is composed of cortex, inner and outer medulla, calyces, pelvis, and ureter.
2. The nephron is the basic unit of the kidney. It is composed of a glomerulus and a series of tubules.
3. The tubules are divided into proximal tubule, loop of Henle, distal convoluted tubule, connecting tubule, initial collecting tubule, and cortical and medullary collecting tubule.
4. Following modification of the glomerular ultrafiltrate by the tubules, urine is sequentially drained into the calyces, renal pelvis, ureter, and bladder.

Renal Circulation

Renal blood flow exceeds most other organs and, on average, the kidneys receive approximately 20% of the cardiac output. This calculates to approximately 1 L/minute of blood and 600 mL of plasma. Of this, 20% of plasma is filtered into Bowman's space, giving a filtration rate of approximately 120 mL/minute. Renal arteries carry blood into the kidney where it passes through serial branches, which include the interlobar, arcuate, and interlobular arteries. Blood enters the glomerulus through the afferent arteriole. A plasma ultrafiltrate is formed within the capillary tuft and passes into Bowman's space. Blood remaining in the capillaries exits the glomerulus via the efferent arteriole. In the cortex, blood in postglomerular capillaries flows adjacent

to the tubules, while branches from the efferent arterioles of juxtamedullary glomeruli enter the medulla and form the vasa recta capillaries. Blood exits the kidney through a venous system into the systemic circulation.

The circulatory anatomy within the kidney determines the final urine composition. First, GFR importantly influences the amount of solute and water that is excreted. Second, peritubular capillaries in cortex modify proximal tubular reabsorption and secretion of solutes and water. They also return reabsorbed solutes and water to the systemic circulation. Third, creation of the countercurrent gradient for water conservation is dependent on vasa recta capillary function. These capillaries also return reabsorbed salt and water to the systemic circulation.

Renal Circulation

1. The kidney receives 20% of the cardiac output or 1 L of blood per minute.
2. Renal circulatory anatomy allows precise modulation of salt and water balance.

Glomerular Anatomy

As stated previously, the glomerulus is comprised of a capillary network with an afferent and efferent arteriolar circulation. This design sets the glomerular circulation apart from other organ systems and allows modification of urine composition to meet the demands of various, often extreme diets. The glomerular capillary tuft sits within the parietal epithelial cell space, known as Bowman's capsule. The parietal epithelium is continuous with the visceral epithelial cells (podocytes), which cover the glomerular capillary tuft. The glomerular capillary loop is comprised of endothelial cell, glomerular basement membrane (GBM), and podocyte, all of which are supported structurally by mesangial cells. The GBM consists of a fusion of endothelial and visceral epithelial cell basement membrane components, which include type IV collagen, laminin, nidogen, and heparan sulfate proteoglycans. It functions to maintain normal glomerular architecture, anchor adjacent cells, and restrict passage of various macromolecules. The podocyte is attached to the GBM by discrete foot processes, which have pores containing slit diaphragms. The slit diaphragm is a thin membrane that acts as the final filtration barrier.

Glomerular Filtration

A key function of the glomerulus is to act as a filtration barrier that permits the passage of water and other solutes and restricts the movement of certain molecules. For example, filtration of water, sodium, urea, and creatinine are integral to proper toxin clearance, volume balance, and electrolyte homeostasis. In contrast, restriction of filtration of large proteins (albumin, immunoglobulin G) prevents the development of hypoalbuminemia, negative nitrogen balance, and infection. The glomerular capillary wall restricts solute movement by using both size and charge selectivity.

Size selectivity is maintained by GBM and podocyte foot process slit diaphragms. The GBM contributes to size selectivity through the creation of functional pores present in the spaces between the cords of type IV collagen. Two populations of pores are present in glomerular capillary wall: a more common small pore (radius 42 Å) and a less numerous larger pore (70 Å). Other capillary loop elements, however, provide additional size selectivity. This is known because isolated GBM studies demonstrate more permeability in GBM than intact glomerulus, suggesting an important role of glomerular epithelial cells. Also, molecules that pass through the GBM are restricted from passage into Bowman's space by epithelial slit diaphragms. A number of podocyte proteins (nephrin, podocin, synaptopodin, podocalyxin, α-actin 3) interact to form the slit diaphragms and maintain podocyte integrity as a filtration barrier.

Mutation in genes that synthesize these proteins, as well as effacement of foot processes by disease states, is associated with filtration barrier loss and the development of proteinuria. Glomerular endothelial cells, however, contribute very little to size selectivity, as their fenestrae are wide and do not restrict macromolecules until they reach a radius larger than 375 Å.

Macromolecule filtration is also prevented by charge selectivity. Electrostatic repulsion is created by anionic sites in the GBM and endothelial cell fenestrae. Heparan sulfate proteoglycans, which are synthesized by glomerular endothelial and epithelial cells, provide the bulk of negative charge. The charge barrier was first noted when the differential effect of similar-sized dextrans with various charges (neutral, cationic, anionic) on filtration was noted. Neutral and cationic dextrans undergo greater filtration than anionic dextrans, despite similar molecular weight (Figure 1.3). This finding supports a glomerular charge barrier. In humans, albumin is restricted from filtration

Figure 1.3

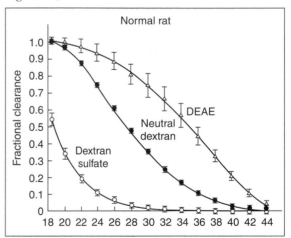

Filtration curves for neutral, cationic (DEAE), and anionic dextrans (dextran sulfate). The curves show that filtration of anionic dextrans is impeded by negative charge in the glomerular capillary wall supporting the conclusion that the glomerular capillary wall impedes protein movement via a charge and size barrier. (From Brenner, B.M., Bohrer, M.P., Baylis, C., and Deen, W.M. *Kidney Int* 12:229–237, 1977, with permission.)

based on both size and charge selectivity. When glomerular injury occurs, impairment of both size and charge selectivity results. An increased number of larger pores, the development of rents and cavities in the GBM, and a defect in charge selectivity allow proteinuria in diseases such as membranous nephropathy, diabetic nephropathy, and focal glomerulosclerosis. Loss of charge selectivity plays a major role in the protein leak that occurs with minimal change disease, although loss of size selectivity may contribute. It is interesting to note that small solute and water clearance are impaired in this setting, likely due to loss of capillary surface area, while protein losses continue through large pores unimpeded because of loss of anionic charge repulsion.

Other Glomerular Functions

In addition to filtration, the glomerulus has other roles in the kidney. Endothelial cells secrete hormones (endothelin, prostacyclin, and nitric oxide) that influence vasomotor tone in the renal circulation. They also participate in inflammation by expressing adhesion molecules that enhance inflammatory cell accumulation. Glomerular epithelial cells remove macromolecules that penetrate the GBM and enter the subepithelial space. As noted previously, they synthesize key components of the GBM.

An area of the glomerulus not discussed previously but nonetheless an important member of the glomerular architecture is the mesangium. Two cell types comprise the mesangium. The mesangial cell has contractile properties that originate from its smooth muscle-like microfilaments. It can also synthesize PGs and react to AII. These properties make the mesangial cell ideally suited to regulate glomerular hemodynamics through changes in glomerular capillary surface area and in the vasomotor tone of the renal microcirculation. Mesangial cells are also involved in immune-mediated glomerular diseases. They produce various cytokines (interleukin [IL]-1, IL-6, chemokines) and proliferate following exposure to platelet

derived growth factor (PDGF) and epithelial growth factor (EGF), leading to mesangial hypercellularity and matrix expansion, as well as glomerular injury. Circulating macrophages and monocytes that enter and exit the mesangium constitute the second cell type. They function primarily as phagocytes to remove macromolecules that cannot pass through the GBM and remain in the capillary wall. They may also, however, contribute to inflammation in immune-mediated diseases.

KEY POINTS
Glomerular Anatomy

1. The glomerular capillary loop is comprised of an endothelial cell and epithelial cell (podocyte) whose basement membranes fuse to form a common GBM.
2. Both size and charge selectivity restrict passage of macromolecules into Bowman's space. Loss of either of these from disease processes results in proteinuria.
3. Size selectivity is determined by the GBM and, most importantly, the podocyte slit diaphragm.
4. Charge selectivity is anionic and provided by heparan sulfate proteoglycans in GBM and endothelial cell fenestrae.
5. Mesangial cells modulate glomerular hemodynamics and participate in phagocytic functions.

Glomerular Filtration Rate

Urine formation requires that an initial separation of ultrafiltrate from plasma occurs across the glomerular capillary wall into Bowman's space. The major determinant of ultrafiltrate formation is

Starling's forces across the capillary wall. These forces are proportional to glomerular capillary permeability and the balance between hydraulic and oncotic pressure gradients. Thus, GFR can be described by the following formulas:

$$GFR = (capillary\ porosity \times surface\ area)$$
$$\times (\Delta\ hydraulic\ pressure$$
$$- \Delta\ oncotic\ pressure)$$

$$GFR = (capillary\ porosity \times surface\ area)$$
$$\times ([P_{GC} - P_{Bs}] - s[\pi_p - \pi_{bs}])$$

$$GFR = (capillary\ porosity \times surface\ area)$$
$$\times (P_{GC} - P_{Bs} - \pi_p)$$

where P_{GC} and P_{Bs} are the hydraulic pressures in glomerular capillary and Bowman's space, respectively. Also, s is the reflection coefficient of proteins across the capillary wall (a measure of permeability) and $\pi_p - \pi_{Bs}$ are the oncotic pressure of plasma in glomerular capillaries and Bowman's space, respectively. Since π_{Bs} is zero (the filtrate is essentially protein free) and the capillary wall is completely permeable (making $s = 1$), the last equation $GFR = (capillary\ porosity \times surface\ area) \times (P_{GC} - P_{Bs} - \pi_p)$ represents the formula for GFR. In general, hydraulic pressure in the capillaries and Bowman's space remains constant while oncotic pressure in plasma rises progressively with formation of a protein-free ultrafiltrate. Thus, at some point along the capillary loop, the net filtration gradient falls to zero and filtration equilibrium occurs (Table 1.1). In contrast to other primates, humans only require a net gradient favoring filtration of approximately 4 mmHg to maintain glomerular filtration. It is also notable that plasma oncotic pressure entering the efferent arteriole and peritubular capillary is elevated, an effect that increases peritubular capillary oncotic pressure and enhances proximal tubular fluid and sodium reabsorption.

As one can see from examining the GFR equation, alterations in renal plasma flow rate (RPF) or any of the factors noted in the formula above can change the GFR. RPF is an important determinant of GFR in the presence of filtration equilibrium, as it influences glomerular capillary oncotic pressure. Thus, GFR rises or falls in proportion to

Table 1.1

Determinants of Glomerular Filtration (Primates)

	GLOMERULAR PRESSURES (MMHG)	
	AFFERENT ARTERIOLE	EFFERENT ARTERIOLE
Hydraulic pressure		
Capillary	46	45
Interstitium	10	10
Mean gradient	36	35
Oncotic pressure		
Capillary	23	35
Interstitium	0	0
Mean gradient	23	35
Mean gradient favoring filtration	+13	0
	(mean = +6 mmHg)	

changes in RPF. Due to the unique design of the glomerulus, capillary hydrostatic pressure is influenced by variables such as the aortic (renal artery) pressure, as well as afferent and efferent arteriolar resistances. Resistance in these vessels is controlled by a combination of myogenic control, tubuloglomerular feedback (TGF) from the macula densa, and vasodilatory/vasoconstrictor hormones (AII, norepinephrine, PGs, endothelin, atrial natriuretic peptide [ANP], nitric oxide). Changes in resistance of these arterioles have opposite effects on P_{GC} and thus allows rapid regulation of P_{GC} and GFR. For example, an increase in afferent arteriolar resistance decreases P_{GC} and GFR, while an increase in efferent resistance increases both. In addition, arteriolar tone affects RPF. An increase in the resistance of either glomerular arteriole will elevate total renal resistance and diminish RPF. Thus, the afferent arteriole regulates RPF and GFR in parallel, while the efferent arteriole regulates them inversely. This will determine the direction of change in the filtration fraction (FF), which is the fraction of RPF that is filtered across the glomerulus (FF = GFR/RPF). Changes in efferent tone change the filtration fraction, whereas changes in afferent tone do not. GFR can then increase, not change or decrease based on the magnitude of efferent constriction.

To be complete, factors considered less important in the regulation of GFR than the systemic arterial pressure, arteriolar tone, and RPF are noted below. In health, changes in capillary permeability are typically minimal and have no effect on GFR. Severe glomerular injury, however, can reduce permeability and impair GFR. Reductions in the capillary surface area by disease (glomerulonephritis) or vasoactive hormones (AII, antidiuretic hormone, PGs) can develop. These effects lead to a net decline in GFR. Alterations in hydrostatic pressure in Bowman's space, as occurs with complete urinary tract or tubular obstruction, initially reduces GFR through an elevation in hydrostatic pressure. Finally, increasing plasma oncotic pressure may counter hydrostatic pressure and reduce GFR. Clinical examples are therapy with hypertonic mannitol and severe intravascular volume depletion with marked hemoconcentration.

KEY POINTS

Glomerular Filtration Rate

> 1. Formation of glomerular ultrafiltrate is dependent on glomerular capillary permeability and the balance between hydrostatic and oncotic pressure gradients.
> 2. Arterial pressure, RPF, and afferent and efferent arteriolar tone importantly influence GFR.
> 3. Changes in resistance of afferent and efferent arterioles have opposite effects on P_{GC}. This allows rapid regulation of GFR.

Regulation of RPF and GFR

Regulation of GFR (and RPF) occurs primarily through changes in arteriolar resistance. In the normal host, autoregulation and TGF interact to maintain RPF and GFR at a constant level. In disease states such as true or effective volume depletion, however, these two intrarenal processes contribute minimally and are superseded by actions of systemic neurohormonal factors. A more detailed description of the regulation of renal hemodynamics follows.

Autoregulation

Autoregulation of the renal circulation serves the purpose of maintaining a relatively constant RPF and GFR. Since GFR is determined primarily by P_{GC}, variations in arterial perfusion pressure would be expected to promote large changes in GFR. The phenomenon of autoregulation, however, prevents large swings in RPF and GFR expected from changes in arterial perfusion pressure. Changes in afferent arteriolar tone likely play a major role in autoregulation, since RPF and GFR vary in parallel (versus changes in efferent tone where RPF and GFR vary inversely). An increase in afferent arteriolar tone prevents the transmission of high arterial pressures to the glomerulus, while low arterial pressure is associated with reduced afferent arteriolar tone. These changes in afferent tone maintain the P_{GC} and GFR constant despite swings in perfusion pressure. In general, autoregulation maintains GFR constant until either the mean arterial pressure exceeds 70 mmHg or falls below 40–50 mmHg.

Myogenic stretch receptors in the afferent arteriolar walls are thought to play an important part in renal autoregulation. Increased wall stretch with high arterial pressure promotes vasoconstriction, perhaps mediated by enhanced cell calcium entry. The absence of voltage-gated calcium channels in efferent arterioles supports the less important or nonexistent role of this arteriole in autoregulation.

Tubuloglomerular Feedback

Changes in GFR are also mediated by alterations in tubular flow rate sensed by the macula densa. Specialized cells in the macula densa, located at the end of the thick ascending limb of Henle, sense changes in tubular fluid chloride entry into the cell. Increases in renal perfusion pressure are associated with an increase in GFR, which is associated with enhanced sodium chloride delivery to the macula densa. To counterbalance this increase in GFR, macula densa cells send signals to the afferent arteriole that promote vasoconstriction. This reduces P_{GC} and returns GFR toward normal and reduces sodium chloride delivery to the macula densa. In contrast, reduced sodium chloride delivery to the macula densa, as occurs with prerenal azotemia, has the opposite effect—afferent arteriolar vasodilatation occurs and GFR increases. This phenomenon is called tubuloglomerular feedback.

The mediator(s) of TGF are not well understood. It is likely that multiple factors act to mediate the signal to the afferent arteriole. Factors that play a role include AII (more as a permissive role), adenosine, thromboxane, and nitric oxide. Adenosine and thromboxane increase when excessive chloride entry is sensed by the macula densa, thereby constricting the afferent arteriole. These substances are reduced when chloride delivery is low, allowing afferent arteriolar vasodilatation. Nitric oxide is also thought to modulate the TGF response to sodium chloride delivery, allowing TGF to be reset by variations in salt intake. For example, low sodium chloride delivery increases nitric oxide, whereas increased sodium chloride delivery reduces nitric oxide.

Neurohumoral Factors

Daily maintenance of renal hemodynamics in normal hosts is subserved primarily by autoregulation and TGF. These factors also participate in regulation of GFR in disease states such as renal artery stenosis (low renal perfusion) and hypertension (increased renal perfusion). In more severe states, however, the sympathetic nervous system (SNS), renin-angiotensin-aldosterone system (RAAS), as well as other vasoconstrictor (endothelin), and vasodilator (prostaglandins, nitric oxide) substances are produced. For example, severe intravascular volume depletion, whether true (vomiting) or effective (congestive heart failure), stimulates the production of catecholamines and the RAAS to maintain circulatory integrity. The net renal effect of an outpouring of these mediators varies based on the severity of the initiating disease process, the degree of stimulation of neurohumoral substances, and other coexisting processes. Stimulation of both the SNS and RAAS reduces renal perfusion pressure but may have no net effect on GFR. As an example, the patient with congestive heart failure who has this type of neurohumoral response maintains relatively normal GFR because the afferent arteriolar constriction induced by the SNS is balanced by the preferential constriction of the efferent arteriole by AII. Also, renal vasoconstriction is balanced by the production of vasodilatory substances such as PGs (PGE_2, PGI_2) and nitric oxide. Administration of an inhibitor of PG synthesis (nonsteroidal anti-inflammatory drugs) tips the balance in favor of vasoconstriction and reduced GFR. Severe states of volume depletion (i.e., hypovolemic and cardiogenic shock) will overcome all attempts by the body at preservation of renal perfusion, resulting in severe renal ischemia and renal failure.

KEY POINTS
Regulation of RPF and GFR

1. Autoregulation and TGF regulate minute-to-minute changes in GFR by modulating afferent arteriolar tone.
2. Neurohumoral substances, such as the SNS, RAAS, nitric oxide, PGs, and endothelin influence GFR in disease states that disturb intravascular volume status.

Clinical Assessment of GFR

Measurement of GFR is essential to the management of patients with kidney disease. Functioning renal mass is best assessed by measuring total kidney GFR, a reflection of the sum of filtration rates of functioning nephron units. Serial GFR measurement allows identification of kidney disease, progression (or improvement) of kidney dysfunction, appropriate drug dosing, and initiation of dialysis when renal failure supervenes. To measure GFR precisely, the substance employed as a marker should be freely filtered by the glomerulus and not reabsorbed, secreted, or metabolized by the kidney. The following formula is used to measure GFR:

$$GFR = \frac{\text{urine concentration A} \times \text{volume}}{\text{plasma concentration A}}$$

where A is the substance that meets the criteria as an ideal marker. The compound that is the best marker of GFR is inulin. Because of its characteristics, inulin clearance accurately reflects GFR. Inulin is not employed as a clinical marker of GFR, however, because it requires intravenous infusion, most clinical laboratories are unable to assay inulin, and it is expensive. Thus, other less optimal markers are employed to measure GFR. They are briefly reviewed.

Creatinine

Endogenously produced creatinine is the marker most commonly employed to measure GFR. Creatinine is produced from the metabolism of skeletal muscle creatine. It is released into plasma at a stable rate in normal subjects and freely filtered at the glomerulus. Unfortunately, creatinine also enters urine via secretion by the organic cation transporter in proximal tubule, overestimating GFR by 10–20%. As kidney function declines, the rate of tubular creatinine secretion increases. In this circumstance creatinine clearance may overestimate true GFR. Administration of cimetidine, which competitively blocks tubular cell creatinine secretion, enhances the accuracy of this test while combining creatinine and urea clearance gives a close estimate of GFR. Nonetheless, creatinine clearance is widely employed in clinical practice. It is calculated by the following formula

that uses a serum sample for creatinine concentration and a 24-hour urine specimen for creatinine concentration and urine volume:

$$CrCl = \frac{UCr \times \text{volume}}{Scr}$$

where Cr is creatinine, Cl is clearance, U is urine, and S is serum. In addition to the inaccuracy of the creatinine clearance method to measure GFR, there are problems with patient collection (undercollection) of the urine sample.

Iothalamate

The inaccuracy of creatinine clearance stimulated a search for other more accurate markers for GFR. Radiolabeled iothalamate provides an accurate estimate of GFR. It correlates tightly with inulin clearance and is used in clinical studies to replace inulin as the marker of choice to assess GFR. As with inulin, however, iothalamate is not widely available in all centers for clinical practice. It is also expensive and somewhat cumbersome to employ.

GFR Estimates

Although serum creatinine concentration is used to assess kidney function, it is a poor marker of GFR. It is more useful when plotted as 1/serum creatinine, when used to follow changes in GFR over time. Serum creatinine concentration is inaccurate for various reasons (reviewed in Chapter 16) and alone is suboptimal to measure GFR. This is illustrated graphically in Figure 1.4. In both men and women serum creatinine concentration rises little as the GFR falls from 120 to 60 mL/minute. Large changes in GFR result in minimal changes in serum creatinine concentration largely due to the fact that creatinine secretion by renal tubules increases. Once GFR has declined to 40–60 mL/minute creatinine secretion cannot increase further and fairly small changes in GFR result in large changes in serum creatinine concentration. Because of this problem,

Figure 1.4

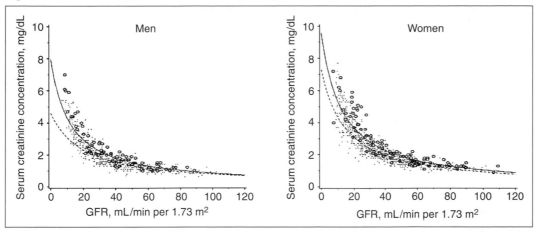

The relationship between serum creatinine concentration and GFR in men (A) and women (B). The relationship between serum creatinine concentration and GFR is not a linear one. Serum creatinine concentration is insensitive to changes in GFR within the range of GFRs between 60 and 120 mL/minute due to increasing tubular secretion. (From Levey, A.S., Bosch, J.P., Lewis, J.B., Greene, T., Rogers, N., Roth, D. *Ann Intern Med* 130:461–470, 1999, with permission.)

formulas were created using serum creatinine concentration, as well as other clinical and laboratory data to more accurately estimate GFR. These include the Cockcroft-Gault formula (estimates creatinine clearance) and both the full and abbreviated forms of the Modification of Diet in Renal Disease (MDRD) formula. These formulas are discussed in Chapter 16.

KEY POINTS
Clinical Assessment of GFR

1. The gold standard measurement of GFR is inulin clearance because of its characteristics as a substance that is freely filtered at the glomerulus and not secreted, reabsorbed, or metabolized in tubules.
2. Endogenous creatinine is employed to estimate GFR, but is inaccurate and overestimates GFR due to its secretion by proximal tubular cells via the organic cation transporter.
3. Iothalamate is an accurate marker but it has limited use in clinical practice.
4. Estimates of GFR using equations such as the Cockcroft-Gault and MDRD formulas are available.

Additional Reading

Abrahamson, D.R. Structure and development of the glomerular capillary wall and basement membrane. *Am J Physiol* 253:F783–F796, 1987.

Brewster, U.C., Perazella, M.A. The renin-angiotensin-aldosterone system and the kidney: effects on kidney disease. *Am J Med* 116:263–272, 2004.

Dworkin, L.D., Ichikawa I., Brenner, B.M. Hormonal modulation of glomerular function. *Am J Physiol* 244:F95–F111, 1983.

Guasch, A., Deen, W.M., Myers, B.D. Charge selectivity of the glomerular filtration barrier in healthy and nephrotic humans. *J Clin Invest* 92:2274–2289, 1993.

Levey, A.S., Bosch, J.P., Lewis, J.B., Greene, T., Rogers, N., Roth, D. A more accurate method to estimate glomerular filtration rate from serum creatinine: a new prediction equation. Modification of Diet in Renal Disease Study Group. *Ann Intern Med* 130:461–470, 1999.

Perrone, R.D., Steinman, T.I., Beck, G.J., Skibinski, C.I., Royal, H.D., Lawlor, M., Hunsicker, L.G. Utility of radioisotopic filtration markers in chronic renal insufficiency: simultaneous comparison of ^{125}I-iothalamate, [169]Yb-DTPA, [99]TC-DTPA, and inulin. *Am J Kidney Dis* 16:224–237, 1990.

Schnermann, J., Briggs, J.P. The macula densa is worth its salt. *J Clin Invest* 104:1007–1009, 1999.

Tischer, C.C., Madsen, K.M. Anatomy of the kidney. In: Brenner, B.M., Rector, F.C. (eds.), *The Kidney*, 4th ed. WB Saunders, Philadelphia, PA, 1991, p. 3.

Robert F. Reilly, Jr.

Disorders of Sodium Balance

Recommended Time to Complete: 2 days

Guiding Questions

1. How does the kidney regulate extracellular fluid (ECF) volume differently from sodium concentration?
2. What effector systems regulate renal sodium excretion?
3. What is effective arterial blood volume (EABV)?
4. Can you describe the forces involved in edema formation?
5. How does edema form in congestive heart failure (CHF), cirrhosis, and nephrotic syndrome?
6. What are the most common renal and extrarenal causes of total body sodium depletion?

Introduction

One of the more difficult concepts to grasp in nephrology is that disorders of ECF volume are the result of disturbances in sodium balance and that disorders of sodium concentration (hypo- and hypernatremia) are the result of disturbances in water balance. The control of ECF volume is dependent on the regulation of sodium balance. Sodium concentration alone is not reflective of ECF volume status. This is illustrated graphically by the cases in Figure 2.1. Patient A has diarrhea (Na concentration of diarrheal fluid is approximately 80 meq/L) but does not have free access to water and the ECF volume as a result is depleted

13

Figure 2.1

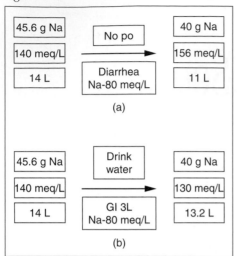

(a)

(b)

Sodium concentration does not reflect ECF volume status. Both of the patients shown have decreased ECF volume but in case A the serum sodium concentration is increased while in case B the serum sodium concentration is decreased. Abbreviations: po, by mouth; GI, gastrointestinal.

3 L from its starting point of 14 L. The serum sodium concentration rises to 156 meq/L. Patient B has an equivalent amount of diarrhea but is awake, alert, and has free access to water. Patient B drinks enough free water to increase the ECF volume from 11 to 13.2 L. Sodium losses in the diarrheal fluid coupled with free water replacement result in a serum sodium concentration of 130 meq/L. The serum sodium concentration is high in case A and low in case B, yet in both patients ECF volume is decreased. These cases illustrate that serum sodium concentration, in and of itself, does not provide information about the state of ECF volume. In both patients sensor mechanisms detect ECF volume depletion and effector mechanisms are activated to increase renal sodium reabsorption.

ECF volume reflects the balance between sodium intake and sodium excretion and is regulated by a complex system acting via the kidney. The average intake of sodium in developed countries is between 150 and 250 meq/day and must be balanced by an equivalent daily sodium excretion.

States where ECF volume is increased are related to a net gain of sodium and often present with edema in the presence or absence of hypertension. States where ECF volume is decreased reflect a total body sodium deficit and are often due to sodium and water losses from the gastrointestinal or genitourinary tracts and commonly present with decreased blood pressure.

A normal person maintains sodium balance without edema, hypertension, or hypotension across a broad range of sodium intake (10–1000 meq/day). A variety of sensors detect alterations in sodium balance and effectors respond by adjusting renal sodium excretion (Table 2.1). Sodium sensors respond to the adequacy of intravascular filling and the effector limb modifies sodium excretion accordingly. When patients are edematous, however, there is sodium retention even in the setting of an expanded ECF volume.

This phenomenon led to the postulation of an important but confusing concept known as the effective arterial blood volume (EABV) that is defined based on the activity of the sodium homeostasis effector mechanisms in the kidney.

Table 2.1

Sensors and Effectors of Sodium Balance

Sodium Sensors	Effectors
Low pressure receptors (atria and veins)	Glomerular filtration rate
High pressure receptors (aortic arch and carotid sinus)	Peritubular physical factors (ionic, osmotic, and hydraulic gradients)
Hepatic volume receptor	Sympathetic nervous system
Cerebrospinal fluid sodium receptor	Renin-angiotensin-aldosterone system
Renal afferent arteriole receptors	Atrial natriuretic factor
	Other natriuretic hormones

Effective arterial blood volume is a concept rather than an objectively measured volume. Since the stimulation of sodium sensors cannot be directly measured, their activity is inferred based on the response of the effector limb. It is an estimate of the net level of stimulation of all sodium sensors. Volume sensors in the arterial and venous circulation including the renal vessels monitor the sense of fullness of the vascular tree. Ultimately, it is the relationship between the cardiac output and peripheral vascular resistance that is sensed. Effective arterial blood volume can also be defined based on how far the mean arterial pressure (equal to the diastolic blood pressure plus one-third of the pulse pressure) is displaced from its set point. In many edematous disorders the set point is normal, as in congestive heart failure and cirrhosis of the liver, and the mean arterial pressure tends to be low. In nephrotic syndrome the set point is increased by kidney disease and the mean arterial pressure is high. Despite the fact that mean arterial pressure is high, it still remains below the set point. In both situations the kidney retains salt and water in an attempt to return blood pressure to its set point. In clinical practice, however, net renal sodium handling determines the state of the EABV. When the kidney retains sodium, it is inferred that the EABV is decreased and when the kidney excretes sodium, it is inferred that the EABV is increased.

KEY POINTS
ECF and Sodium Concentration

1. Disorders of ECF volume result from disturbances in sodium balance and disorders of serum sodium concentration (hypo- and hypernatremia) result from alterations in water balance.
2. Extracellular fluid volume control is dependent on the regulation of sodium balance. Regulation of ECF volume reflects the balance between sodium intake and sodium excretion.

3. Serum sodium concentration is not reflective of ECF volume status.
4. Extracellular fluid volume expansion is related to a net gain of sodium and often presents as edema.
5. A variety of sensors detect alterations in sodium balance and effectors respond by modifying renal sodium excretion. Sodium sensors respond to the adequacy of intravascular filling and the effector limb adjusts renal sodium excretion accordingly.
6. Effective arterial blood volume is a concept and not a volume that is objectively measured. It is an estimate of the net level of activation of all sodium sensors. It is inferred that the EABV is decreased when the kidney retains sodium and that the EABV is increased when the kidney excretes sodium.

Effector Systems

Regulation of Sodium Transport in the Kidney

When ECF volume is decreased, renal sodium excretion is minimized by decreasing the amount of sodium filtered and increasing tubular sodium reabsorption. Extracellular fluid volume depletion stimulates the release of angiotensin II (AII), aldosterone, and arginine vasopressin (AVP), as well as activates the sympathetic nervous system resulting in salt and water retention. Thirst and the craving for salt are also stimulated. Angiotensin II and aldosterone act synergistically to stimulate salt appetite and AII is a strong stimulator of thirst. Extrarenal losses of salt are minimized by decreased sweating and fecal losses. Decreased ECF volume decreases intravascular volume and results in decreased renal perfusion. The resultant decline in glomerular filtration rate (GFR) decreases the filtered load (amount presented to the proximal tubule) of sodium. Tubular sodium reabsorption is increased by activation of the renin-angiotensin-aldosterone system (RAAS), changes in peritubular physical forces, and suppression of natriuretic peptides.

The filtered load of sodium chloride is 1.7 kg/day. This is 11 times the amount of sodium chloride in the ECF. Less than 1% of the filtered load is excreted in the final urine under the control of a complex system of effector mechanisms that regulate sodium reabsorption along the nephron. The cellular and molecular mechanisms of action of these effector systems in each nephron segment are discussed below.

Proximal Tubule

The proximal tubule reabsorbs 60–70% of the filtered sodium chloride load. Physical factors, the sympathetic nervous system, and the RAAS regulate sodium reabsorption in this segment. The principal pathway for sodium entry into the proximal tubular cell is the Na$^+$-H$^+$ exchanger (isoform NHE3).

Physical factors regulate sodium reabsorption through changes in filtration fraction (FF) that create hydrostatic and oncotic gradients for water movement. The filtration fraction is the ratio of GFR to renal plasma flow (RPF) shown in the equation below:

$$FF = \frac{GFR}{RPF}$$

Efferent arteriolar constriction by AII increases the FF via two mechanisms. It reduces renal blood flow (decreases RPF) and increases glomerular capillary pressure, which is the main determinant of GFR (raises GFR). The resultant increase in FF increases oncotic pressure and decreases hydrostatic pressure in the peritubular capillary. These changes promote the movement of salt and water from the tubular lumen to the interstitial space and finally into the peritubular capillary. In addition, AII reduces medullary blood flow, which has similar effects on driving forces in medullary nephron segments.

The RAAS also has direct effects on tubular transport mediated via NHE3 and the Na$^+$-K$^+$-ATPase. Angiotensin II and aldosterone both upregulate NHE3. The AII effect may be mediated via protein kinase C, whereas aldosterone was recently shown to increase the insertion of preformed transporter proteins into the apical membrane. The Na$^+$-K$^+$-ATPase, which is present in the basolateral membrane of all nephron segments and is the major pathway by which sodium exits tubular cells, is also stimulated by AII. The sympathetic nervous system and insulin also stimulate the movement of NHE3 into the apical membrane and increase proximal tubular sodium reabsorption.

Systemic blood pressure itself also plays a key role in proximal tubular sodium reabsorption. As blood pressure rises the renal excretion of NaCl increases in an attempt to reduce ECF fluid volume and normalize blood pressure. This phenomenon is known as pressure natriuresis. Pressure natriuresis is not mediated by an increase in filtered sodium load. An acute rise in blood pressure does not change the amount of sodium filtered by the glomerulus due to autoregulation of the renal microvasculature. As blood pressure increases, the afferent arteriole constricts in order to maintain glomerular capillary hydrostatic pressure constant. Afferent arteriolar constriction results from both a direct myogenic reflex and tubuloglomerular feedback (discussed below). Acute rises in blood pressure are sensed in the vasculature and a signal is transmitted to the proximal tubule to reduce sodium chloride reabsorption. This is mediated by removal of NHE3 from the luminal membrane of proximal tubule via a two-step internalization process regulated in part by AII shown in Figure 2.2. NHE3 first moves from the microvillar membrane to the intermicrovillar cleft (first step) and then from the intermicrovillar cleft to subapical endosomes (second step). A fall in AII concentration plays a role in the first step. Na$^+$-K$^+$-ATPase activity is also decreased via a similar process of internalization.

Increased delivery of NaCl to the thick ascending limb of Henle is sensed by macula densa cells. The macula densa is a specialized region near the junction of the cortical thick ascending

Figure 2.2

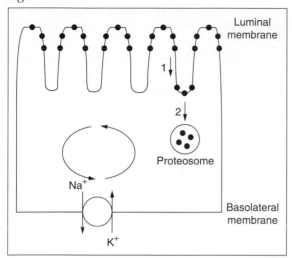

Sodium transporters in proximal tubule and pressure natriuresis. NHE3 (filled circles) is internalized in two steps in response to elevated blood pressure. In step 1, NHE3 moves from microvilli to the intermicrovillar cleft, a process that is regulated by angiotensin II. In step 2, NHE3 moves from the intermicrovillar cleft to proteosomes and is degraded. The Na⁺-K⁺-ATPase is regulated in a similar fashion.

limb and distal convoluted tubule (DCT). The macula densa is in close proximity to the granular renin-producing cells in the afferent arteriole and together this region is referred to as the juxtaglomerular (JG) apparatus. The JG apparatus mediates a process known as tubuloglomerular feedback. When increased sodium chloride delivery is sensed by the macula densa a signal is transmitted to the afferent arteriole to constrict and the single-nephron GFR decreases. Renin release by the JG apparatus is suppressed and AII levels fall. Conversely, when decreased sodium chloride is sensed by the macula densa, renin release is stimulated and the RAAS activated. Tubuloglomerular feedback serves two purposes. First, it maintains sodium chloride delivery to distal nephron segments (distal convoluted tubule and collecting duct) relatively constant over a wide range of conditions in the short term. It is in distal nephron where the final fine-tune regulation of sodium and water balance occurs. Additionally, in the

long term the JG apparatus is responsible for controlling renin secretion at a rate that is optimal in order to maintain sodium balance.

Thick Ascending Limb of Henle

The thick ascending limb of Henle reabsorbs 20–30% of the filtered sodium chloride load. Sodium and chloride enter the thick ascending limb cell via the Na⁺-K⁺-2Cl⁻ cotransporter, which is inhibited by loop diuretics. Since sodium and chloride concentration in urine are much higher than potassium, in order for the transporter to operate maximally there must be a mechanism present for potassium to recycle back into the tubular lumen. A ROMK potassium channel in the luminal membrane mediates potassium recycling. Sodium exits on the Na⁺-K⁺-ATPase and chloride exist via a chloride channel.

The rate of NaCl absorption in this segment is load dependent. The higher the delivered load of NaCl the higher the absorption. Sodium reabsorption is increased by β-adrenergic agonists, arginine vasopressin in some species, parathyroid hormone, calcitonin, and glucagon. Prostaglandin E₂ inhibits sodium reabsorption.

Distal Convoluted Tubule

The DCT reabsorbs 5–10% of the filtered sodium load. Sodium and chloride enter the DCT cell via the thiazide-sensitive Na⁺-Cl⁻ cotransporter (NCC) and sodium exits through the Na⁺-K⁺-ATPase. Aldosterone upregulates NCC expression. In order for mineralocorticoids to play a role in the regulation of sodium transport in any nephron segment that segment must also express the mineralocorticoid receptor and the type 2 11 β-hydroxysteroid dehydrogenase (HSD). The mineralocorticoid receptor is expressed in DCT, while type 2 11 β-HSD is expressed in the later half (DCT2) of the DCT. DCT2 also contains the epithelial sodium channel (ENaC). Type 2 11 β-HSD degrades cortisol to the inactive cortisone in mineralocorticoid target tissues. This is required in order to maintain mineralocorticoid specificity, given the facts that the mineralocorticoid receptor can also bind glucocorticoids and that glucocorticoids circulate at much higher concentrations than mineralocorticoids.

Genetic studies of a rare monogenic disorder provided insight into NCC regulation. Pseudohypoaldosteronism type II (PHA II) is an autosomal dominant disease characterized by hypertension, hyperkalemia, and extreme sensitivity to thiazide diuretics. Mutations in two members of the WNK (with no lysine[K]) kinase family, WNK1 and WNK4, cause the disease. WNK4 is expressed in DCT and reduces expression of NCC in the cell membrane. It does this via a kinase-dependent mechanism that does not involve changes in the synthesis of NCC. Mutations in WNK4 lead to NCC overactivity. WNK4 also inhibits the ROMK potassium channel. ROMK inhibition is not dependent on WNK4 kinase activity but occurs through clathrin-dependent endocytosis of the channel. Interestingly, WNK4 mutations of PHA II increase NCC activity but decrease ROMK activity. This not only explains the hypertension and hyperkalemia of PHA II but also shows that WNK4 can differentially regulate NCC and ROMK.

WNK4 may be the master switch that regulates the balance between NaCl reabsorption and potassium excretion in distal nephron. Aldosterone is stimulated by decreased ECF volume and hyperkalemia. Yet when aldosterone concentrations are elevated, how does the distal nephron know whether to reabsorb sodium (stimulate NCC and inhibit ROMK) or excrete potassium (stimulate ROMK and inhibit NCC)? The answer to this question, which remains unknown, may lie in the regulation of WNK4 kinase activity.

WNK1 is expressed in a variety of chloride transporting epithelia including kidney, colon, sweat ducts, pancreas, and bile ducts. WNK1 does not appear to bind NCC but rather interacts with WNK4 and inhibits its ability to downregulate NCC. In PHA II, mutations in WNK1 increase its expression and further augment its ability to inhibit WNK4 resulting in increased NCC activity. In the model of DCT sodium transport shown in Figure 2.3 delivery of NCC to the luminal membrane is inhibited by WNK4, while WNK1 inhibits the activity of WNK4. Mutations in either WNK1 or WNK4 result in increased NCC expression in the cell membrane and the PHA II phenotype.

Cortical Collecting Duct

The collecting duct reabsorbs 1–3% of the filtered sodium load. The RAAS is the major regulator of NaCl reabsorption in this segment. Sodium enters

Figure 2.3

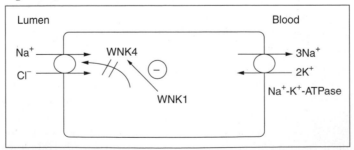

Model of DCT sodium transport and PHA II. The PHA II phenotype is caused by mutations in both WNK4 and WNK1. WNK4 impairs the delivery of the Na⁺-Cl⁻ cotransporter (NCC) to the luminal membrane and mutations that decrease its activity increase NCC expression in the cell membrane. Wildtype WNK1 interacts with WNK4 and decreases its activity.

Figure 2.4

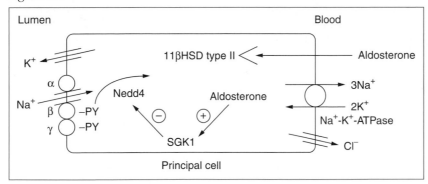

Model of CCD sodium transport and Liddle's syndrome. In Liddle's syndrome mutations in β and γENaC subunits increase ENaC activity. Mutations occur in a PY motif involved in protein-protein interaction. The PY motif interacts with Nedd4 that ubiquitinates ENaC and leads to its internalization and proteosome-mediated degradation. Nedd4 is inactivated via phosphorylation by SGK1, which is upregulated by aldosterone. After phosphorylation Nedd4 no longer interacts with ENaC resulting in increased ENaC expression in the cell membrane.

the cortical collecting duct (CCD) cell via ENaC and exits through the basolateral Na^+-K^+-ATPase (shown in Figure 2.4). The epithelial sodium channel is composed of three subunits (α, β, γ). Aldosterone and possibly AII increase ENaC abundance in CCD. Aldosterone also upregulates the Na^+-K^+-ATPase and the mitochondrial enzyme citrate synthetase.

As in the DCT, studies of monogenic disorders causing hypertension led to important insights into ENaC regulation. Liddle's syndrome is an autosomal dominant disorder characterized by the onset of hypertension at an early age, hypokalemia, and metabolic alkalosis. Linkage studies revealed that Liddle's syndrome resulted from mutations in β and γ ENaC subunits that increased ENaC activity. The mutations clustered in a PY motif, which is involved in protein-protein interaction, at the C-terminus of the protein. The PY motif of ENaC interacts with Nedd4. Nedd4 ubiquitinates ENaC that leads to its internalization and proteosome-mediated degradation. Nedd4 is inactivated via phosphorylation by the serum and glucocorticoid-stimulated kinase (SGK1), which is upregulated by aldosterone. Once Nedd4 is

phosphorylated it no longer interacts with ENaC. In summary, these studies revealed that aldosterone upregulates SGK1, SGK1 phosphorylates, and inactivates Nedd4, Nedd4 does not ubiquitinate ENaC and ENaC remains active in the cell membrane. Aldosterone increases the synthesis of SGK1 mRNA within 30 minutes, after several hours it also increases synthesis of the α subunit of ENaC and Na^+-K^+-ATPase mRNA.

Medullary Collecting Duct

In the inner medullary collecting duct (IMCD) there are two transport pathways whereby sodium enters the cell (Figure 2.5). The first is ENaC also expressed in CCD and the second is a cyclic GMP-gated cation channel that transports sodium, potassium, and ammonium. Sodium exits the cell via the Na^+-K^+-ATPase.

The cyclic GMP-gated cation channel is inhibited by natriuretic peptides, the major effector pathway regulating sodium transport in IMCD. Although natriuretic peptides also increase GFR (via dilation of the afferent arteriole and constriction

Figure 2.5

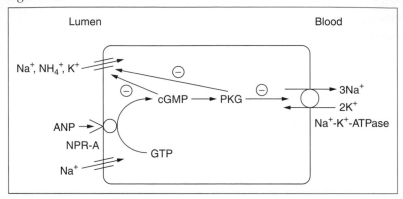

Sodium transport in the inner medullary collecting duct. Sodium enters the cell via either ENaC or a cyclic GMP-gated cation channel that transports sodium, potassium, and ammonium and exits through the Na^+-K^+-ATPase. Natriuretic peptides such as ANP bind to their receptors (NPR A-C) and catalyze the conversion of GTP to cyclic GMP (cGMP). Cyclic GMP inhibits the cation channel directly and indirectly through the protein kinase G (PKG). Natriuretic peptides also inhibit the Na^+-K^+-ATPase either through protein kinase G (ANP) or prostaglandin E_2.

of the efferent arteriole), their major natriuretic effect is in IMCD. Natriuretic peptides are a family of proteins that include atrial natriuretic peptide (ANP), long-acting atrial natriuretic peptide, vessel dilator, kaliuretic peptide, brain-type natriuretic peptide (BNP), C-type natriuretic peptide (CNP), and urodilatin. They act on target cells by binding to three types of receptors, natriuretic peptide receptors (NPR) A, B, and C. Natriuretic peptide receptors A and B are isoforms of particulate guanylate cyclase that catalyze the conversion of GTP to cyclic GMP after ligand binding. NPR B may be a specific receptor for CNP. Atrial natriuretic peptide acts through NPR A. The primary sites of production of these peptides are: ANP—cardiac atrium, BNP—cardiac ventricles, CNP—endothelial cells, and urodilatin—distal tubule of the kidney. Atrial natriuretic peptide also inhibits the basolateral Na^+-K^+-ATPase. All of the other effector systems discussed above are antinatriuretic; these peptides constitute the major effector system that results in natriuresis. They are important in protecting against ECF volume expansion, especially in congestive heart failure.

KEY POINTS
Effector Systems

1. As ECF volume decreases, renal sodium excretion is minimized by reducing the filtered sodium load and increasing tubular sodium reabsorption. This is mediated via release of A-II, aldosterone, and arginine vasopressin, as well as activation of the sympathetic nervous system.
2. In proximal tubule physical factors, the sympathetic nervous system and the RAAS regulate sodium reabsorption. Physical factors operate through changes in FF, thereby altering hydrostatic and oncotic pressure gradients for sodium and water movement. The RAAS also has direct effects on tubular sodium transport mediated via NHE3 and Na^+-K^+-ATPase.
3. Systemic blood pressure itself also plays a key role in proximal tubular sodium reabsorption through pressure natriuresis that involves internalization of NHE3. The resultant

increase in NaCl delivery to the macula densa activates tubuloglomerular feedback reducing single-nephron GFR.

4. The thick ascending limb of Henle reabsorbs 20–30% of the filtered sodium chloride load and reabsorption is load dependent.

5. The DCT reabsorbs 5–10% of the filtered sodium load. Activity of NCC is regulated via WNK1 and WNK4. WNK4 reduces NCC expression in the cell membrane.

6. WNK4 may function as a master switch that integrates aldosterone action in distal nephron.

7. The CCD reabsorbs 1–3% of the filtered sodium load under regulation by the RAAS. Aldosterone acts on both sodium entry (ENaC) and exit (Na$^+$-K$^+$-ATPase) pathways.

8. Aldosterone increases ENaC activity through the phosphorylation of SGK1. SGK1 phosphorylates and blocks the activity of Nedd4, a protein that ubiquitinates ENaC causing its removal from the cell membrane.

9. Natriuretic peptides constitute the major effector system resulting in natriuresis. They act primarily by inhibiting the IMCD cyclic GMP-gated nonspecific cation channel and the Na$^+$-K$^+$-ATPase.

Disorders Associated with Increased Total Body Sodium (ECF Volume Expansion)

Hypervolemic states (increased ECF volume) are associated with increased total body sodium and commonly present with edema with or without hypertension. Edema is the accumulation of excess interstitial fluid. Interstitial fluid is that part of the ECF not contained within blood vessels.

Edema fluid resembles plasma in terms of its electrolyte content and has a variable protein concentration. Edema may be localized due to local vascular or lymphatic injury or can be generalized as in congestive heart failure, cirrhosis, and nephrotic syndrome. On physical examination, edema is detected by applying pressure with the thumb or index finger on the skin of the lower extremities or presacral region. If edema is present an indentation or "pitting" results.

Edema is generated by an alteration in physical forces originally described by Starling that determine the movement of fluid across the capillary endothelium. Alterations in these forces explain the development of both localized and generalized edema. Major causes of edema are classified according to the mechanisms responsible and are illustrated in Table 2.2. The interaction between hydrostatic and oncotic pressure governs the movement of water across the capillary wall. An increase in hydrostatic pressure or a decrease in oncotic pressure within the capillary favors the movement of fluid out of the blood vessel and into the interstitium resulting in edema formation. Increases in capillary permeability also favor edema formation. The final common pathway maintaining generalized edema is the retention of excess salt and water by the kidney.

The pathophysiology of ECF volume expansion based on the presence or absence of hypertension and edema is shown in Table 2.3.

Hypertension Present, Edema Present

With kidney disease and a decreased GFR hypertension and edema are often present. The decrease in renal function results in sodium retention and ECF volume expansion. If the expansion is severe enough, hypertension and edema result.

In acute glomerulonephritis the renal lesion results in a primary retention of NaCl. The stimulus for NaCl retention and the molecular mechanisms whereby it occurs remain unknown. Studies in children with acute poststreptococcal glomerulonephritis showed that renin activity is low

Table 2.2
Pathophysiology of Edema Formation

INCREASED FORMATION	DECREASED REMOVAL	ILL-DEFINED MECHANISMS
Increased capillary hydrostatic pressure	Decreased plasma colloid osmotic pressure	Idiopathic cyclic edema
Venous obstruction	Nephrotic syndrome	Pregnancy
Congestive heart failure	Malabsorption	Hypothyroidism
Cirrhosis of the liver	Cirrhosis of the liver	
Primary salt excess (nephrotic syndrome)		
Increased capillary permeability	Impaired lymphatic outflow	
Trauma—burns		
Allergic reactions		

Abbreviations: ARF, acute renal failure; CKD, chronic renal failure.

supporting the conclusion that ECF volume is expanded. In addition, studies of patients with acute nephritis also showed increased concentration of atrial natriuretic peptides, as would be expected if ECF volume were expanded. Expansion of ECF volume induces hypertension and edema that in turn suppresses renin production and stimulates release of atrial natriuretic peptides.

Hypertension Present, Edema Absent (Excess Aldosterone or Aldosterone-Like Activity)

These disorders are due to sodium retention by the kidney stimulated by excess mineralocorticoids (primary aldosteronism due to an aldosterone-producing tumor, renal artery stenosis, and renin-producing tumors of the JG apparatus), glucocorticoids binding to the mineralocorticoid receptor (Cushing's syndrome, licorice, and apparent mineralocorticoid excess), or genetic diseases that result in increased sodium reabsorption in the distal nephron (Liddle's syndrome and pseudohypoaldosteronism type II). Liddle's syndrome is due to overactivity of the sodium channel in CCD. Pseudohypoaldosteronism type II is due to

overactivity of the thiazide-sensitive Na-Cl cotransporter in DCT caused by mutations in WNK kinases.

In all of these conditions the kidney is able to maintain ECF volume homeostasis but at the cost of hypertension. The relationship between defects in renal salt excretion and the subsequent development of hypertension is best explained by the computer models of Guyton and his collaborators. In order for long-term increases in blood pressure to occur there must be a reduction in the kidney's ability to excrete salt and water. In normal individuals, raising arterial pressure results in increased sodium excretion and a return of blood pressure to normal. This effect is mediated via pressure natriuresis (discussed earlier). A steady state is reestablished where sodium intake equals sodium excretion at a normal blood pressure. Increases in salt intake may transiently raise blood pressure but if the pressure natriuresis mechanism is intact blood pressure must always return to normal as shown in Figure 2.6. Pressure natriuresis is the key component of a feedback system that stabilizes blood pressure and ECF volume. Activation of neurohumoral systems, especially the RAAS, shifts the curve to the right blunting the pressure natriuresis response.

Table 2.3

Pathophysiology of ECF Volume (Total Body Sodium) Expansion

Hypertension-present, edema-present
Kidney disease
Hypertension-present, edema-absent
Mineralocorticoid excess
    Primary hyperaldosteronism
    Renal artery stenosis
    Renin-producing tumors
Glucocorticoids binding to the mineral-
    ocorticoid receptor
    Cushing's disease
    Licorice
    AME
Increased distal sodium reabsorption
    Liddle's syndrome
    Pseudohypoaldosteronism type II
Hypertension-absent, edema-present
Decreased cardiac output
    Congestive heart failure
    Constrictive pericarditis
    Pulmonary hypertension
Decreased oncotic pressure
    Nephrotic syndrome
Peripheral vasodilation
    Cirrhosis
    High-output heart failure
    Pregnancy
Increased capillary permeability
    Burns
    Sepsis
    Pancreatitis

Abbreviation: AME, apparent mineralocorticoid excess.

Suppression of the RAAS increases the ability of the kidney to excrete sodium with minimal to no change in blood pressure. Long-term increases in blood pressure can only occur if the curve is shifted to the right. This rightward shift results in sustained hypertension that is a "trade-off" that allows the kidney to excrete normal amounts of sodium but at the expense of hypertension.

Rightward shifts of the curve are caused by diseases that increase preglomerular resistance, increase tubular reabsorption of sodium, or reduce the number of functional nephrons.

With nephron loss remaining nephrons must excrete greater amounts of sodium to maintain balance. Compensatory changes that must occur in order to achieve this include increased single-nephron GFR and decreased tubular sodium reabsorption. Decreased sodium reabsorption leads to increased NaCl delivery to the macula densa and suppression of renin release. In this situation since renin is already maximally suppressed, the kidney's ability to excrete a salt load (such as with a high-salt diet) is impaired and will require a higher blood pressure. This explains the higher prevalence of "salt-sensitive" hypertension in patients with kidney disease. Renal arteriolar vasodilation and a sustained increase in single-nephron GFR damage surviving nephrons and lead to glomerulosclerosis. When this process becomes severe the pressure natriuresis curve shifts to the right and hypertension develops. Damage to surviving nephrons is key in shifting the pressure natriuresis curve to the right. Studies in dogs with surgically induced nephron loss (five-sixths nephrectomy) show that sustained increases in sodium intake shift the curve to the right and induce "salt-sensitive" hypertension that resolves when sodium is restricted.

Hypertension Absent, Edema Present (Decreased EABV)

Congestive heart failure, nephrotic syndrome, and cirrhosis of the liver are characterized by edema; however, hypertension is absent. In these disorders a primary abnormality results in decreased EABV that stimulates effector mechanisms resulting in renal sodium retention. The primary abnormality varies depending on the disease.

In CHF the primary abnormality is a decreased cardiac output. There is a secondary increase in peripheral vascular resistance to maintain

Figure 2.6

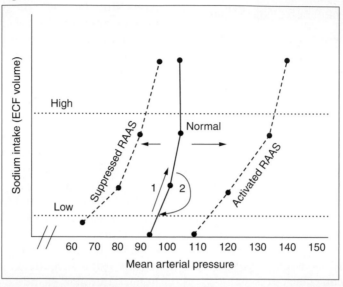

Pressure volume regulation in hypertension. Increases in sodium intake may transiently raise blood pressure (shown by the arrow at number 1) but if the pressure natriuresis mechanism is intact blood pressure must always return to normal (illustrated by the curved line at number 2). Activation of the RAAS shifts the curve to the right blunting the pressure natriuresis response. Suppression of the RAAS shifts the curve to the left of normal and increases the kidney's ability to excrete sodium with minimal change in blood pressure even at high sodium intakes. Hypertension can only occur if the pressure natriuresis (pressure volume) curve is shifted to the right. Sustained hypertension is the "trade-off" that allows the kidney to excrete ingested sodium but at the cost of hypertension.

blood pressure. Plasma volume is expanded. Since most of this increase is on the venous side of the circulation, however, arterial underfilling is sensed by baroreceptors. Effector systems are activated resulting in stimulation of the sympathetic nervous system and the RAAS, as well as the nonosmotic release of AVP. Plasma concentrations of renin, aldosterone, AVP, and norepinephrine are increased. The net effect is the renal retention of salt and water in order to compensate for arterial underfilling. The intensity of the neurohumoral response is proportional to the severity of the heart failure. Sodium concentration correlates inversely with AVP concentration and the severity of the hyponatremia is a predictor of cardiovascular mortality. Despite the fact that atrial natriuretic

peptide concentrations are elevated in patients with CHF, there is resistance to their action. This is likely related to an increase in sodium reabsorption in nephron segments upstream of the inner medullary collecting duct. Natriuresis is restored by renal denervation, probably due to decreased proximal tubular sodium reabsorption and increased distal sodium delivery.

In cirrhosis of the liver the primary abnormality is decreased peripheral vascular resistance that leads to a secondary increase in cardiac output. Plasma volume in cirrhotic patients is increased and the increase occurs before the development of ascites. Splanchnic vasodilation is present early in the course of cirrhosis and results in arterial underfilling and activation of neurohumoral mechanisms that lead to salt and water retention. There is a direct correlation between the degree of decrease in peripheral vascular resistance and the increase in plasma volume. As in CHF the severity of hyponatremia is a predictor of clinical outcome. Splanchnic vasodilation may be mediated by nitric oxide. Shear forces in splanchnic arteriovenous shunts stimulate nitric oxide production. Studies in cirrhotic rats showed that endothelial nitric oxide was increased in the aorta and mesenteric arteries. When nitric oxide synthase inhibitors were administered to these animals there was a reversal of the increase in nitric oxide, the hyperdynamic circulation, and neurohumoral activation. Water excretion increased and the serum sodium concentration rose.

Two hypotheses were proposed to explain the edema of nephrotic syndrome, the underfill hypothesis, and the overflow hypothesis. The underfill hypothesis, which is most commonly taught, states that edema forms in nephrotic syndrome as a result of decreased EABV. The decreased EABV is secondary to decreased capillary oncotic pressure that results from proteinuria. The reduced oncotic pressure leads to increased fluid movement into the interstitium (edema) and reduces the ECF volume. Effector mechanisms are activated increasing renal salt and water reabsorption that maintain the edema.

The overflow hypothesis argues that edema in nephrotic syndrome is due to a primary increase in renal sodium reabsorption as occurs with glomerulonephritis. This would result in ECF volume expansion and suppression of the RAAS. Although measurement of ECF volume would be expected to resolve this issue, ECF volume determinations are often not reproducible and controversy exists as to whether the measurement should be normalized per kilogram of dry or wet weight.

Studies of counterregulatory hormone activity show conflicting results. Approximately one-half of nephrotic patients have elevated plasma renin activity (underfill subgroup). Plasma and urinary catecholamine concentrations are often increased compatible with the underfill hypothesis.

Plasma vasopressin concentrations correlate with blood volume and are reduced by albumin infusion (underfill subgroup). Other authors point out that natriuresis precedes the increase in plasma albumin concentration in patients with minimal change disease that respond to corticosteroid therapy, blood pressure is often increased and falls with clinical remission in children with nephrotic syndrome, renin and angiotensin activity are suppressed in many patients, and in animal models of unilateral nephrosis, sodium is retained in the affected kidney arguing that there is a primary defect in sodium reabsorption supporting the overfill hypothesis.

One analysis of 217 nephrotic patients showed that plasma volume was reduced in 33%, normal in 42%, and increased in 25%. Based on this study it is likely that subgroups of patients exist, some with decreased ECF volume (underfill hypothesis) and others with increased ECF volume (overfill hypothesis). The underfilled nephrotic patient will have decreased EABV, activation of the RAAS, and lack hypertension. The overfilled nephrotic patient will demonstrate hypertension, suppression of the RAAS, and may be more likely to have a lower GFR. Attempts to better subdivide these groups may have important implications regarding therapy. The overfilled patient is likely to respond well to diuretics, whereas diuretics may further reduce renal perfusion in the underfilled patient.

Disorders that increase capillary permeability, such as burns and sepsis, may also cause edema in the absence of hypertension, although other mechanisms may also play a role. Burns can result in localized or generalized edema. Localized edema is the result of thermal injury and the release of vasoactive substances that cause capillary vasodilation and increased permeability. This effect may persist for 24–48 hours. Diffuse edema occurs when full thickness burns involve more than 30% of body surface area. This is due to reduced capillary oncotic pressure resulting from loss of plasma proteins into the wounds. Extensive third-degree burns can result in the loss of as much as 350–400 g of protein per day.

In addition, there are increased insensible losses from damaged skin that may be as high as 300 mL/hour/m² of burned skin. All of these factors contribute to decreased EABV that leads to increased renal salt and water reabsorption further increasing the edema.

Septic patients with severe inflammatory response syndrome (SIRS) due to increased release of inflammatory mediators may develop edema. There is an increase in capillary permeability, as well as precapillary vasodilation. The resultant increase in capillary hydrostatic pressure associated with increased capillary permeability, which increases interstitial oncotic pressure, results in edema formation. In addition, large amounts of intravenous fluids are often administered to maintain systemic blood pressure, which may worsen the edema. Positive pressure ventilation and positive end expiratory pressure (PEEP) ventilation may also worsen edema by decreasing venous return and reducing cardiac output. This results in activation of the sympathetic nervous system and the RAAS leading to increased renal salt and water reabsorption. Lymphatic drainage through the thoracic duct is also impeded by increased intrathoracic pressure.

Approach to the Edematous Patient

A careful history, physical examination, and selected laboratory tests will reveal the cause of edema. The clinician encountering the edematous patient should first ask whether edema is generalized or localized. Localized edema is often due to vascular or lymphatic injury. One next searches for evidence of heart, liver, or kidney disease in the patient's history. The location of the edema may help narrow the differential diagnosis. Left-sided CHF results in pulmonary edema. In right-sided CHF and cirrhosis of the liver edema may accumulate in the lower extremities or abdomen (ascites).

On physical examination the presence of an S3 gallop suggests CHF. One also looks for stigmata of chronic liver disease, such as palmar erythema, spider angiomas, hepatomegaly, and caput medusae. Laboratory studies that should be obtained include serum blood urea nitrogen (BUN) and creatinine concentrations, liver function tests, serum albumin concentration, urinalysis for protein excretion, chest radiograph, and electrocardiogram.

Treatment of the Edematous Patient

Treatment is first directed at halting the progression of the underlying disease. Therapies that aid in reversing the underlying pathophysiology, such as angiotensin converting enzyme inhibitors in CHF should be used when possible. A low-salt diet is critical to the success of any regimen. If these measures are unsuccessful a diuretic may be required. The clinical use of diuretics is discussed in detail in chapter 4.

KEY POINTS
Disorders Associated with Increased Total Body Sodium

1. Hypervolemic states (increased ECF volume) are associated with increased total body sodium and commonly present with edema with or without hypertension.
2. Edema is the accumulation of excess interstitial fluid and is detected by noting an indentation or "pitting" of the skin after applying pressure with the thumb or index finger on the skin of the lower extremities or presacral region.
3. Edema is generated by an alteration in Starling's forces that govern the movement of fluid across the capillary endothelium. An increase in hydrostatic pressure or a decrease in oncotic pressure favors movement of fluid out of the capillary resulting in edema formation.
4. The pathophysiology of ECF volume expansion is divided into three general categories based on the presence or absence of edema and hypertension.

5. Kidney disease is the major cause of ECF volume expansion with both hypertension and edema.

6. Extracellular fluid volume expansion associated with hypertension and the absence of edema occurs with excess concentrations of mineralocorticoids, when glucocorticoids bind to the mineralocorticoid receptor, and with genetic diseases that increase sodium reabsorption in distal nephron.

7. Disorders characterized by a decreased EABV such as CHF, nephrotic syndrome, and cirrhosis of the liver are major causes of ECF volume expansion associated with edema in the absence of hypertension.

Table 2.4

Manifestations of ECF Volume (Total Body Sodium) Depletion

SYMPTOMS	SIGNS
Increased thirst	Orthostatic fall in blood pressure
Weakness and apathy	Orthostatic rise in pulse
Headache	Decreased pulse volume
Muscle cramps	Decreased jugular venous pressure
Anorexia	Dry skin and decreased sweat
Nausea	Dry mucous membranes
Vomiting	Decreased skin turgor

Disorders Associated with Decreased Total Body Sodium (ECF Volume Depletion)

Sodium is the most abundant extracellular ion. As a result it determines the osmolality and volume of the ECF. Sodium depletion means ECF volume depletion. Sodium depletion does not imply hyponatremia and conversely hyponatremia does not imply sodium depletion. The serum sodium concentration is primarily determined by changes in water metabolism (Chapter 3). Manifestations of sodium and ECF volume depletion are illustrated in Table 2.4.

When sodium excretion exceeds input, negative sodium balance and decreased ECF volume results. Given the fact that the normal kidney can rapidly lower sodium excretion to near zero, decreased sodium intake alone never causes decreased ECF volume. Sodium depletion results from ongoing sodium losses from the kidney, skin, or the gastrointestinal tract. If the kidney is the source of sodium loss then urine sodium concentration exceeds 20 meq/L. If losses are from skin or gastrointestinal

tract and the kidney is responding normally, the urine sodium concentration is less than 20 meq/L.

Renal sodium losses are due either to intrinsic kidney disease or external influences on renal function. Kidney diseases associated with sodium wasting include nonoliguric acute renal failure, the diuretic phase of acute renal failure, and "salt-wasting nephropathy." Salt-wasting nephropathy occurs after relief of urinary tract obstruction, with interstitial nephritis, medullary cystic disease, or polycystic kidney disease. External factors causing natriuresis include solute diuresis from sodium bicarbonate, glucose, urea, and mannitol; diuretic administration; and mineralocorticoid deficiency as a result of hypoaldosteronism or decreased renin secretion.

Gastrointestinal losses are external or internal. External losses occur with diarrhea, vomiting, gastrointestinal suction, or external fistulas. Internal losses or so-called "third spacing" result from peritonitis, pancreatitis, and small bowel obstruction. Skin losses also are external or internal. External losses result from excessive sweating, cystic fibrosis, and adrenal insufficiency. Burns cause excessive internal and external losses.

In order to protect blood pressure and tissue perfusion during ECF volume depletion a variety of compensatory mechanisms are activated. These mechanisms maintain blood pressure, minimize renal sodium excretion, and in the process maintain ECF volume.

Approach to the Patient with Decreased ECF Volume

As in the patient with an increased ECF volume, a careful history, physical examination, and selected laboratory tests often reveal the cause and extent of ECF volume depletion. Clinical signs and symptoms of total body sodium deficit are shown in Table 2.4. The history focuses on identification of potential sources of sodium loss. The patient is questioned regarding polydipsia and diuretic use (kidney), diarrhea and vomiting (gastrointestinal tract), and sweating (skin). Physical examination can reveal the extent of ECF volume depletion (postural changes in blood pressure and pulse, degree of hypotension), as well its cause (intestinal obstruction or gastrointestinal fistula). Laboratory tests also aid in determining whether the sodium loss is renal or extrarenal. The presence of a decreased urine sodium concentration, concentrated urine, and a BUN to creatinine ratio greater than 20:1 suggests that sodium losses are extrarenal and the kidney is responding appropriately. The one exception to this caveat is the patient in whom diuretics were recently discontinued. Even though sodium losses occurred via the kidney, once the diuretic effect has dissipated, the kidneys reabsorb salt and water appropriately in order to restore ECF volume. Conversely, an elevated urine sodium concentration suggests that the kidney is the source of the sodium loss.

Treatment of the Patient with Decreased ECF Volume

In mild depletion states treatment of the underlying disorder and replacement of normal dietary salt and water intake are sufficient to correct deficits. When blood pressure and tissue perfusion are compromised or the oral route of replacement cannot be used, intravenous fluid administration

is required. The use of intravenous fluids is reviewed in more detail in Chapter 5 and only general guidelines are discussed here.

The amount and rate of repletion depend on the clinical situation. Cerebral perfusion and urine output are used as markers of tissue perfusion. Response of blood pressure and pulse to postural changes are adequate noninvasive indicators of ECF volume status. Response to a rapid infusion of normal saline or direct measures of cardiovascular pressures are also used.

Fresh frozen plasma and packed red cells are the most effective initial intravascular volume expander because they remain within the intravascular space (5% of total body weight). Increased cost and potential infectious complications limit their use. Isotonic sodium chloride (normal saline) is an effective volume expander. Its space of distribution is confined to the ECF (20% of total body weight). Because of its widespread availability, low cost, and lack of infectious complications normal saline is often used when rapid increases in ECF volume are required. Five percent dextrose in water (D_5W) is a poor intravascular volume expander. Once the glucose is metabolized, which happens quickly, the remaining water is distributed in total body water (60% of total body weight). It should never be used to expand the intravascular space since only approximately 8% of the administered volume remains intravascular.

Depending on the source of sodium loss other electrolyte deficiencies may also need to be corrected. Potassium is lost with gastrointestinal causes such as diarrhea or vomiting. Magnesium may be deficient with thiazide diuretic use and diarrheal illnesses.

KEY POINTS
Disorders Associated with Decreased Total Body Sodium

1. Total body sodium determines ECF volume. Sodium depletion is synonymous with ECF volume depletion.
2. Sodium depletion results from kidney, skin, or gastrointestinal tract losses.

3. If the kidney is the source of sodium loss, urine sodium concentration exceeds 20 meq/L.
4. Urine sodium concentration is less than 20 meq/L if losses are from skin or gastrointestinal tract and the kidneys are responding appropriately.
5. Renal sodium loss is caused by intrinsic kidney disease or external influences on the kidney.
6. Treatment of the underlying disorder and replacement of normal dietary salt and water intake are sufficient to correct deficits with mild sodium depletion. Intravenous fluid administration is required when blood pressure and tissue perfusion are compromised or oral replacement cannot be used.

Additional Reading

Beltowski, J., Wojcicka, G. Regulation of renal tubular sodium transport by cardiac natriuretic peptides: two decades of research. *Med Sci Monit* 8:RA39–RA52, 2002.

De Santo, N.G., Pollastro, R.M., Saviano, C., Pascale, C., Di Stasio, V., Chiricone, D., Cirillo, E., Molino, D., Stellato, D., Frangiosa, A., Favazzi, P., Capodicasa, L., Bellini, L., Anastasio, P., Perna, A., Sepe, J., Cirillo, M. Nephrotic edema. *Semin Nephrol* 21:262–268, 2001.

Greger, R. Physiology of renal sodium transport. *Am J Med Sci* 319:51–62, 2000.

Guyton, A.C. Blood pressure control—special role of the kidneys and body fluids. *Science* 252:1813–1816, 1991.

Guyton, A.C., Coleman, T.G. Quantitative analysis of the pathophysiology of hypertension. *J Am Soc Nephrol* 10:2248–2258, 1999.

Hall, J.E., Guyton, A.C., Brands, M.W. Pressure-volume regulation in hypertension. *Kidney Int* 49(S55):S35–S41, 1996.

Kahle, K.T., Wilson, F.H., Leng, Q., Lalioti, M.D., O'Connell, A.D., Dong, K., Rapson, A.K., MacGregor, G.G., Giebisch, G., Hebert, S.C., Lifton, R.P. WNK4 regulates the balance between renal NaCl reabsorption and K⁺ secretion. *Nat Genet* 35:372–376, 2003.

Kahle, K.T., Gimenez, I., Hassan, H., Wilson, F.H., Wong, R.D., Forbush, B., Aronson, P.S., Lifton, R.P. WNK4 regulates apical and basolateral Cl⁻ flux in extrarenal epithelia. *Proc Natl Acad Sci USA* 101:2064–2069, 2004.

Krug, A.W., Papavassiliou, F., Hopfer, U., Ullrich, K.J., Gekle, M. Aldosterone stimulates surface expression of NHE3 in renal proximal brush borders. *Pflugers Arch* 446:492–496, 2003.

Kurtzman, N.A. Nephritic edema. *Semin Nephrol* 21:257–261, 2001.

McDonough, A.A., Biemesderfer, D. Does membrane trafficking play a role in regulating the sodium/hydrogen exchanger isoform 3 in the proximal tubule? *Curr Opin Nephrol Hypertens* 12:533–541, 2003.

McDonough, A.A., Leong, P.K., Yang, L.E. Mechanisms of pressure natriuresis: how blood pressure regulates renal sodium transport. *Ann NY Acad Sci* 986:669–677, 2003.

O'Shaughnessy, K.M., Karet, F.E. Salt handling and hypertension. *J Clin Invest* 113:1075–1081, 2004.

Schafer, J.A. Abnormal regulation of ENaC: syndromes of salt retention and salt wasting by the collecting duct. *Am J Physiol Renal Physiol* 283:F221–F235, 2002.

Schnermann, J., Traynor, T., Yang, T., Arend, L., Huang, Y.G., Smart, A., Briggs, J.P. Tubuloglomerular feedback: new concepts and developments. *Kidney Int* 54(S67):S40–S45, 1998.

Schnermann, J. The expanding role of aldosterone in the regulation of body Na content. *Pflugers Arch* 446:410–411, 2003.

Schrier, R.W., Fassett, R.G. A critique of the overfill hypothesis of sodium and water retention in the nephrotic syndrome. *Kidney Int* 53:1111–1117, 1998.

Schrier, R.W., Ecder, T. Gibbs memorial lecture. Unifying hypothesis of body fluid volume regulation: implications for cardiac failure and cirrhosis. *Mt Sinai J Med* 68:350–361, 2001.

Skott, O. Body sodium and volume homeostasis. *Am J Physiol Regul Integr Comp Physiol* 285:R14–R18, 2003.

Yang, C.L., Angell, J., Mitchell, R., Ellison, D.H. WNK kinases regulate thiazide-sensitive Na-Cl cotransport. *J Clin Invest* 111:1039–1045, 2003.

Robert F. Reilly, Jr.

Chapter 3

Disorders of Water Balance (Hypo- and Hypernatremia)

Recommended Time to Complete: 2 days

Guiding Questions

1. What is the difference between tonicity and osmolality?
2. How does the kidney excrete free water and defend against hyponatremia?
3. How does one formulate a clinical approach to the patient with hyponatremia?
4. What is the definition of SIADH?
5. Can you outline a treatment approach for the correction of hyponatremia that minimizes potential complications?
6. How does the body defend against the development of hypernatremia?
7. What is the differential diagnosis of the hypernatremic patient?
8. How does one treat the patient with hypernatremia?

Introduction

One of the more difficult concepts to grasp in nephrology is that changes in serum sodium concentration result from derangements in water balance, while disorders of extracellular fluid (ECF) volume regulation are related to total body sodium balance. This is best explained by the fact that serum sodium is a concentration term and reflects only the relative amounts of sodium and water present in the sample. Low serum sodium concentration (shown in the equation below) denotes a relative deficit of sodium and/or a relative excess of water. Sodium concentration is not a measure of total body sodium content.

$$[\text{Serum Na}^+] = \frac{\text{ECF Na}^+}{\text{ECF H}_2\text{O}}$$

As seen in the formula above, hyponatremia may result from either a decrease in the numerator or an increase in the denominator. Although one might conclude that hyponatremia is more likely the result of a decrease in the numerator, in clinical practice a relative excess of water most commonly causes hyponatremia. Nonosmotic release of arginine vasopressin (AVP) is the key pathophysiologic process in most cases. The regulation of water homeostasis is dependent on (1) an intact thirst mechanism, (2) appropriate renal handling of water, and (3) intact AVP release and response.

Renal free water excretion is the major factor controlling water metabolism, and the major factor controlling renal free water excretion is AVP. Above a plasma osmolality (P_{osm}) of 283, AVP increases by 0.38 pg/mL per 1 mOsm/kg increase in P_{osm}. In turn, urine osmolality (U_{osm}) responds to increments in AVP. A rise in AVP of 1 pg/mL increases U_{osm} about 225 mOsm/kg. The two major afferent stimuli for thirst are an increase in plasma osmolality and a decrease in ECF volume. Thirst is first sensed when plasma osmolality increases to 294 mOsm/kg (the osmolar threshold for thirst). At this osmolality AVP is maximally stimulated (concentration > 5 pg/mL) and is sufficient to maximally concentrate urine. Arginine vasopressin and angiotensin II directly stimulate thirst.

Osmolality is an intrinsic property of a solution and is defined as the number of osmoles of solute divided by the number of kilograms of solvent. It is independent of a membrane. Tonicity or "effective osmolality" is equal to the sum of the concentration of solutes with the capacity to exert an osmotic force across a membrane. It is a property of a solution relative to a membrane. The tonicity of a solution is less than osmolality by the total concentration of "ineffective solutes" that it contains. Solutes that are freely permeable across cell membranes such as urea are ineffective osmoles. From a cellular viewpoint, tonicity determines the net osmolar gradient across the cell membrane that acts as a driving force for water movement.

Sodium is the most abundant cation in ECF and its concentration is the major determinant of tonicity and osmolality. Furthermore, water moves freely across cell membranes allowing the maintenance of osmotic equilibrium between various compartments, therefore ECF tonicity reflects tonicity of the intracellular fluid (ICF). Plasma osmolality is calculated from the following formula:

$$P_{osm} \text{ (mOsm/kg)} = \frac{2 \times \text{Na(meq/L)} + \text{BUN(mg/dL)}}{2.8} + \frac{\text{glucose (mg/dL)}}{18}$$

To calculate tonicity one includes only the sodium and glucose terms in the equation. It is measured directly by freezing point depression or vapor pressure techniques.

Body tonicity, measured as plasma osmolality, is maintained within a narrow range (285–295 mOsm/kg). This is achieved via regulation of water intake and excretion. Disturbances in body tonicity are reflected by alterations in serum sodium concentration and clinically present as either hypo- or hypernatremia.

Tonicity and Osmolality

> 1. Changes in serum sodium concentration are indicative of a problem in water balance, while changes in ECF volume are related to total body sodium.
> 2. Renal excretion of free water is the major factor controlling water metabolism.
> 3. The most abundant cation in ECF is sodium, therefore its concentration is the major determinant of ECF tonicity and osmolality.

Hyponatremia

Hyponatremia, defined as a serum sodium concentration <135 meq/L, is the most frequent electrolyte abnormality and is seen in up to 10–15% of hospitalized patients. It is especially common in critical care units. Hyponatremia is caused by either (1) excess water intake (water intoxication) with normal renal function or (2) continued solute-free water intake with a decreased renal capacity for solute-free water excretion. It occurs whenever free water intake exceeds free water excretion.

In subjects with normal renal function excessive water intake alone does not cause hyponatremia unless it exceeds about 1 L/hour. As a general rule one's maximal free water excretion is equal to about 10–15% of glomerular filtration rate (GFR). With a GFR of 180 L/day, maximal free water excretion equals approximately 24 L/day or 1 L/hour. In patients with a normal GFR, hyponatremia due to excessive water intake is observed only rarely, such as in psychotic patients who drink from faucets or showers. A reduction in GFR, however, will limit free water excretion. An individual whose GFR is 20% of normal will become hyponatremic on drinking over 3.6 L/day. Often patients with psychogenic polydipsia have some degree of renal impairment.

Almost all hyponatremic patients have impaired renal free water excretion. An understanding of how the kidney excretes free water is critical for understanding the pathophysiology of hyponatremia.

The essential features of renal free water excretion are the following:

1. **Normal delivery of tubular fluid to distal diluting segments of the nephron.** An adequate GFR without excessive proximal tubular reabsorption is required in order to deliver tubular fluid to the diluting segments of the kidney (thick ascending limb of the loop of Henle and distal convoluted tubule [DCT]). Although tubular fluid remains isotonic in the proximal tubule, proximal fluid reabsorption is an important determinant of water excretion. Normally 70% of glomerular filtrate is absorbed in the proximal tubule and the remaining 30% is isotonic to plasma as it enters the loop of Henle. Thus, if proximal tubular reabsorption increases, as in volume depletion, free water excreted is limited. To use an extreme example, a patient with acute renal failure and a GFR of 5 mL/minute forms only 7.2 L of glomerular filtrate daily. If 30% is delivered to the diluting segments that means a total of only 2.2 L is delivered daily. Even if the distal nephron were completely impermeant to water only 2.2 L of urine is excreted (only part of this total is free water).

2. **Normal function of the diluting segments (ascending limb of Henle's loop and DCT).** Tubular fluid is diluted in the water-impermeable ascending limb of Henle's loop and DCT by the reabsorption of sodium chloride. Sodium is transported on the Na^+-K^+-$2Cl^-$ cotransporter in the thick ascending limb of Henle and the thiazide-sensitive Na-Cl cotransporter in DCT. It is in the diluting segments where U_{osm} declines to less than P_{osm} that free water is generated.

3. **Absence of AVP.** Arginine vasopressin must be suppressed in order to prevent solute-free water reabsorption in the collecting duct. This factor is of primary importance since the renal

interstitium remains slightly hypertonic even during a water diuresis. Therefore, if the collecting duct were water-permeable, osmotic equilibration of fluid between the tubular lumen and interstitium would concentrate the urine and impair water excretion.

Arginine vasopressin is released from the posterior pituitary, enters the blood stream, binds to its receptor (V_2) in the basolateral membrane of the collecting duct, and increases water permeability. Arginine vasopressin is released in response to osmotic and nonosmotic stimuli. An increase in ECF osmolality as little as 1% stimulates AVP release and the relationship of AVP to plasma osmolality is linear (Figure 3.1). Nonosmotic stimuli are associated with changes in autonomic neural tone such as physical pain, stress, hypoxia, and decreases in effective circulating volume. The nonosmotic pathway is less sensitive and requires a 5–10% decrement in blood volume to stimulate AVP release. Once the threshold is reached, however, the rise in AVP concentration is exponential

(Figure 3.1). Defense of volume has priority. Arginine vasopressin concentration increases and stimulates renal water reabsorption protecting volume at the expense of hyponatremia. It is more important for the body to maintain blood volume than to maintain tonicity. The volume-depleted patient may become profoundly hyponatremic because nonosmotic stimuli for AVP release predominate over osmotic stimuli. Arginine vasopressin also has a pressor effect mediated via the V_1 receptor, contributing perhaps 10% to mean arterial pressure during volume depletion. Thus, AVP is normally osmoregulatory, but during stress becomes a volume regulatory hormone. As a general principle the kidney will always act to preserve blood and ECF volume at the expense of electrolyte and acid-base homeostasis. The nonosmotic release of AVP is the key pathophysiologic process in the majority of patients with hyponatremia.

AVP binds to the V_2 receptor in the basolateral membrane of collecting duct. Adenylate cyclase is activated, cyclic AMP generated, and water channels (aquaporins—AQP2) insert into the apical membrane increasing its water permeability.

4. **Adequate solute intake.** Although the kidney has an enormous capacity to generate free water, it cannot excrete pure water. The lowest U_{osm} attainable in humans is 50 mOsm/kg. One of the main roles of the kidney is to eliminate the osmolar load contained in the diet (approximately 10 mOsm/kg). The volume of urine required to achieve this is expressed in the equation below:

$$\text{urine volume} = \frac{\text{osmolar intake or excretion}}{U_{osm}}$$

In the steady state, osmolar intake and excretion are equal and either can be used. In theory a 70-kg person with a standard osmolar dietary load and a maximally dilute urine could generate 14 L of free water per day (700 mOsm/50 mOsm). If solute intake is very low, however, as in someone drinking only beer (beer drinker's potomania),

Figure 3.1

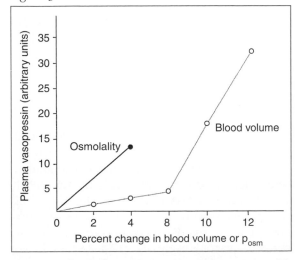

The changes in plasma AVP induced by alterations in osmolality or blood volume. Note that response to changes in osmolality are linear, whereas response to changes in blood volume approximates an exponential curve.

hyponatremia could develop despite the fact that urine is maximally dilute. For example, if solute intake were only 150 mOsm/day with a maximally dilute urine, urine volume would be only 3 L. In this situation water intake could exceed renal-free water excretion and hyponatremia will develop.

KEY POINTS
Hyponatremia

1. Hyponatremia is defined as a serum sodium concentration <135 meq/L and is the most common electrolyte abnormality in hospitalized patients.
2. Hyponatremia occurs whenever free water intake exceeds free water excretion.
3. Almost all patients with hyponatremia have impaired renal free water excretion.
4. The essential features of renal free water excretion are delivery of tubular fluid to distal diluting segments of the nephron, normal function of the diluting segments, suppression of AVP, and adequate solute intake.

Etiology

Hyponatremia most commonly results from an inability to maximally dilute the urine coupled with continued water intake. Before implicating a defect in renal free water excretion as the cause of hyponatremia, the presence of hypoosmolality must be documented because hyponatremia can occur with an elevated or normal serum osmolality.

Hyponatremia with a normal serum osmolality or "pseudohyponatremia" is a laboratory artifact. Serum is made up of two fractions, an aqueous fraction and a particulate fraction. Pseudohyponatremia results from a decrease in the aqueous

fraction. The flame photometry method of sodium analysis measures sodium per liter of total serum. Conditions that reduce the aqueous fraction below the usual 93% of serum (the remaining 7% is the particulate fraction made up of proteins and lipids) decrease the total amount of sodium per aliquot of serum. Sodium concentration, however, in the aqueous fraction is normal. Three conditions that reduce the aqueous fraction are hyperlipidemia, hypercholesterolemia, and hyperproteinemia. This is not a common problem. A clue to the presence of hyperlipidemia is a report from the lab of lipemic serum. Lipemic serum means that after centrifugation of whole blood the supernatant is cloudy. Elevations in cholesterol concentration do not result in lipemic serum. Excess production of paraproteins as in multiple myeloma and the administration of intravenous immunoglobulin also increase the particulate fraction and may result in pseudohyponatremia. Measurement of serum sodium concentration by ion-sensitive electrodes yields a normal value provided the sample is not diluted prior to measurement. If the sample is diluted (indirect potentiometry), the error is reintroduced and pseudohyponatremia can occur. For each 100 mg/dL rise in glycine concentration the serum sodium concentration falls by 3.8 meq/L.

Translocational hyponatremia is due to a shift of water out of cells in response to a nonsodium solute. Serum osmolality is elevated. Water moves down an osmotic gradient from ICF to ECF when nonsodium solute increases ECF osmolality and creates a driving force for water movement. The most common cause is hyperglycemia. Mannitol and glycine infusion also cause translocational hyponatremia. For each increase in serum glucose of 100 mg/dL above its normal concentration, serum sodium concentration falls by 1.6 meq/L. This is a calculated correction factor. In practice this rule of thumb works well for glucose concentrations up to 400 mg/dL. At higher concentrations the correction factor is likely larger (2.4–2.8 meq/L). For each 460 mg/dL increase in triglyceride concentration the serum sodium concentration falls by 1 meq/L.

The remaining causes of hyponatremia alter the external balance of water and are associated with low serum osmolality (*true hyponatremia*). True hyponatremia is caused by either (1) excess water intake (water intoxication) with normal renal function or (2) continued solute-free water intake with a decreased renal capacity for solute-free water excretion. The most common pathophysiologic mechanism is the nonosmotic release of AVP that prevents maximal urinary dilution. Rarely, severely depressed urine flow rate, as with low GFR, increased proximal tubule fluid reabsorption, or decreased solute intake limits urine dilution resulting in positive water balance and hyponatremia.

A clue to the source of the increased AVP concentration lies in the evaluation of the patient's volume status. Common causes are edematous states, extrarenal and renal sodium and water losses, syndrome of inappropriate ADH (SIADH), and psychogenic polydipsia. The presence of edema is indicative of increased total body sodium. Hyponatremia results because the increase in total body water exceeds the increase in total body sodium. In these circumstances, effective circulating volume is decreased and volume/pressure receptors are activated releasing AVP. Thus a decreased effective circulating volume is sensed despite an absolute increase in total body salt and water. The increase in AVP is "appropriate" to the sensed signal. Major causes of hyponatremia with increased total body sodium are congestive heart failure, hepatic cirrhosis, nephrotic syndrome, and advanced chronic or acute renal failure. The hallmark of these disorders on physical examination is dependent edema.

Renal and extrarenal salt and water losses are characterized by signs and symptoms of decreased ECF volume such as thirst, orthostatic hypotension, tachycardia, and decreased skin turgor. In this setting AVP release is "appropriate" to defend ECF volume. Loss of total body sodium exceeds the loss of total body water. Common etiologies of hyponatremia with decreased ECF volume include gastrointestinal losses (excessive salt and water loss causes sufficient hypovolemia to stimulate baroreceptors to increase AVP release); third spacing of fluids; burns; pancreatitis; diuretic overuse or abuse; salt-wasting nephropathy; adrenal insufficiency; and osmotic diuresis. With extrarenal fluid loss the sodium concentration of the lost fluid is less than the serum sodium concentration. If this is the case, how does the patient become hyponatremic? The answer lies in the fact that thirst is intact and that the replacement fluid has a lower sodium concentration than the fluid lost.

Hyponatremia from diuretics is almost always a result of thiazide rather than loop diuretics, since thiazides interfere with dilution of urine but not urinary concentrating ability. By contrast, loop diuretics interfere with both diluting and concentrating ability, and result in medullary washout of solute and diminished AVP-induced free water reabsorption. Diuretic-induced volume depletion decreases GFR and increases proximal tubular salt and water reabsorption, thereby decreasing water delivery to distal segments. Potassium depletion may result in intracellular shifts of sodium, and alters the sensitivity of the osmoreceptor mechanism leading to AVP release. Most patients have an associated hypokalemic metabolic alkalosis. Older women are at highest risk and this generally occurs in the first 2–3 weeks of therapy. Mineralocorticoid and glucocorticoid deficient states lead to volume depletion with enhanced proximal tubular reabsorption and nonosmotic stimulation of AVP release.

Hyponatremia in the presence of a clinically normal ECF volume is most commonly the result of SIADH or psychogenic polydipsia. The term "clinically normal" should be stressed. If total body sodium and total body water were truly normal then serum sodium concentration must also be normal. In reality, total body water is increased as a result of the "inappropriate" release of AVP. "Inappropriate" implies that AVP is released despite the absence of the two physiologic stimuli for its release: increased serum osmolality and decreased effective circulating volume. This state of mild volume expansion results in

Table 3.1

Disease Processes Causing SIADH

CARCINOMAS	PULMONARY DISEASES	CNS DISORDERS
Lung (small cell)	Viral pneumonia	Encephalitis
Duodenum	Bacterial pneumonia	Meningitis
Pancreas	Pulmonary abscess	Acute psychosis
	Tuberculosis	Stroke
	Aspergillosis	Porphyria (AIP)
	Mechanical ventilation	Tumors
		Abscesses
		Subdural injury
		Guillain-Barre syndrome
		Head trauma

Abbreviations: CNS, central nervous system; AIP, acute intermittent porphyria.

urinary sodium wasting and a clinically unde-tectable decrease in total body sodium. SIADH is characterized by hyponatremia, a low serum osmolality, and an inappropriately concentrated urine (less than maximally dilute). Urine sodium concentration is generally increased but it can be low if the patient develops ECF volume depletion. The patient must be clinically euvolemic with no evidence of adrenal, renal, or thyroid dysfunc-tion; and not taking a drug that stimulates AVP release or action. SIADH is caused by malignan-cies, pulmonary, or central nervous system dis-ease (Table 3.1). This is an important disorder to diagnose because hyponatremia will worsen if normal saline is administered.

A variety of drugs impair renal free water excretion by potentiating the action or release of AVP. A partial list is shown in Table 3.2. In hypothyroidism the ability of the kidney to excrete free water is impaired by a decrease in GFR, an increase in proximal tubular reabsorp-tion, and an increase in AVP secretion. In second-ary adrenal insufficiency hyponatremia results since glucocorticoids are required to maximally suppress AVP release.

Psychogenic polydipsia or water intoxication is the result of excess water intake with normal renal function. It is differentiated from SIADH in that the U_{osm} is maximally or near maximally dilute.

Table 3.2

Drugs That Result in Arginine Vasopressin (AVP) Release

STIMULATE AVP RELEASE	OTHER MECHANISMS
Nicotine	Chlorpropamide: enhance renal effect of AVP
Clofibrate	
Vincristine	Tolbutamide
Isoproterenol	Cyclophosphamide
Chlorpropamide	Morphine
Antidepressants (SSRIs)	Barbiturates
	Carbamazepine
Antipsychotic agents	Acetaminophen
	NSAIDs: inhibits PG which antagonize AVP
Ecstacy	

Abbreviations: PG, prostaglandins; SSRI, selective serotonin reuptake inhibitors; NSAIDs, nonsteroidal anti-inflammatory drugs.

This commonly occurs in patients with psychiatric disease on psychotropic medications that result in dry mouth and increased water intake. It is also seen in those with beer drinker's potomania whose renal free water excretion is limited by solute intake.

KEY POINTS

Etiology of Hyponatremia

1. Hyponatremia with a normal serum osmolality is known as "pseudohyponatremia" and is a laboratory artifact.
2. Translocational hyponatremia is due to a shift of water out of cells in response to a nonsodium solute. Serum osmolality is elevated. Hyperglycemia is the most common cause.
3. The remaining causes of hyponatremia are associated with a low serum osmolality (*true hyponatremia*). True hyponatremia is caused by either (1) excess water intake with normal renal function or (2) continued solute free water intake with a decreased renal capacity for solute free water excretion.
4. The most common pathophysiologic mechanism is the nonosmotic release of AVP.
5. Edematous states, extrarenal and renal sodium and water losses, SIADH, and psychogenic polydipsia are the most common causes of true hyponatremia.
6. Hyponatremia from diuretics is almost always a result of thiazide diuretics since thiazides interfere with urinary dilution but not urinary concentrating ability.
7. SIADH is characterized by hyponatremia, low serum osmolality, and an inappropriately concentrated urine (less than maximally dilute) in the absence of renal, adrenal, or thyroid disease.

Signs and Symptoms

Gastrointestinal complaints of anorexia, nausea, and vomiting occur early, as do headaches, muscle cramps, and weakness. Thereafter, altered sensorium develops. There may be impaired response to verbal and painful stimuli. Inappropriate behavior, auditory and visual hallucinations, asterixis, and obtundation can be seen. Seizures develop with severe or acute hyponatremia. In far advanced hyponatremia the patient may exhibit decorticate or decerebrate posturing, bradycardia, hyper- or hypotension, respiratory arrest, and coma. The severity of symptoms correlates both with the magnitude and rapidity of the fall in serum sodium concentration and the rapidity of its onset. Central nervous system pathology is due to cerebral edema.

Central nervous system symptoms result from a failure in cerebral adaptation. When plasma osmolality falls acutely, osmotic equilibrium is maintained by either extrusion of intracellular solutes (regulatory volume decrease, RVD) or water influx into the brain. Neurologic symptoms result when osmotic equilibrium is achieved via the latter process. Since the brain is surrounded by a rigid case small increases in its volume result in substantial morbidity and mortality. If solute extrusion is successful and osmotic equilibrium maintained, the patient remains asymptomatic despite low serum sodium concentration and osmolality. Sodium extrusion from the brain by Na^+-K^+-ATPase and sodium channels is the first pathway activated (minutes) in regulatory volume decrease. If this is not adequate to lower brain osmolality then calcium-activated stretch receptors are stimulated. This activates a potassium channel that leads to potassium extrusion (hours).

In contrast to acute hyponatremia, chronic hyponatremia is characterized by fewer and milder neurologic symptoms. This is due to additional regulatory mechanisms. Studies in rats after 21 days of hyponatremia show that brain water content is normal. In this setting loss of organic osmolytes from the brain such as glutamate, glutamine, taurine, and myoinositol play an important role.

KEY POINTS
Signs and Symptoms of Hyponatremia

> 1. The severity of hyponatremic symptoms correlates with the magnitude and rapidity of the fall in serum sodium concentration.
> 2. Central nervous system pathology is due to cerebral edema and a failure in cerebral adaptation.
> 3. Chronic hyponatremia is characterized by fewer and milder neurologic symptoms.

Diagnosis

The diagnostic approach to the hyponatremic patient is divided into three steps.

STEP 1: WHAT IS THE SERUM OSMOLALITY? The first question one needs to answer in the evaluation of the hyponatremic patient is: What is the serum osmolality? This does not necessarily mean that one needs to directly measure serum osmolality but one at least needs to think of the question. The answer divides hyponatremic patients into three broad categories.

a. Isoosmolar or pseudohyponatremia results when the aqueous fraction of plasma is decreased and the particulate fraction is increased. This may result from hyperlipidemia (TG > 1500 mg/dL), hypercholesterolemia, or hyperproteinemia (multiple myeloma, Waldenstrom's macroglobulinemia, administration of intravenous immunoglobulin).
b. Hyperosmolar or translocational hyponatremia due to infusions of glucose, mannitol, or glycine.

The most common cause of translocational hyponatremia is hyperglycemia.
c. Hypoosmolar or "true hyponatremia" makes up the vast majority of cases, further subdivided by Steps 2 and 3.

STEP 2: WHAT IS THE ECF VOLUME (TOTAL BODY SODIUM CONTENT)? IS DEPENDENT EDEMA PRESENT? In the patient with true hyponatremia the second question one asks is what is the apparent ECF volume status. An approach to the evaluation of true hyponatremia is shown in Figure 3.2. States of increased ECF volume are relatively easy to identify on physical examination because they are characterized by the presence of dependent edema. If edema is present then the diagnosis must be congestive heart failure, cirrhosis, nephrotic syndrome, acute renal failure, or chronic kidney disease.

STEP 3: WHAT IS THE URINE SODIUM CONCENTRATION? In the absence of dependent edema the next step is to determine if the patient's ECF volume is decreased or normal. States of severe ECF volume depletion are often clinically apparent. Milder degrees of ECF volume depletion, however, may be difficult to distinguish from euvolemia on physical examination. In the patient with decreased ECF volume a urine sodium concentration less than 20 meq/L and a urine osmolality greater than 400 mOsm/kg suggests extrarenal sodium loss. The fractional excretion of sodium (FE_{Na}) can also be used to assess renal sodium handling. The FE_{Na} is that fraction of the filtered sodium load that is excreted by the kidney. It is calculated using the formula:

$$FE_{Na} = \frac{urine\ [Na] \times serum\ [Cr]}{serum\ [Na] \times urine\ [Cr]} \times 100$$

Sodium concentrations are expressed in meq/L and creatinine concentrations are expressed in mg/dL. A FE_{Na} less than 1% suggests ECF volume depletion. A urine sodium concentration greater than 20 meq/L, a FE_{Na} greater than 2%, and a urine osmolality less than 400 mOsm/kg suggests renal

Figure 3.2

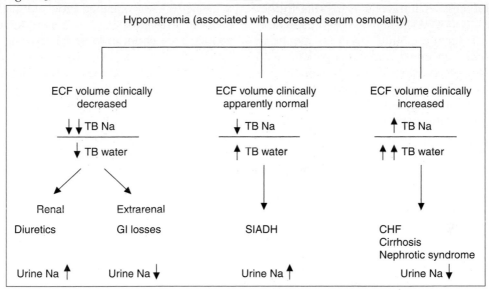

Hyponatremia (associated with decreased serum osmolality)

ECF volume clinically decreased	ECF volume clinically apparently normal	ECF volume clinically increased
↓↓ TB Na	↓ TB Na	↑ TB Na
↓ TB water	↑ TB water	↑↑ TB water
Renal Extrarenal		
Diuretics GI losses	SIADH	CHF Cirrhosis Nephrotic syndrome
Urine Na ↑ Urine Na ↓	Urine Na ↑	Urine Na ↓

Clinical approach to the patient with true hyponatremia. Patients with true hyponatremia (associated with a low serum osmolality) can be subdivided into three categories based on ECF volume status.

sodium loss. If the patient appears euvolemic one should consider SIADH, drugs, psychogenic polydipsia, and hypothyroidism.

KEY POINTS

Diagnosis of Hyponatremia

1. Hyponatremia may be associated with a normal, elevated, or decreased serum osmolality.
2. In patients with decreased serum osmolality (true hyponatremia) an evaluation of ECF volume status subdivides patients into three groups: increased; normal; or decreased ECF volume (total body sodium).
3. Increased ECF volume and total body sodium is identified by the presence of dependent edema on physical examination.
4. Patients with decreased ECF volume are further subdivided based on urinary sodium excretion into those with renal and extrarenal losses of salt and water.

5. The most common cause of hyponatremia in the "clinically euvolemic" patient is SIADH.

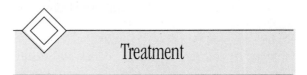

Treatment

The major sequelae of hyponatremia are neurologic. Neurologic injury is secondary to either hyponatremic encephalopathy or improper therapy (too rapid or overcorrection). Clinical studies show that in >90% of cases neurologic injury is secondary to hyponatremic encephalopathy. Hypoxia is the major factor contributing to neurologic injury. Since RVD involves active ion transport that is ATP-dependent, it is blunted by hypoxia. As a result sodium accumulates in the brain and worsens cerebral edema. Hypoxia is also a major stimulus for AVP secretion. Arginine vasopressin directly stimulates water entry into neurons. In addition, AVP decreases ATP generation and decreases intracellular pH that further decreases Na^+-K^+-ATPase activity. Respiratory arrest and seizures often occur suddenly in hyponatremic encephalopathy and patients who suffer a hypoxic event rarely survive without permanent neurologic injury. Predictive factors for neurologic injury include young age, female sex, reproductive status (premenopausal women), and the presence of encephalopathy.

Premenopausal women are at 25-fold increased risk for permanent neurologic injury from hyponatremic encephalopathy compared to postmenopausal women or men. This led to speculation that RVD is not as efficient in young women. Both estrogen and progesterone inhibit brain Na^+-K^+-ATPase. In addition, AVP decreases brain ATP in women but not men. In one study, premenopausal women had a respiratory arrest at higher serum sodium concentrations compared to postmenopausal women, 117 ± 7 meq/L versus 107 ± 8 meq/L, respectively.

Treatment is dependent on the acuity and severity of hyponatremia, as well as the patient's ECF volume status. Caution is exercised not to raise the serum sodium concentration too quickly as a devastating neurologic syndrome, central pontine myelinolysis (CPM), can result from over-aggressive correction. Destruction of myelin sheaths of pontine neurons results in flacid quadriplegia, dysarthria, dysphagia, coma, and death. The consequences are catastrophic and no treatment is currently available. Demyelination may be the result of excessive neuronal dehydration. Oligodendrocytes in the pons are particularly susceptible to osmotic stress. It is associated with increases in serum sodium concentration to normal within 24–48 hours, an increase in the serum sodium concentration greater than 25 meq/L in the first 48 hours, and elevation of serum sodium concentration to hypernatremic levels in patients with liver disease.

Since the neurologic insult may result from a rapid shift of water out of brain cells, it is possible that it could be interrupted at an early stage by shifting water back into brain cells. This was done

successfully in an animal model. The optimal protective effect was obtained provided that the final sodium correction gradient was reduced below 25 meq/L/24 hours and was effective up to 12–24 hours after the onset of osmotic injury. The quickest way to do this is through the administration of dD-AVP (a synthetic analogue of AVP, 1-deamino-8-D-arginine vasopressin, also known as desmopressin). The risk of relowering the serum sodium concentration may be low in the first few days of the correction process. As serum sodium concentration rises during the correction phase, the brain regains extruded osmolytes. This process takes up to 5–7 days to complete.

Severe symptomatic hyponatremia with or without seizures is treated emergently with the goal of raising serum sodium concentration above 120 meq/L. Serum sodium concentration should not be raised faster than 1 meq/L/hour in the absence of seizures or signs of increased intracranial pressure. If seizures are present the serum sodium concentration can be increased by 4–5 meq/L in the first hour. One should admit the symptomatic patient to the intensive care unit and precautions should be taken to ensure a secure airway. Serum sodium concentration is increased with either the infusion of 3% saline (513 meq Na/L) or a combination of a loop diuretic and normal saline. Hypertonic saline is discontinued when the serum sodium concentration increases above 120 meq/L or when symptoms resolve. Serum electrolytes are monitored every 2 hours. In the first 48 hours the clinician should avoid increasing the serum sodium concentration more than 25 meq/L and correcting the serum sodium concentration to or above normal. Water restriction alone has no role in the management of the symptomatic patient since it corrects the serum sodium concentration too slowly. In the absence of severe symptoms, serum sodium concentration is raised more slowly (0.5 meq/L/hour) until above 120 meq/L, and then slowly thereafter.

The patient evolving hyponatremia chronically (>48 hours) is not corrected faster than 8–12 meq/L in the first 24 hours. If liver disease and hypokalemia are present the rate of correction should be closer to 6 meq/day because these patients are at high risk for CPM.

A variety of formulas can be used to calculate the sodium requirement. They allow one to calculate the amount of sodium that would need to be added or water that would need to be removed in order to return the serum sodium concentration to normal. Although both sodium and water have either been removed or added in the process of generating the hyponatremia, these formulas work well in clinical practice. The most commonly employed formula is

[Na] requirement = total body water × (desired serum [Na]
− current serum [Na])

Total body water is equal to 0.6 times the body weight in men and 0.5 times the body weight in women. Based on the requirement one then calculates the infusion rate of 3% saline solution. Alternatively, one can estimate the effect on serum sodium concentration of 1 L of any infused solution using the following formula:

$$\frac{\text{infusate } [Na^+] - \text{serum } [Na^+]}{\text{total body water} + 1}$$

One can then adjust the rate of infusate to achieve the desired increase in serum sodium concentration.

In the hypovolemic patient one discontinues diuretics, corrects gastrointestinal fluid losses, and expands the ECF with normal saline. Replacing the ECF volume deficit is important because this eliminates the stimulus for the nonosmotic release of AVP and leads to the production of a maximally dilute urine. To calculate the sodium deficit one can use the following equation:

Na deficit = (total body water) × (140
− current serum sodium concentration)

One can replace one-third of the deficit over the first 12–24 hours and the remainder over the ensuing 48–72 hours. If vomiting, diarrhea, or diuretics caused the volume depletion, potassium deficits also must be corrected.

In the asymptomatic euvolemic patient one often begins treatment by restricting water. The following example illustrates the degree of reduction in total body water required to restore the serum sodium concentration to normal. A 75-kg man has a total body water of 45 L and a serum sodium concentration of 115 meq/L. The formula below is used to calculate the desired total body water.

$$\frac{\text{Actual serum } [Na]}{\text{Normal serum } [Na]} \times \text{current TBW} = \text{desired TBW}$$

The desired total body water is 36.9 L. Subtracting the desired from the current total body water reveals that 8.1 L of water must be removed to restore the serum sodium concentration to 140 meq/L. Fluid restriction rarely increases the serum sodium concentration by more than 1.5 meq/L/day. When the cause of SIADH is not reversible, demeclocycline can be used (600–1200 mg/day) providing that the patient has normal liver function.

The hypervolemic patient is managed with salt and water restriction. Negative water balance is achieved if daily fluid intake is less than the excretion of free water in urine. If congestive heart failure is the cause, an increase in cardiac output will suppress AVP release.

Common management errors in the treatment of the hyponatremic patient and recommendations include the following:

1. A fear of CPM often leads to a delay in correction or too slow a rate of correction of hyponatremia. Neurologic sequelae are far more commonly related to too slow a rate of correction rather than rapid correction.
2. The belief that 3% saline can be used only in a patient who is seizing. Hypertonic saline should be employed in hyponatremic encephalopathy. Every effort should be made to prevent seizure and respiratory arrest, once these sequelae develop permanent neurologic injury is the rule.
3. Be cognizant of patients at high risk for CPM especially those with abrupt withdrawal of a

stimulus that inhibits free water excretion such as liver transplantation, and elderly women on thiazides (diuretic is discontinued and ECF volume repleted). Magnetic resonance imaging is the study of choice to diagnose CPM but may take up to 1–2 weeks after the onset of signs and symptoms to show characteristic abnormalities.

4. Be aware of patients at high risk for hyponatremic encephalopathy such as premenopausal women in the postoperative setting. Postoperative patients should never receive free water. The intravenous fluid of choice in this setting is normal saline or Ringers lactate. Electrolytes are monitored daily.

5. Patients with SIADH should never be treated with normal saline alone. Normal saline administration in this setting results in a further fall in serum sodium concentration. The kidney is capable of generating free water from normal saline. For example, a patient with SIADH and a urine osmolality of 600 mOsm/kg, who is administered 1 L of normal saline (approximately 300 mOsm), will excrete that osmolar load in 500 mL of urine (300 mOsm given/600 mOsm/kg—urine osmolality = 500 mL final urine volume). This results in the generation of 500 mL of free water (the remainder of the 1 L given) and a further fall in serum sodium concentration.

KEY POINTS

Treatment of Hyponatremia

1. The morbidity and mortality of hyponatremia are related to neurologic injury that occurs as a result of hyponatremic encephalopathy or improper therapy (too rapid or overcorrection).
2. The major factor contributing to neurologic injury is hypoxia. Premenopausal women are at highest risk.
3. Treatment is dependent on the acuity and severity of hyponatremia, and the patient's ECF volume status.

4. Severe symptomatic hyponatremia is treated emergently with the goal of raising serum sodium concentration above 120 meq/L. The clinician should avoid increasing the serum sodium concentration more than 25 meq/L and correcting the serum sodium concentration to or above normal in the first 48 hours.
5. Every effort should be made to prevent seizure and respiratory arrest, once these sequelae develop permanent neurologic injury is the rule.
6. Chronic hyponatremia (>48 hours) is not corrected faster than 8–12 meq/L in the first 24 hours. If liver disease and hypokalemia are present the rate of correction should be closer to 6 meq/day because these patients are at high risk for CPM.
7. Postoperative patients should not receive free water.
8. Patients with SIADH should never be treated with normal saline alone.

Hypernatremia

Pathophysiologic Mechanisms

Hypernatremia is defined as a serum sodium concentration greater than 145 meq/L. It occurs when AVP concentration or effect is decreased or water intake is less than insensible, gastrointestinal and renal water losses. Therefore, hypernatremia results when there is a failure to take in enough free water in either the presence or absence of a urinary concentrating defect. This is most commonly seen in those patients who depend on others for access to water or lack thirst sensation. Infrequently, hypernatremia results from salt ingestion or administration of hypertonic saline solutions.

With free water loss the serum osmolality and sodium concentration increase as shown in

Figure 3.3

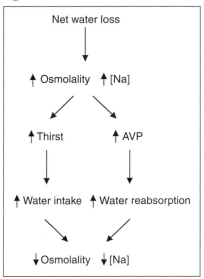

Net water loss

↑ Osmolality ↑ [Na]

↑ Thirst ↑ AVP

↑ Water intake ↑ Water reabsorption

↓ Osmolality ↓ [Na]

Normal response to water loss. The normal response to water loss involves the stimulation of thirst and increased renal water reabsorption.

Figure 3.3. The rise in serum osmolality stimulates thirst and AVP release from the posterior pituitary. Stimulation of thirst results in increased free water intake. Arginine vasopressin binds to its receptor in the basolateral membrane of collecting duct and stimulates water reabsorption.

The normal renal concentrating mechanism in humans allows for excretion of urine that is as much as four times as concentrated as plasma (1200 mOsm/kg H_2O). Since the average daily solute load is approximately 600 mOsm, this solute is excreted in as little as 0.5 L of urine. Note that even under maximal antidiuretic conditions, one must drink at least this volume of water per day in order to maintain water balance. Thirst is an integral component of the water regulatory system. The normal function of the renal concentrating mechanism requires that its various components be intact. These include the following:

1. **The ability to generate a hypertonic interstitium.** Henle's loop acts as a countercurrent multiplier with energy derived from active chloride transport in the water-impermeable thick ascending limb of the loop (mediated via the Na^+-K^+-$2Cl^-$ cotransporter). The transporter serves the dual process of diluting tubular fluid and rendering the interstitium progressively hypertonic from cortex to papilla.

2. **AVP secretion.** This hormone renders the collecting duct permeable to water and allows fluid delivered from the distal tubule to equilibrate with the concentrated interstitium. Arginine vasopressin is a nonapeptide produced by neurons originating in the supraoptic and paraventricular nuclei of the hypothalamus. These neurons cross the pituitary stalk and terminate in the posterior pituitary. Arginine vasopressin is processed and stored in neurosecretory granules along with neurophysin and copeptin.

3. **Normal collecting duct responsiveness to arginine vasopressin.** Abnormalities in the renal concentrating process obligate excretion of a larger volume of urine to maintain solute balance, e.g., with 600 mOsm of solute to be excreted and the inability to increase urine osmolality above plasma, a urine flow of 2 L/day is obligated. Failure to replace these water losses orally leads to progressive water depletion and hypernatremia.

KEY POINTS
Hypernatremia

1. Hypernatremia results when there is a failure to take in enough free water in either the presence or absence of a concentrating defect. It is most commonly seen in those who depend on others for access to water or who lack thirst.
2. Thirst is an integral component of the water regulatory system.
3. Normal concentrating mechanism function requires the ability to generate a hypertonic interstitium, AVP secretion, and normal collecting duct responsiveness to AVP.

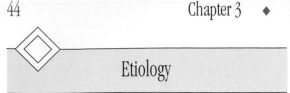

Etiology

Diabetes insipidus (DI) is the result of decreased pituitary production of AVP (central) or decreased renal responsiveness to AVP (nephrogenic). Central DI does not occur until greater than 80% of vasopressin-producing neurons are destroyed.

Central DI may be idiopathic or secondary to head trauma, surgery, or neoplasm. Urine volume ranges from 3 to 15 L/day. Patients tend to be young with nocturia and a preference for cold water. The kidneys should respond to exogenous AVP with a rise in urine osmolality of 100 mOsm/kg above the value achieved following water deprivation. Patients with complete central DI are unable to concentrate urine above 200 mOsm/kg with dehydration, whereas patients with partial DI are able to concentrate urine but not maximally. Treatment consists of administering AVP. The best therapy is long-acting, nasally administered dD-AVP. An important point is that thirst is stimulated by the increased P_{osm} so effectively that serum sodium concentration is only slightly elevated and the most common clinical presentation is polyuria. Psychogenic polydipsia also presents with polyuria; however, the serum sodium concentration is often mildly decreased rather than increased.

One-third to one-half of central DI cases are idiopathic. A lymphocytic infiltrate is present in the posterior pituitary and pituitary stalk. Some of these patients have circulating antibodies directed against vasopressin-producing neurons.

Familial central DI is rare and inherited in three ways. The most common is an autosomal dominant disorder resulting from mutations in the coding region of the AVP gene. The mutant protein fails to fold properly and accumulates in the endoplasmic reticulum resulting in neuronal death. Because neurons die slowly vasopressin deficiency is not present at birth but develops over years. It often gradually progresses

from a partial to complete defect. A similar clinical presentation is seen with X-linked inheritance, although the evidence for this mode of inheritance is weak. Autosomal recessive central DI is a very rare disorder caused by a single amino acid substitution resulting in the production of an AVP with little to no antidiuretic activity.

In nephrogenic DI the collecting duct does not respond appropriately to AVP. The most common inherited form of nephrogenic DI is an X-linked disorder in which cyclic AMP is not generated in response to AVP. It is caused by a number of mutations in the V_2 receptor. Aquaporin-2 gene mutations also result in nephrogenic DI and may be inherited in an autosomal dominant or recessive fashion. In dominant cases heterotetramers form between mutant and wild type aquaporin-2 water channels that are unable to traffic to the plasma membrane. This usually results in complete resistance to the effects of AVP.

Acquired nephrogenic DI is much more common but often less severe. Chronic renal failure, hypercalcemia, lithium treatment, obstruction, and hypokalemia are its causes. Aquaporin-2 expression in principal cells of the collecting duct is markedly reduced. Lithium is the most common treatment for manic-depressive psychosis. Approximately 0.1% of the population is receiving lithium and 20–30% develop severe side effects. In rats administered lithium for 25 days, aquaporin-2 and -3 expression decreases to 5% of control levels. Both hypokalemia and hypercalcemia are associated with a significant downregulation of aquaporin-2. Rats treated with a potassium-deficient diet for 11 days show a 30% decrease in aquaporin-2 expression. Aquaporin-2 expression normalizes after 7 days of a normal potassium diet. Hypercalcemia induced by excessive vitamin D administration in rats results in a concentrating defect that is caused by downregulation of both aquaporin-2 and the Na^+-K^+-2Cl^- cotransporter.

A number of drugs may cause a renal concentrating defect. Ethanol and phenytoin impair AVP release resulting in a water diuresis. Lithium and demeclocycline cause tubular resistance to AVP while amphotericin B and methoxyflurane injure the renal medulla. Thus, a concentrating defect (inability to conserve water) can be secondary to a lack of AVP, unresponsiveness to AVP, or renal tubular dysfunction. Other specific causes and mechanisms for concentrating defects include sickle cell anemia or trait (medullary vascular injury), excessive water intake or primary polydipsia (decreased medullary tonicity), severe protein restriction (decreased medullary urea), and a variety of disorders affecting renal medullary vessels and tubules.

Recently, DI caused by peripheral degradation of AVP was reported in peripartum women. Vasopressinase is an enzyme produced by the placenta that degrades AVP and oxytocin. It appears in plasma of women early in pregnancy and increases in activity throughout gestation. After delivery, which is curative due to loss of the placenta, vasopressinase rapidly becomes undetectable. Although only case reports of diabetes insipidus from vasopressinase are published to date, it is unclear how frequently this condition actually occurs. These patients often respond to desmopressin (dD-AVP), which is not degraded by vasopressinase.

KEY POINTS

Etiology of Hypernatremia

> 1. Diabetes insipidus may be central due to decreased pituitary production and release of AVP or nephrogenic secondary to decreased renal responsiveness to AVP.
> 2. Central DI is idiopathic or secondary to head trauma, surgery, or neoplasm.
> 3. Acquired nephrogenic DI occurs most commonly with lithium administration. Aquaporin-2 expression in principal cells of collecting duct is markedly reduced.
> 4. A variety of drugs cause renal concentrating defects.

Signs and Symptoms

Cellular dehydration occurs as water shifts out of cells. This results in neuromuscular irritability with twitches, hyperreflexia, seizures, coma, and death. In children, severe acute hypernatremia (serum sodium concentration >160 meq/L) has a mortality rate of 45%. Two-thirds of survivors have permanent neurologic injury. In adults, acute hypernatremia has a reported mortality as high as 75% and chronic hypernatremia 60%. Hypernatremia is often a marker of serious underlying disease. Of note, the brain protects itself from the insult of hypernatremia by increasing its own osmolality, in part due to increases in free amino acids. The mechanism is unclear, but the phenomenon is referred to as the generation of "idiogenic osmoles." The therapeutic corollary is that water repletion must be slow with chronic hypernatremia to allow inactivation of these solutes and thus avoid cerebral edema.

KEY POINTS

Signs and Symptoms of Hypernatremia

> 1. Symptoms of hypernatremia result from a shift of water out of brain cells.
> 2. In chronic hypernatremia the brain generates "idiogenic osmoles" that reduce the gradient for water movement.

Diagnosis

Although hypernatremia can occur in association with hypovolemia, hypervolemia, and euvolemia, patients most commonly present with hypovolemia. Those that are euvolemic may be mildly

Figure 3.4

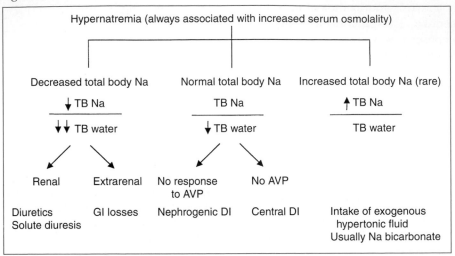

Clinical approach to the patient with hypernatremia. Patients with hypernatremia can also be categorized based on ECF volume status. The majority have decreased or normal ECF volume (total body sodium).

hypernatremic but their most common complaint is polyuria. Many disorders may result in hypernatremia; however, decreased thirst, inability to gain access to water, and drugs are the most common causes (Figure 3.4).

A high serum sodium concentration results from free water loss that is not compensated for by an increase in free water intake. Free water loss may be renal or extrarenal in origin. Extrarenal losses originate from skin, respiratory tract, or from the gastrointestinal tract. Renal losses are the result of a solute (osmotic) or water diuresis. A solute or osmotic diuresis most commonly results from excretion of glucose in uncontrolled diabetes mellitus. A water diuresis is secondary to central or nephrogenic DI. If thirst is intact, patients with renal losses present with the chief complaint of polyuria, defined as the excretion of more than 3 L of urine daily.

An increased serum sodium concentration is a potent stimulus for thirst and AVP release. After a thorough history and physical examination are performed the clinician must answer several

questions in the hypernatremic patient. First, is thirst intact? If the serum sodium concentration is elevated above 147 meq/L the patient should be thirsty. Second, if the patient is thirsty, is he capable of getting to water? The next step is to evaluate the hypothalamic-pituitary-renal axis. This involves an examination of urine osmolality. If the hypothalamic-pituitary-renal axis is intact a rise in serum sodium concentration above 147 meq/L maximally stimulates AVP release and results in a urine osmolality greater than 700 mOsm/kg. If urine osmolality is greater than 700 mOsm/kg then free water losses are extrarenal. A urine osmolality less than plasma indicates that the kidney is the source of free water loss as a result of either central or nephrogenic DI. These disorders are differentiated by the response to exogenous AVP. Either 5 units of aqueous vasopressin subcutaneously or 10 μg of dD-AVP intranasally increases urine osmolality by 50% or more in central DI but has no effect on urine osmolality in nephrogenic DI. In central DI the onset is generally abrupt, urine volume remains fairly constant over the course of the day, nocturia is common, and patients have a preference for drinking cold water.

Urine osmolality in the intermediate range (300–600 mOsm/kg) may be secondary to psychogenic polydipsia, an osmotic diuresis, and partial central or nephrogenic DI. Psychogenic polydipsia is generally associated with a mildly decreased rather than increased serum sodium concentration. Partial central and nephrogenic DI may require a water deprivation test to distinguish. In the water deprivation test water is prohibited and urine volume and osmolality measured hourly and serum sodium concentration and osmolality every 2 hours. The test is stopped if either the urine osmolality reaches normal levels, the plasma osmolality reaches 300 mOsm/kg, or the urine osmolality is stable on two successive readings despite a rising serum osmolality. In the last two circumstances exogenous vasopressin is administered and the urine osmolality and volume measured. In partial central DI the urine osmolality generally increases by greater than 50 mOsm/kg. In partial nephrogenic DI the urine osmolality may increase slightly but generally remains below serum osmolality. An osmotic diuresis is suspected if the total osmolar excretion exceeds 1000 mOsm/day. Total osmolar excretion is calculated by multiplying the urine osmolality by the urine volume in a 24-hour collection.

KEY POINTS

Diagnosis of Hypernatremia

1. Hypernatremia occurs most commonly in association with hypovolemia.
2. The euvolemic patient is only mildly hypernatremic but will complain of polyuria.
3. A high serum sodium concentration results from free water loss that is not compensated for by an increase in free water intake. Free water loss is renal or extrarenal in origin.
4. The clinician should first examine whether thirst and access to free water are intact.

5. The next step is to evaluate the hypothalamic-pituitary-renal axis. This involves an examination of the urine osmolality. If urine osmolality is greater than 700 mOsm/kg then free water losses are extrarenal.
6. A urine osmolality less than plasma indicates that the kidney is the source of free water loss from either central or nephrogenic DI. These disorders are differentiated by the response of urine osmolality to exogenous AVP.

Treatment

Treatment of hypernatremia is divided into two parts: restoring plasma tonicity to normal and correcting sodium imbalances, and providing specific treatment directed at the underlying disorder.

When restoring plasma tonicity to normal and correcting sodium imbalances, sodium may need to be added or removed while providing water. A formula to calculate the total amount of water needed to lower serum sodium concentration from one concentration to another can be used. This does not take into account, however, changes in sodium balance as it is based on a rough estimate of total body water as 60% of weight (kg) in men and 50% of weight (kg) in women:

water needed (L) = (total body water)
$$\times ((\text{actual sodium/desired sodium}) - 1)$$

Water deficits are restored slowly in order to avoid sudden shifts in brain cell volume. Water deficits are corrected preferably with increased oral intake or with intravenous administration of hypotonic solution. The serum sodium concentration should not be lowered faster than 8–10 meq/day. The formula above calculates the amount of free water replacement needed at the time the patient is first seen. It does not take into account ongoing free water losses that may be occurring from the kidney while one is attempting to correct the deficit. If urine volume is high or urine osmolality low then one must add ongoing renal free water losses to the replacement calculation.

In order to determine ongoing renal free water losses one must calculate the electrolyte-free water clearance. For this purpose urine is divided into two components: an isotonic component (the volume needed to excrete sodium and potassium at their concentration in serum),and an electrolyte-free water component. This is shown in the formula below:

$$\text{urine volume} = C_{\text{Electrolytes}} + C_{\text{H}_2\text{O}}$$

$$C_{\text{Electrolytes}} = \frac{\text{urine [Na]} + [K]}{\text{serum [Na]}} \times \text{urine volume}$$

where $C_{\text{H}_2\text{O}}$ is the volume of urine from which the electrolytes were removed during the elaboration of a hypotonic urine.

◆ CASE 3.1

This is best illustrated with a case. A 70 kg male with a history of nephrogenic DI is found unconscious at home and is brought to the Emergency Department. The serum sodium concentration is 160 meq/L. A Foley catheter is placed and urine output is 500 mL/hour. Urine electrolytes reveal a sodium concentration of 60 meq/L, a potassium concentration of 20 meq/L, and a urine osmolality of 180 mOsm/kg. How much water must be administered in order to correct the serum sodium concentration to 140 meq/L?

Water needed (L) = (0.6 × body weight in kg)
$\qquad$ × ((actual [Na]/desired [Na])
$\qquad$ − 1)
$\qquad$ = (0.6 × 70) × ((160/140) − 1)
$\qquad$ = 42 × 0.14 or 6 L

One next determines the time frame over which the deficit will be corrected. If the serum sodium concentration were decreased by 8 meq/L in the first 24 hours, then 2.4 L of water is administered at a rate of 100 mL/hour. If water were given at this rate in the form of D5W, serum sodium concentration would increase not decrease. The

reason for this is that the replacement calculation did not include the large ongoing free water loss in urine.

To include renal free water losses one must calculate the electrolyte-free water clearance as illustrated below:

$$C_{\text{Electrolytes}} = \frac{\text{urine [Na]} + [K]}{\text{serum [Na]}} \times \text{urine volume}$$

$$= \frac{60 + 20}{160} \times 500 \text{ mL/hour}$$

$$= \frac{80}{160} \times 500 = 250 \text{ mL/hour}$$

$$C_{\text{H}_2\text{O}} = \text{urine volume} - C_{\text{Electrolytes}}$$

$$C_{\text{H}_2\text{O}} = 500 - 250 = 250 \text{ mL/hour}$$

The ongoing renal free water losses of 250 mL/hour must be added to the replacement solution, 100 mL/hour, in order to correct the serum sodium concentration.

Treatment is also directed at the underlying disorder. In the patient with nephrogenic DI significant hypernatremia will not develop unless thirst is impaired or the patient lacks access to water. The goal of treatment is to reduce urine volume and renal free water excretion. As discussed earlier, urine volume is equal to osmolar excretion or intake (they are the same in the steady state) divided by the urine osmolality. Urine volume can be reduced by decreasing osmolar intake with protein or salt restriction or by increasing urine osmolality. Thiazide diuretics inhibit urinary dilution and increase urine osmolality. Nonsteroidal anti-inflammatory agents (NSAIDs) by inhibiting renal prostaglandin synthesis increase concentrating ability. Prostaglandins normally antagonize the action of AVP. Their effects are partially additive to those of thiazide diuretics. Electrolyte disturbances such as hypokalemia or hypercalcemia should be corrected. Early in the course of lithium-induced nephrogenic DI, amiloride may be of some benefit. Amiloride prevents the entry of lithium into the cortical collecting duct principal cell and can limit its toxicity.

The patient with central DI and a deficiency of AVP secretion is treated with hormone replacement

Table 3.3

Treatment of Central DI

CONDITION	DRUG	DOSE
Complete		
	dD-AVP	5–20 µg intranasally q 12–24 hours
		0.1–0.4 mg orally q 12–24 hours
Incomplete		
	Chlorpropamide	125–500 mg/day
	Carbamazepine	100–300 mg bid
	Clofibrate	500 mg qid

Abbreviations: bid, twice a day; qid, four times a day.

(Table 3.3). Intranasal desmopressin is most commonly used. The initial dose is 5 µg at bedtime and is titrated upward to a dose of 5–20 µg once or twice daily. Desmopressin can also be administered orally. In general a 0.1 mg tablet is equivalent to 2.5–5.0 µg of the nasal spray. Serum sodium concentration must be followed carefully during dose titration to avoid hyponatremia. Desmopressin is expensive. As a consequence drugs that increase AVP release or enhance its effect can be added to reduce cost. These drugs can also be used in patients with partial central DI. Chlorpropamide and carbamazepine enhance the renal action of AVP. Clofibrate may increase AVP release. As with nephrogenic DI thiazide diuretics and NSAIDs can also be employed.

KEY POINTS

Treatment of Hypernatremia

1. Treatment of hypernatremia is directed at restoring plasma tonicity to normal, correcting sodium imbalances, and providing specific treatment directed at the underlying disorder.
2. Water deficits are restored slowly to avoid sudden shifts in brain cell volume. The serum sodium concentration is not lowered faster than 8–10 meq/day.
3. If urine volume is high or urine osmolality low then one must account for ongoing renal free water losses.
4. In the patient with nephrogenic DI urine volume is reduced by decreasing osmolar intake with protein or salt restriction or by increasing urine osmolality with thiazide diuretics.
5. Hormone replacement therapy with desmopressin (dD-AVP) is the cornerstone of treatment of central DI.

Additional Reading

Adrogue, H.J., Madias, N.E. Hypernatremia. *N Engl J Med* 342:1493–1499, 2000.

Adrogue, H.J., Madias, N.E. Hyponatremia. *N Engl J Med* 342:1581–1589, 2000.

Bedford, J.J., Leader, J.P., Walker, R.J. Aquaporin expression in normal human kidney and in renal disease. *J Am Soc Nephrol* 14:2581–2587, 2003.

Calakos, N., Fischbein, N., Baringer, J.R., Jay, C. Cortical MRI findings associated with rapid correction of hyponatremia. *Neurology* 55:1048–1051, 2000.

Fraser, C.L., Arieff, A.I. Epidemiology, pathophysiology, and management of hyponatremic encephalopathy. *Am J Med* 102:67–77, 1997.

Goldszmidt, M.A., Iliescu, E.A. DDAVP to prevent rapid correction in hyponatremia. *Clin Nephrol* 53:226–229, 2000.

Kumar, S., Berl, T. Sodium. *Lancet* 352:220–228, 1998.

Milionis, H.J., Liamis, G.L., Elisaf, M.S. The hyponatremic patient: a systematic approach to laboratory diagnosis. *CMAJ* 166:1056–1062, 2002.

Moran, S.M., Jamison, R.L. The variable hyponatremic response to hyperglycemia. *West J Med* 142:49–53, 1985.

Nielsen, S., Froklaer, J., Marples, D., Kwon, T.-H., Agre, P., Knepper, M.A. Aquaporins in the kidney: from molecules to medicine. *Physiol Rev* 82:205–244, 2002.

Zarinetchi, F., Berl, T. Evaluation and management of severe hyponatremia. *Adv Intern Med* 41:251–283, 1996.

Mark A. Perazella

Diuretics

Recommended Time to Complete: 1 day

Guiding Questions

1. What is the difference between diuresis and natriuresis?
2. How do diuretics reach their site of action?
3. Where do diuretics act in the nephron?
4. Which diuretics act in the proximal tubule and what is their mechanism of action?
5. What transporter in the loop of Henle reabsorbs NaCl?
6. Which diuretics act in the distal convoluted tubule (DCT)?
7. How do diuretics that act in cortical collecting duct (CCD) induce natriuresis?
8. What are some of the common adverse effects of various diuretics?
9. What is diuretic resistance and how does one assess for the cause of resistance?
10. How does diuretic resistance develop in the setting of chronic loop diuretic therapy?
11. How does one treat various causes of diuretic resistance?

Introduction

The primary renal effect of diuretics is to increase the amount of urine formed or diuresis (water, sodium, urea, and other substances). A large part of this effect is due to enhanced natriuresis, which is defined as an increase in renal sodium excretion. Diuretics were initially described as a useful therapy to reduce edema in the sixteenth century. The first agent known to increase urine output was mercurous chloride. In 1930, the antimicrobial sulfanilamide was noted to increase renal Na^+ excretion and reduce edema formation in patients with congestive heart failure (CHF). It is interesting that most diuretics were discovered serendipitously when they were noted to increase urine output and change urine composition. These changes in urine were considered an adverse effect of drugs intended for other purposes. Targeted disruption of various renal transporters was not part of the development of these drugs as the mechanism of transport was unknown; rather diuretics were developed empirically. Diuretics are the most commonly prescribed medications in the United States. They are used to treat a variety of clinical disease states including hypertension, edema, congestive heart failure, hyperkalemia, and hypercalcemia.

To understand the actions of diuretics, one must first appreciate renal handling of sodium and water. This subject is reviewed in detail in Chapter 2, but will be briefly reviewed here. The kidneys regulate extracellular fluid (ECF) volume by modulating NaCl and water excretion. Sodium intake is balanced by the renal excretion of sodium. A normal glomerular filtration rate (GFR) is important for the optimal excretion of sodium and water. Following formation and passage of glomerular ultrafiltrate into Bowman's space, delivery of sodium and water to the proximal tubule is the first site of tubular handling. Along the nephron sodium is reabsorbed by several different transport mechanisms. Sodium absorption is regulated by a number of different factors. For example, various hormones

(renin, angiotensin II, aldosterone, atrial natriuretic peptide (ANP), prostaglandins, and endothelin) and physical properties (mean arterial pressure, peritubular capillary pressure, and renal interstitial pressure) modify renal handling of sodium and water. Direct effects on tubular transport along the nephron underlie the major influence of these factors on renal sodium and water handling. Sodium reabsorption is driven primarily by Na^+-K^+-ATPase located on the basolateral membrane of all tubular epithelial cells. This pump provides energy required by transporters located on the apical (luminal) membrane that reabsorb sodium from glomerular filtrate. Cell-specific transporters are present on these tubular cells.

Diuretics act to enhance renal sodium and water excretion by inhibiting these transporters at different nephron sites (Figure 4.1). They act to reduce sodium entry into the tubular cell. With the exception of spironolactone and eplerenone, all diuretics exert their effects from the luminal side of the cell. Thus, most diuretics must enter tubular fluid to be effective. Secretion across the proximal tubule via either organic acid or base transport pathways is the primary mode of entry (except for mannitol, which undergoes glomerular filtration). Diuretic potency depends significantly on drug delivery to its site of action, as well as the nephron site where it acts. Other factors that influence diuretic action are level of kidney function (glomerular filtration rate), state of the effective arterial blood volume (congestive heart failure, cirrhosis, and nephrosis), and treatment with certain medications such as nonsteroidal anti-inflammatory drugs (NSAIDs) and probenecid. Diuretics may also have a variety of adverse effects, some that are common to all diuretics and others that are unique to specific agents (Table 4.1).

KEY POINTS

Diuretics

> 1. Diuretics increase renal sodium and water excretion.

Figure 4.1

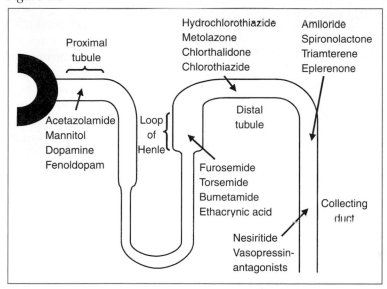

Sites of diuretic action in the nephron. Sodium chloride reabsorption is reduced by various diuretics in proximal tubule, loop of Henle, distal tubule, and collecting duct.

2. Diuretics were developed empirically based on observed effects on urine volume and change in urine composition.
3. Several hormones control renal sodium and water excretion through effects on tubular transport.
4. The majority of diuretics enter the urine by tubular secretion and act on the luminal surface to reduce sodium reabsorption.

Sites of Diuretic Action in the Kidney

Proximal Tubule

The initial site of diuretic action in the kidney is the proximal tubule. Transport of sodium in the proximal tubular cell is driven by Na^+-K^+-ATPase activity, which drives sodium reabsorption by the Na^+-H^+ exchanger on the apical membrane. The Na^+-K^+-ATPase uses energy derived from ATP to extrude three Na^+ ions in exchange for two potassium ions. This results in a reduction of intracellular Na^+ concentration. Sodium can then move down its electrochemical gradient from tubular lumen into the cell via the Na^+-H^+ exchanger in exchange for an H^+ that moves out of the cell against its electrochemical gradient. Secretion of H^+ by this exchanger is associated with reclamation of filtered bicarbonate. Two diuretics that impair sodium reabsorption in this nephron segment are mannitol and acetazolamide. Each acts differently to reduce sodium reclamation. Mannitol, an osmotic diuretic, is mainly employed for prophylaxis to prevent ischemic or nephrotoxic renal injury and to reduce cerebral edema. It is a nonmetabolizable osmotic agent that is freely filtered by the glomerulus and enters the tubular space where it raises intratubular fluid osmolality. This effect drags water, which is accompanied by sodium from tubular cells into the tubular fluid. Mannitol is poorly absorbed with oral administration and is

Table 4.1

Table 4.1

Adverse Effects of Diuretic Drugs

Proximal tubule diuretics
Carbonic anhydrase inhibitors (acetazolamide)
Hypokalemia, metabolic acidosis
Drowsiness, fatigue, lethargy, paresthesias
Bone marrow suppression
Osmotic diuretics (mannitol)
Hypokalemia, hyperkalemia (cell shift)
Expansion of the ECF, CHF
Nausea and vomiting, headache
Loop diuretics (furosemide, bumetanide, torsemide, ethacrynic acid)
Hypokalemia, hypomagnesemia, hyponatremia
Metabolic alkalosis, hypovolemia
Ototoxicity, diarrhea
Blood dyscrasia (thrombocytopenia, agranulocytosis)
DCT diuretics (thiazides, metolazone)
Hypokalemia, hypomagnesemia, hyponatremia
Hypercalcemia, hyperuricemia
Metabolic alkalosis, hypovolemia
Mild hyperglycemia, hyperlipidemia
Hypersensitivity, interstitial nephritis
Leukopenia, thrombocytopenia, aplastic and hemolytic anemia
CCD diuretics
Mineralocorticoid receptor antagonists (spironolactone*, eplerenone)
Hyperkalemia
Gynecomastia*, hirsutism*, menstrual irregularities*, testicular atrophy*
Sodium channel inhibitors (amiloride#, triamterene◆)
Hyperkalemia
Glucose intolerance#, megaloblastic anemia◆, urinary crystals◆

Abbreviations: ECF, extracellular fluid; CHF, congestive heart failure.

active only when given intravenously. It acts in the kidney within 10 minutes and has a $t_{1/2}$ of approximately 1.2 hours in patients with normal renal function. Toxicity develops when filtration of mannitol is impaired, as in renal failure.

Retained mannitol causes increased plasma osmolality, which can exacerbate CHF, induce hyponatremia, and causes a hyperoncotic syndrome. As a result of these effects, mannitol is contraindicated in patients with CHF and moderate-to-severe kidney disease.

The carbonic anhydrase (CA) inhibitor acetazolamide is prescribed to alkalinize the urine (certain drug overdoses), prevent and treat altitude sickness, and decrease intraocular pressure in certain forms of glaucoma. The CA inhibitors disrupt bicarbonate reabsorption by impairing the conversion of carbonic acid (H_2CO_3) into CO_2 and H_2O in tubular fluid. Excess bicarbonate in the tubular lumen associates with Na^+, the most abundant cation in tubular fluid, and exits the proximal tubule. Acetazolamide and other CA inhibitors exert their effect within half an hour and maintain a $t_{1/2}$ of approximately 13 hours. Over time, the effect of these drugs diminishes due to the reduction in plasma and filtered bicarbonate. Metabolic consequences of CA inhibitors include metabolic acidosis and hypokalemia. Hypokalemia results from enhanced delivery of sodium and bicarbonate to the principal cell, which promotes potassium secretion through a change in membrane potential. These drugs should be avoided in patients with cirrhosis (increases serum NH_3) and those with uncorrected hypokalemia. Because downstream nephron segments such as the loop of Henle, distal convoluted tubule (DCT), and CCD avidly reabsorb sodium, these two drugs are relatively weak diuretics.

Thick Ascending Limb of the Loop of Henle

In this nephron segment, the Na^+-K^+-$2Cl^-$ cotransporter on the apical surface of tubular cells, powered by Na^+-K^+-ATPase on the basolateral membrane reabsorbs significant amounts of NaCl (20–30% of the filtered sodium load). In addition to NaCl, potassium, calcium, and magnesium are reclaimed in this tubular segment. It is not surprising that the most potent diuretics, the loop diuretics, retard the action of this transporter. Loop diuretics consist of those that are sulfonamide derivatives (furosemide, bumetanide, and torse-mide) and ethacrynic acid, a non-sulfa-containing loop diuretic. These drugs are used primarily to treat states of volume overload refractory to other diuretics including CHF, cirrhosis-associated ascites and edema, and nephrotic syndrome. Other indications are hypercalcemia and hypertension associated with moderate-to-severe kidney disease, which is often a sodium retentive state. Rarely, these drugs are employed to help correct hyponatremia in patients with the syndrome of inappropriate antidiuretic hormone (SIADH).

Loop diuretics can be administered as either oral or intravenous (IV) preparations. They are well absorbed orally, unless significant bowel edema is present as in severe CHF, cirrhosis, and nephrotic syndrome. Loop diuretics act within 20–30 minutes and have a $t_{1/2}$ of approximately 1–1.5 hours. In healthy subjects given intravenous furosemide or an oral dose twice the IV dose, there was no difference in cumulative urine volume, natriuresis, or potassium and chloride excretion. The major difference between the two modes of administration was a 30-minute peak natriuretic action with IV furosemide compared with a 75-minute peak for oral therapy. This difference is likely due to the rapid increase in plasma levels with IV dosing. In patients with chronic kidney disease, the dose of loop diuretic to promote effective natriuresis is higher than patients with normal kidney function. This is due

to several factors. Most important is that a reduced GFR is associated with a reduction in filtered sodium load. For example, the filtered sodium for a patient with a GFR of 100 mL/minute is 15 meq/minute, whereas it is only 0.15 meq/minute in a patient with kidney disease and a GFR of 10 mL/minute. In advanced chronic kidney disease (creatinine clearance = 17 mL/minute), the maximal diuretic response to intravenous furosemide occurs at 160–200 mg, much higher than required in subjects with normal renal function. Decreased delivery of loop diuretic to its site of action is another factor in renal failure that limits efficacy at lower administered doses.

In normal subjects, the dose equivalency for the various loop diuretics is as follows:

$$\text{bumetanide } 1 \text{ mg} = \text{torsemide } 10 \text{ mg}$$
$$= \text{furosemide } 40 \text{ mg}$$

The maximum dose of each drug varies based on the indication and the underlying disease state. Table 4.2 notes the approximate ceiling doses for the loop diuretics based on the associated clinical condition. Ceiling dose is defined as the dose that provides maximal inhibition of NaCl reabsorption, reaching a plateau in the diuretic dose-response curve. Adverse effects from loop diuretics are related in part to their therapeutic effect on natriuresis and changes in urine composition. These include hypokalemia, hypocalcemia, hypomagnesemia, volume contraction (which can

Table 4.2

Ceiling Doses of Intravenous and Oral Loop Diuretics in Various Clinical Conditions

CLINICAL CONDITION	FUROSEMIDE (MG)		BUMETANIDE (MG)		TORSEMIDE (MG)	
	IV	PO	IV	PO	IV	PO
Kidney disease						
GFR 20–50 mL/minute	80	60–80	2–3	2–3	20–50	20–50
GFR <20 mL/minute	200	240	8–10	8–10	50–100	50–100
Congestive heart failure	40–80	160–240	2–3	2–3	20–50	20–50
Nephrotic syndrome	120		3		50	50
Cirrhosis	40–80	80–160	1	1–2	10–20	20–50

Abbreviations: IV, intravenous; PO, oral; GFR, glomerular filtration rate.

result in hypotension and shock), and metabolic alkalosis. Groups most susceptible to these untoward effects, in particular volume contraction, are the elderly and patients with hypertension who lack clinical edema. Loop diuretics must also be used cautiously in patients with cirrhosis, to avoid precipitation of the hepatorenal syndrome and in patients treated with digoxin that are at high risk for lethal arrhythmias when hypokalemia develops. Ototoxicity is another complication of high plasma drug levels. Ethacrynic acid is associated with severe ototoxicity and is rarely employed except in patients with sulfonamide allergy. Furosemide, torsemide, and bumetanide are contraindicated in patients with sulfonamide allergy. Rarely, mild hyperglycemia occurs in patients due to inhibition of insulin release by loop diuretics.

Distal Convoluted Tubule

The DCT contains the thiazide-sensitive Na^+-Cl^- cotransporter (NCC), which reabsorbs sodium and chloride delivered from the loop of Henle. This segment reabsorbs approximately 5–10% of the filtered sodium load. Thiazide and thiazide-like diuretics inhibit NCC. Common drugs include hydrochlorothiazide (HCTZ), metolazone, and the intravenous preparation chlorothiazide. Through inhibition of NCC, this class of drugs is used primarily to treat hypertension, particularly in patients with salt-sensitive hypertension. Additional uses include treatment of osteoporosis and nephrolithiasis. While not intuitively obvious as a therapy for these states, thiazide-type diuretics increase calcium reabsorption in proximal tubule and DCT. This increases total body calcium to enhance bone density in patients with osteoporosis and decreases urinary calcium concentration, thereby reducing renal stone formation. Finally, as will be discussed later, thiazides are used in combination with loop diuretics to enhance diuresis and natriuresis in patients who develop diuretic resistance.

Thiazide diuretics are less potent than loop diuretics. They are available as both oral (HCTZ and metolazone) and intravenous (chlorothiazide) preparations. They are well absorbed following oral administration with an onset of action within approximately 1 hour. The $t_{1/2}$ is variable between drugs and they have a duration of action from 6 to 48 hours depending on the drug. The HCTZ dose ranges from 12.5 to 50 mg/day, however, most of the benefit occurs with 25 mg/day. Adverse effects develop more frequently with higher doses. Metolazone dosing ranges from 2.5 mg/day up to 10 mg twice daily. Patients treated with metolazone should measure their weight daily to avoid excessive diuresis and volume contraction. Bioavailability is reduced in patients with kidney disease, liver disease, and CHF. Patients with kidney disease, especially those with a GFR less than 25–40 mL/minute, have limited drug delivery to its site of action. Metolazone, however, appears to maintain efficacy at lower levels of GFR.

Adverse effects associated with thiazide-type diuretics include hypokalemia, hypomagnesemia, hyponatremia, and metabolic alkalosis. As with loop diuretics, hypokalemia can be life threatening in patients with heart disease and those on digoxin. Patients with cirrhosis are at risk for encephalopathy from associated hypokalemia and elevated plasma NH_3 levels. Hypercalcemia can develop in patients at risk such as those with primary hyperparathyroidism and bed bound patients. Hyponatremia occurs in patients with excessive ADH concentrations that are treated with a thiazide diuretic. This results from the thiazide's effect to diminish the kidney's diluting capacity without affecting concentrating ability, allowing ADH to enhance water reabsorption. Hypersensitivity reactions are noted including pancreatitis, hemolytic anemia, and thrombocytopenia. Finally, due to increased proximal uric acid reabsorption promoted by thiazide diuretics, patients can develop hyperuricemia and clinical gout.

Cortical Collecting Duct

The CCD reabsorbs approximately 1–3% of the filtered sodium load. Reabsorption of NaCl and secretion of potassium is controlled primarily by aldosterone and the prevailing plasma potassium concentration. Intratubular flow rate and sodium concentration also participate in this process. The CCD principal cell is constructed to perform this function based on the presence of an apical epithelial Na$^+$ channel (ENaC) and potassium channel (ROMK) and a basolateral Na$^+$-K$^+$-ATPase. Sodium is reabsorbed through ENaC and potassium secreted through ROMK following stimulation of the Na$^+$-K$^+$-ATPase (and opening of ENaC and ROMK) by aldosterone and an increased plasma potassium concentration. Medications that inhibit either ENaC transport or Na$^+$-K$^+$-ATPase function increase NaCl excretion while minimizing potassium loss. Potassium-sparing diuretics such as spironolactone and eplerenone competitively inhibit the mineralocorticoid receptor and blunt aldosterone-induced NaCl reabsorption and potassium secretion. These drugs are indicated to treat hypertension, especially due to either primary or secondary aldosteronism. They are also useful to reduce edema and ascites in patients with cirrhosis and improve cardiac dysfunction in patients with CHF characterized by an ejection fraction less than 40%. In contrast, amiloride and triamterene reduce NaCl reabsorption and potassium secretion by blocking ENaC. They are employed to reduce potassium losses associated with non-potassium-sparing diuretics and thereby prevent hypokalemia. Most often, they are given in combination with thiazide diuretics (HCTZ and amiloride, HCTZ and triamterene). They may also be added to a regimen that includes loop diuretics.

The potassium-sparing diuretics, in particular spironolactone and eplerenone, work best when aldosterone concentrations are elevated. Spironolactone, which is available only in oral form, is well absorbed. The drug undergoes hepatic metabolism. It has a $t_{1/2}$ of approximately 20 hours and requires up to 2 days to become effective. The dose range is 25–200 mg/day. Eplerenone is a relatively new oral potassium-sparing diuretic that has similar renal effects as spironolactone. It differs from spironolactone in that it has a shorter $t_{1/2}$ (4–6 hours), is metabolized by the liver (CYP3A4),

and excreted primarily (67%) by the kidneys. It is most effective when dosed twice per day. The dose range is 25–100 mg/day. Amiloride is well absorbed with oral administration. It has a $t_{1/2}$ of 6 hours and is excreted by the kidney. Triamterene is similar to amiloride except for a shorter $t_{1/2}$ (3 hours). All drugs that act in the CCD are weak diuretics, not unexpected due to the limited Na$^+$ reabsorption that occurs in this nephron segment.

The most common and concerning adverse effect of these drugs is hyperkalemia. The groups at highest risk are patients with moderate-to-severe kidney disease and those taking either potassium supplements or medications that impair potassium homeostasis such as the angiotensin converting enzyme (ACE) inhibitors, angiotensin receptor blockers (ARBs), and NSAIDs. Other patients at risk include those with diabetes mellitus (hyporeninemic hypoaldosteronism) and tubulointerstitial kidney disease. Spironolactone therapy is complicated by gynecomastia and amenorrhea. This occurs because it binds to estrogen and androgen receptors, especially when the dose equals or exceeds 100 mg/day. Eplerenone is specific for the mineralocorticoid receptor and is free of these adverse effects. In addition to hyperkalemia, amiloride causes a mild metabolic acidosis. Nausea and vomiting can also develop with either amiloride or triamterene therapy. Rarely, hyponatremia may occur in the elderly.

KEY POINTS
Sites of Diuretic Action

1. Mannitol and acetazolamide reduce sodium reabsorption in proximal tubule. Due to increases in sodium reabsorption at downstream sites, they are weak diuretics.
2. In thick ascending limb of Henle, loop diuretics induce a significant natriuresis by inhibiting the Na$^+$-K$^+$-2Cl$^-$ cotransporter. Loop diuretics are employed to treat volume

overload (CHF, cirrhosis, and nephrotic syndrome), hypertension complicated by chronic kidney disease, hypercalcemia, and some forms of hyponatremia.

3. Hypokalemia, volume contraction, and metabolic alkalosis are relatively common adverse effects of loop diuretics.

4. Thiazide-type diuretics are used primarily to treat hypertension; however, they are also useful for osteoporosis, nephrolithiasis, and combination therapy for patients with loop diuretic resistance.

5. Hypokalemia, hyponatremia, hypomagnesemia, and hyperuricemia are common side effects of the thiazide diuretics.

6. In CCD, the principal cell reabsorbs sodium and secretes potassium under the stimulation of aldosterone, plasma potassium concentration, urinary flow rate, and sodium delivery.

7. Spironolactone and eplerenone reach the mineralocorticoid receptor from the peritubular (blood) side, while amiloride and triamterene block apical ENaC from the urinary space. Despite different mechanisms of action, these drugs ultimately enhance NaCl excretion and inhibit potassium excretion.

8. Hyperkalemia is the primary adverse effect of diuretics that act in CCD. Patients with moderate-to-severe kidney disease and diabetes mellitus, as well as patients on medications that impair renal potassium excretion are at highest risk.

Diuretic Resistance

The desired goal of diuretic therapy is typically to reduce ECF volume in disorders such as CHF (peripheral and pulmonary interstitial edema), cirrhosis (ascites and peripheral edema), and

nephrotic syndrome (peripheral and renal edema) and control blood pressure in patients with hypertension. Inability to achieve these goals despite appropriate diuretic therapy (standard doses) is the definition of diuretic resistance. Identification of the problem is the first step. Assessing diuretic resistance requires a logical approach to the problem (Table 4.3). The second step requires appropriate diagnosis of the cause of edema. It is essential to ensure that the patient has generalized renal-related edema rather than localized edema from venous or lymphatic obstruction. Cyclic edema, a problem generally found only in women and interstitial edema due to fluid

Table 4.3

Approach to Patients with Diuretic Resistance

Step 1: Define diuretic resistance as failure to resolve edema or hypertension with standard diuretic doses.

Step 2: Identify cause of edema as renal-related edema vs. edema due to other causes (obstruction of veins or lymphatics, cyclic edema, calcium channel blocker therapy).

Step 3: Examine for incomplete therapy of the primary disorder requiring diuretic therapy.

Step 4: Assess patient compliance with salt restricted diet and diuretic regimen.

Step 5: Consider pharmacokinetic alterations of the diuretic including incomplete or delayed medication absorption and/or impaired kidney function (acute or chronic renal failure).

Step 6: Consider pharmacodynamic alterations of the diuretic regimen including severity of the edema state, activation of the renin-angiotensin-aldosterone system and sympathetic nervous system, and compensatory hypertrophy of distal nephron sites (particularly the DCT).

Step 7: Explore for adverse drug interactions including concurrent traditional NSAID or selective COX-2 inhibitor therapy.

Abbreviations: DCT, distal convoluted tubule; NSAID, nonsteroidal anti-inflammatory drug; COX-2, cyclooxygenase-2.

redistributed from the plasma compartment, as seen with calcium channel blocker therapy, are other forms of edema not amenable to diuretic treatment.

The next step (step 3) is to examine whether the primary disorder requiring diuretic therapy is adequately treated. Clinical disorders associated with impaired diuretic response include CHF, cirrhosis with ascites, nephrotic syndrome, hypertension, and kidney disease. These disease states and their specific causes of diuretic resistance are covered in more detail later in the chapter, but an example of resistance due to inadequate therapy of the primary disorder includes suboptimal management of CHF. These patients often require afterload reduction with an antagonist of the renin-angiotensin-aldosterone system (RAAS) in addition to diuretic therapy. In patients with severe congestive cardiomyopathies and decompensated heart failure, an intravenous inotropic agent such as dobutamine or milrinone may be indicated to improve cardiac pump function and renal perfusion. Excessive reductions in arterial blood pressure may also induce diuretic resistance. Allowing the blood pressure to increase can be beneficial in this situation.

A common cause of diuretic resistance that should not be overlooked is poor compliance with dietary salt restriction or the actual diuretic regimen. Step 4 mandates a thorough history to identify either of these problems. Direct questioning about diet, in particular ingestion of canned foods or fast foods, is often illuminating. Many patients also believe that drinking large amounts of certain beverages (gatorade, powerade) is healthy. This behavior can overcome diuretic effect on edema formation. Adverse effects from diuretics, such as impotence and muscle cramps, may promote noncompliance. These symptoms should be inquired about in all patients.

Step 5 requires a search for alterations in pharmacokinetics as the source of diuretic resistance. One common cause of ineffective diuresis is poor absorption of the agent. Patients with edematous states may also have bowel edema. This hampers gastrointestinal absorption of the oral diuretic, causing incomplete or delayed drug absorption. In patients with poor cardiac output, vascular disease of the intestinal tree, and advanced cirrhosis, blood flow to the intestinal absorptive sites may be inadequate to allow appropriate drug absorption. The presence of kidney disease (reduced GFR) decreases the concentration of diuretic that is secreted in active form into the tubular lumen, the site of their action. It also increases the fraction that is eliminated by hepatic excretion or glycosylation.

Pharmacodynamic causes of diuretic resistance are included in step 6. The most important cause in this category is extreme renal sodium retention from various mechanisms. Pronounced activation of the RAAS and sympathetic nervous system (SNS) reduces diuretic response by lowering GFR (reduced filtered load of sodium) and increasing NaCl reabsorption along all nephron segments. Angiotensin II enhances NaCl reabsorption in proximal tubule, loop of Henle, and DCT, while aldosterone increases NaCl reabsorption in DCT and CCD. Stimulation of the RAAS and SNS occurs for two basic reasons. First, the underlying disease state, which includes conditions such as CHF, cirrhosis, and nephrotic syndrome, decreases effective arterial blood volume. This activates the RAAS, SNS, and other pathways that enhance renal sodium reabsorption. Second, diuretics also may reflexively activate the RAAS and SNS, perpetuating diuretic resistance. An important participant in the development of diuretic resistance is compensatory changes in distal nephron tubular cells following chronic therapy with loop diuretics. Increased delivery of NaCl to the DCT induces hypertrophy and hyperplasia of tubular cells (Figure 4.2) and increases the density of both Na^+-K^+-ATPase pump sites and NCC cotransporters. This intranephronal adaptation enhances the intrinsic capacity of the DCT to reabsorb Na^+ and Cl^-. Experimental animal data suggests that treatment with loop diuretics increases reabsorption of NaCl threefold in DCT. As will be discussed later, these changes in the DCT underlie the enhanced natriuretic response noted when a thiazide diuretic is added to a loop diuretic.

Figure 4.2

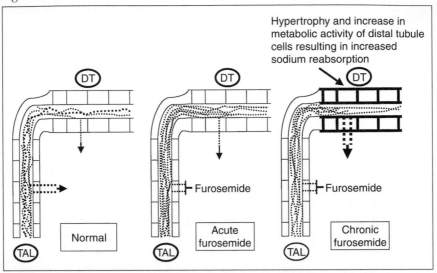

Intranephronal adaptation of distal tubular (DT) cells with chronic loop diuretic therapy. Hypertrophy and hyperplasia of DT cells and increased density of Na^+-K^+-ATPase pump sites and NCC cotransporters induce diuretic resistance. Abbreviation: TAL, thick ascending limb.

The final step in the assessment of diuretic resistance is to inquire about use of medications that may blunt diuretic action. Two particularly important culprits are the traditional NSAIDs and selective cyclooxygenase-2 inhibitors (COX-2). These drugs impair intrarenal prostaglandin synthesis by the COX-2 isoenzyme, which is important in the kidney to maintain renal blood flow and GFR and to block NaCl reabsorption in all nephron segments. Reduced natriuresis and increased blood pressure, as well as diuretic resistance results in patients with at risk physiology (hypertension, CHF, cirrhosis, nephrotic syndrome, and chronic kidney disease). Other drugs that impair diuretic response do so by reducing delivery of active diuretic to the site of action by competing for secretion through proximal tubular cell transport pathways. Probenecid, cimetidine, and trimethoprim are examples of drugs that compete for these pathways and reduce secretion of diuretic into urine, where they reach their site of action.

All of these factors need to be considered to adequately diagnose and successfully treat the patient suffering from either uncontrolled hypertension or refractory edema (or both) associated with diuretic resistance.

KEY POINTS
Diuretic Resistance

1. Diuretic resistance is defined as the inability to control blood pressure or reduce edema formation despite appropriate diuretic therapy (standard doses).
2. The logical approach to diuretic resistance includes assessment of variables such as verification of renal-related edema, appropriate therapy of the primary disorder, dietary and diuretic compliance, pharmacokinetic and pharmacodynamic issues, and therapy with antinatriuretic medications.

3. Activation of the RAAS and SNS promote renal sodium retention, while intranephronal adaptation by DCT cells with chronic loop diuretic therapy blunts diuretic response.
4. Concomitant therapy with NSAIDs and selective COX-2 inhibitors reduce prostaglandin-induced NaCl excretion and perpetuate diuretic resistance.

Clinical Conditions Associated with Specific Causes of Diuretic Resistance

In addition to the previously noted general causes of diuretic resistance, certain clinical conditions that can be associated with poor diuretic response are encountered in practice. Each of these disease states induces diuretic resistance through effects on circulatory and renal hemodynamics and/or tubular transport function in various nephron segments.

Congestive Heart Failure

The hemodynamics associated with CHF results in sodium and water retention from reduced renal perfusion, activated RAAS and SNS, and enhanced arginine vasopressin (AVP) release. The severity of cardiac dysfunction dictates the degree of tubular NaCl and fluid reabsorption. It is therefore intuitive that the ideal treatment of CHF is directed at improving cardiac function. When this fails or is only partially successful, assessment of other factors of diuretic resistance in this clinical condition need to be considered. Impaired absorption of diuretic across the gastrointestinal (GI) tract contributes to suboptimal response to the drug. A 50% decrease in peak urinary diuretic concentrations

following oral administration was noted in patients with CHF. Bowel edema, reduced bowel wall perfusion, and disturbed GI motility can alter GI tract absorption.

Nephrotic Syndrome

Sodium and fluid retention in patients with nephrotic syndrome develops from activated RAAS and SNS, increased concentrations of AVP, and direct stimulation of NHE3 transport activity in proximal tubule by excessive urinary protein concentration. The presence of renal dysfunction exacerbates nephrotic syndrome as it reduces the filtered load of NaCl. Primary renal sodium retention is an important cause of edema formation in a subgroup of these patients. Either complete or partial remission of the primary renal lesion (reduce proteinuria) and ACE inhibitors or ARBs are basic steps to improve renal sodium and fluid excretion. Diuretic resistance occurs by several mechanisms. Because loop and thiazide diuretics are highly protein bound, the volume of distribution of drug increases due to hypoalbuminemia. This reduces the concentration of drug in the circulation and the amount delivered to the kidney. Also, albumin directly stimulates the organic anion transport pathway that transports these drugs from blood into the proximal tubular cell. Thus, hypoalbuminemia hampers urine diuretic concentrations independent of renal delivery. Collecting duct resistance to ANP-associated natriuresis also contributes to diuretic resistance. Finally, since albumin binds diuretics, excessive concentrations of albumin in the tubule fluid blunt the ability of these drugs to inhibit NaCl transport in the loop of Henle.

Cirrhosis

Edema formation and ascites occur most commonly with advanced cirrhosis or during acute decompensation of chronic liver disease. Enhanced proximal tubular NaCl and fluid reabsorption, stimulated by an activated RAAS and SNS, reduces NaCl delivery to more distal sites where loop diuretics act. In addition, secondary aldosteronism stimulates avid NaCl uptake by the DCT and CCD. These mechanisms are integral to reduced diuretic response in patients with early cirrhosis. Patients with advanced cirrhosis and gross ascites have, in addition to the aforementioned factors, other causes of diuretic resistance. Intestinal edema limits drug absorption, while the volume of distribution of drug is increased significantly with hypoalbuminemia and a markedly expanded ECF volume. Unrecognized reductions in GFR also contribute to suboptimal diuresis. Finally, spontaneous bacterial peritonitis, hypotension, and bleeding from varices can exacerbate the tenuous hemodynamics in the cirrhotic and underlie the development of diuretic resistance.

Hypertension

Essential hypertension remains primarily a disturbance in renal salt handling. Thereby, salt restriction and diuretic therapy are the most appropriate initial management options. While dietary sodium restriction and diuretics are successful in many patients, as much as a third of patients remain resistant to therapy. In this situation, a lapse in dietary salt restriction, usually from ingestion of processed, canned, or fast foods that contain excessive amounts of sodium, is present. In some patients, the RAAS is activated prior to diuretic therapy. Treatment of these patients with a diuretic further activates the RAAS as well as the SNS, promoting renal NaCl retention and peripheral vasoconstriction. These effects can induce hypertension resistant to standard diuretic therapy. The addition of moderate-to-severe kidney disease to hypertension is a frequent cause of diuretic resistance. Salt restriction alone or with a diuretic is typically insufficient to control blood pressure. This is particularly true if the GFR is below the 25–40 mL/minute and the patient is receiving a thiazide diuretic. Reduced drug delivery and limited diuretic effect on natriuresis

underlies resistance to thiazides, although metolazone maintains fairly good efficacy in these patients.

Kidney Disease

As GFR declines, the diuretic and natriuretic effect of diuretics diminishes. Thiazide diuretics with the exception of metolazone are generally ineffective with a GFR below 30 mL/minute, while escalating doses of loop diuretics are required to promote an adequate, albeit reduced diuresis. Reduction in filtered sodium, reduction in delivered drug, and accumulation of endogenous organic anions with uremia are responsible for diuretic resistance. Endogenous organic anions compete with diuretics for the organic anion transport pathway, thereby reducing secretion of drug into tubular fluid. Thus, the diuretic can't reach its site of action in a concentration sufficient to inhibit NaCl reabsorption.

KEY POINTS
Clinical Conditions Associated with Specific Causes of Diuretic Resistance

> 1. Diuretic resistance in CHF is due to multiple factors. The hemodynamics of cardiac dysfunction, as well as reduced drug absorption from bowel wall edema, GI dysmotility, and reduced perfusion contribute to NaCl retention and impaired diuretic response.
> 2. Nephrotic syndrome promotes diuretic resistance due to hypoalbuminemia and albuminuria. Activation of the RAAS and SNS, as well as direct stimulation of NH_3 in proximal tubule induces NaCl retention. Reduced drug delivery to renal sites of action, decreased collecting duct responsiveness to ANP, and binding of diuretic in tubular fluid reduces efficacy.
> 3. Extreme activation of the RAAS and SNS promote diuretic resistance in cirrhosis.

> Bowel edema, an expanded volume of distribution, and reduced GFR also contribute to NaCl retention and diuretic resistance.
>
> 4. Renal failure causes suboptimal response to diuretics from a reduction in filtered sodium and impaired delivery of diuretics to their respective sites of action. Thiazide diuretics with the exception of metolazone become ineffective at a GFR less than 30 mL/minute.

Treatment of Diuretic Resistance

Once diuretic resistance is identified and appropriate steps to assess the cause of the resistant state are undertaken, a number of maneuvers can be used to improve diuretic response. Therapy is based on the recognized cause of diuretic resistance and the underlying clinical condition.

Intravenous Diuretic Therapy

Initial treatment of patients with diuretic resistance is escalation of the oral dose of loop diuretic (assuming the patient was switched from a thiazide-type diuretic previously). Ceiling doses for oral loop diuretics are noted in Table 4.2. The dosing interval for loop diuretics must be no longer than 8 hours (based on time of drug effect), or a rebound increase in sodium reabsorption (postdiuretic NaCl retention) will occur. Intravenous therapy is often required to restore diuretic efficacy in patients with absorptive problems such as bowel edema, altered GI motility, and reduced bowel perfusion. Ceiling doses for IV diuretics are also noted in Table 4.2. The major limitation of high-dose loop diuretic therapy is drug-related toxicity. Ototoxicity occurs in patients receiving very high-dose or prolonged high-dose therapy. This adverse effect is typically reversible, but is rarely associated with an irreversible defect. Myalgias may complicate high-dose bumetanide therapy; while thiamine deficiency was described in patients receiving chronic furosemide for CHF.

Continuous Diuretic Infusion

Patients who are failing or responding marginally to high-dose IV loop diuretics may benefit from continuous diuretic infusion. This therapy has several potential advantages. Trough concentrations of loop diuretic are avoided and postdiuretic NaCl retention is averted. Continuous infusions are also more efficient, achieving approximately 30% more natriuresis for the same IV bolus dose. The efficacy is greatest for bumetanide (which has the shortest $t_{1/2}$) and least for torsemide (which has the longest $t_{1/2}$). Titration of diuretic dose is more easily achieved with continuous infusion. Finally, toxicity is reduced with continuous infusion as the spike in peak concentrations is obviated. Thus, the occurrence of ototoxicty and myalgias is lessened. Table 4.4 reviews the starting bolus dose and continuous infusion dose range for loop diuretics. Careful observation to avoid overdiuresis and other electrolyte abnormalities is required.

Table 4.4

Dosing Guidelines for Continuous Infusions of Loop Diuretics

DIURETIC	BOLUS DOSE (MG)	INFUSION RATE (MG/HOUR)
Furosemide	20–80	2–100 (up to 1.0 mg/kg/hour)
Torsemide	25	1–50 (up to 0.5 mg/kg/hour)
Bumetanide	1.0	0.2–2 (up to 0.02 mg/kg/hour)

Combination Diuretic Therapy

The addition of a second class of diuretics can often overcome diuretic resistance. In general, the patient who is failing the ceiling dose of a loop diuretic benefits from addition of a thiazide diuretic. While the combination of a loop and proximal tubule diuretic increases efficacy, addition of a DCT diuretic to a loop diuretic is synergistic and more potent. This enhanced efficacy results from several effects, none of which is due to a change in the bioavailability or pharmacokinetics of either drug. The longer half-life of thiazide diuretics attenuates the postdiuretic NaCl retention of loop diuretics. High-dose IV chlorothiazide improves delivery of sodium from the proximal tubule to the loop of Henle by inhibiting carbonic anhydrase. The most important effect of thiazides in improving loop diuretic efficacy is their ability to blunt NaCl reabsorption by the hypertrophic and hyperplastic DCT cells (Figure 4.3). Patients with CHF, cirrhosis, and nephrotic syndrome are likely to gain benefit from a CCD

diuretic like spironolactone or eplerenone. This diuretic class modulates the activated RAAS in these patients and reduces the development of potentially harmful hypokalemia.

Thiazide diuretics should be added to loop diuretics that are at their ceiling dose. Also, either proximal tubule or CCD diuretics can be added depending on the underlying clinical condition and desired effect. For example, patients with a severe metabolic alkalosis and edema may benefit from acetazolamide, as long as hypokalemia is corrected prior to administration. In patients with an activated RAAS and concurrent hypokalemia (without advanced kidney disease), a CCD diuretic should be considered. Patients with CHF have improved heart failure management and survival with the addition of spironolactone or eplerenone. Table 4.5 notes the diuretic doses that are appropriate for use in combination with a loop diuretic. Combination diuretic therapy can promote vigorous diuresis with severe hypovolemia, as well as electrolyte disturbances. Cautious prescription and close monitoring for adverse effects is

Figure 4.3

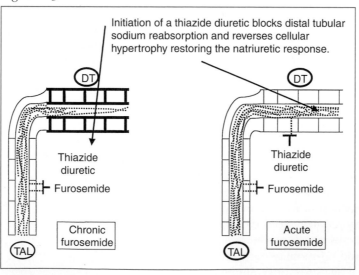

Combination therapy with a thiazide-type diuretic and loop diuretic improves diuretic response. Enhanced NaCl reabsorption by hypertrophic and hyperplastic distal tubular (DT) cells is inhibited by the addition of a thiazide-type diuretic to a loop diuretic. Abbreviation: TAL, thick ascending limb.

Table 4.5

Dosing Guidelines for Diuretics Added to Loop Diuretics for Combination Therapy

CLASS OF DIURETIC	DOSE RANGE (MG/DAY)
Proximal tubule diuretics	
Acetazolamide	250–375; up to 500 (IV)
Distal convoluted tubule diuretics	
Chlorothiazide	500–1000 (IV)
Metolazone	2.5–10 (oral)
Hydrochlorothiazide	25–100 (oral)
Collecting tubule diuretics	
Amiloride	5–10 (oral)
Spironolactone	100–200 (oral)
Eplerenone	25–100 (oral)

Abbreviation: IV, intravenous.

required. Patients should be counseled to perform daily weights and contact their physician with any changes greater than 2 lb/day. In addition, electrolytes and renal function should be measured within 5–7 days of initiating combination therapy.

Cardiovascular Agents

Several drugs available as an infusion increase renal blood flow, GFR, and natriuresis through both cardiovascular and direct renal effects. Acute dopamine infusion at very low doses (1–3 µg/kg/minute) stimulates renal dopamine receptors (DA_1 and DA_2) and stimulates natriuresis. A dose of 5 µg/kg/minute stimulates beta-adrenergic receptors and increases cardiac output, thereby enhancing renal perfusion and diuresis. Doses greater than 5 µg/kg/minute are associated with tachycardia and increased systemic vascular resistance, and potentially reduce natriuresis. After 24 hours of dopamine infusion, however, natriuresis wanes. The addition of dopamine to diuretics is of limited benefit and is associated with potentially serious tachyarrhyth-

mias. Fenoldopam is a selective DA_1 receptor agonist that is approved to treat severe (urgent or malignant) hypertension. It lowers blood pressure by vasodilating the vasculature. It also induces a natriuresis by binding renal DA_1 receptors and inhibiting the action of NHE3. Its renal effects are six times more potent than dopamine.

Dobutamine is an inotropic agent and dopamine derivative that does not cause systemic or mesenteric vasoconstriction. It increases cardiac output and reflexively reduces systemic vascular resistance. These effects improve renal blood flow in the patient with congestive cardiomyopathy and enhance urinary sodium and fluid excretion following diuretic administration. The combination of dopamine and dobutamine produces synergistic effects, providing a rationale for combining low doses of dopamine (2–5 µg/kg/minute) and dobutamine in critically ill patients with impaired cardiac pump function.

Atrial natriuretic peptide (ANP) is a hormone produced by myocardial atrial (and ventricular less commonly) cells when volume expansion increases cardiac wall stress. Brain natriuretic peptide (BNP) is similar to ANP. Although it was initially identified in the brain, it is also synthesized in the heart, particularly the ventricles. Both peptides are released in response to the high filling pressures associated with heart failure. These hormones have natriuretic and diuretic effects and also lower blood pressure by reducing RAAS, SNS, and endothelin activity. Diuresis and natriuresis occurs through increases in GFR (increased Na^+ filtration), stimulation of cyclic GMP in the inner medullary collecting duct (closing nonspecific cation channels), stimulation of dopamine secretion in the proximal tubule, and inhibition of AII and aldosterone production. Based on these characteristics, ANP and in particular, BNP (nesiritide) are infused intravenously to treat heart failure resistant to other medical management. Nesiritide is administered as an IV bolus of 2 µg/kg, followed by a continuous infusion of 0.01 µg/kg/minute titrated up to a maximum dose of 0.03 µg/kg/minute. This therapy often increases natriuresis, increases cardiac index, lowers cardiac filling pressure, and reduces blood pressure. The major adverse effect is hypotension, which is reversible with drug discontinuation.

Vasopressin (V_2) receptor antagonists represent a class of agents that target the AVP receptor in kidney. Since AVP increases water reabsorption in CCD by increasing the number of aquaporins (water channels) in the apical membrane, V_2 antagonists facilitate a water diuresis. Orally active V_2 antagonists are available for experimental use. They will likely be beneficial to enhance free water clearance and treat various forms of hyponatremia, including that induced by diuretics.

KEY POINTS
Treatment of Diuretic Resistance

1. High-dose intravenous diuretics overcome decreased GI absorption that can occur with oral agents. Ototoxicity needs to be monitored in patients receiving high-dose loop diuretics.
2. Combining a loop diuretic with an agent that acts at another nephron segment effectively overcomes diuretic resistance. Certain clinical conditions warrant choice of one class of diuretic over another. For example, a patient with edema and metabolic alkalosis may benefit from the addition of acetazolamide to a loop diuretic.
3. Combination diuretic therapy must be monitored closely for hypovolemia and electrolyte disturbances. Hypokalemia is a particular concern when loop diuretics are combined with either proximal tubule diuretics or DCT diuretics.
4. Dopamine and fenoldopam increase diuresis and natriuresis through increases in renal blood flow, GFR, and direct tubular effects. Low doses are effective, while higher doses add little benefit but are associated with dangerous tachyarrhythmias.
5. Dobutamine is an inotropic agent that improves cardiac output and lowers

systemic vascular resistance. These effects improve renal blood flow and GFR, thereby enhancing response to diuretics. The combination of dobutamine and dopamine is more effective in increasing natriuresis than either drug alone.
6. Atrial natriuretic peptide and nesiritide increase diuresis and natriuresis through multiple effects along the nephron. They are used in CHF refractory to routine medical management.
7. V_2 antagonists are experimental agents with great potential for treatment of hyponatremia from SIADH and diuretic therapy. They act by blocking the binding of antidiuretic hormone to the V_2 receptor, reducing the number of aquaporins available to reabsorb water in CCD.

Additional Reading

Denton, M.D., Chertow, G.M., Brady, H.M. "Renal-dose" dopamine for the treatment of acute renal failure: scientific rationale, experimental studies and clinical trials. *Kidney Int* 49:4–14, 1996.

Ellison, D.H. The physiologic basis of diuretic synergism: its role in treating diuretic resistance. *Ann Intern Med* 114:886–894, 1991.

Ellison, D.H. Diuretic drugs and the treatment of edema: from clinic to bench and back again. *Am J Kidney Dis* 23:623–643, 1994.

Ellison, D.H., Okusa, M.D., Schrier, R.W. Mechanisms of diuretic action. In: Schrier, R.W. (ed.), *Diseases of the Kidney and Urinary Tract*, 7th ed. Lippincott Williams & Wilkins, Philadelphia, PA 2001, pp. 2423–2454.

Martin, S.J., Danziger, L.H. Continuous infusion of loop diuretics in the critically ill: a review of the literature. *Crit Care Med* 22:1323–1329, 1994.

Rose, B.D. Diuretics. *Kidney Int* 39:336–352, 1991.

Wilcox, C.S. Diuretics. In: Brenner, B.M. (ed.), *The Kidney*, 5th ed. W.B. Saunders, Philadelphia, PA, 1996, pp. 2299–2330.

Robert F. Reilly, Jr.

Chapter 5

Intravenous Fluid Replacement

Recommended Time to Complete: 1 day

Guiding Questions

1. How are sodium and water distributed across body fluid compartments and what forces govern their distribution?
2. What options are available for volume resuscitation?
3. What are the guiding principles behind intravenous fluid replacement?
4. How does one assess the degree of intravascular and extracellular fluid volume depletion?
5. How does one manage the critically ill patient with extracellular fluid (ECF) volume depletion?

Introduction

Every physician and physician in training must master the ability to use intravenous solutions for the expansion of the intravascular and ECF volume. Proper understanding of solutions available

(colloid vs. crystalloid), their space of distribution, their cost and potential adverse effects, as well as an assessment of the patient's volume status are essential for their proper use. Mistakes are made when there is improper understanding of the patient's volume and electrolyte status.

Hypovolemia is a common problem in hospitalized patients, especially those in critical care units. It can occur in a variety of clinical settings

67

including those characterized by obvious fluid loss as with hemorrhage or diarrhea, as well as in patients without obvious fluid loss as a result of vasodilation with sepsis or anaphylaxis. In one study, inadequate volume resuscitation was viewed as the most common management error in patients who died in the hospital after admission for treatment of injuries.

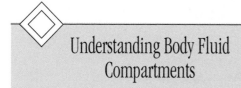

Understanding Body Fluid Compartments

Total body water constitutes 60% of lean body weight in men and 50% of lean body weight in women. It is distributed between intracellular fluid (ICF) (66.7%) and ECF (33.3%) compartments (see Figure 5.1). The ECF compartment is further subdivided into intravascular and interstitial spaces. Twenty-five percent of the ECF compartment consists of the intravascular space, with the remaining 75% constituted by the interstitial space.

Osmotic forces govern the distribution of water between ICF and ECF. The ECF and ICF are in osmotic equilibrium, and if an osmotic gradient is established, water will flow from a compartment of low osmolality to a compartment of high osmolality. For example, if a solute is added to the ECF such as glucose that raises its osmolality, water will flow out of the ICF until the osmotic gradient is dissipated. Water movement into and out of cells, particularly in the brain, with resultant cell swelling or shrinking is responsible for the symptoms of hyponatremia and hypernatremia.

Urea distributes rapidly across cell membranes and equilibrates throughout total body water and is with one exception, an ineffective osmole. Equilibration of urea across the blood-brain barrier can take several hours. If urea is rapidly removed from the ECF with the initiation of hemodialysis in a patient with end-stage renal disease, the potential exists for the development of "dialysis disequilibrium syndrome." Patients at increased risk are those with a blood urea nitrogen (BUN) >100 mg/dL that have rapid rates of urea removal during their first or second hemodialysis session. As urea concentration falls during hemodialysis a transient osmotic gradient

Figure 5.1

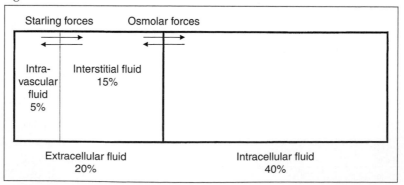

Body fluid compartments. Total body water consists of intracellular fluid and extracellular fluid. Intracellular fluid is 40% of lean body weight and extracellular fluid is 20% of lean body weight. The major driving force for fluid movement between these compartments is osmosis. The extracellular fluid can be further subdivided into the intravascular and interstitial spaces that constitute 5 and 15% of total body weight, respectively. The major driving force for fluid movement between these compartments are Starling's forces.

for water movement into the brain is established. This results in headache, nausea, vomiting, and in some cases generalized seizures. Dialysis disequilibrium can be minimized by initiating hemodialysis with low blood flow rates and for short periods of time.

Each compartment has one major solute that acts to hold water within it: ECF—Na salts; ICF—K salts; and intravascular space—plasma proteins. It is important to appreciate that the serum sodium concentration is a function of the ratio of the amounts of sodium and water present and does not correlate with ECF volume, which is a function of total body sodium. This is illustrated by the three examples below where ECF volume is increased in all three cases but serum sodium concentration is high, low, and normal.

If one adds NaCl to the ECF, it remains within the ECF increasing its osmolality resulting in water movement out of cells. Equilibrium is characterized by hypernatremia, an increase in ECF osmolality (NaCl addition), and ICF osmolality (water loss). As a result ECF volume increases and ICF volume decreases. Therefore, even though sodium is restricted to the ECF, its administration results in an increase in osmolality of both ECF and ICF, and a reduction in ICF volume. The osmolar effects of NaCl administration are distributed throughout total body water even though NaCl is confined to the ECF. If one adds 1 L of water to the ECF there is an initial fall in ECF osmolality promoting water movement into cells. Equilibrium is characterized by hyponatremia and an expansion of both ECF and ICF volumes. One-third of the water remains in the ECF and only 8% in the intravascular space.

Finally, if one adds 1 L of isotonic saline to the ECF, the saline is confined to the ECF and it will increase by 1 L. The intravascular volume will increase by 250 mL. Since there is no change in osmolality there is no shift of water between the ECF and ICF and serum sodium concentration remains unchanged.

Starling's forces govern movement of water between intravascular and interstitial spaces (Figure 5.2). Expansion of the interstitial space results in the clinical finding of edema. Edema fluid resembles plasma in electrolyte content, although its protein content may vary. The interstitial

Figure 5.2

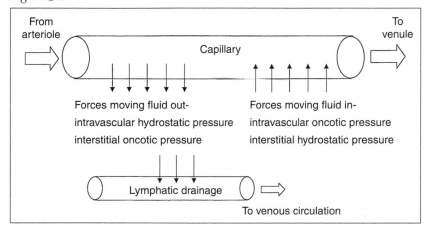

Starling's forces across the capillary bed. Starling's forces that move fluid out of the capillary are intravascular hydrostatic pressure (most important) and interstitial oncotic pressure. Forces acting to move fluid into the capillary are the intravascular oncotic pressure (most important) and interstitial hydrostatic pressure. Fluid in the interstitial space drains back to the venous system via lymphatics.

Table 5.1

Mechanism of Edema Formation

INCREASED HYDROSTATIC PRESSURE	DECREASED CAPILLARY ONCOTIC PRESSURE
Venous obstruction	Nephrotic syndrome
Congestive heart failure	Malabsorption
Cirrhosis of the liver	Cirrhosis of the liver

space must be expanded by 3–5 L before edema in dependent areas is detected. Edema may be localized due to vascular or lymphatic injury or it may be generalized as in congestive heart failure. Forces governing edema formation are summarized by the equation below where K_c reflects the surface area and permeability of the capillary. LR is the lymphatic return. P_c and P_t are the hydrostatic pressures in the capillary and tissue, respectively, whereas π_c and π_t are the oncotic pressures in the capillary and tissue, respectively.

$$\text{Net accumulation} = K_c \times [(P_c - \pi_c) - (P_t - \pi_t)] - \text{LR}$$

The most common abnormalities leading to edema formation are an increase in capillary hydrostatic pressure or a decrease in capillary oncotic pressure. In CHF, for example, the P_c increases. In cirrhosis, the P_c increases (secondary to portal hypertension) and the π_c declines. The major specific causes of edema, classified according to the major mechanism(s) responsible are shown in Table 5.1. The final common pathway maintaining generalized edema is renal retention of excess sodium and water.

KEY POINTS

Body Fluid Compartments

1. Total body water constitutes 60% of lean body weight in men and 50% of lean body weight in women. It is distributed between ICF (67.7%) and ECF (33.3%) compartments.

2. Twenty-five percent of the ECF compartment consists of the intravascular space, with the remaining 75% constituted by the interstitial space.
3. Osmotic forces determine the distribution of water between ICF and ECF.
4. Each compartment has one major solute that acts to hold water within it: ECF-Na salts; ICF-K salts; and intravascular space-plasma proteins.
5. The serum sodium concentration is a function of the ratio of sodium to water and does not correlate with ECF volume, which is a function of total body sodium.
6. Starling's forces govern movement of water between intravascular and interstitial spaces.
7. The most common abnormalities leading to edema formation are an increase in capillary hydrostatic pressure or a decrease in capillary oncotic pressure.

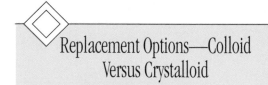

Replacement Options—Colloid Versus Crystalloid

Despite the fact that adequate volume replacement is essential in the management of critically ill patients, the optimal replacement fluid remains a focus of considerable debate. The clinician can choose between a wide array of crystalloids and colloids. Crystalloid solutions consist of water and dextrose and may or may not contain other electrolytes. The composition varies depending on the type of solution. Some of the more commonly used crystalloid solutions and their components are shown in Table 5.2 and include dextrose in water (D_5W), normal saline (0.9%), one-half normal saline (0.45%), and Ringer's lactate. Ringer's lactate is used more commonly on surgical services and normal saline on medical services.

Table 5.2

Commonly Used Crystalloid Solutions

Preparation	Osmolality (mOsm/L)	Glucose (g/L)	Sodium (meq/L)	Chloride (meq/L)	Lactate (meq/L)
D₅W	252	50	—	—	—
0.9% NS	308	—	154	154	—
0.45% NS	154	—	77	77	—
Ringer's lactate	272	—	130	109	28

Abbreviations: D₅W, 5% dextrose in water; NS, normal saline.

Colloid solutions consist of large molecular weight molecules such as proteins, carbohydrates, or gelatin. Colloids increase osmotic pressure and remain in the intravascular space longer compared to crystalloids. Osmotic pressure is proportional to the number of particles in solution. Colloids do not readily cross normal capillary walls and result in fluid translocation from interstitial space to intravascular space.

Colloids are referred to as monodisperse, like albumin, if the molecular weight is uniform, or polydisperse, if there is a range of different molecular weights, as with starches. This is important because molecular weight determines the duration of colloidal effect in the intravascular space. Smaller molecular weight colloids have a larger initial oncotic effect but are rapidly renally excreted and, therefore, have a shorter duration of action. Hydroxyethyl starch (HES), dextran, and albumin are the most commonly used colloids. Gelatins are not commercially available in the United States.

Hydroxyethyl starch is a glucose polymer derived from amylopectin. Hydroxyethyl groups are substituted for hydroxyl groups on glucose. The substitution results in slower degradation and increased water solubility. Naturally occurring starches are degraded by circulating amylases and are insoluble at neutral pH. Hydroxyethyl starch has a wide molecular weight range. Duration of action is dependent on rates of elimination and degradation. Smaller molecular weight species

are eliminated rapidly by the kidney. The rate of degradation is determined by the degree of substitution (the percentage of glucose molecules having a hydroxyethyl group substituted for a hydroxyl group). Substitution occurs at positions C2, C3, and C6 of glucose and the location of the hydroxyethyl group also affects the rate of degradation. Characteristics associated with a longer duration of action include larger molecular weight, a high degree of substitution, and a high C2/C6 ratio.

Hetastarch is a HES with a large molecular weight (670 kDa), slow elimination kinetics, and is associated with an increase in bleeding complications after cardiac and neurosurgery. The larger the molecular weight and the slower the rate of elimination, the more likely that HES will cause clinically significant bleeding. Newer HES preparations with lower molecular weights and more rapid elimination kinetics may be associated with fewer complications. Hetastarch use is also associated with an increased risk of acute renal failure in septic patients and in brain-dead kidney donors. Given these findings, Hetastarch cannot be recommended in patients with impaired kidney function. The threshold level of glomerular filtration rate below which Hetastarch should be avoided is unknown. A comparison between albumin and Hetastarch is shown in Table 5.3. Hetastarch is available as a 6% solution in normal saline. One liter of Hetastarch will initially expand the intravascular space by 700–1000 mL.

Table 5.3

Albumin vs. Hetastarch

	ALBUMIN	HETASTARCH
MW	69,000	670,000
Made from	Human sera	Starch
Compound	Protein	Amylopectin
Preparations	25 and 5%	6%

Abbreviation: MW, molecular weight.

Dextrans are glucose polymers with an average molecular weight of 40–70 kDa produced by bacteria grown in the presence of sucrose. In addition to expanding the intravascular volume, dextrans also have anticoagulant properties. Several studies show that they decrease the risk of postoperative deep venous thrombosis and pulmonary embolism. Dextran infusion decreases levels of von Willebrand factor and factor VIII:c more than can be explained by plasma dilution alone. Dextrans also enhance fibrinolysis and protect plasmin from the inhibitory effects of α-2 antiplasmin. In clinical studies comparing dextran to unfractionated heparin, low-molecular weight heparin, and heparinoids in the prophylaxis of postoperative deep venous thrombosis, dextran was associated with increased blood loss after transurethral resection of the prostate and hip surgery. Dextran 40 use is also associated with acute renal failure in the setting of acute ischemic stroke.

Two large meta-analyses by the Cochrane Injuries group and by Wilkes and Navickis evaluated albumin as an intravascular volume expander. The Cochrane group compared albumin to crystalloid in critically ill patients with hypovolemia, burns, and hypoalbuminemia. The pooled relative risk of death was increased by 68% in the albumin group. The authors found no evidence that albumin reduced mortality and a strong suggestion that it increased risk of death. Wilkes and Navickis showed that the relative risk of death was increased with albumin administration in patients with trauma, burns, and hypoalbuminemia but the increase in all cases was not statistically significant. Given these concerns and the higher cost of albumin compared to crystalloids and other synthetic colloids, routine use of albumin as a plasma volume expander cannot be supported. Albumin is available in two concentrations. A 5% solution that contains 12.5 g of albumin in 250 mL of normal saline and has a colloid osmotic pressure of 20 mmHg and a 25% solution that contains 12.5 g of albumin in 50 mL of normal saline and has a colloid osmotic pressure of 100 mmHg. After 1 L of 5% albumin is infused the intravascular space is expanded by 500–1000 mL.

Advocates of colloids argue that crystalloids excessively expand the interstitial space and predispose patients to pulmonary edema. Crystalloid advocates point out that colloids are more expensive, have the potential to leak into the interstitial space in clinical conditions where capillary walls are damaged, as in sepsis, and increase tissue edema. Despite decades of research, however, in most clinical situations there is no difference in pulmonary edema, mortality, or length of hospital stay between colloids and crystalloids.

KEY POINTS

Replacement Options

1. Crystalloids contain water and dextrose and may or may not contain other electrolytes. The most commonly used crystalloids are normal saline and Ringer's lactate.
2. Colloid solutions consist of large molecular weight molecules. Colloids increase osmotic pressure and remain in the intravascular space longer compared to crystalloids.
3. Hetastarch is associated with an increased risk of acute renal failure in septic patients and in brain-dead kidney donors. Its use cannot be recommended in patients with impaired kidney function. Further studies are needed to establish the threshold level of glomerular filtration rate below which Hetastarch should be avoided.

4. Given the higher cost of albumin compared to crystalloids and other synthetic colloids and the possible association with higher mortality rates, the routine use of albumin as an intravascular plasma volume expander cannot be recommended.
5. In critically ill patients there is no difference in pulmonary edema, mortality, or length of hospital stay with either colloid or crystalloid use.

General Principles

One must first decide on the amount of sodium and volume to be replaced based on the physical examination and clinical situation. As a general rule the fluid deficit is 3–5 L in the patient with a history of volume loss, 5–7 L in the patient with orthostatic hypotension, and 7–10 L in the septic patient. Since colloids are initially confined to the intravascular space, about one-fourth of these volumes are required if colloids are used. For most clinical indications crystalloids and colloids are equivalent. In the bleeding patient crystalloids are preferred. In the patient with total body salt and water excess (CHF, cirrhosis, nephrosis) colloids minimize sodium overload. Albumin should only be used in specialized situations such as large volume paracentesis.

In the hypotensive patient a solution must be employed that will remain in the intravascular and/or extracellular space. Dextrose in water (D_5W) should not be used since only 8% of the administered volume remains intravascularly. Crystalloids such as normal saline and Ringer's lactate or colloids are the replacement fluid of choice.

In patients with identifiable sources of fluid loss, it is important to be aware of the electrolyte content of body fluids (shown in Table 5.4). Of note, sweat and gastric secretions are relatively low in sodium and potassium, whereas colonic fluids are high in potassium and bicarbonate.

Normal maintenance requirements for fluids and electrolytes must also be considered and added to deficits. Insensible water losses average 500–1000 mL/day or approximately 10 mL/kg/day. Insensible water losses are less in the ventilated patient breathing humidified air. The average maintenance requirements for sodium, potassium, and glucose are 50–100 meq/day; 40–80 meq/day; and 150 g/day, respectively. Potassium should be repleted carefully in patients with chronic kidney disease.

KEY POINTS
General Principles

1. The amount of sodium and fluid replaced is based on the physical examination and clinical situation.

Table 5.4

Electrolyte Content of Body Fluids

	SODIUM (MEQ/L)	POTASSIUM (MEQ/L)	CHLORIDE (MEQ/L)	BICARBONATE (MEQ/L)
Sweat	30–50	5	50	—
Gastric	40–60	10	100	0
Pancreatic	150	5–10	80	70–80
Duodenum	90	10–20	90	10–20
Ileum	40	10	60	70
Colon	40	90	20	30

2. For most clinical indications crystalloids and colloids are equivalent.
3. Dextrose in water must not be used in the hypotensive patient.
4. One needs to be aware of normal daily losses of water and electrolytes.
5. Caution should be exercised in repleting potassium in patients with chronic kidney disease.

Assessing ECF Volume

ECF volume is notoriously difficult to assess based on history and physical examination. Signs and symptoms such as dry mouth, thirst, diminished axillary sweat, decreased capillary refill, and decreased skin turgor are often unreliable. Axillary sweat is more commonly related to the patient's anxiety level than volume status. Decreased skin turgor is also seen with aging and rapid loss of body weight, as well as the rare genetic disorder pseudoxanthoma elasticum. Perhaps the most reliable physical finding of ECF volume depletion is orthostatic hypotension. The American Autonomic Society and the American Academy of Neurology define orthostatic hypotension as a decline in systolic blood pressure of greater than or equal to 20 mmHg or a decrease in diastolic blood pressure of greater than or equal to 10 mmHg. An increase in pulse was not included in their definition, although this commonly occurs in patients without autonomic dysfunction.

Fluid resuscitation is initiated with boluses of crystalloid or colloid with periodic reassessment of clinical end points such as heart rate, urine output, and blood pressure. In patients with advanced chronic kidney disease or end-stage renal disease one cannot use urine output as a measure of the adequacy of fluid resuscitation. Patients who do not respond or who have severe comorbid illness of the heart or lungs are considered for invasive monitoring. Central venous pressure and pulmonary artery occlusion pressure measurements via a central venous or pulmonary artery catheter are used as the gold standard of left ventricular preload and response to fluid therapy. In most patients cardiac output is optimized at filling pressures of 12–15 mmHg.

This approach, however, has several limitations especially in ventilated patients. In the mechanically ventilated patient pulmonary artery occlusion pressure and left ventricular end diastolic pressure are affected by factors other than left ventricular end diastolic volume such as intrathoracic pressure and myocardial compliance. This has led to a search for more reliable markers of intravascular volume status. Although these approaches may be more accurate, they are also more invasive. For example, measurement of intrathoracic blood volume, total end diastolic volume, and extravascular lung water require an intraaortic fiberoptic catheter in addition to a pulmonary artery catheter. Analysis of changes in aortic blood velocity requires transesophageal echocardiography and heavy sedation to suppress spontaneous ventilation. The measurement of respiratory changes in arterial pulse pressure in response to volume repletion appears promising but also requires sedation to completely suppress spontaneous respiratory activity. A less invasive method to predict the response of the critically ill ventilated patient to volume resuscitation is needed.

KEY POINTS
Assessing ECF Volume

1. ECF volume is difficult to assess based on history and physical examination.
2. Orthostatic hypotension may be the most reliable sign of volume depletion.
3. Volume repletion is initiated with boluses of crystalloid or colloid with periodic reassessment of clinical end points such as heart

rate, urine output, and blood pressure. Nonresponders or those with severe comorbid illness of the heart or lungs are candidates for invasive monitoring.

4. Pulmonary artery occlusion pressure measurement via a pulmonary artery catheter is used as the gold standard of left ventricular preload and response to fluid therapy. In most patients cardiac output is optimized at filling pressures of 12–15 mmHg. This approach, however, has several limitations, especially in ventilated patients.

The Septic Patient

In septic shock cardiac output is generally high and systemic vascular resistance low. Tissue perfusion is compromised by both systemic hypotension and maldistribution of blood flow in the microcirculation. Septic shock is more complex than other forms of shock that are related to global hypoperfusion. With global hypoperfusion, as in cardiogenic shock or hypovolemic shock, a decrease in cardiac output results in anaerobic metabolism. In septic shock, however, maldistribution of a normal or increased cardiac output impairs organ perfusion, and inflammatory mediators disrupt cellular metabolism. In this setting adenosine triphosphate (ATP) stores are depleted despite maintenance of tissue oxygenation and lactic acid levels can be elevated despite normal tissue PO_2.

Shock is characterized by hypotension, which is defined as a mean arterial pressure <60 mmHg. The primary goals of fluid resuscitation in septic shock are normalization of tissue perfusion and oxidative metabolism. Large fluid deficits are present in the septic patient. As many as 2–4 L of colloid and 5–10 L of crystalloid are required. Survival in the septic patient is associated with increased cardiac output, and blood and plasma volumes.

Volume repletion significantly improves cardiac output and enhances tissue perfusion. Fluid resuscitation alone, in the absence of inotropic agents, increases cardiac index by 25–40%. In as many as 50% of septic patients with hypotension, shock is reversed with volume replacement alone. When crystalloids and colloids are titrated to the same filling pressure they are equally effective.

Acute respiratory distress syndrome develops in one-third to two-thirds of patients with septic shock. A major challenge for the clinician managing the patient with septic shock is balancing the potential benefits of intravascular volume expansion on vital organ perfusion, such as the brain and kidney, with the potentially adverse impact of worsening pulmonary edema. On theoretical grounds both crystalloids and colloids could worsen pulmonary edema. With crystalloid infusion plasma oncotic pressure may fall acting as a driving force for water movement out of the intravascular space and lung water accumulation. With colloid infusion if microvascular permeability is increased, colloid particles could migrate into the interstitium, thereby acting as a driving force for water movement, and worsen pulmonary edema. Despite these potential problems studies have shown that there is no significant difference in the development of pulmonary edema between crystalloids and colloids when lower filling pressures are maintained.

KEY POINTS
The Septic Patient

1. In septic shock tissue perfusion is compromised by systemic hypotension and maldistribution of blood flow.
2. Large fluid deficits are present in the septic patient. As many as 2–4 L of colloid and 5–10 L of crystalloid may need to be administered in the first 24 hours.
3. Fluid resuscitation is initiated with boluses of crystalloid or colloid with periodic reassessment of clinical end points.

4. When crystalloids and colloids are titrated to the same filling pressure they are equally effective.
5. A major challenge for the clinician managing the patient with septic shock is balancing the benefits of intravascular volume expansion on vital organ perfusion with the potential adverse impact of worsening pulmonary edema.

The Cardiac Surgery Patient

Patients undergoing cardiac surgery are at risk for intraoperative and postoperative bleeding. Cardiopulmonary bypass induces multiple platelet abnormalities including decreased platelet count, decreased von Willebrand factor receptor, and desensitization of platelet thrombin receptors. Several studies indicate that increased postcardiopulmonary bypass blood loss requiring reoperation is an independent risk factor for prolonged intensive care unit stay and death.

Trials comparing HES to albumin show increased postoperative bleeding and higher transfusion requirements in those receiving HES. One large retrospective study revealed a 25% lower mortality in those receiving albumin versus HES. In this study, the authors estimated that albumin use would save 5–6 lives per 1000 patients undergoing cardiopulmonary bypass. Other studies showed increased blood loss with HES even in low-risk patients.

Whether this is related to a beneficial effect of albumin or a deleterious effect of HES is unknown. Cardiopulmonary bypass activates inflammatory mediators and complement. There is an increase in free radical generation and lipid peroxidation. Albumin has significant antioxidant properties and inhibits apotosis in microvascular endothelium. Free fatty acid production contributes to erythrocyte crenation that in turn inhibits platelet

function. This process is inhibited by albumin. Albumin also coats the surface of the extracorporeal circuit decreasing the polymer surface affinity for platelets and reducing platelet granule release. HES reduces von Willebrand factor more than can be explained by hemodilution alone. Platelet dysfunction is mediated in part by the HES-induced fall in von Willebrand factor coupled with the decrease in von Willebrand receptor function induced by cardiopulmonary bypass.

KEY POINTS
The Cardiac Surgery Patient

1. There is an increased risk of bleeding in patients undergoing cardiopulmonary bypass.
2. Cardiopulmonary bypass induces multiple platelet abnormalities.
3. Increased postoperative bleeding and higher transfusion requirements are noted in cardiopulmonary bypass patients receiving HES. Whether this is related to a beneficial effect of albumin or a deleterious effect of HES remains to be determined.

Additional Reading

Boldt, J. New light on intravascular volume replacement regimens: what did we learn from the past three years? *Anesth Analg* 97:1595–1604, 2003.

Boussat, S., Jacques, T., Levy, B., Laurent, E., Gache, A., Capellier, G., Neidhardt, A. Intravascular volume monitoring and extravascular lung water in septic patients with pulmonary edema. *Intensive Care Med* 28:712–718, 2002.

Choi, P.T., Yip, G., Quinonez, L.G., Cook, D.J. Crystalloids vs. colloids in fluid resuscitation: a systematic review. *Crit Care Med* 27:200–210, 1999.

Cittanova, M.L., Leblanc, I., Legendre, C., Mouquet, C., Riou, B., Coriat, P. Effect of hydroxyethylstarch in brain-dead kidney donors on renal function in kidney-transplant recipients. *Lancet* 348:1620–1622, 1996.

Cochrane Injuries Group Albumin Reviewers. Human albumin administration in critically ill patients: systematic review of randomized controlled trials. *BMJ* 317:235–240, 1998.

de Jonge, E., Levi, M. Effects of different plasma substitutes on blood coagulation: a comparative review. *Crit Care Med* 29:1261–1267, 2001.

Evans, P.A., Heptinstall, S., Crowhurst, E.C., Davies, T., Glenn, J.R., Madira, W., Davidson, S.J., Burman, J.F., Hoskinson, J., Stray, C.M. Prospective double-blind randomized study of the effects of four intravenous fluids on platelet function and hemostasis in elective hip surgery. *J Thromb Haemost* 1:2140–2148, 2003.

Feissel, M., Michard, F., Mangin, I., Ruyer, O., Faller, J.P., Teboul, J.L. Respiratory changes in aortic blood velocity as an indicator of fluid responsiveness in ventilated patients with septic shock. *Chest* 119:867–873, 2001.

Kramer, G.C. Hypertonic resuscitation: physiologic mechanisms and recommendations for trauma care. *J Trauma* 54(5 Suppl.):S89–S99, 2003.

Matejovic, M., Krouzecky, A., Rokyta, R. Jr., Novak, I. Fluid challenge in patients at risk for fluid loading-induced pulmonary edema. *Acta Anaesthesiol Scand* 48:69–73, 2004.

Michard, F., Boussat, S., Chemla, D., Anguel, N., Mercat, A., Lecarpentier, Y., Richard, C., Pinsky, M.R., Teboul, J.L. Relation between respiratory changes in arterial pulse pressure and fluid responsiveness in septic patients with acute circulatory failure. *Am J Respir Crit Care Med* 162:134–138, 2000.

Schortgen, F., Lacherade, J.C., Bruneel, F., Cattaneo, I., Hemery, F., Lemaire, F., Brochard, L. Effects of hydroxyethylstarch and gelatin on renal function in severe sepsis: a multicentre randomised study. *Lancet* 357:911–916, 2001.

Sedrakyan, A., Gondek K., Paltiel, D., Elefteriades, J.A. Volume expansion with albumin decreases mortality after coronary artery bypass graft surgery. *Chest* 123:1853–1857, 2003.

Task Force of the American College of Critical Care Medicine, Society of Critical Care Medicine. Practice parameters for hemodynamic support of sepsis in adult patients in sepsis. *Crit Care Med* 27:639–660, 1999.

Treib, J., Baron, J.F., Grauer, M.T., Strauss, R.G. An international view of hydroxyethyl starches. *Intensive Care Med* 25:258–268, 1999.

Wilkes, M.M., Navickis, R.J. Patient survival after human albumin administration. A meta-analysis of randomized, controlled trials. *Ann Intern Med* 135:149–164, 2001.

Wilkes, M.M., Navickis, R.J., Sibbald, W.J. Albumin versus hydroxyethyl starch in cardiopulmonary bypass surgery: a meta-analysis of postoperative bleeding. *Ann Thorac Surg* 72:527–533, 2001.

Mark A. Perazella

Potassium Homeostasis

Recommended Time to Complete: 2 days

Guiding Questions

1. What role does potassium (K⁺) play in cellular function?
2. How does the body avoid a lethal cardiac arrhythmia following the ingestion of a potassium rich meal?
3. What are the major factors that influence cellular shift of potassium and how do they accomplish their effect?
4. What is the major site of K⁺ secretion by the kidney?
5. What are the four key factors that modulate renal K⁺ excretion?
6. Does diet play a major role in the development of either hypo- or hyperkalemia?
7. What are the general categories of causes of hypokalemia?
8. What are the three general categories of causes of hyperkalemia?
9. Treatment of clinical disorders of potassium balance is best guided by what two factors?
10. What is the most appropriate method of potassium supplementation in patients with severe hypokalemia?
11. What three treatment steps are employed to treat patients with severe hyperkalemia?

Introduction

Potassium (K^+) is found in nearly all food sources. It is the predominant intracellular cation in the body. A high cellular concentration is required to maintain normal function of a number of cellular processes. These include nucleic acid and protein synthesis, regulation of cell volume and pH, cell growth, and enzyme activation. In particular, a high intracellular K^+ concentration is necessary for the maintenance of the resting membrane potential. The resting membrane potential, in concert with the threshold membrane potential, sets the stage for generation of the action potential. This process is ultimately required for proper functioning of excitable tissues. Hence, these actions allow normal functioning of cardiac and skeletal muscles. Regulation of K^+ homeostasis is achieved mainly through cellular shifts of potassium, as well as renal K^+ excretion. These two regulatory mechanisms are under the control of a variety of factors that are reviewed in subsequent sections. Disturbances in these homeostatic mechanisms result in either hypokalemia or hyperkalemia. Both of these disturbances in K^+ balance promote a variety of clinical symptoms and physical findings that are predominantly caused by disruption of action potential formation, leading to neuromuscular dysfunction and inhibition of normal cell enzymatics. Rapid recognition and treatment of these disorders are required to avoid serious morbidity and mortality.

Potassium Homeostasis

Total body K^+ stores in an adult are between 3000 and 4000 meq (50–60 meq/kg body weight). Total body K^+ content is also influenced by age and sex. As compared with a young male, an elderly man

has 20% less total body K^+ content. Also, age-matched females have 25% less total body K^+ than males. Potassium is readily absorbed from the gastrointestinal (GI) tract and subsequently distributed in cells of muscle, liver, bone, and red blood cells. Maintenance of total body K^+ stores within narrow limits is achieved by zero net balance between input and output, as well as by regulation of K^+ between the extracellular fluid (ECF) and intracellular fluid (ICF). The bulk (90%) of dietary potassium is excreted in urine and the rest in feces (10%) in an adult. In contrast to sodium (Na^+), K^+ is predominantly an intracellular cation, with 98% of body K^+ located inside the cell. Hence, only 2% of K^+ is present in the ECF. As a result, there is a dramatic difference in K^+ concentration intracellularly (145 meq/L) versus extracellularly (4–5 meq/L). Despite this fact, however, the serum K^+ concentration is employed as an index of potassium balance, since it is the most readily available clinical test. In general, it is a reasonably accurate reflection of total body potassium content. In disease states, however, the serum potassium concentration may not always represent total body K^+ stores. The clinician must keep this in mind when assessing patients with abnormal laboratory values.

KEY POINTS
Potassium (K^+)

1. Potassium is the most abundant intracellular cation in the body. It plays a key role in cell growth, nucleic acid, and protein synthesis.
2. Proper functioning of these various cellular processes depends on maintenance of high K^+ concentration within cells.
3. Generation of an action potential in neuromuscular tissue is a key function of K^+ movement between ICF and ECF.
4. Total body K^+ stores range between 3000 and 4000 meq and are determined by age, sex, and body size.

5. To maintain net zero K⁺ balance, approximately 90% of K⁺ is excreted by the kidneys, while 10% is excreted by the GI tract.
6. Serum K⁺ concentration is the marker used to estimate total body K⁺ balance.

potential. Any change in serum K⁺ concentration alters the action potential and excitability of the cell. Thus, regulation of K⁺ distribution must be efficient, since a small movement of K⁺ from the ICF or ECF results in a potentially fatal change in serum K⁺ concentration. Physiologic and pathologic factors influence K⁺ distribution between ICF and ECF.

Role of K⁺ in the Resting Membrane Potential

Movement of cations, such as K⁺ and Na⁺, into their respective compartments requires active and passive cellular transport mechanisms. The location of K⁺ and Na⁺ in their respective fluid compartments is maintained predominantly by the action of the Na⁺-K⁺-ATPase pump in the cell membrane. This enzyme hydrolyzes ATP to create the energy required to pump Na⁺ out of the cell and K⁺ into the cell in a 3:2 ratio. Potassium moves out of the cell at a rate dependent on the electrochemical gradient, this creates the resting membrane potential (E_m). As seen below, the Goldman-Hodgkin-Katz equation calculates the membrane potential on the inside of the membrane using Na⁺ and K⁺ concentrations. Three factors determine the E_m: (1) the electrical charge of each ion; (2) the membrane permeability to each ion; and (3) the concentration of the ion on each side of the membrane. Inserting the intracellular K⁺ (145) and Na⁺ (12) concentrations and extracellular K⁺ (4.0) and Na⁺ (140) concentrations into the formula results in a resting membrane potential of –90 mV. The cell interior is –90 mV, largely due to the movement of Na⁺ out of the cell via the Na⁺-K⁺- ATPase pump.

$$E_m = -61 \log \frac{3/2\,(140) + 0.01\,(12)}{3/2\,(4.0) + 0.01\,(145)} = -90 \text{ mV}$$

The resting potential sets the stage for membrane depolarization and generation of the action

Cellular Distribution of K⁺

Many foods have a high K⁺ content that can raise serum K⁺ concentration, sometimes to levels that significantly disturb cell function and, as a result, are potentially lethal. In order to maintain the serum K⁺ concentration within a safe range, movement of K⁺ into cells is the first response of the body following ingestion of a potassium rich meal. This is a key feature of K⁺ homeostatic mechanisms because renal excretion of K⁺ requires several hours. The critical importance of this process is illustrated in the following case.

◆ CASE 6.1

A 70-kg man drinks three glasses of orange juice (40 meq of K⁺). In the absence of cellular shift, the K⁺ would remain in the ECF (17 L) and raise the serum K⁺ concentration by 2.4 meq/L. The excess K⁺, however, is rapidly shifted into cells and gradually excreted by the kidneys over the next several hours. This prevents a potentially lethal acute rise in serum K⁺ concentration.

Not surprisingly, insulin, which is secreted following a meal to maintain proper glucose balance, is also integral to cellular K⁺ homeostasis. As such, serum K⁺ concentration is maintained in the normal range by the physiologic effects of insulin. This role of insulin to move K⁺ into cells is well suited since renal K⁺ excretion does not occur immediately following ingestion of a meal containing large amounts of potassium. Movement of K⁺

into cells allows rapid lowering of the serum K^+ concentration until the K^+ load is fully excreted by the kidneys. Insulin stimulates K^+ uptake into cells by increasing the activity and number of Na^+-K^+-ATPase pumps in the cell membrane. Two K^+ ions are transported into the cell while three Na^+ ions are moved out of the cell by this energy-requiring transporter. The intracellular shift of K^+ is independent of glucose transport. A deficiency of insulin, as occurs in many patients with type 1 diabetes mellitus, is associated with hyperkalemia from impaired cellular uptake of K^+. The following clinical experiment illustrates the effect of insulin on cellular K^+ homeostasis.

Infusion of somatostatin, an inhibitor of pancreatic insulin release, in normal subjects reduced basal insulin concentrations to very low levels. Serum K^+ concentrations were measured with KCl infusion during baseline, infusion with somatostatin, and infusion with somatostatin plus insulin. An exaggerated rise in serum K^+ concentration developed with somatostatin, this effect was completely reversed by insulin infusion.

As noted with insulin, endogenous catecholamines and β_2-adrenergic agonists promote K^+ movement into cells through stimulation of the Na^+-K^+-ATPase. Activation of the β_2 receptor underlies the effect on this active enzyme pump to move K^+ into cells. Receptor activation is signaled through adenylate cyclase to generate cyclic AMP. This second messenger system ultimately stimulates the Na^+-K^+-ATPase pump to shift K^+ into cells. Medications such as albuterol, a β_2-adrenergic agonist used for asthma, can lower serum K^+ concentration through stimulation of cell uptake while propranolol, an antihypertensive medication which blocks β_2-adrenergic receptors, may cause hyperkalemia through inhibition of K^+ movement into cells. Intoxication with a medication such as digoxin may raise serum K^+ concentration by disrupting the Na^+-K^+-ATPase, thereby blocking cellular K^+ uptake. The clinical observation described below demonstrates the effect of digoxin on Na^+-K^+-ATPase function and serum K^+ concentration.

An elderly male with a history of heart disease presents to the emergency department with severe weakness, nausea, and vomiting. Severe digoxin intoxication is documented on blood testing. Serum K^+ concentration is 7.1 meq/L, previous serum K^+ concentration was 4.9 meq/L. This case shows the effect of digoxin intoxication on cellular K^+ balance, an effect mediated through inhibition of the Na^+-K^+-ATPase.

Other physiologic factors that modulate cellular K^+ movement include exercise, changes in extracellular pH, in particular metabolic acidosis and alkalosis, as well as changes in plasma osmolality. Exercise has a dual effect on cellular K^+ movement. A transient rise in serum K^+ concentration occurs primarily to increase blood flow to muscle. This homeostatic effect occurs because local release of K^+ vasodilates vessels and improves perfusion of ischemic muscles (provides more oxygen). A counterbalancing effect of endogenous catecholamine secretion also develops with exercise; this moves K^+ back into the ICF (activation of β_2-adrenergic receptors) and restores the serum K^+ concentration to normal. The level of exercise influences the cellular release of K^+. For example, a 0.3–0.4 meq/L rise with slow walking, a 0.7–1.2 meq/L rise with moderate exercise, and as much as a 2.0 meq/L rise with exercise to the point of exhaustion. Rest is associated with rapid correction of the rise in serum K^+ concentration, mainly through the actions of the Na^+-K^+-ATPase. Physical conditioning reduces the rise in K^+ concentration presumably through an improvement in pump activity.

Changes in pH also influence serum K^+ concentration. Metabolic acidosis is associated with an exit of K^+ from cells in exchange for protons (H^+) as the cells attempt to buffer the ECF pH. The exchange of K^+ for H^+ maintains electroneutrality across membranes. In this setting, up to 60% of excess protons are buffered within cells. An opposite effect is observed with metabolic alkalosis as K^+ enters the ICF to allow H^+ to enter the ECF and reduce alkalemia. In general, the serum K^+ concentration increases or decreases by 0.4 meq/L for every 0.1 decrease or increase in pH. There is a wide variability, however, in the change in serum K^+ concentration with pH change in metabolic acidosis (0.2–1.7 meq/L for every 0.1 fall in pH). Furthermore, this effect is more prominent with mineral (nonanion gap) metabolic acidoses than organic anion acidoses. The explanation for the differential effects of these types of acidoses on cellular K^+ movement is based on the ability of the accompanying anion to cross cell membranes. In mineral metabolic acidosis, the anion chloride is unable to cross the membrane, therefore K^+ must exit the cell to maintain electroneutrality. In contrast, the anion lactate is able to cross the membrane and less K^+ is required to exit the cell to maintain electroneutrality.

An increase in plasma osmolality, as occurs with hyperglycemia in diabetes mellitus, raises serum K^+ concentration as a result of a shift of K^+ out of cells. Potassium movement from cells is induced by solvent drag as K^+ accompanies water that is diffusing from the ICF into the ECF. Also, as water leaves the cell, the intracellular K^+ concentration rises, resulting in an increased driving force for passive diffusion of K^+ out of the cell. In general, the serum K^+ concentration rises by 0.4–0.8 meq/L for every 10 mOsm/kg increase in the effective osmolality. As will be discussed later, other hyperosmolar substances can cause a shift of K^+ out of cells. There exists a small amount of data suggesting that aldosterone may increase cellular uptake of K^+ through stimulation of the Na^+-K^+-ATPase pump. The role of aldosterone on cellular K^+ movement, however, is controversial and probably of only minor importance. As will be noted later, aldosterone has its major effect to enhance renal K^+ excretion.

KEY POINTS
Cellular Distribution of K^+

1. Potassium is distributed between ECF and ICF by a number of physiologic factors.
2. Insulin and β_2-adrenergic agonists act to move K^+ into cells by stimulating the activity of Na^+-K^+-ATPase.
3. Metabolic alkalosis and acidosis shift K^+ into and out of cells in exchange for H^+ to buffer pH changes.

4. Hyperosmolality increases serum K^+ concentration through the effects of both solvent drag on intracellular K^+ and creation of a diffusional driving force for K^+ to exit the cell.

K^+ Handling by the Kidney

Proximal Tubule

Potassium handling in the kidney occurs through the processes of glomerular filtration and both tubular reabsorption and secretion. In proximal nephron, 100% of K^+ reaches the tubule as K^+ is freely filtered by the glomerulus. Approximately 60–80% of filtered K^+ is reabsorbed by proximal tubule. Uptake of K^+ occurs via passive rather than active transport mechanisms. Potassium is reabsorbed by a K^+ transporter and through paracellular pathways coupled with Na^+ and water. Any process that affects Na^+ and water movement in the proximal tubule will also influence K^+ reabsorption. For example, volume depletion will increase Na^+ and water reabsorption, also increasing K^+ uptake while volume expansion will inhibit passive diffusion of K^+.

Loop of Henle

In the loop of Henle, K^+ is both secreted and reabsorbed. Ultimately, 25% of the filtered K^+ is reabsorbed in this nephron segment. Potassium is secreted into the lumen and the K^+ concentration at the tip of the loop of Henle may exceed the amount filtered. In contrast, K^+ is actively and passively reabsorbed in the medullary thick ascending limb. Active K^+ transport occurs by the $1Na^+$-$1K^+$-$2Cl^-$ cotransporter (Figure 6.1), which is powered by the enzymatic activity of Na^+-K^+-ATPase on the basolateral membrane. Secondary active cotransport is driven by the steep Na^+

Figure 6.1

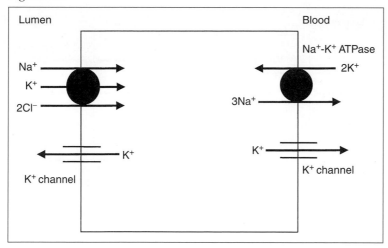

Cell model of the thick ascending limb of Henle. The Na^+-K^+-ATPase on the basolateral membrane provides the energy required to drive secondary active K^+ transport by the $1Na^+$-$1K^+$-$2Cl^-$ cotransporter in the thick ascending limb of Henle.

gradient across the apical membrane created by this enzyme pump. To allow continued cotransport, K^+ must recycle across the apical membrane from the cell into the tubular lumen. This provides a continuous supply of K^+ ions for cotransport with Na^+ and Cl^-, and negates the limiting effect of low luminal K^+. Medications such as loop diuretics and certain genetic disorders impair the transport function of this cotransporter resulting in Na^+ and K^+ wasting.

Distal Nephron

Following K^+ handling in the previously described nephron segments, approximately 10% of filtered K^+ reaches the distal tubule. In contrast to the other nephron segments, net K^+ secretion occurs in the distal tubule. This develops because of the high luminal Na^+ concentration and low luminal Cl^- concentration, which stimulates the K^+-Cl^- cotransporter to secrete K^+. In cortical collecting duct (CCD), K^+ is both secreted and reabsorbed. The CCD is the major site of K^+ secretion in the kidney. Two major cell types modulate K^+ movement in

this nephron segment. The principal cell is uniquely designed to secrete K^+ (Figure 6.2). The apical membrane of this cell contains epithelial Na^+ channels (ENaC) and K^+ channels, which act in concert with basolateral Na^+-K^+-ATPase to reabsorb Na^+ and secrete K^+. Reabsorption of Na^+ through ENaC increases K^+ secretion through its channel by creating an electrochemical gradient for K^+ movement from cell to tubular lumen. An electrical gradient develops as a result of Na^+ entry into the principal cell without an accompanying anion, creating a lumen negative charge that stimulates K^+ secretion. Also, the entry of Na^+ into cells increases basolateral Na^+-K^+-ATPase activity to lower intracellular Na^+. Transporting three Na^+ ions out of the cell and two K^+ ions into the cell increases intracellular K^+ concentration and creates a diffusional gradient favoring K^+ exit from cells through apical K^+ channels into the tubular lumen. Blockade of the Na^+ channel (amiloride, trimethoprim) reduces renal K^+ excretion by blocking generation of the electrochemical gradient. Administration of an aldosterone receptor antagonist (spironolactone, eplerenone) reduces apical Na^+ channel function, as well as Na^+-K^+-ATPase

Figure 6.2

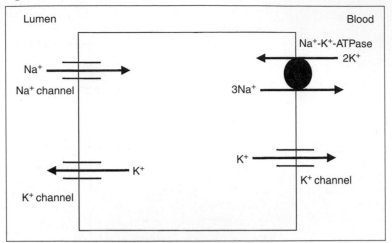

Cell model of the principal cell. The principal cell functions to regulate renal K^+ excretion. Reabsorption of Na^+ through ENaC increases K^+ secretion via ROMK by creating an electrochemical gradient for K^+ movement from cell to tubular lumen.

activity, which limits K^+ secretion from cells to urine. The other cell in the distal nephron involved in K^+ movement is the intercalated cell. There are two types of intercalated cells α and β. The α intercalated cell pictured below (Figure 6.3) excretes K^+. An H^+-K^+-ATPase on the apical surface of this cell reabsorbs K^+ in exchange for H^+. The β intercalated cell excretes HCO_3^- and is not pictured.

Figure 6.3

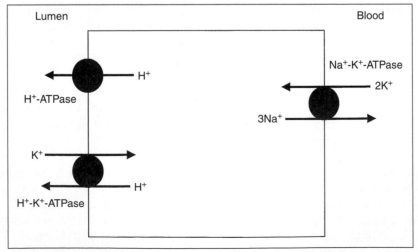

Cell model of the α intercalated cell. The intercalated cell promotes K^+ reabsorption via the H^+-K^+-ATPase located on the apical surface. This action stimulates K^+ reabsorption in exchange for H^+ ion.

Table 6.1

Factors That Influence Renal Potassium Excretion

Aldosterone
Plasma potassium concentration
Tubular flow rate
Tubular sodium concentration
Antidiuretic hormone
Glucocorticoids
Metabolic alkalosis
Metabolic acidosis
Impermeant anions in the urine (sulfate, bicarbonate, carbenicillin)

Factors Controlling Renal K⁺ Excretion

Although a number of factors influence renal K^+ excretion (Table 6.1), this discussion focuses on four clinically relevant factors that control K^+ secretion in principal cells. Most important is the mineralocorticoid aldosterone, which acts through binding its steroid receptor. This hormone stimulates Na^+ entry through apical channels and enhances basolateral Na^+-K^+-ATPase activity. This dual effect on the cell creates both an electrical potential for K^+ secretion (lumen negative charge stimulates K^+ movement from cell to urine), as well as a diffusional gradient for K^+ secretion (raising intracellular K^+ concentration). The plasma K^+ concentration also influences K^+ secretion by the kidney. As the plasma K^+ concentration rises above 5 meq/L, it produces effects on the principal cell that are similar to aldosterone as described above. This likely represents a protective mechanism to maintain renal K^+ excretion even when aldosterone is deficient or absent. On the luminal side (urinary space), both urine flow rate and Na^+ delivery influence K^+ secretion. High flow rates enhance K^+ secretion by maintaining a low urine K^+ concentration and a favorable diffusional gradient for intracellular K^+. Urinary Na^+ delivery to the principal cell promotes K^+ secretion by enhancing the entry of Na^+ ions through ENaC and creating a favorable electrochemical gradient. Thus, an increase in urine flow rate and Na^+ delivery, as created by use of a loop diuretic will increase K^+ excretion. In contrast, disease states such as congestive heart failure or true intravascular volume depletion reduce urine flow rate or Na^+ delivery, and as a result impair renal K^+ excretion. The impact of urine flow rates and Na^+ delivery on renal K^+ excretion are less important, however, than aldosterone or the plasma K^+ concentration.

KEY POINTS

K⁺ Handling by the Kidney

1. Potassium is freely filtered by the glomerulus.
2. The proximal tubule reabsorbs 60–80% of filtered K^+, the loop of Henle reabsorbs approximately 25%, while the distal nephron is the primary site of renal K^+ secretion.
3. In distal nephron, the principal cell in CCD is the primary regulator of K^+ excretion.
4. Several factors modulate K^+ excretion.
5. Aldosterone and plasma K^+ concentration primarily influence K^+ secretion by the principal cell.
6. Urinary Na^+ concentration and urine flow rate also regulate K^+ secretion by the principal cell, but are less important than aldosterone and plasma K^+ concentration.

Clinical Disorders of K⁺ Homeostasis

Clinical disorders of potassium balance are common problems in patients with a variety of medical conditions, especially those that require therapy with certain medications. In general, the causes of these disturbances promote K^+ imbalance by interrupting cell shift or renal excretion of K^+. Other factors that contribute include variations in dietary K^+ intake and disturbed gastrointestinal K^+ handling.

Hypokalemia

Hypokalemia is typically defined as a serum (or plasma) K^+ concentration less than 3.5 meq/L. Causes of hypokalemia (Table 6.2) can be broadly categorized as (1) reduced dietary intake, (2) increased cellular uptake, (3) increased renal excretion, and (4) excessive GI losses. Inadequate ingestion of K^+ alone is rarely a cause of hypokalemia due to the ubiquitous presence of this cation in foods. More often, diet only contributes to another primary cause of serum K^+ deficiency and rarely causes hypokalemia alone. Hypokalemia may develop from a shift of K^+ into cells from the effects of excessive production of endogenous insulin or catecholamines. Exogenous administration of insulin induces shift of K^+ into cells and precipitates hypokalemia. A classic example is the patient with diabetes mellitus who presents with ketoacidosis and is administered a continuous insulin infusion. Serum K^+ concentration often falls dramatically due to the effect of insulin on cellular K^+ uptake, as well as correction of the hyperosmolar state. β_2-adrenergic agonists used for asthma (albuterol) or labor (ritodrine) can lower serum K^+ concentration through cell uptake mediated by β_2 receptors. A clinical scenario where hypokalemia may develop from a β_2-adrenergic agonist is the patient with severe asthma who requires frequent nebulized treatments to correct bronchospasm. Metabolic alkalosis may also promote cell shift of K^+ and precipitate hypokalemia. Typically, this acid-base disorder is precipitated by vomiting and diuretic use, both of which contribute to hypokalemia through renal K^+ losses. Hypokalemic periodic paralysis is an inherited disorder associated with severe hypokalemia from cellular uptake of K^+, a phenomenon often precipitated by stress, exercise, or a large carbohydrate meal. The mutation is in the α_1 subunit of the dihydropyridine-sensitive calcium channel.

Table 6.2

Causes of Hypokalemia

Reduced dietary intake
Inadequate oral intake (in combination with other factors)
Increased cellular uptake
Insulin
Catecholamines (β_2 adrenergic)
  Endogenous catecholamines
  Epinephrine
  Dopamine
  Aminophylline
  Isoproterenol
Chloroquine intoxication
Metabolic alkalosis
Hypokalemic periodic paralysis
Hypothermia
Cell growth from B_{12} therapy
Increased renal excretion
Aldosteronism (primary or secondary)
Corticosteroid excess
High urine flow rate from diuretics
High distal delivery of sodium
Renal tubular acidosis
Drugs
  Amphotericin B
  Diuretics
  Aminoglycosides
  Lithium
  Cisplatinum
  Some penicillins
Genetic renal diseases
  Bartter's syndrome
  Gitelman's syndrome
  Liddle's syndrome
  Apparent mineralocorticoid excess syndrome
Gastrointestinal potassium loss
Vomiting
Diarrhea
Ostomy losses
Skin loss of potassium
Strenuous exercise
Severe heat stress

Hypothermia and chloroquine intoxication are rare causes of hypokalemia secondary to the shift of potassium into cells. Finally, rapid synthesis of red blood cells induced by B_{12} or iron therapy may cause hypokalemia. This phenomenon occurs because newly formed cells use available K^+ to develop the high intracellular K^+ concentration common to all cells.

Renal K^+ losses contribute significantly to the development of hypokalemia. A number of medications promote K^+ excretion by the kidney via actions in various nephron segments. In proximal tubule, K^+ reabsorption is impaired by different mechanisms. For example, acetazolamide, through blocking carbonic anhydrase induces bicarbonaturia and promotes K^+ wasting. Osmotic diuretics increase flow through the proximal tubule, reducing Na^+ and water reabsorption and thus paracellular K^+ reabsorption. Drugs such as aminoglycosides and cisplatin injure proximal tubular cells and cause K^+ wasting. The loop of Henle reabsorbs K^+ via the $1Na^+-1K^+-2Cl^-$ transporter. Loop diuretics inhibit the function of this transporter and reduce K^+ reabsorption significantly. In distal tubule, thiazide diuretics block the activity of the Na^+-Cl^- cotransporter, thereby increasing delivery of Na^+ and urine volume to principal cells in CCD. As discussed previously, these luminal effects increase K^+ secretion. Fludrocortisone, a mineralocorticoid agonist, binds the aldosterone receptor and stimulates renal K^+ secretion in principal cells. The antifungal agent amphotericin B causes K^+ loss from the kidney through a rather unique mechanism. Through interactions with membrane sterols, it disrupts cell membranes and allows K^+ to leak out of the principal cell into the urinary space following its diffusional gradient. Primary or secondary aldosteronism, as well as corticosteroid excess, may induce severe hypokalemia through stimulation of mineralocorticoid receptors and associated K^+ secretion in CCD. Primary or acquired forms of renal tubular acidosis (RTA) cause hypokalemia through tubular dysfunction proximally (type 2 RTA) or distally (type 1 RTA). Nonreabsorbable anions, by increasing lumen negative charge, increase the driving force for K^+

secretion in the CCD. These include carbenicillin, hippurate in patients who sniff glue (toluene), and β-hydroxybutyrate in patients with diabetic ketoacidosis. Inherited renal disorders also cause hypokalemia. In the loop of Henle, various mutations cause dysfunction of the $1Na^+-1K^+-2Cl^-$ cotransporter, the apical K^+ channel, the basolateral Cl^- channel, or the β subunit (Barttin) that traffics the Cl^- channel to the basolateral membrane. An activating mutation in the calcium sensing receptor on the basolateral membrane of the loop of Henle causes inhibition of ROMK and renal Na^+ and K^+ wasting. Various Bartter's syndrome phenotypes accompany each mutation, ultimately leading to K^+ wasting and hypokalemia. A mutation of the gene encoding the thiazide sensitive Na^+-Cl^- cotransporter causes the inherited disorder known as Gitelman's syndrome. As seen with a thiazide diuretic, Gitelman's syndrome causes renal K^+ wasting and hypokalemia. Liddle's syndrome promotes severe hypokalemia by causing overactivity of the epithelial Na^+ channel in the principal cell, an effect that favors unregulated renal potassium secretion. Mutations in subunits of the epithelial Na^+ channel (β and γ) underlies this genetic disorder.

Hypomagnesemia causes renal potassium wasting for unknown reasons. Gastrointestinal losses of K^+, such as vomiting, diarrhea, and excessive ostomy output may cause excessive K^+ losses from the body. In rare cases, excessive skin K^+ losses from extreme heat or strenuous exercise may cause hypokalemia.

A practical algorithm to assess the cause of hypokalemia is described in Figure 6.4. After excluding pseudohypokalemia and cell shift, hypokalemia is first evaluated by measuring the patient's blood pressure. Hypokalemia associated with hypertension is then classified based on concentrations of renin and aldosterone. In patients with hypokalemia that is associated with normal or low blood pressure, the next step in evaluation entails measuring urinary K^+ concentration to identify renal or extrarenal causes. Finally, acid-base status determines further classification of hypokalemia. Most have hypokalemia that is

Figure 6.4

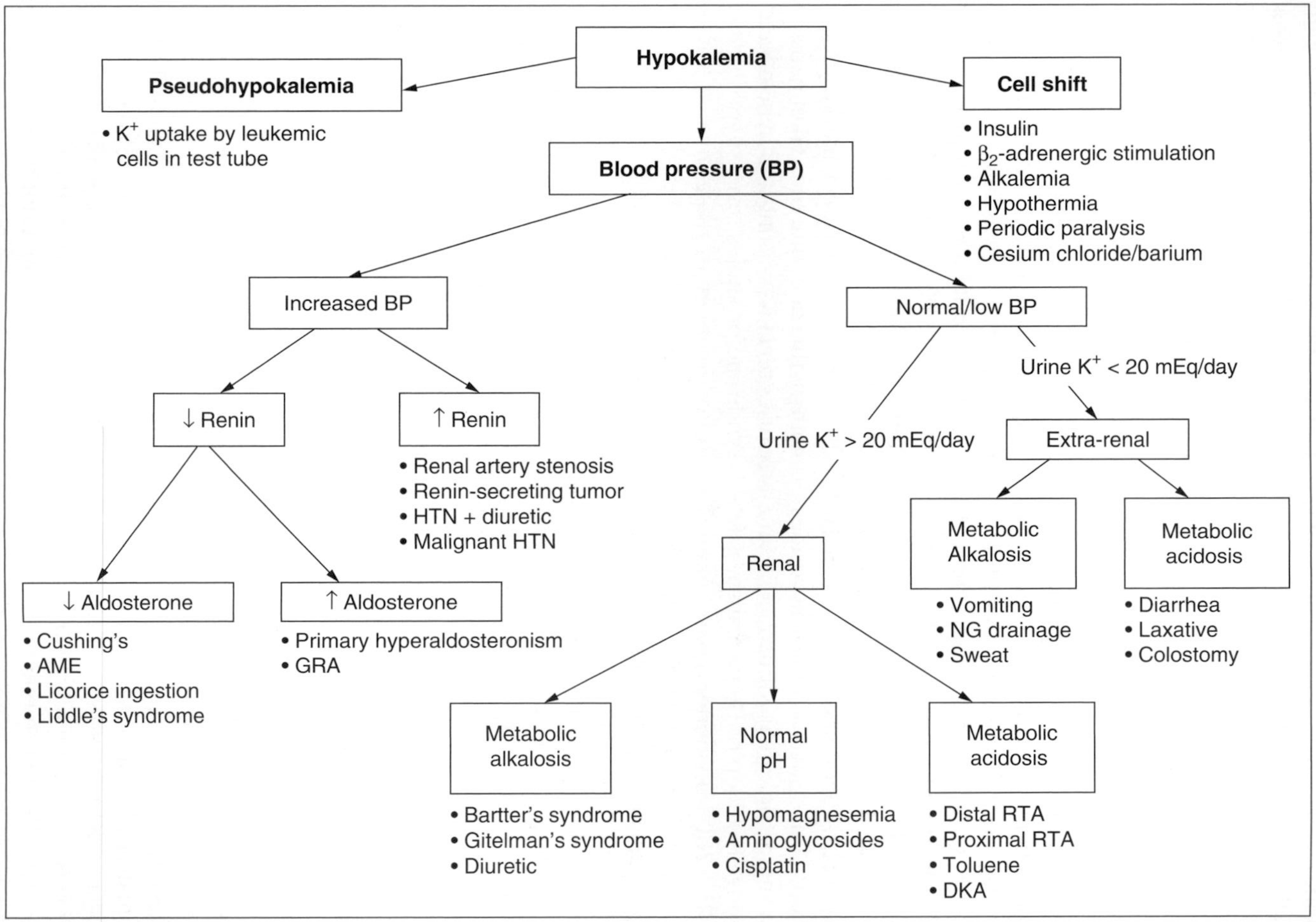

Clinical algorithm to evaluate hypokalemia. After excluding pseudohypokalemia and cell shift, blood pressure and various serum and urine tests are employed to classify hypokalemia. Abbreviations: HTN, hypertension; NG, nasogastric; AME, apparent mineralocorticoid excess; GRA, glucocorticoid remediable aldosteronism; RTA, renal tubular acidosis; DKA, diabetic ketoacidosis.

associated with either a metabolic acidosis or alkalosis.

The clinical manifestations of hypokalemia represent the effects of serum K^+ deficits on action potential generation in excitable tissues, protein synthesis, enzyme function, and regulation of cell pH and volume. Impaired neuromuscular function precipitates a spectrum of clinical findings ranging from muscle weakness to frank paralysis. Respiratory failure results from diaphragmatic muscle weakness while ileus is a GI manifestation of disturbed smooth muscle contractility. Cardiac disturbances include a variety of atrial and ventricular arrhythmias, as well as abnormal myocardial contractile function. Arrhythmias that develop from hypokalemia are a major clinical concern as they may be fatal in patients on digoxin or in those with underlying cardiac disease. Renal manifestations of hypokalemia include impaired urinary concentration (polyuria), increased renal ammonia production and bicarbonate reabsorption (perpetuating metabolic alkalosis), and renal failure from either tubular vacuolization (hypokalemic nephropathy) or myoglobinuria (rhabdomyolysis). Finally, other metabolic perturbations associated with hypokalemia include hyperglycemia from decreased insulin release, and impaired hepatic glycogen and protein synthesis.

Treatment of hypokalemia is guided by two factors. First, the physiologic effects of the K^+ deficit need to be determined and second, the cause of hypokalemia (cell shift versus renal or GI excretion) and approximate K^+ deficit need to be estimated. Physiologic effects of hypokalemia are best judged by (1) physical examination of neuromuscular function and (2) electrocardiographic (ECG) interrogation of the cardiac conduction system. Muscle weakness is often present with significant hypokalemia, while paralysis signals severe hypokalemia. The presence of prominent u waves on ECG (Figure 6.5) suggests a serum K^+ concentration in the 1.5–2.0 meq/L range. The K^+ deficit is approximated by the knowledge of the underlying mechanism of hypokalemia (less with cell shift, more with renal/GI losses) and the prevailing serum K^+ concentration. Potassium

concentrations in the 3.0–3.5 meq/L range usually represent a total body deficit in the 200–400 meq range. Correction with oral potassium chloride (KCl—40–80 meq/day) is preferred with mild-to-moderate deficits such as these. In the 2.0–3.0 meq/L range, K^+ deficits can reach 400–800 meq. Intravenous KCl (20–40 meq/L in 1 L of 0.45 normal saline) at a rate of no more than 20 meq/hour, in addition to oral KCl, is often required to correct severe K^+ deficits. Faster rates may injure veins (sclerosis) and cause cardiac dysrhythmias and must be avoided. Obviously, correction of the underlying etiology of hypokalemia is part of the treatment strategy.

KEY POINTS
Hypokalemia

1. The multiple causes of hypokalemia are related to both disturbances in cellular K^+ homeostasis and renal K^+ excretion. Reduced dietary K^+ intake rarely causes hypokalemia.
2. Clinical manifestations of hypokalemia are due primarily to neuromuscular and cardiac effects of potassium on excitable cells. Findings include muscle weakness and cardiac arrhythmias.
3. The significance of the total K^+ deficit is determined by the combination of the mechanism of hypokalemia (cell shift versus renal/GI K^+ loss) and the serum (or plasma) K^+ concentration.
4. Electrocardiographic evidence of hypokalemia is confirmed by the presence of u waves.
5. Treatment of hypokalemia is determined by severity of the K^+ deficit. Intravenous KCl is given with severe deficits, while oral KCl is employed for mild-to-moderate deficits.

Hyperkalemia

Hyperkalemia is defined as a serum (or plasma) K^+ concentration greater than 5.5 meq/L. Rarely, the

Figure 6.5

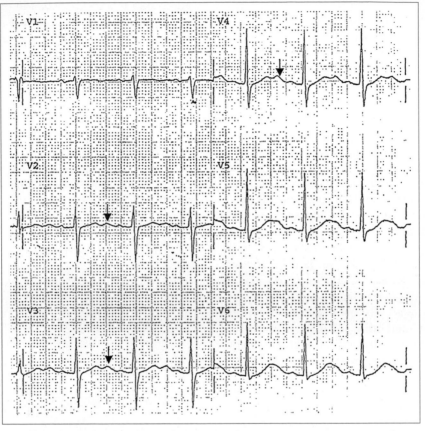

ECG of a patient with hypokalemia. The presence of prominent u waves on ECG signals profound hypokalemia. The u waves are illustrated by the arrows.

serum K^+ concentration may be falsely elevated (pseudohyperkalemia) due to release of K^+ from cells in the test tube. Lysis of cells following prolonged tourniquet application during venipuncture, and release of K^+ from large cell numbers (white blood cells >100,000 cells/mm^3; platelets >1,000,000 cells/mm^3) are examples of spurious hyperkalemia. As with hypokalemia, causes of hyperkalemia (Table 6.3) are broadly categorized as (1) increased dietary intake, (2) decreased cellular uptake, and (3) decreased renal excretion. Excessive K^+ intake alone does not cause hyperkalemia but does contribute to other more important causes of K^+ overload, such as those with

renal excretory defects. Shift of K^+ from the intracellular space to the ECF occurs in a variety of clinical states. As will be seen, disturbances in insulin, β_2-adrenergic actions, acidemia, and elevations in plasma osmolality all promote the shift of K^+ from ICF to ECF. Deficient concentration of either endogenous or exogenous insulin reduces K^+ entry into cells. This is a frequent cause of hyperkalemia in patients with insulin-dependent diabetes mellitus. Therapy with β_2-adrenergic antagonists (propranolol, carvedilol) to treat hypertension and heart disease can raise serum K^+ concentration through inhibition of β_2-receptor-mediated cell uptake. Nonanion gap (mineral)

Table 6.3

Causes of Hyperkalemia

Increased dietary intake
Excessive oral or intravenous intake (in combination with other factors)

Cellular release of potassium
Lack of insulin (fasting, diabetes mellitus)
β_2-adrenergic blockade
  Propranolol
  Labetolol
  Carvedilol
Metabolic acidosis
Hyperkalemic periodic paralysis
Succinylcholine
Hyperosmolality
  Hyperglycemia
  Mannitol
Aminocaproic acid, lysine
Digoxin toxicity
Cell lysis (hemolysis, rhabdomyolysis, tumor lysis)
Severe exercise

Decreased renal excretion
Hypoaldosteronism
  Hypoadrenalism
  Hyporeninemic hypoaldosteronism
  Heparin
  ACE-inhibitors, angiotensin receptor blockers
  NSAIDs
Low urine flow rate
Low distal delivery of sodium
Renal tubular resistance to aldosterone
  Obstructive uropathy
  Systemic lupus erythematosis
  Sickle cell disease
Drugs
  Amiloride
  Triamterene
  Spironolactone
  Trimethoprim
  Pentamidine
  Calcineurin inhibitors
Genetic renal diseases
  Pseudohypoaldosteronism type 1
  Pseudohypoaldosteronism type 2 (Gordon's syndrome)
Reduced GFR

Abbreviations: ACE, angiotensin-converting enzyme; NSAIDS, non-steroidal anti-inflammatory drugs.

metabolic acidosis also promotes shift of K^+ out of cells and hyperkalemia. Hyperkalemic periodic paralysis is an inherited disorder associated with impaired cellular uptake of K^+ and hyperkalemia. The mutation is in the α subunit of the skeletal muscle sodium channel. Hyperosmolality, as develops in diabetes mellitus with hyperglycemia and in patients treated with certain hyperosmolar substances (mannitol, dextran, hydroxyethyl-starch), can shift K^+ out of cells via solvent drag and elevate serum K^+ concentration. Severe lysis of red blood cells (hemolysis), muscle cells (rhabdomyolysis), and tumor cells (tumor lysis) causes hyperkalemia from massive release of K^+ from these cells.

Decreased K^+ excretion by the kidneys contributes significantly to the development of hyperkalemia. Several medications reduce renal K^+ excretion. The major action of these drugs is to blunt the kaliuretic mechanisms of the principal cell. Drugs such as the nonsteroidal anti-inflammatory drugs (including selective cyclooxygenase-2 inhibitors), angiotensin-converting enzyme inhibitors, angiotensin receptor antagonists, and heparin reduce aldosterone synthesis. Spironolactone and eplerenone compete with aldosterone for its steroid receptor and diminish K^+ secretion. Amiloride, triamterene, trimethoprim, and pentamidine all block the apical Na^+ channel on the principal cell and reduce the electrochemical gradient for K^+ secretion. Inhibition of Na^+-K^+-ATPase by digoxin, cyclosporine, and tacrolimus also impair renal K^+ secretion. Several clinical diseases affect the ability of the kidneys to excrete potassium. Advanced renal failure limits K^+ secretion by reduction in the number of functioning nephrons. Aldosterone deficiency from adrenal dysfunction, diabetes mellitus, or other forms of hyporeninemic hypoaldosteronism also impairs renal K^+ excretion. This has been called a type 4 renal tubular acidosis. Hyperkalemia also develops from tubular resistance to aldosterone or cellular defects in tubular K^+ secretion (obstructive uropathy, systemic lupus erythematosis, and sickle cell nephropathy). Inherited renal disorders such as pseudohypoaldosteronism types 1 and 2 manifest a K^+ secretory defect, hyperkalemia, and hypertension. Finally, limited distal delivery of Na^+ and sluggish urine flow rates, as seen with severe volume depletion may impair K^+ secretion by the principal cell.

A practical clinical algorithm to assess the cause of hyperkalemia is described in Figure 6.6. After excluding pseudohyperkalemia and shift of K^+ out of cells, hyperkalemia is evaluated by measuring urinary K^+ excretion and the transtubular K^+ gradient (TTKG). The TTKG provides a more accurate assessment of the tubular fluid K^+ concentration at the end of the cortical collecting tubule and whether hyperkalemia is due to a defect in renal excretion or other process. The TTKG is calculated by measuring urinary and serum K^+ and osmolality (osm), respectively and plugging the values into the following formula:

$$TTKG = Urine\ [K]^+ \div (urine\ osm/serum\ osm)$$
$$\div serum\ [K]^+$$

Reduced urine K^+ excretion and a TTKG less than 5 suggest a renal defect in K^+ excretion. Patients who fall into this category are evaluated further by measuring serum aldosterone and renin concentrations to determine the ultimate cause of hyperkalemia. Those with an elevated K^+ excretion and TTKG greater than 5 are categorized as non-renal causes of hyperkalemia as noted in Figure 6.6.

The clinical manifestations of hyperkalemia are derived from the pathologic effects of high serum K^+ concentration on the generation of action potentials in excitable tissues, in particular heart and neuromuscular tissues. Hyperkalemia promotes various cardiac conduction disturbances that ultimately affect the rate and rhythm of the heart. These include various AV nodal blocks, ventricular tachycardia and fibrillation, and asystole. Myocardial contractility is also impaired in this setting and contributes to hypotension and shock. Various degrees of muscle weakness and paralysis are also important clinical signs of hyperkalemia.

Hyperkalemia is potentially lethal and must be promptly identified and treated. As with hypokalemia, treatment of hyperkalemia should be guided by two factors. First, the physiologic effects of the excess K^+ state need to be determined and second, the cause of hyperkalemia (cell shift versus impaired renal excretion) should be identified and aggressively treated. Physiologic effects of hyperkalemia are noted by signs of neuromuscular dysfunction and ECG evidence of the cardiac conduction disturbances. Significant hyperkalemia often manifests as muscle weakness of varying severity. Well-characterized ECG changes suggest the presence of hyperkalemia. One of the earliest changes is tenting of the t waves. As the serum K^+ concentration increases, the QRS complex widens (Figure 6.7), the p wave disappears, and a sine wave pattern develops, ultimately leading to ventricular fibrillation or asystole. Aggressive therapy is required to prevent a fatal outcome (Table 6.4). Treatment of hyperkalemia should include three main objectives: stabilize excitable tissues; shift K^+ into cells to lower serum K^+ concentration; and remove K^+ from the body. Stabilization of excitable membranes, in particular cardiac tissues, is the first priority. This is best accomplished by administering intravenous calcium (Ca^{2+}) as either Ca^{2+} gluconate or Ca^{2+} chloride under cardiac monitoring. For patients on digoxin, the calcium should be given as a slower drip. Following Ca^{2+} therapy, the serum K^+ concentration is lowered rapidly employing methods to shift K^+ into cells. Effective therapies include intravenous regular insulin (10–20 units) with 25–50 g of glucose in nondiabetics (to prevent hypoglycemia). Insulin acts within 30 minutes and lasts approximately 4–6 hours. It lowers the serum K^+ concentration by approximately 0.5–1.0 meq/L. High-dose β_2-adrenergic agonists (albuterol 20 mg nebulized) will lower serum K^+ concentration by approximately 0.6 meq/L within 30 minutes. Its effect lasts for 1–2 hours. In patients who can tolerate a sodium load and have a severe nonanion gap metabolic acidosis, sodium bicarbonate shifts K^+ into cells. The cation-exchange resin, sodium polystyrene sulfonate, mixed with sorbitol and given either orally or as a retention enema is used to increase GI K^+ excretion. High-dose loop diuretics increase renal K^+ excretion in patients with reasonably good kidney

Figure 6.6

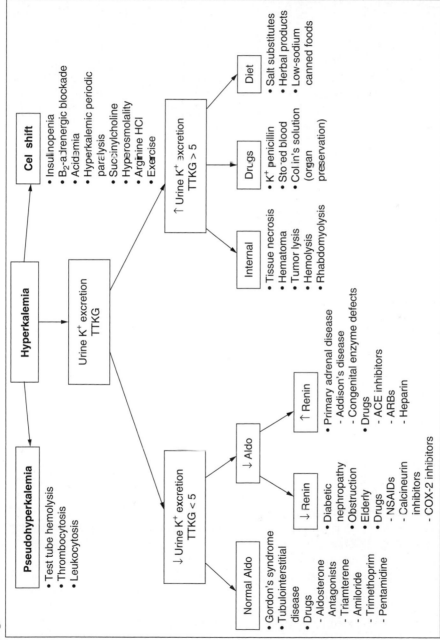

Clinical algorithm to evaluate hyperkalemia. After excluding pseudohyperkalemia and cell shift, urine K⁺ excretion and TTKG are used to initially classify hyperkalemia. Renin and aldosterone are used to further classify renal causes of hyperkalemia. Abbreviations: Aldo, aldosterone; NSAIDs, nonsteroidal antiinflammatory drugs; COX-2, cyclooxygenase-2; ACE, angiotensin converting enzyme; ARBs, angiotensin receptor blockers.

Figure 6.7

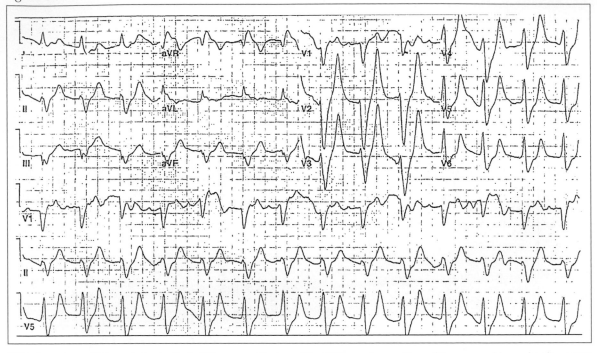

ECG of a patient with hyperkalemia. Peaked T waves, widening of the QRS complex, and loss of the p wave (shown here) are ECG changes consistent with hyperkalemia. The development of a sine wave indicates imminent cardiac arrest.

Table 6.4

Treatment of Hyperkalemia

TREATMENT	DOSE	ONSET	DURATION	MECHANISM
Calcium gluconate (10%)	10–20 mL IV	1–5 minutes	30–60 minutes	Stabilize excitable membranes
Insulin and glucose	10 U of IV insulin and 25 g of glucose	30 minutes	4–6 hours	Cell uptake
Albuterol (β_2 agonist)	20 mg in 4 mL of normal saline for nebulization	30 minutes	1–2 hours	Cell uptake
Sodium bicarbonate	50–75 meq IV	30–60 minutes	1–6 hours	Cell uptake
Sodium polystyrene sulfonate	30–45 g oral 50–100 g enema	2–4 hours	4–12 hours	GI excretion
Hemodialysis	1–2 meq/L potassium bath	Immediate	2–8 hours	Removal from the blood

Abbreviations: IV, intravenous; U, units; GI, gastrointestinal.

function. Hemodialysis is an efficient modality to quickly remove K^+ from the body in patients with significant renal impairment. Correction of the primary cause of hyperkalemia and adjustment in dietary K^+ intake should also be undertaken.

KEY POINTS
Hyperkalemia

1. Hyperkalemia is caused principally by the combination of disturbances in cellular K^+ uptake and impaired renal K^+ excretion. Excessive dietary K^+ intake contributes to hyperkalemia when renal K^+ excretion is decreased.
2. Clinical manifestations of hyperkalemia are due primarily to the disruption of the normal generation of the resting membrane potential in excitable tissues. Thus, neuromuscular and cardiac functions are impaired, resulting in muscle weakness and life-threatening cardiac arrhythmias.
3. Electrocardiographic evidence of hyperkalemia is confirmed by the presence of peaked (tented) t waves, widening of the QRS, loss of the p wave, and formation of the ominous sine wave.
4. Treatment of hyperkalemia is based on the principles of stabilization of excitable cell membranes, shifting of K^+ into cells, and removal of K^+ from the body using renal excretion, colonic excretion, or dialysis.
5. Rapid recognition and treatment of hyperkalemia is required to avoid serious morbidity and mortality.

Additional Reading

Biswas, P., Perazella, M.A. Acute hyperkalemia associated with intravenous epsilon-aminocaproic acid therapy. *Am J Kidney Dis* 33:782–785, 1999.

Cruz, D.N, Perazella, M.A. Hypertension and hypokalemia: unusual syndromes. *Conn Med* 61:67–75, 1997.

Giebisch, G.H. A trail of research on potassium. *Kidney Int* 62:1498–1512, 2002.

Good, D.W, Wright, F.S. Luminal influences on potassium secretion: sodium concentration and fluid flow rate. *Am J Physiol* 236:F192–F205, 1979.

Perazella, M.A., Brown, E. Electrolyte and acid-base disorders associated with AIDS: an etiologic review. *J Gen Intern Med* 9:232–236, 1994.

Perazella, M.A., Mahnensmith, R.L. Hyperkalemia in the elderly: drugs exacerbate impaired potassium homeostasis. *J Gen Intern Med* 12:646–656, 1997.

Perazella, M.A. Hyperkalemia in the end-stage renal disease patient in the emergency department. *Conn Med* 63:131–136, 1999.

Perazella, M.A. Drug-induced hyperkalemia: old culprits and new offenders. *Am J Med* 109:307–314, 2000.

Perazella, M.A., Rastegar, A. Disorders of potassium and acid-base metabolism in association with renal disease In: Schrier, R.W. (ed.)., *Diseases of the Kidney*, 7th ed. Little, Brown & Company, New York, NY, 2001, pp. 2577–2605.

Smith, J.D., Perazella, M.A., DeFronzo, R.A. Hypokalemia: clinical disorders. In: Arief, A.A., DeFronzo R.A. (eds.), *Fluid, Electrolyte and Acid-Base Disorders*, 2nd ed. Churchill Livingstone, New York, NY, 1995, pp. 387–426.

Dinkar Kaw and
Joseph I. Shapiro

Chapter 7

Metabolic Acidosis

Recommended Time to Complete: 2 days

Guiding Questions

1. Why is evaluation of acid-base status important?
2. What is "buffering?"
3. What determines the pH in the intracellular and extracellular spaces?
4. How does one assess acid-base balance?
5. What processes are involved in renal acid excretion?
6. What stepwise approach can be used to identify acid-base disturbances?
7. What is metabolic acidosis and how does it occur?
8. What are the compensatory mechanisms for metabolic acidosis?
9. What are the biochemical and physiologic effects of metabolic acidosis?
10. What is the serum anion gap (SAG) and how is it used in the differential diagnosis of metabolic acidosis?
11. What is the urine anion gap and what is it used for?
12. How does one diagnostically approach metabolic acidosis?
13. What is the treatment of metabolic acidosis?

Acid-Base Chemistry and Biology

Acid-base disorders are one of the most common problems encountered by the clinician. Although the degree of acidosis or alkalosis that results is rarely life threatening, careful evaluation of the patient's acid-base status often provides insight into the underlying medical problem. Moreover, the pathophysiology and differential diagnosis of these disorders can be approached logically with a minimum of laboratory and clinical data.

Acid-base homeostasis consists of the precise regulation of CO_2 tension by the respiratory system and plasma bicarbonate (HCO_3^-) concentration [HCO_3^-] by the kidney. The kidney regulates the plasma [HCO_3^-] by altering HCO_3^- reabsorption and elimination of protons (H^+). The pH of body fluids is determined by CO_2 tension and [HCO_3^-]. These body fluids can generally be readily sampled and analyzed with a blood gas instrument that determines CO_2 tension (in arterial blood, $PaCO_2$), pH, and [HCO_3^-], the latter is generally calculated (see below). Primary abnormalities of CO_2 tension are considered respiratory disturbances, whereas primary derangements of [HCO_3^-] are referred to as metabolic disturbances.

Understanding clinical acid-base chemistry requires an appreciation of buffers. For diagnostic purposes, we can define an acid as a chemical that donates a H^+, and a base as a H^+ acceptor. For an acid (HA) and its conjugate base (A^-), we describe its strength (or tendency to donate a H^+) by its dissociation constant K_{eq} and the formula:

$$[HA] = K_{eq} \times [H^+][A^-] \qquad (1)$$

If we rearrange this equation and apply a log transformation, we arrive at the following:

$$pH = pK + \log_{10} \frac{[A^-]}{[HA]} \qquad (2)$$

We use the term *buffering* to describe the capacity of a solution to resist a change in pH when a strong (i.e., highly dissociated) acid or alkali is added. As a concrete example, say we added 100 mL of 0.1 M HCl to 900 mL of distilled water. The [H^+] of what was previously distilled water would increase from 10^{-7} to 10^{-2} M. In other words, the pH would fall from 7.0 to 2.0. In contrast, if we added 100 mL of 0.1 M HCl to 900 mL of a 1 M phosphate *buffer* (pK = 6.9 at pH 7.0), most of the dissociated H^+ from HCl would associate with dibasic phosphate ($HPO_4^=$) and the ratio of dibasic to monobasic ($H_2PO_4^-$) phosphate would only be slightly changed. As a result, the pH would fall by only 0.1. In this latter example, the hydrochloric acid (HCl) was *buffered* by the phosphate solution, whereas in the case where hydrochloric acid was added to distilled water, no such buffering occurred.

In higher animals such as mammals, the most important buffer in the extracellular space is the bicarbonate buffer system. Inorganic phosphate and proteins are less important buffers in the extracellular space. Inorganic phosphate is quantitatively the most important buffer followed by bicarbonate and intracellular proteins in the intracellular or cytosolic space (Figure 7.1).

Figure 7.1

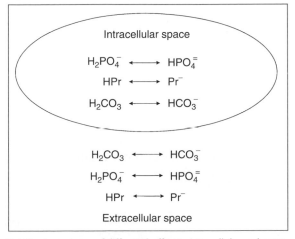

Relative importance of different buffers in intracellular and extracellular spaces. Note that in the intracellular space, phosphate and proteins play a greater role than they do in the extracellular space where the bicarbonate buffer system is most important.

While cytosolic or intracellular pH (pHi) is probably more important in predicting physiologic and clinical consequences than extracellular pH, it is extremely difficult to measure in vivo. Because extracellular acid-base status is still informative, we focus our clinical efforts on classifying disease states using this information that can readily be obtained. Specifically, we focus our attention on the bicarbonate buffer system (Figure 7.1). It is generally assumed that equilibrium conditions apply to the bicarbonate buffer system in blood because of the abundance of carbonic anhydrase (CA) in red blood cells and the high permeability of the red blood cell membrane to components of the bicarbonate buffer system. Therefore, we can express the following equations:

$$H^+ + HCO_3^- \xrightarrow{K_{eq}} H_2CO_2 \tag{3}$$

or

$$[H^+] = K_{eq} \times \frac{[H_2CO_3]}{[HCO_3^-]} \tag{4}$$

Furthermore, H_2CO_3 is defined by the partial pressure of CO_2 and the solubility of CO_2 in physiologic fluids that is, for all intents and purposes, a constant S. We can, therefore, rearrange equation (4) to read

$$[H^+] = K \times \frac{S \times PCO_2}{[HCO_3^-]} \tag{5}$$

Taking the antilog of both sides we get

$$pH = pK + \log_{10} \frac{[HCO_3^-]}{S \times PCO_2} \tag{6}$$

that is called the Henderson-Hasselbalch equation. In blood (at 37°C), the pK referred to in equation (6) is 6.1 and the solubility coefficient for CO_2 (S) is 0.03. Therefore, we can simplify this expression to

$$pH = 6.1 + \log_{10} \frac{[HCO_3^-]}{0.03 \times PaCO_2} \tag{7}$$

This formula allows us to view acid-base disorders as being attributable to the numerator of the ratio (metabolic processes), the denominator (respiratory processes), or both (mixed or complex acid-base disorders).

KEY POINTS
Acid-Base Chemistry and Biology

1. Evaluation of acid-base status provides insight into underlying medical problems.
2. Many cellular functions are dependent on optimum pH of body fluids.
3. The pH is defined as the negative logarithm of $[H^+]$.
4. Interplay among body buffers, lungs, and kidneys is responsible for maintaining pH within normal limits.
5. The most important buffer in the extracellular space is bicarbonate and in the intracellular space is inorganic phosphate.
6. Lungs excrete CO_2 and kidneys excrete H^+ to maintain serum bicarbonate and pH in the normal range.

Assessing Acid-Base Balance

A myriad of enzymatic reactions involve the loss or gain of protons that occur with ongoing catabolism and anabolism. To understand whether acid or base is produced; however, one simply examines the initial substrates and final products. To do this, it is helpful to think of acids and bases as "Lewis" acids and bases; in other words, to consider acids as electron acceptors rather than as proton donors. In concrete terms, when a substrate is metabolized to something more anionic (e.g., glucose is metabolized to lactate through the Embden-Meyerhoff glycolytic pathway), acid is generated. Conversely, if a substrate is metabolized to something more cationic

Figure 7.2

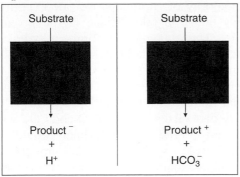

Substrate	Substrate
Product$^-$ + H$^+$	Product$^+$ + HCO$_3^-$

"Black box" approach to acid-base metabolism. The left panel shows that when a substrate is metabolized to a more electronegative product, a proton is generated. Conversely, the right panel demonstrates that when a substrate is metabolized to a more electropositive product, a proton is consumed and bicarbonate is generated.

KEY POINTS

Assessing Acid-Base Balance

1. When a substrate is metabolized to something more anionic (e.g., glucose is metabolized to lactate through the Embden-Meyerhoff glycolytic pathway), acid is generated.
2. If a substrate is metabolized to something more cationic (e.g., lactate is metabolized to CO_2 and H_2O via the TCA cycle), acid is consumed.
3. The kidneys regulate serum [HCO$_3^-$] and acid-base balance by reclaiming filtered HCO$_3^-$ and generating new HCO$_3^-$ to replace that lost internally (in titrating metabolic acid) and externally (e.g., from the gastrointestinal tract).

(e.g., lactate is metabolized to CO_2 and H_2O via the tricarboxylic acid [TCA] cycle), acid is consumed (Figure 7.2). Because of the importance of the bicarbonate buffer system in overall acid-base homeostasis, we generally consider the addition of a proton as equivalent to the decrease in total body HCO$_3^-$ and loss of a proton as a gain in HCO$_3^-$.

The classic normal values for an arterial blood gas are pH: 7.4; [HCO$_3^-$]: 24 meq/L; and PaCO$_2$: 40 mmHg. The kidneys regulate serum [HCO$_3^-$] and acid-base balance by reclaiming filtered HCO$_3^-$ and generating new HCO$_3^-$ to replace that lost internally (in titrating metabolic acid) and externally (e.g., from the gastrointestinal tract). Approximately 1 mmol of H$^+$/kg body weight per day is generated from the metabolism of a normal "Western diet." To maintain acid-base homeostasis the kidney must excrete this acid load. The role of the kidney in acid-base homeostasis can be divided into two basic functions: (1) the reabsorption of filtered bicarbonate and (2) the excretion of the acid load derived from dietary metabolism.

Acid Excretion by the Kidney

Our understanding of renal acid excretion has evolved considerably in the past decade. In particular, we have identified the specific ion pumps and transporters that are involved in tubular proton secretion in different portions of the nephron. It is clear that the major ion transporters and pumps include the sodium-proton exchanger (Na$^+$-H$^+$ exchanger, which exchanges one H$^+$ for one sodium ion), the sodium-phosphate cotransporter (which transports three sodium ions with one dibasic phosphate molecule), and the vacuolar H$^+$ ATPase (which pumps H$^+$ directly into the tubular lumen). Other important transport proteins include the chloride-bicarbonate exchanger, the "colonic" H$^+$-K$^+$ ATPase, and the Na$^+$-K$^+$ ATPase. These transport proteins are expressed to varying degrees in different cell types and nephron segments of the kidney, depending on the specific functions of these cells.

Regarding overall acid-base handling by the kidney, there is a strong relationship between acid secretion and the reclamation of filtered bicarbonate, as well as the production of new bicarbonate by the kidney as one would anticipate based on our earlier discussion. First, plasma is filtered at the glomerulus and HCO_3^- enters the tubular lumen. Each HCO_3^- molecule that is reclaimed requires the epithelial secretion of one H^+. This H^+ secretion occurs via the Na^+-H^+ exchanger on the luminal membrane or through an electrogenic H^+ ATPase. On an integrated physiologic level, we can think of the HCO_3^- reabsorption processes establishing a *plasma threshold* for bicarbonate, i.e., that level of plasma HCO_3^- at which measurable HCO_3^- appears in urine. This concept of a *plasma threshold* is well established for renal glucose handling, historically, the appearance of glucose in urine was used as a surrogate for elevated blood glucose levels before blood glucose monitoring became widespread. Continuing this analogy to renal glucose handling, we can also define the maximal net activity of tubular HCO_3^- reabsorption as the T_{max}. The T_{max} and *plasma threshold* for HCO_3^- are, of course, intimately related. As the T_{max} for HCO_3^- increases, the *plasma threshold* for HCO_3^- increases. Conversely, decreases in T_{max} result in decreases in the *plasma threshold*. Quantitatively, to eliminate HCO_3^- from urine with a glomerular filtration rate of 100 mL/minute and a plasma $[HCO_3^-]$ of 24 meq/L, the tubules must secrete about 2.4 mmol of H^+ per minute. Ergo, HCO_3^- reclamation by the tubules involves a considerable amount of H^+ secretion.

Bicarbonate reclamation is closely related to sodium reabsorption and is, therefore, sensitive to a number of other influences that impact sodium reabsorption. In particular, states of extracellular fluid (ECF) volume expansion and decreases in $PaCO_2$ decrease the apparent T_{max} for HCO_3^-, whereas ECF volume contraction and increases in $PaCO_2$ increase the apparent T_{max} for HCO_3^-. Parathyroid hormone inhibits proximal tubule HCO_3^- reabsorption and lowers the apparent T_{max} and plasma threshold for HCO_3^-. The majority of HCO_3^- reabsorption (approximately 80–90%) takes place in the proximal tubule. The enzyme carbonic anhydrase is expressed intracellularly, as well as on the luminal membrane of the proximal tubule cell, which allows the secreted H^+ to combine with tubular fluid HCO_3^- to form H_2CO_3. This H_2CO_3 rapidly dissociates to form H_2O and CO_2, which then can reenter the proximal tubule cell. Intracellularly, water dissociates into H^+ and OH^-. Intracellular carbonic anhydrase catalyzes the formation of HCO_3^- from CO_2 and OH^-. Bicarbonate leaves the cell via several bicarbonate transport proteins including the sodium-bicarbonate cotransporter, as well as the Cl^--HCO_3^- exchanger. In the proximal tubule, where the reclamation of HCO_3^- filtered from the blood occurs, HCO_3^- is formed inside the renal tubular cells when either H^+ secretion or ammonium (NH_4^+) synthesis occurs. The HCO_3^- is then transported back into blood predominantly via the basolateral Na^+-$3HCO_3^-$ cotransporter.

Proton secretion by the distal nephron is aided by the production of an electrogenic gradient. This gradient, which is produced by removal of sodium from the luminal fluid in excess to anion reabsorption, favors H^+ secretion. There is also direct pumping of H^+ into the tubular lumen. Na^+-H^+ exchange, as well as the activities of the vacuolar H^+ ATPase and the Na^+-K^+ ATPase in intercalated and principal cells, accomplish these tasks. Chloride exchange with bicarbonate on the basolateral side of these distal tubular cells allows for proton secretion to be translated into bicarbonate addition to blood as discussed earlier. The epithelial membrane in the distal nephron must not allow backleak of H^+ or loss of the electrogenic gradient. Under normal circumstances, urine pH can be as low as 4.4. This represents a 1000:1 gradient of $[H^+]$ between tubular and extracellular fluids.

Net acid excretion (NAE) is the total amount of H^+ excreted by the kidneys. Quantitatively, we can calculate NAE to be the amount of H^+ (both buffered and free) excreted in urine minus the amount of HCO_3^- that failed to be reclaimed and was lost in the urine. Because H^+ secretion into the tubule lumen results in a 1:1 HCO_3^- addition to the ECF, NAE equals the amount of new HCO_3^- generated.

Net acid excretion is accomplished through two processes that are historically separated on the basis of a colorimetric indicator (phenolphthalein) that detects pH changes effectively between pH 5 and 8. That acid, which can be detected by titrating sufficient alkali into urine to achieve color changes with this indicator, is called titratable acid and is mostly phosphate in the monobasic ($H_2PO_4^-$) form. Nontitratable acid excretion occurs primarily in the form of NH_4^+. This form of acid excretion is not detected by phenolphthalein since the pK (approximately 9) for ammonium is too high. Even though most clinicians equate NAE with an acidic urine, it is important to recognize that a low urine pH does not necessarily mean that NAE is increased. For example, at a urine pH of 4.0 the free H^+ concentration is only 0.1 mmol. In a 70-kg person on an average Western diet one can see that free protons would make up only a small fraction of the approximately 70 mmol of net acid that need to be excreted per day. The majority of NAE is in the form of protons bound to buffers, either phosphate or ammonium. This makes it possible to elaborate a much less acid urine but still achieve adequate NAE. In fact, there are several pathologic conditions (discussed later) in which the urine pH is relatively acid but NAE is insufficient. In subjects that consume a typical Western diet, adequate NAE occurs through the functions of both the proximal tubule to synthesize NH_4^+ (which generates HCO_3^-) and distal and collecting tubules where H^+ and NH_4^+ secretion occur.

Net acid excretion is influenced by several factors including the serum potassium concentration (serum K^+ elevations decrease NH_4^+ excretion, while decreases enhance distal nephron H^+ secretion), $PaCO_2$, and the effects of aldosterone. Quantitatively, NAE is usually evenly divided between titratable acid and ammonium excretion, however, our capacity to increase NAE is mostly dependent on enhanced ammoniagenesis and NH_4^+ excretion. The older view that NH_4^+ excretion was accomplished by simple passive trapping of NH_4^+ in the tubular lumen has been revised. We now understand that the excretion of NH_4^+ is more "active." First, in proximal tubule cells, there is deamination of glutamine to form alphaketoglutarate (αKG) and two NH_4^+. The further metabolism of αKG to CO_2 and H_2O generates two new HCO_3^- molecules as discussed earlier. Proximal tubule cells actively secrete NH_4^+ into the lumen, probably via the luminal Na^+-H^+ exchanger. NH_4^+ can substitute for H^+ and be transported into the urine in exchange for sodium. NH_4^+ is subsequently reabsorbed in the medullary thick ascending limb of Henle where it can be transported instead of K^+ via the Na^+-K^+-$2Cl^-$ cotransporter. This increases medullary interstitial concentrations of NH_4^+. Interstitial NH_4^+ enters the collecting duct cell, substituting for K^+ on the basolateral Na^+-K^+ ATPase. The NH_4^+ is next secreted into the tubular lumen, possibly by substitution for H^+ in the apical Na^+-H^+ exchanger or H^+-K^+ ATPase and is ultimately excreted into the final urine. It is important to note that the net generation of any HCO_3^- from αKG metabolism is dependent on this excretion of NH_4^+. Quite simply, if this NH_4^+ molecule is not excreted in urine, it is returned via the systemic circulation to the liver, where it will be used to form urea at the expense of generating two protons. In this case, the HCO_3^- molecules that were generated by the metabolism of αKG are neutralized and no net generation of HCO_3^- will result.

Because routine clinical measurement of urinary NH_4^+ concentrations never became standard, our appreciation of NH_4^+ in net acid-base balance during pathophysiologic conditions was delayed until recently, however, assessment of NH_4^+ is key in understanding NAE. It turns out that urinary $[NH_4^+]$ is estimated by calculations based on urinary electrolyte concentrations (either urinary anion gap or urinary osmolar gap) that are routinely measured. This will be discussed later.

KEY POINTS

Acid Excretion by the Kidney

1. Each HCO_3^- reclaimed from the proximal tubular lumen requires the epithelial secretion of one H^+. Largely, a Na^+-H^+ exchanger on the luminal membrane accomplishes this, although an electrogenic H^+ ATPase is also involved.
2. Net acid excretion by the kidney is the amount of H^+ (both buffered and free) excreted in the urine minus the amount of HCO_3^- excreted in the urine.
3. Net acid excretion is accomplished primarily through elimination of titratable acid (which is mostly phosphate) and nontitratable acid (in the form of NH_4^+).
4. An acidic urine (low urine pH) does not necessarily mean that NAE is increased.
5. Proton secretion by distal nephron is facilitated by the production of an electrogenic gradient that is produced by removal of sodium from the luminal fluid.

◇ Clinical Approach to the Patient with an Acid-Base Disorder

The approach to acid-base disorders often confounds practitioners of medicine, however, if one follows a fairly standard algorithm, acid-base disorders can be dissected fairly easily. We suggest the following seven steps when confronting a suspected acid-base disorder. The information necessary to approach a suspected acid-base disorder involves a blood gas (which gives pH, PaO_2, $PaCO_2$, and calculated $[HCO_3^-]$ values) and serum chemistry panel (which gives serum Na^+, K^+, Cl^-, and total CO_2 content). It is these data on which subsequent decisions are based. The total

CO_2 content (TCO_2), which is the sum of the serum $[HCO_3^-]$ and dissolved CO_2 (usually determined on a venous serum sample) is often referred to as the "CO_2", however, it must not be confused with the $PaCO_2$, which refers to the partial pressure of CO_2 in arterial blood. Since the serum $[HCO_3^-]$ or TCO_2 includes a component of dissolved CO_2, it is often 1–2 meq/L higher than the calculated $[HCO_3^-]$ derived from arterial blood gases.

1. What is the blood pH (is the patient acidemic or alkalemic)? Based on a normal sea level pH of 7.40 ± 0.02, a significant decrease in pH or acidemia means that the primary ongoing process is an acidosis. Conversely, an increase in pH or alkalemia indicates that the primary ongoing process is an alkalosis.
2. Identify the primary disturbance. In order to accomplish this one must examine the directional changes of $PaCO_2$ and serum $[HCO_3^-]$ from normal. If pH is low and $[HCO_3^-]$ is low, then metabolic acidosis is the primary disturbance. Conversely, if pH is high and $[HCO_3^-]$ is high, then metabolic alkalosis is the primary disturbance.
3. Is compensation appropriate? This step is essential for one to understand whether the disturbance is simple (compensation appropriate) or complex (mixed). With metabolic acidosis, the $PaCO_2$ (in mmHg) must decrease, conversely, with metabolic alkalosis the $PaCO_2$ must increase. Inadequate compensation is equivalent to another primary acid-base disturbance. It is important to recognize that compensation is never complete. Compensatory processes cannot return one's blood pH to what it was before one suffered a primary disturbance.
4. What is the serum anion gap (discussed in detail later in this chapter)? Calculating the serum anion gap provides insight into the differential diagnosis of metabolic acidosis (anion gap and non-anion gap metabolic acidosis) and can also indicate that metabolic acidosis is present in the patient with metabolic alkalosis.

5. Compare the change in serum anion gap to the change in serum bicarbonate concentration (discussed more fully in Chapter 9). If the change in the serum anion gap is much larger than the fall in serum bicarbonate concentration, one can infer the presence of both an anion gap metabolic acidosis and metabolic alkalosis. If the fall in serum bicarbonate concentration is, however, much larger than the increase in the serum anion gap (and the serum anion gap is significantly increased), one can infer the presence of both an anion gap and non-anion gap metabolic acidosis.

6. Identify the underlying cause of the disturbance. This is the whole purpose of analyzing acid-base disorders. One must remember that acid-base disorders are merely laboratory signs of an underlying disease. The pathologic cause of the acid-base disorder is usually obvious once the individual primary disturbances are identified.

7. Initiate appropriate therapy. The acid-base disturbance must be directly addressed in several clinical situations. Ultimately, treatment of the underlying cause is most important.

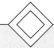

Metabolic Acidosis

Pathophysiologic Mechanisms and Compensation

Metabolic acidosis is characterized by a primary decrease in [HCO_3^-]. This systemic disorder may occur in several ways:

1. Addition of a strong acid that consumes HCO_3^-.
2. Loss of HCO_3^- from the body (usually through the gastrointestinal [GI] tract or kidneys).
3. Rapid addition of non-bicarbonate-containing solutions to ECF, also called dilutional acidosis.

In the latter two situations where HCO_3^- is lost or diluted, an organic anion is not generated. In this case, electroneutrality is preserved by reciprocal increases in serum chloride concentration. These forms of metabolic acidosis are generally referred to as hyperchloremic or non-anion gap metabolic acidosis, however, when an organic acid consumes HCO_3^-, the organic anion that is produced is often retained in ECF and serum. In this circumstance, the serum chloride concentration does not increase. This important concept is discussed in detail below.

The first line of defense against the fall in pH resulting from metabolic acidosis is the participation of buffer systems. This always occurs to some degree. As a general rule, nonbicarbonate buffers buffer about one-half of an acid load, however, with more severe acidosis, the participation of nonbicarbonate buffers can become even more important. Bone contributes importantly to buffering in chronic metabolic acidosis. The attendant loss of calcium from bone that results in reduced bone density and increased urinary calcium excretion are major deleterious consequences of chronic metabolic acidosis.

The second line of defense is the respiratory system. The $PaCO_2$ declines in the setting of metabolic acidosis. This is a normal, compensatory response. Failure of this normal adaptive response indicates the concomitant presence of respiratory acidosis. An excessive decline in $PaCO_2$, producing a normal pH, indicates the presence of concomitant respiratory alkalosis. Both situations are considered to be complex or mixed acid-base disturbances (Chapter 9). The respiratory response to metabolic acidosis is mediated primarily by pH receptors in the central nervous system (CNS). Peripheral pH receptors probably play a smaller role. This explains the small time delay prior to the establishment of respiratory compensation observed in animals and humans subjected to experimental metabolic acidosis. The normal, compensatory fall in $PaCO_2$ (in mmHg) should be between 1 and 1.5 times the fall in serum [HCO_3^-] (in meq/L). Even with extremely severe metabolic acidosis, however, the $PaCO_2$ cannot be maintained below 10–15 mmHg.

The kidney provides the third and final line of pH defense. This mechanism is, however, relatively slow compared to the immediate effect of buffering and respiratory compensation, which begins within 15–30 minutes. In contrast, the renal response requires 3–5 days to become complete. In the presence of normal renal function, acidosis induces increases in NAE by the kidney. This increase in NAE is due primarily to increases in NH_4^+ excretion rather than the minimal changes in phosphate (titratable acid) excretion. Acidosis increases the deamination of glutamine that generates NH_4^+. Excretion of the NH_4^+ and the ultimate catabolism of αKG, leads to generation of new HCO_3^-. In fact, there is both transcriptional and translational upregulation of key enzymes involved in glutamine metabolism that are induced by acidosis. Chronic metabolic acidosis also increases renal endothelin-1 that activates the Na^+-H^+ exchanger on the proximal tubule brush border. Therefore, acidosis induces both the generation of new HCO_3^- via the glutamine system and the enhancement of HCO_3^- reabsorption and titratable acid formation. Interestingly, the decreases in $PaCO_2$ that occur from respiratory compensation, actually limit renal correction in metabolic acidosis.

KEY POINTS
Metabolic Acidosis

1. Metabolic acidosis is a systemic disorder characterized by a primary decrease in serum $[HCO_3^-]$.
2. This occurs in three ways: the addition of strong acid that is buffered by (i.e., consumes) HCO_3^-; the loss of HCO_3^- from body fluids, usually through the GI tract or kidneys; and the rapid addition to the ECF of nonbicarbonate-containing solutions (dilutional acidosis).
3. In hyperchloremic or normal anion gap metabolic acidosis no organic anion is generated.
4. Organic anions are generated when an organic acid consumes bicarbonate leading to increased anion gap metabolic acidosis.
5. Fall in $PaCO_2$ is a normal compensatory response to simple metabolic acidosis.
6. Increases in NAE by the kidney develop in response to metabolic acidosis. The increase in NAE is due mostly to increases in NH_4^+ excretion that take up to 5 days to become maximal.

Biochemical and Physiologic Effects of Metabolic Acidosis

In the short term, mild degrees of acidemia are often well tolerated. In fact, some physiologic benefit such as increased P_{50} for hemoglobin favoring O_2 delivery to tissues occurs. If acidosis is severe (pH less than 7.10), however, myocardial contractility and vascular reactivity are depressed; in this setting, hypotension often progresses to profound shock. These consequences of acidosis result from well-described molecular mechanisms. First, acidosis depresses both vascular and myocardial responsiveness to catecholamines. In the case of the vasculature, supraphysiologic concentrations of catecholamines may restore reactivity, but the myocardial depression created by acidosis will eventually overcome this effect as pH continues to fall.

Metabolic acidosis induces an intracellular acidosis, and this appears to be particularly deleterious to physiologic function in cardiac myocytes. In addition, metabolic acidosis impairs the ability of cardiac myocytes to use energy. Some of this results from a blockade of glycolysis at the level of phosphofructokinase, but direct inhibition of mitochondrial respiratory function also occurs. On a physiologic level, intracellular acidosis impairs contractile responses to normal and elevated cytosolic calcium concentrations. Specifically, intracellular acidosis significantly shifts the sensitivity of Troponin C to calcium. Perhaps even more important, acidosis induces impairment of actin-myosin cross-bridge cycling. This results directly from increases in inorganic phosphate concentration in the monovalent form ($H_2PO_4^-$). This increase in $H_2PO_4^-$ results both from the acidic environment, as well as an impairment of myocardial energy production that increases the total intracellular concentration of inorganic phosphate. Metabolic acidosis and hypoxia synergistically impair myocardial myocyte metabolism, a phenomenon consistent with the monovalent inorganic phosphate hypothesis.

With mild degrees of acidosis, it may be difficult to discern an increase in ventilatory effort. More severe metabolic acidosis, pH < 7.20, increases the ventilatory effort. This is readily apparent as respirations become extremely deep and rapid, a clinical sign known as Kussmaul respiration. Mild degrees of acidosis do not markedly impair hemodynamic stability in subjects with otherwise normal cardiovascular function, but severe metabolic acidosis often leads to hypotension, pulmonary edema, and ultimately, ventricular standstill. Bone effects of even mild chronic metabolic acidosis are prominent. This acid-base disturbance leaches calcium from bone, resulting in hypercalciuria and bone disease. Treatment of renal tubular acidosis (RTA) or the acidosis of chronic kidney disease hinges on these important effects.

Decreased blood pH (acidemia), serum [HCO_3^-] (primary response), and $PaCO_2$ (compensatory response) are the laboratory findings that are the hallmark of simple metabolic acidosis. We reiterate that if the $PaCO_2$ does not fall by 1–1.5 times the decline in serum [HCO_3^-], this implies the coexistence of respiratory acidosis. We would argue that the profound clinical implications of this make this more than a semantic argument. It is, in fact, common for subjects with profound metabolic acidosis to eventually tire of their extraordinary respiratory effort. In this setting, the $PaCO_2$ rises to a level consistent with inadequate compensation, often just prior to respiratory arrest. Ergo, this must be considered as respiratory acidosis in order to mobilize the appropriate, emergent clinical response (Chapter 9). Normal or increased serum potassium in the face of decreased total body potassium stores occurs commonly with metabolic acidosis. This occurs because acidosis shifts potassium from the intracellular fluid to the extracellular fluid and renal potassium excretion increases in many states of metabolic acidosis. As is discussed in the next section, metabolic acidosis is classified as an anion gap (organic) or non-anion gap (hyperchloremic) metabolic acidosis. In general, metabolic acidosis states are characterized by the retention of an organic anion generated in concert with HCO_3^- consumption (organic acidosis) and others are not (hyperchloremic). As screening of serum for such organic anions is not practical on a routine, immediate basis, a calculation performed on the serum electrolytes called the anion gap is employed.

KEY POINTS
Biochemical and Physiologic Effects of Metabolic Acidosis

1. With marked acidemia (pH less than 7.10), myocardial contractility is depressed and peripheral resistance falls.
2. Acidosis depresses both vascular and myocardial responsiveness to catecholamines, as well as innate myocardial contractility. Both myocardial beta-receptor density, as well as physiologic responses to beta-agonists, are decreased by metabolic acidosis.
3. Decreased myocardial calcium sensitivity results in contractile dysfunction.
4. Metabolic acidosis and hypoxia act synergistically to impair myocardial function, a phenomenon consistent with the monovalent inorganic phosphate hypothesis.
5. Chronic metabolic acidosis causes hypercalciuria and bone disease.

Use of the Serum and Urine Anion Gap in the Differential Diagnosis of Metabolic Acidosis

The serum anion gap is used to determine whether an organic or mineral acidosis is present. This very simple concept that we will discuss in some detail allows the clinician to use simple electrolyte determinations to accurately infer whether an organic anion is present in high concentration. We calculate the serum anion gap as

$$SAG = [Na^+] - [Cl^-] - [TCO_2] \qquad (8)$$

In this equation, we use the TCO_2 as an index of serum $[HCO_3^-]$. We rather arbitrarily define "unmeasured" as not being in the equation (8). In other words, unmeasured cations (UC) are those cations that are not Na^+ (e.g., K^+, Mg^{2+}, Ca^{2+}) and unmeasured anions (UA) as anions that are not Cl^- or HCO_3^- (e.g., SO_4^-, $H_2PO_4^-$, HPO_4^-, albumin, and organic anions). The SAG, UA, and UC are expressed in units of meq/L. Equation (9) is written as such to maintain electroneutrality.

$$[Na^+] + UC = [Cl^-] + [TCO_2] + UA \qquad (9)$$

When we combine equations (8) and (9), the following equation for SAG is derived:

$$SAG = UA - UC \qquad (10)$$

For ease of computation, we consider a normal SAG to be about 10 meq/L; actually it is somewhere between 6 and 10 meq/L. We further assume that every proton generated causes a stoichiometric reduction in serum $[HCO_3^-]$. With these assumptions, it is clear that the addition of organic acid will cause an increase in the SAG, whereas addition of mineral acid (HCl) will not (Figure 7.3). The SAG is extremely useful in the differential diagnosis of metabolic acidosis. We stress, however, that it must be interpreted with some caution. While an organic acidosis should theoretically produce anions in concert with protons (discussed

Figure 7.3

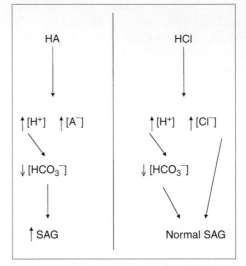

Organic acidosis is associated with an increase in serum anion gap (SAG) (left panel) whereas mineral acidosis is not (right panel). Note that addition of organic acid (HA) causes an increase in $[H^+]$ which, in turn, results in a decrease in $[HCO_3^-]$. Since $[Cl^-]$ and $[Na^+]$ do not change, the SAG defined as $[Na^+] - [Cl^-] - [HCO_3^-]$ increases. In contrast, when HCl is added, the decrease in $[HCO_3^-]$ is matched by an increase in $[Cl^-]$ and the SAG does not change.

above), note that the relationship between the increase in SAG and fall in bicarbonate concentration depends primarily on the clearance mechanisms for the anion and the volume of distribution for both bicarbonate and the anion. In general, the SAG is most useful when it is extremely elevated. A major increase in the anion gap (e.g. SAG >25 meq/L) always reflects the presence of an organic acidosis.

Unmeasured anions include SO_4^{2-}, $H_2PO_4^-$, HPO_4^{2-}, albumin and organic anions. Unmeasured cations include K^+, Mg^{2+}, and Ca^{2+}. A low SAG is seen in four clinical circumstances: (1) a reduction in the concentration of unmeasured anions (primarily albumin); (2) underestimation of the serum sodium concentration; (severe hypernatremia); (3) overestimation of the serum chloride concentration (bromide intoxication and marked hyperlipidemia); and (4) increased non-sodium cations (hyperkalemia, hypermagnesemia, hypercalcemia, lithium toxicity, or a cationic paraprotein). For each 1 g/dL decrease in serum albumin concentration the SAG will decrease by 2.5 meq/L. Therefore, in patients with hypoalbuminemia the SAG should be adjusted upward based on this correction factor.

As discussed earlier, one cannot routinely measure urinary ammonium concentration. Therefore, we must use the same type of reasoning employed for the SAG to develop a method to estimate NH_4^+ concentration based on the electrolyte content of urine. Because of electroneutrality we presume

$$[Na^+] + [K^+] + UC = [Cl^-] + UA \qquad (11)$$

Furthermore, when urine pH is <6, the urine does not contain appreciable amounts of bicarbonate. More relevant, the UC is made up mostly of NH_4^+. Therefore, we can define the urinary anion gap (UAG) as

$$UAG = [Na^+] + [K^+] - [Cl^-] \qquad (12)$$

It is clear that the UAG will be negative when urinary $[NH_4^+]$ is high. It turns out that low concentrations of urinary NH_4^+ are associated with a positive UAG. While the SAG is useful in many settings of clinical acid-base diagnosis and therapy, we must stress that the UAG is limited to a few clinical situations, specifically, it is used to differentiate renal (principally tubular acidosis) from non-renal causes of non-anion gap metabolic acidosis (such as diarrhea).

KEY POINTS

Use of the Serum and Urine Anion Gap in the Differential Diagnosis of Metabolic Acidosis

1. The serum anion gap is a concept used in acid-base pathophysiology to infer whether an organic or mineral acidosis is present.
2. Venous serum electrolytes are used to calculate the serum anion gap as

$$SAG = [Na^+] - [Cl^-] - [TCO_2]$$

3. The addition of organic acid will cause an increase in the SAG, whereas addition of mineral acid (HCl) will not.
4. The urinary anion gap is used to estimate the quantity of NH_4^+ in urine.
5. The UAG is used in the differentiation of renal from non-renal causes of non-anion gap metabolic acidosis.

Differential Diagnosis of Metabolic Acidosis

The first step in the differential diagnosis of metabolic acidosis is examination of the SAG. An anion gap metabolic acidosis is characterized by retention of an organic anion (elevated anion gap). In contrast, a hyperchloremic or non-anion gap metabolic acidosis is not associated with retention of an organic anion (normal anion gap).

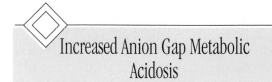

Increased Anion Gap Metabolic Acidosis

There are three forms of anion gap metabolic acidosis that are characterized by ketonemia or ketonuria and these include diabetic ketoacidosis, starvation ketosis, and alcoholic ketoacidosis (AKA) (Table 7.1). In all of these disorders, impaired lipid metabolism leads to generation and accumulation of short chain fatty ketoacids, specifically, beta-hydroxybutyric and acetoacetic acids. These ketoacids are relatively strong acids that produce acidosis, as well as an increase in the anion gap. The initial step in the evaluation of the patient with anion gap metabolic acidosis is an examination of blood and urine for ketones.

Table 7.1

Causes of Increased Anion Gap (Organic) Metabolic Acidosis

Increased acid production
Lactic acidosis
Ketoacidosis
Diabetic ketoacidosis
Starvation
Alcoholic ketoacidosis
Inborn errors of metabolism
Toxic alcohol ingestions
Salicylate overdose
Other intoxications (e.g., toluene, isoniazid)
Failure of acid excretion
Acute renal failure
Chronic kidney disease

Diabetic Ketoacidosis

Diabetic ketoacidosis is a common form of anion-gap metabolic acidosis. This entity results from a nearly absolute deficiency of insulin along with increases in glucagon. We should stress that the amount of insulin needed for catabolism of short chain fatty acids is significantly less than that necessary for glucose homeostasis, ergo, DKA is a common presentation in patients with insulin dependent diabetes mellitus but is rather unusual in patients with non-insulin dependent diabetes mellitus. Patients with non-insulin dependent diabetes mellitus present with marked increases in serum glucose concentrations without ketosis (non-ketotic hyperglycemic coma). This entity is also associated with an increase in the anion gap, but the chemical nature of the accumulated anion(s) has, surprisingly, not yet been well characterized.

DKA is diagnosed by the combination of anion gap metabolic acidosis, hyperglycemia, and demonstration of increased serum (or urine) ketones, however, the presence of serum and urine ketones is not specific for DKA. In fact, elevated ketones may accompany starvation and alcoholic ketoacidosis, where there may be some associated acidosis (see below), as well as isopropyl alcohol intoxication that is characterized by ketosis without significant acidosis.

Starvation

Starvation produces some metabolic processes that are similar to those seen with DKA. As carbohydrate availability becomes limited, hepatic ketogenesis is accelerated and tissue ketone metabolism is reduced. This produces increases in the serum (and urine) concentration of ketoacids and ketones. At first, there is minimal associated acidosis as renal NAE maintains balance. With more prolonged starvation the serum [HCO_3^-] often declines, however, it does not generally fall below 18 meq/L since ketonemia promotes insulin release.

Alcoholic Ketoacidosis

AKA is a relatively common form of acidosis seen in inner city hospitals. The acid-base disturbance results from the combination of alcohol toxicity and starvation. Ethanol itself leads to an increase in cytosolic NAD^+, but without glucose (the starvation component), ketogenesis and decreased ketone usage results. The serum glucose concentrations can actually range over a wide spectrum. In some cases they are very low (i.e., <50 mg/dL), but occasionally they may be moderately high (e.g., 200–300 mg/dL). In the latter circumstance, clinicians may confuse AKA with DKA. Patients with AKA often present with complex acid-base disorders (Chapter 9) rather than simple metabolic acidosis. A marked increase in the SAG is a hallmark of this disorder.

Alcoholic ketoacidosis may be a difficult diagnosis to make. Sometimes it is confused with DKA (discussed above). When the acidosis is severe, however, the majority of ketoacids circulating in the serum may not be detected by the Acetest assay, which is relatively insensitive to β-hydroxybutyric acid. Therefore, a high index of suspicion must be held in the appropriate clinical setting.

Lactic Acidosis

Anaerobic metabolism results in the production of lactic acid. Aerobic tissues metabolize carbohydrates to pyruvate that then enters an oxidative metabolic pathway (TCA) in mitochondria. This results in the regeneration of NAD^+ that was consumed in the TCA cycle, as well as in the glycolytic pathway. When tissues perform anaerobic glycolysis, however, NAD^+ cannot be regenerated from electron transport. In order to regenerate NAD^+, the reaction catalyzed by lactate dehydrogenase (LDH),

$$H^+ + pyruvate + NADH \rightarrow lactate + NAD^+ \quad (13)$$

must proceed and lactate is generated. Despite consumption of an H^+, the net effect of glycolysis is to generate lactic acid from carbohydrates and as discussed earlier, generate H^+. Normally, lactate (L isomer) production is closely matched by lactate metabolism to glucose (Cori cycle) or aerobic metabolism to CO_2 and H_2O, and circulating concentrations are maintained in a very low range. Under certain pathologic conditions, there may be a substantial increase in lactate concentrations and a concomitant development of metabolic acidosis, known as lactic acidosis. These include those with local or systemic decreases in oxygen delivery, impairments in oxidative metabolism, or impaired hepatic clearance. Of these, local or systemic decreases in O_2 delivery as a result of hypotension are most common.

Lactic acidosis is one of the most common forms of anion gap metabolic acidosis. It must be considered as a possible cause of any anion gap metabolic acidosis, particularly if the clinical circumstances include hemodynamic compromise, sepsis, tissue ischemia, or hypoxia. Measurement of the serum lactate concentration employs a spectrophotometric assay using the LDH reaction. Please note that D-lactic acidosis will be missed with this approach since LDH does not recognize D-lactate. D-lactic acidosis occurs with blind intestinal loops colonized with D-lactate-producing organisms. The clinician must suspect this diagnosis in the appropriate clinical setting and confirm D-lactic acidosis with alternate measurement methods (e.g., ^{1}H NMR spectroscopy, HPLC, specific enzymatic method for D-lactate).

Renal Failure

After eliminating ketoacidosis and lactic acidosis as potential causes for an anion gap metabolic acidosis one next examines the serum blood urea nitrogen (BUN) and creatinine concentrations to determine if organic anion accumulation is the result of kidney failure. Normally, the kidney is responsible for excretion of the approximately 1 meq/kg/day of H^+ generated by dietary protein. If the kidney fails to do this, one develops metabolic acidosis. With both acute and chronic renal failure, there is some retention of anions (including phosphate, sulfate, and some poorly characterized organic anions), and the SAG is typically elevated, however, it is common to find that the increase in SAG is less than the fall in bicarbonate concentration. In short, renal failure typically gives a mixed anion gap and non-anion gap metabolic acidosis. Metabolic acidosis in the setting of acute and chronic renal failure is generally not severe unless a marked catabolic state occurs, or another acidotic condition (e.g., non-anion gap acidosis from diarrhea) supervenes.

Toxic Alcohol Ingestions

Toxic alcohol ingestion should be considered in all patients with an unexplained anion gap metabolic acidosis. Delays in diagnosis and therapy of these intoxications are likely to be accompanied by permanent organ damage and death. These entities are also important to recognize because they often require hemodialysis to remove the offending agent and their metabolites. The most important toxic alcohols include methanol and ethylene glycol. These are often taken as a suicide attempt, but they may be inadvertently ingested by children or inebriated adults. While the clinical syndrome ultimately results in very severe metabolic acidosis, it must be stressed that the patient's acid-base status may initially be normal if they present to the hospital early after ingestion.

Because these toxic alcohols are osmotically active, the serum osmolar gap (defined as the difference between measured serum osmolarity and calculated serum osmolarity) is used to identify these patients.

$$\text{Calculated serum osmolarity} = 2\,[Na^+] + \frac{[\text{glucose}]}{18}$$
$$+ \frac{[\text{BUN}]}{2.8}$$

where $[Na^+]$ is in meq/L and [glucose] and [BUN] are in mg/dL.

This osmolar gap is generally elevated soon after ingestion because of the presence of the toxic alcohol in serum, however, if the ingestion is remote, it may not be substantially elevated. Although useful in suggesting this diagnosis, elevations in serum osmolar gap are neither sensitive nor specific for toxic alcohol ingestions. In fact, ethanol is the most common cause of an elevated serum osmolar gap. Therefore, it should be measured and its contribution to the osmolar gap calculated. The contribution of ethanol to the osmolar gap is estimated by dividing its concentration in mg/dL by 4.6.

Methanol intoxication typically presents with abdominal pain, vomiting, headache, and visual disturbances. This latter symptom derives from the toxicity of formic acid, a methanol metabolite to the optic nerve. Metabolism is folic acid dependent. Methanol toxicity can be seen with ingestions as small as 30 mL, and more than 100 mL of methanol is generally fatal unless treated promptly. Ethylene glycol is a major component of antifreeze. It apparently has a sweet taste that makes it appealing to children and inebriated adults. Ethylene glycol intoxication presents very similarly to that of methanol; both produce CNS disturbances and severe anion gap metabolic acidosis. In contrast to methanol, however, ethylene glycol does not usually produce retinitis, but it may cause both acute and chronic renal failure. The clinical presentation often consists of three

stages: (1) CNS depression that lasts for up to 12 hours associated with metabolic acidosis; (2) cardiopulmonary failure; and (3) oliguric acute renal failure that may be heralded by flank pain. Detection of oxalate crystals in urine is common in cases of ethylene glycol ingestion but may take up to 8 hours to appear. Oxalate monohydrate crystals may be erroneously interpreted as hippurate crystals by the clinical laboratory. The lethal dose may be as little as 100 mL.

Consideration of either ethylene glycol or methanol ingestion is important because they require very similar and immediate treatment. Neither ethylene glycol nor methanol are particularly toxic in their own right. It is the metabolism of these agents through the enzyme alcohol dehydrogenase that produces toxic metabolites. Therefore, blockade of their metabolism by the administration of agents that block alcohol dehydrogenase (ethanol or fomepizole) should be considered early. Moreover, since both the parent compounds and metabolites are low molecular weight and have small volumes of distribution, hemodialysis is generally employed. It is important to note that if ethanol is used to block metabolism of the parent compound and dialysis is also prescribed, the dose of ethanol must be adjusted to compensate for its concomitant removal by the dialysis procedure. As with ethanol, fomepizole requires dose adjustment during hemodialysis. With ethylene glycol intoxication pyridoxine and thiamine promote the conversion of glyoxalate to the less toxic metabolites glycine and beta hydroxyketoadipate, respectively.

Salicylate Intoxication

Salicylate overdoses are also common. Salicylate intoxication may occur as a suicide attempt, but often, especially in the elderly, may result from routine use. Aspirin or methylsalicylate intoxication may lead to serious and complex acid-base abnormalities. In younger subjects with salicylate intoxication, metabolic acidosis may be simple, whereas in older subjects a complex acid-base disturbance involving respiratory alkalosis and metabolic acidosis is more likely. Elderly subjects often demonstrate a major discordance between blood concentrations and symptoms. CNS toxicity almost always accompanies extremely elevated blood concentration (serum salicylate concentrations >50 mg/dL).

Salicylates stimulate respiration and produce a component of respiratory alkalosis, especially early in the course of toxicity in adults. The acids responsible for the metabolic acidosis and increase in the SAG are primarily endogenous acids (e.g., lactate and ketoanions) whose metabolism is affected by toxic amounts of salicylates that uncouple oxidative phosphorylation. Salicylic acid contributes to a minor degree.

The diagnosis of salicylate toxicity should be considered when a history of aspirin use, nausea, and tinnitus are present. Suspicion should also be raised by clinical findings of unexplained respiratory alkalosis, anion gap metabolic acidosis, or noncardiogenic pulmonary edema. Advanced age and a delay in the diagnosis of salicylate toxicity are associated with significant morbidity and mortality. Efforts to remove the salicylate include urine alkalinization to a urine pH of 8.0 with sodium bicarbonate in milder cases. Systemic pH should be carefully monitored and kept below 7.6. Hemodialysis is indicated if the salicylate level is >100 mg/dL, or if the patient has altered mental status, a depressed GFR, is fluid overloaded, or has pulmonary edema. Glucose should be administered because CSF glucose concentrations are often low despite normal serum glucose concentration. Acetazolamide should be avoided because it is highly protein bound and may increase free salicylate concentration.

Other Intoxications

Several other intoxications produce anion gap metabolic acidosis. These include toluene, strychnine, paraldehyde, iron, isoniazid, papaverine, tetracyclines (outdated), hydrogen sulfide, and carbon monoxide. These substances interfere with oxidative metabolism and produce lactic acidosis. Citric acid (present in toilet bowl cleaner) is an exception; the citrate itself causes an increase in SAG. Citric acid toxicity is associated with marked hyperkalemia. Toluene is another exception; it may produce a distal renal tubular acidosis in concert with an elevation of serum hippuric acid (a metabolite of toluene) concentration. Hippurate is rapidly eliminated from the body by the kidney, and as a consequence the anion does not accumulate, leading to a non-anion gap metabolic acidosis. This—rather than a distal renal tubular acidosis is—the likely mechanism of the normal SAG metabolic acidosis seen with toluene ingestion.

Inborn Errors of Metabolism

Inborn errors of metabolism represent an unusual but important cause of organic acidosis. In some cases (e.g., mitochondrial myopathies, some glycogen storage diseases), lactic acidosis develops without evidence for hypoxia or hypoperfusion. In other conditions (e.g., maple syrup urine disease, methylmalonic aciduria, propionic acidemia, and isovaleric acidemia), the accumulation of other organic acids occurs in concert with metabolic acidosis. Although many of these diseases present shortly after birth, some conditions may be first suspected in adulthood.

KEY POINTS
Causes of Anion Gap Metabolic Acidosis

1. The diagnosis of lactic acidosis must be considered in all forms of metabolic acidosis associated with an increased anion gap, particularly those cases associated with local or systemic decreases in oxygen delivery, impairments in oxidative metabolism, or impaired hepatic clearance.
2. Diabetic ketoacidosis results from lack of sufficient insulin necessary to metabolize glucose and excess glucagon that causes the

generation of short chain fatty ketoacids. The diagnosis of diabetic ketoacidosis is made by finding the combination of anion gap metabolic acidosis, hyperglycemia, and demonstration of serum (or urine) ketoacids.

3. Ethylene glycol and methanol ingestion are important causes of an anion gap metabolic acidosis that are associated with an elevated osmolar gap.

4. Metabolic acidosis in the setting of acute and chronic renal failure is generally not severe.

Hyperchloremic Metabolic Acidosis

Table 7.2

Causes of Hyperchloremic Metabolic Acidosis

Gastrointestinal loss of HCO_3^-
Diarrhea
Gastrointestinal drainage and fistulas
Urinary diversion to bowel
Chloride containing anion-exchange resins
$CaCl_2$ or $MgCl_2$ ingestion
Renal loss of HCO_3^-
Renal tubular acidosis
Carbonic anhydrase inhibitors
Potassium sparing diuretics
Miscellaneous causes of hyperchloremic acidosis
Recovery from ketoacidosis
Dilutional acidosis
Addition of HCl
Parenteral alimentation
Sulfur ingestion

In contrast to SAG acidosis, hyperchloremic metabolic acidosis is not associated with accumulation of organic anions (Table 7.2). Rather, loss of HCO_3^- (renal or GI), as well as some miscellaneous causes, add HCl to blood and lower serum HCO_3^- and raise serum Cl^- concentration. The urinary anion gap can be used to differentiate renal from GI causes of non-anion gap metabolic acidosis if the diagnosis is not obvious based on history and physical examination. The urinary anion gap is equal to the sum of urinary sodium and potassium concentrations minus urine chloride concentration. It will be negative in situations where urinary $[NH_4^+]$ is elevated and the kidney is responding appropriately to metabolic acidosis (nonrenal causes). The urinary anion gap is negative because NH_4^+ when excreted in urine is accompanied by Cl^- to maintain charge neutrality. In situations where the kidney is responsible for the metabolic acidosis the urinary anion gap will be positive. This may occur with either renal tubular acidosis or renal failure. Renal failure is identified by elevated serum concentrations of BUN and creatinine. The urinary anion gap can be misleading in two clinical circumstances. The first is when decreased sodium delivery compromises distal acid excretion. Therefore, in order to use the urinary anion gap urine sodium concentration must be greater than 20 meq/L. Decreased distal sodium delivery impairs collecting duct H^+ secretion and the UAG cannot be used if delivery of sodium to this segment is decreased. The second occurs when an anion (usually a ketoanion or hippurate) is excreted with sodium or potassium. Urinary sodium and potassium may be elevated leading to a positive urine anion gap and the impression that the kidney is not responding appropriately. The urinary osmolar gap (UOG) is not affected by the excretion of other anions and may need to be used in this situation.

$$UOG = 2(Na + K) + [BUN]/2.8 + [glucose]/18$$

The UOG is not affected by unmeasured anions in the urine since they are associated with cations (sodium or potassium). Dividing the UOG by 2 will approximate the urinary $[NH_4^+]$. A value less than 20 implies that the kidney is not responding appropriately to metabolic acidosis.

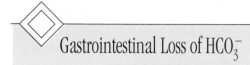

Gastrointestinal Loss of HCO_3^-

Diarrhea

The concentration of HCO_3^- in diarrheal fluid is usually greater than the concentration of HCO_3^- in serum. Although it seems like it should be obvious, the diagnosis of diarrhea to explain non-anion gap metabolic acidosis may be difficult in the very young or very old who are unable to provide historical details. In children, the distinction between diarrhea and an underlying RTA may be very important. In this situation, the UAG provides helpful information. When diarrhea causes metabolic acidosis, a significantly negative UAG (i.e., <10 meq/L) reflecting the presence of ample urinary NH_4^+ concentrations is present. In contrast, patients with all forms of distal RTA have positive UAGs reflecting the relatively low urinary $[NH_4^+]$ present in these conditions. Some patients with GI bicarbonate losses will have a urine pH >6.0 due to complete titration of NH_3 to NH_4^+. The urine anion gap in these patients will be negative, helping to distinguish those with renal tubular acidosis.

Gastrointestinal Drainage and Fistulas

Intestinal, pancreatic, and biliary secretions have high HCO_3^- and relatively low Cl^- concentrations. The intestine produces approximately 600–700 mL of fluid per day, but this may be increased in states of disease. Biliary secretions amount to more than 1L/day. This fluid usually contains HCO_3^- concentrations as high as 40 meq/L. Pancreatic secretions are an even greater potential source of bicarbonate loss, as the volume may exceed 1–2 L/day and contain $[HCO_3^-]$ up to 100 meq/L.

Because of the high $[HCO_3^-]$, drainage of these fluids or fistulas can cause significant metabolic acidosis. One interesting variation to this phenomenon occurs with kidney pancreas transplantation when the exocrine pancreas is drained through the bladder. This procedure almost universally leads to substantial metabolic acidosis as the NAE of the transplanted kidney is essentially nullified by the combination with pancreatic secretions. For this reason, most kidney pancreas transplants are now performed with intestinal drainage of the exocrine pancreas.

Urinary Diversion to Bowel

Surgical approaches to bladder and ureteral disease include creation of alternative drainage of urine through in situ bowel and or conduits produced from excised bowel. In both of these settings, active Cl^-/HCO_3^- exchange by bowel mucosa can impair renal NAE. Because of this, a non-anion gap metabolic acidosis may complicate both of these procedures. In fact, metabolic acidosis is almost certain when an ureterosigmoidostomy is performed. It is less common with ureteroileostomies and is generally only seen when contact time between the urine and the intestinal mucosa is increased, as occurs with stomal stenosis.

Chloride Containing Anion-Exchange Resins

Cholestyramine, a resin used to bind bile acids, can also bind HCO_3^-. Because of this, Cl^-/HCO_3^- exchange across bowel mucosa may be facilitated, and metabolic acidosis may develop. This is most likely in conditions of chronic kidney disease where new HCO_3^- generation is impaired.

$CaCl_2$ or $MgCl_2$ Ingestion

Calcium and magnesium are not absorbed completely in the gastrointestinal tract. As was the case for cholestyramine, unabsorbed Ca^{2+} or Mg^{2+} may bind HCO_3^- in the intestinal lumen and facilitate

Cl^-/HCO_3^- exchange. In this way, a non-anion gap metabolic acidosis may result.

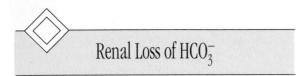

Renal Loss of HCO_3^-

Renal Tubular Acidosis

There is no topic in nephrology that confuses students and clinicians more than RTA. The RTAs are a group of functional disorders that are characterized by impaired renal HCO_3^- reabsorption and H^+ excretion. We distinguish these conditions from the acidosis of renal failure by requiring that the impairment in NAE is out of proportion to any reduction in glomerular filtration rate (GFR) that may be present. In most cases, RTAs occur in patients with a completely normal or near normal GFR.

Renal tubular acidoses can be approached in several different ways. We prefer to separate them based on whether the proximal (bicarbonate reabsorption) or distal (NAE) nephron is primarily involved. From a clinical standpoint, it is then most simple to divide the distal RTAs into those that are associated with hypokalemia and those that are associated with hyperkalemia. The hyperkalemic type can then be further divided into those due to hypoaldosteronism and those characterized by a general defect in sodium reabsorption. We prefer this approach to the confusing numbering system that has been used: proximal RTA (type II); distal RTA (type I) and distal RTA secondary to hypoaldosteronism (type IV).

Proximal RTA

Proximal RTA is a relatively uncommon disease. In proximal RTA, bicarbonate reabsorption in proximal tubule is impaired, and the *plasma threshold* for HCO_3^- is decreased. When plasma $[HCO_3^-]$ exceeds the *plasma threshold* for HCO_3^-, the delivery of HCO_3^--rich fluid to distal nephron

sites leads to substantial bicarbonaturia. This is associated with profound urinary losses of both potassium and sodium. When plasma $[HCO_3^-]$ falls below the *plasma threshold* for HCO_3^-, however, NAE increases and a steady state is achieved. Thus, patients with proximal RTA typically manifest a mild metabolic acidosis with hypokalemia. The serum $[HCO_3^-]$ is generally between 14 and 20 meq/L. If one treats patients with sodium bicarbonate, however, bicarbonaturia recurs, and urinary potassium losses become severe. Diagnostically, patients with suspected proximal RTA undergo an infusion with bicarbonate to correct the serum $[HCO_3^-]$. Proximal RTA can be diagnosed in this setting when fractional HCO_3^- excretion (i.e., the fraction of filtered HCO_3^- that is excreted in the urine) exceeds 15%.

Proximal RTA may occur as an isolated disturbance of HCO_3^- reabsorption, but more commonly coexists with other defects in proximal nephron function (e.g., reabsorption of glucose, amino acids, phosphate, and uric acid). In the situation where proximal tubule function is deranged for these other substances, the term "Fanconi's syndrome" is used. In addition to the mild metabolic acidosis usually associated with proximal RTA, Fanconi's syndrome is complicated by osteomalacia and malnutrition. Proximal RTA may occur as an inherited disorder (Lowe's syndrome, cystinosis, and Wilson's disease) and present in infancy. Alternatively, it may be acquired in the course of other diseases, following exposure to proximal tubular toxins (heavy metals), or in the setting of drug therapy. In the past, mercurial diuretics were commonly associated with the development of Fanconi's syndrome. Now the most common acquired causes include medications (nucleotide analogues) and multiple myeloma (light chains cause proximal tubular dysfunction).

Distal RTAs

Although classic hypokalemic distal RTA was initially characterized by an impairment in urinary acidification, all distal RTAs result in an impairment in NAE. This impairment in NAE is largely due to reduced urinary NH_4^+ excretion. Distal RTA may be associated with either hypokalemia or hyperkalemia. Distal RTA associated with hyperkalemia is the most common form of RTA, and generally results from hypoaldosteronism. All distal RTAs are characterized by a positive UAG in the setting of acidosis, reflecting inadequate NH_4^+ excretion.

Hypokalemic distal RTA is best considered a disorder of collecting duct capacity for effective proton secretion such that patients cannot achieve the necessary NAE to maintain acid-base balance. Patients with hypokalemic distal RTA usually present with hyperchloremic metabolic acidosis but are unable to acidify their urine (below pH 5.5) despite systemic acidosis. We stress that the failure to acidify the urine does not fully explain the defect in NAE, which is primarily due to an associated defect in NH_4^+ excretion. The two mechanisms that were suggested for impaired acidification by distal nephron in hypokalemic distal RTA are (1) backleak of acid through a "leaky" epithelium and (2) proton pump failure (i.e., the H^+ ATPase cannot pump sufficient amounts of H^+). Hypokalemic distal RTA may be inherited or may be associated with other acquired disturbances. Some of the same conditions that can cause hypokalemic distal RTA (e.g., urinary obstruction, autoimmune disorders) can also cause hyperkalemic distal RTA due to a defect in sodium reabsorption, suggesting that the mechanistic analysis discussed above might be somewhat artificial. In its primary form, hypokalemic distal RTA is quite unusual, and generally is diagnosed in young children. The afflicted children typically present with extremely severe metabolic acidosis, growth retardation, nephrocalcinosis, and nephrolithiasis. Hypokalemia, which is usually present, may actually be caused by the associated sodium depletion and stimulation of the renin-angiotensin-aldosterone axis. Therefore, renal potassium losses decrease considerably when appropriate therapy with sodium bicarbonate is instituted. This is completely different from patients with proximal RTA where urinary potassium losses increase during therapy because of the bicarbonaturia associated urinary potassium losses.

Hyperkalemic distal RTAs can develop from several mechanisms. These include (1) a defect in sodium reabsorption where a favorable transepithelial voltage cannot be generated and/or maintained, and (2) hypoaldosteronism. Hyperkalemic distal RTA from decreased sodium reabsorption is more common than either classic hypokalemic distal RTA or proximal RTA. Urinary obstruction is the most common cause of this form of distal RTA. Other causes include cyclosporin nephrotoxicity, renal allograft rejection, sickle cell nephropathy, and many autoimmune disorders such as lupus nephritis and Sjögren's syndrome. In contrast to hypoaldosteronism, urinary acidification is impaired in these subjects. Also, hyperkalemia plays a less significant role in the pathogenesis of the impaired NH_4^+ excretion that is more closely tied to impaired distal nephron function.

Hyperkalemic distal RTA from hypoaldosteronism results from either selective aldosterone deficiency or complete adrenal insufficiency. Probably the most common form of RTA is a condition called hyporeninemic hypoaldosteronism that is most often seen in patients afflicted with diabetic nephropathy. In patients with this form of RTA, urinary acidification assessed by urine pH is normal but NAE is not. The defect in NAE in some of these patients can be explained by impaired NH_4^+ synthesis in the proximal nephron resulting directly from the hyperkalemia. Hyperkalemia also interferes with NH_4^+ recycling in the thick ascending limb of Henle where it competes with NH_4^+ for transport on the potassium site of the Na-K-2Cl cotransporter. Other patients with hyporeninemic hypoaldosteronism have a more complex pathophysiology.

Another contrasting point between proximal RTA and hypokalemic distal RTA is the amount of alkali therapy needed. Patients with hypokalemic distal RTA only need enough alkali to account for the amount of acid generated from diet and metabolism. Therefore, approximately 1 mmol/kg/day is generally sufficient in these patients, whereas patients with proximal RTA require enormous amounts of bicarbonate and potassium supplementation. Some authors actually discourage trying to treat such patients with alkali.

Carbonic Anhydrase Inhibitors

CA inhibitors (e.g., acetazolamide) inhibit both proximal tubular luminal brush border and cellular carbonic anhydrase. This disruption of CA results in impaired HCO_3^- reabsorption similar to that of proximal RTA. Topiramate is an anti-seizure medication used in children that causes a mild-to-moderate proximal RTA through this mechanism.

Potassium Sparing Diuretics

Aldosterone antagonists (e.g., spironolactone and eplerenone) or sodium channel blockers (e.g., amiloride and triamterene) may also produce a hyperchloremic acidosis in concert with hyperkalemia. Trimethoprim and pentamidine may also function as sodium channel blockers and cause hyperkalemia and hyperchloremic metabolic acidosis. This is most often seen in human immunodeficiency virus (HIV)-infected patients.

KEY POINTS
Causes of Hyperchloremic Acidosis

1. Gastrointestinal loss of bicarbonate and renal tubular acidosis are two main causes of non-anion gap metabolic acidosis.
2. In the setting of non-anion gap metabolic acidosis, a negative urine anion gap would reflect gastrointestinal bicarbonate loss, whereas, in all forms of distal renal tubular acidosis the urine anion gap will be positive.
3. Proximal renal tubular acidosis is due to impairment in proximal tubular reabsorption of bicarbonate.
4. Distal renal tubular acidosis is due to impaired net acid excretion and can be either hypokalemic or hyperkalemic.

Miscellaneous Causes of Hyperchloremic Acidosis

Recovery from Ketoacidosis

Patients with DKA generally present with a "pure" anion gap metabolic acidosis. In other words, the increase in the anion gap roughly parallels the fall in bicarbonate concentration, however, during therapy, renal perfusion is often improved, and substantial loss of ketoanions in urine may result. Therefore, many patients afflicted with DKA may eliminate the ketoanions faster than they correct their acidosis, leaving them with a non-anion gap or hyperchloremic metabolic acidosis. Rarely, this phenomenon may even occur in patients who drink enough fluid to maintain glomerular filtration rate (GFR) close to normal as they develop DKA.

Dilutional Acidosis

The rapid, massive expansion of ECF volume with fluids that do not contain HCO_3^- (e.g., 0.9% saline) can dilute the plasma and cause a mild, non-anion gap metabolic acidosis. This is occasionally seen with trauma resuscitation or during treatment of right ventricular myocardial infarction.

Addition of Hydrochloric Acid (HCl)

Therapy with HCl or one of its congeners (e.g., ammonium chloride or lysine chloride) will rapidly consume HCO_3^-, and thus, cause a hyperchloremic metabolic acidosis.

Parenteral Alimentation

Amino acid infusions may produce a hyperchloremic metabolic acidosis in a manner similar to addition of HCl. In fact, this is actually quite common if alkali-generating compounds (e.g., acetate or lactate) are not administered concomitantly with amino acids, however, replacement of the chloride salt of these amino acids with an acetate salt easily avoids this problem. It turns out that it is metabolism of sulfur containing amino acids that obligates excretion of acid since neutrally charged sulfur is excreted as sulfate. In general, 1 g of amino acid mixture generally requires 1 meq of acid to be excreted. Ergo, the acetate content of parenteral alimentation should probably match the amino acid content on a meq/g basis.

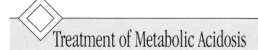

Treatment of Metabolic Acidosis

As stated earlier, the reason we analyze acid-base disorders is to obtain information as to the clinical condition underlying the acid-base abnormality. The fundamental principles of acid-base therapy are that a *diagnosis must be made* and *treatment of the underlying disease state* initiated. That said, some direct therapy of the acidosis is sometimes indicated. With most of the hyperchloremic states of metabolic acidosis, gradual correction of the acidosis is effective and beneficial. Oral bicarbonate or an anion that can be metabolized to bicarbonate is generally preferred. One gram of sodium bicarbonate is equivalent to 12 meq of HCO_3^-. In order to administer 1 meq/kg/day, doses will generally exceed 5 g/day in adults. Commercially available sodium or mixed sodium and potassium citrate solutions (e.g., Shohl's solution, Bicitra or Polycitra) contain 1–2 meq of HCO_3^- equivalent per mL. Citrate solutions may be better tolerated than sodium bicarbonate tablets or powder (baking soda), however, citrate can increase GI absorption of aluminum and should, therefore, not be administered along with aluminum-based phosphate binders.

The acute treatment of metabolic acidosis associated with an increased anion gap with intravenous sodium bicarbonate is controversial. Unfortunately, there is little in the form of randomized clinical data to guide us. Based primarily on experimental models, it appears that bicarbonate therapy may actually be deleterious in this setting, especially if the acidosis is associated with impaired tissue perfusion. The so-called "paradoxical" intracellular acidosis which results when bicarbonate is infused during metabolic acidosis probably accounts for a portion of these deleterious effects. This "paradoxical" intracellular acidosis is a direct consequence of the greater permeability of cell membranes to CO_2 than HCO_3^-. The addition of HCO_3^- to blood (or an organism) produces CO_2. When metabolic acidosis is present, more CO_2 is produced for a given dose of sodium bicarbonate than if there were no acidosis. In fact, recent studies performed in a closed, human blood model demonstrate that the production of CO_2 from administered HCO_3^- is directly dependent on the initial pH. When ventilation is normal, the lungs rapidly eliminate this extra CO_2. When pulmonary ventilation, or more commonly tissue ventilation however, is impaired (by poor tissue perfusion) this CO_2 generated by infused HCO_3^- may diffuse into cells (far more rapidly than the original HCO_3^- molecule) and paradoxically decrease the intracellular pH (Figure 7.4). Experimentally, administration of sodium bicarbonate in models of metabolic acidosis is associated with a fall in intracellular pH in several organs including the heart. Bicarbonate infusion in these settings also causes hemodynamic compromise. In addition to this "paradoxical" intracellular acidosis, hypertonic sodium bicarbonate therapy in the form of 50 mL ampules of 1 M $NaHCO_3$ may promote hypertonicity. The hypertonic state itself may impair cardiac function, especially in patients undergoing resuscitation for cardiac arrest. Based on these data, we do not support therapy with intravenous sodium bicarbonate for acute anion gap metabolic acidosis in the emergency situation. This area, however, remains controversial.

Figure 7.4

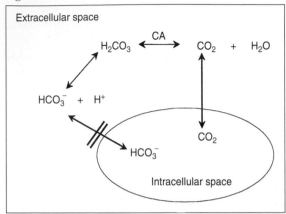

Mechanism of "paradoxical" intracellular acidosis following administration of sodium bicarbonate. Note that the sudden addition of bicarbonate causes increases in $PaCO_2$ accompanying the increase in $[HCO_3^-]$. This occurs, in part, because abundant carbonic anhydrase (CA) allows for the virtually instantaneous dehydration of H_2CO_3 in blood. Because most cell membranes are permeable to CO_2 but are not nearly as permeable to HCO_3^-, the intracellular PCO_2 increases faster than $[HCO_3^-]$ and the intracellular pH transiently falls.

To address the concerns for sodium bicarbonate discussed above, alternatives have been developed including non-CO_2 generating buffers such as trishydroxymethyl aminomethane (THAM) and Carbicarb (a 1:1 mixture of disodium carbonate and sodium bicarbonate). Dichloroacetate, which is specifically designed to decrease lactate production in lactic acidosis, was used in animals with some success. Clinical data with these agents are limited, and these agents are not Food and Drug Administration (FDA) approved for routine clinical use. Perhaps, more concerning is that none of these agents are still protected by patents, and it is unclear who (if anyone) will bear the cost of studies necessary to demonstrate their clinical safety and efficacy.

KEY POINTS
Treatment of Metabolic Acidosis

1. Hyperchloremic metabolic acidosis is usually effectively treated by gradual correction of acidosis with administration of bicarbonate.

2. Acute treatment of an anion gap metabolic acidosis with intravenous sodium bicarbonate may be deleterious, especially in conditions associated with impaired tissue perfusion.

3. The administration of sodium bicarbonate in animals with metabolic acidosis is associated with a fall in intracellular pH in several organs, as well as additional hemodynamic compromise.

Additional Reading

Adrogue, H.J., Madias, N.E. Management of life-threatening acid-base disorders. Second of two parts. *N Engl J Med* 338:107–111, 1998.

Adrogue, H.J., Eknoyan, G., Suki, W.K. Diabetic ketoacidosis: role of the kidney in the acid-base homeostasis re-evaluated. *Kidney Int* 25:591–598, 1984.

Adrogue, H.J., Madias, N.E. Management of life-threatening acid-base disorders. First of two parts. *N Engl J Med* 338:26–34, 1998.

Batlle, D.C., Arruda, J.A.L., Kurtzman, N.A. Hyperkalemic distal renal tubular acidosis associated with obstruction. *N Engl J Med* 304:373–379, 1981.

Batlle, D.C., Hizon, M., Cohen, E., Gutterman, C., Gupta, R. The use of the urinary anion gap in the diagnosis of hyperchloremic metabolic acidosis. *N Engl J Med* 318:594–599, 1988.

Filley, G.F. *Acid-Base and Blood Gas Regulation*. 1st edition. Lea & Febiger, Philadelphia, PA, 1971.

Gabow, P.A., Kaehny, W.D., Fennessey, P.V., Goodman, S.I., Gross P.A., Schrier, R.W. Diagnostic importance of an increased serum anion gap. *N Engl J Med* 303:854–858, 1980.

Halperin, M.L., Bear, R.A., Hannaford, M.C., Goldstein, M.B. Selected aspects of the pathophysiology of metabolic acidosis in diabetes mellitus. *Diabetes* 30:781–787, 1981.

Oh, M.S., Carroll, H.J. The anion gap. *N Engl J Med* 297:814–817, 1977.

Reilly, R.F., Anderson, R.J. Interpreting the anion gap. *Crit Care Med* 26:1771–1772, 1998.

Shapiro, J.I. Pathogenesis of cardiac dysfunction during metabolic acidosis: therapeutic implications. *Kidney Int Suppl* 61:S47–S51, 1997.

Dinkar Kaw and
Joseph I. Shapiro

Chapter 8

Metabolic Alkalosis

Recommended Time to Complete: 1 day

Guiding Questions

1. What is metabolic alkalosis and how does it occur?
2. What are the compensatory mechanisms for metabolic alkalosis?
3. How is metabolic alkalosis maintained?
4. What are the clinical features of metabolic alkalosis?
5. How does one differentiate various causes of metabolic alkalosis?
6. How does one treat metabolic alkalosis?

Pathophysiology of Metabolic Alkalosis

Metabolic alkalosis is an acid-base disorder that occurs as the result of a process that increases pH (alkalemia) from a primary increase in serum $[HCO_3^-]$. The primary elevation of serum $[HCO_3^-]$ is caused by the pathophysiologic processes outlined below.

Net H^+ Loss from ECF

A loss of protons from the body occurs primarily through either the kidneys or the gastrointestinal (GI) tract. When H^+ losses exceed the daily H^+ load produced by metabolism and diet a net negative H^+ balance results. Because the loss of H^+ results in the generation of a HCO_3^-, increases in serum $[HCO_3^-]$ result. Gastrointestinal loss of protons generally occurs in the stomach; in this setting, H^+ secretion by the luminal gastric parietal cell H^+ ATPase leaves a HCO_3^- to be reclaimed at the basolateral surface.

119

In the kidney, the coupling between net acid excretion (NAE) and bicarbonate generation was discussed at length in Chapter 7. Finally, shifting of H^+ into cells may accompany significant potassium depletion. Again, this should produce a rise in extracellular fluid (ECF) [HCO_3^-]. Regarding this last mechanism, we should point out that evidence of intracellular acidosis developing during experimental potassium depletion has not been consistently observed in experimental settings.

Net Bicarbonate or Bicarbonate Precursor Addition to ECF

HCO_3^- administration or addition of substances that generate HCO_3^- (e.g., lactate, citrate) at a rate greater than that of metabolic H^+ production also leads to an increase in ECF [HCO_3^-]. In the presence of normal kidney function, however, ECF [HCO_3^-] will not increase significantly. This occurs because as serum [HCO_3^-] exceeds the plasma threshold for HCO_3^- reabsorption, the kidney excretes the excess HCO_3^-. As a result serum bicarbonate concentration will not rise unless there is a change in renal bicarbonate handling (maintenance factor). The need for maintenance factors in the pathogenesis of metabolic alkalosis is discussed in more detail below.

Loss of Fluid From the Body That Contains Chloride in Greater Concentration and Bicarbonate in Lower Concentration Than Serum

If this type of fluid is lost ECF volume must contract. If this contraction is substantial enough, a measurable increase in serum [HCO_3^-] develops. Protons are not lost in this setting in contrast to losses noted with vomiting or nasogastric suction. Bicarbonate is now distributed in a smaller volume, however, resulting in an absolute increase in ECF [HCO_3^-]. This is referred to as contraction alkalosis.

KEY POINTS
Pathophysiology of Metabolic Alkalosis

1. Metabolic alkalosis is a systemic disorder characterized by increased pH due to a primary increase in serum bicarbonate concentration.
2. Primary elevation of serum bicarbonate concentration is due to net H^+ loss or net addition of bicarbonate precursors to the ECF.

Compensatory Mechanisms for Metabolic Alkalosis

The normal kidney has a powerful protective mechanism against the development of significant increases in ECF [HCO_3^-], namely the plasma threshold for [HCO_3^-] above which proximal reabsorption fails and HCO_3^- losses in urine begin. Because of this, in almost all cases of metabolic alkalosis, the kidney must participate in the pathophysiology of the metabolic alkalosis. Exceptions to this rule occur when renal function is dramatically impaired (e.g., renal failure) and/or when the ongoing alkali load truly overwhelms the renal capacity for bicarbonate elimination. These exceptional situations are both uncommon and easily identified. Therefore, we usually approach the pathophysiology of metabolic alkalosis by addressing initiation factors (i.e., factors that initiate the process) and maintenance factors (those that prevent renal excretion of excess bicarbonate). In some cases, as will be seen, the same factor may be responsible for both initiation and maintenance.

The first line of pH defense during metabolic alkalosis is, again, buffering. When HCO_3^- is added to ECF, protons react with some of this HCO_3^- to produce CO_2 that is normally exhaled by the lungs. Through this chemical reaction, the increase in serum and ECF [HCO_3^-] is attenuated.

It has been shown that the ICF contributes the majority of H⁺ used in this buffering process.

Respiratory compensation also occurs with metabolic alkalosis. Under normal conditions, control of ventilation occurs in the brainstem and is most sensitive to interstitial H⁺ concentration (Chapter 9). Respiratory compensation to metabolic alkalosis follows the same principles as respiratory compensation to metabolic acidosis. Of course, the direction of the change of $PaCO_2$ is different (i.e., hypercapnia due to hypoventilation rather than hypocapnia due to hyperventilation occurs) and constraints regarding oxygenation must limit the magnitude of this hypoventilatory response. With metabolic alkalosis, the $PaCO_2$ should increase 0.6–1.0 times the increase in serum [HCO_3^-]. Absence of compensation in the setting of metabolic alkalosis constitutes the coexistence of a secondary respiratory disturbance.

The third line of defense is kidney. In a manner analogous to tubular reabsorption of glucose, we can consider the maximal amount of tubular bicarbonate reabsorption (T_{max}) as the *plasma threshold* (PT) above which bicarbonaturia occurs. Once the PT is exceeded, bicarbonate excretion in urine is proportional to the glomerular filtration rate (GFR). If a patient has a GFR of 100 mL/minute and the bicarbonate concentration is 10 meq/L above the PT, bicarbonate will be lost in the urine initially at a rate of 1 meq/minute! Therefore, the corrective response by the kidney to excrete excessive HCO_3^- in urine will usually correct metabolic alkalosis unless there is a maintenance factor that prevents this.

KEY POINTS
Compensatory Mechanisms for Metabolic Alkalosis

1. The first line of defense is buffering. When HCO_3^- is added to ECF, H⁺ reacts with HCO_3^- to produce CO_2 that is normally exhaled in expired gas. Most of the H⁺ used in this buffering comes from the ICF.

2. Rise in $PaCO_2$ is the normal compensatory response to simple metabolic alkalosis.

3. In virtually all cases of metabolic alkalosis, the kidney participates in the pathogenesis by not excreting the excess bicarbonate.

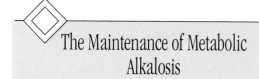

The Maintenance of Metabolic Alkalosis

A number of factors increase the apparent T_{max} for HCO_3^-. As a result, they increase net HCO_3^- reabsorption by the kidney. This is shown schematically in Figure 8.1.

Arterial Blood Volume Decrease

Volume depletion either absolute (e.g., salt losses through vomiting or bleeding) or effective (e.g.,

Figure 8.1

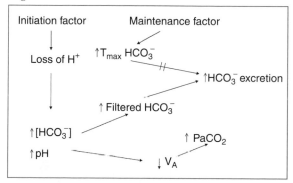

Importance of maintenance factors in the pathophysiology of metabolic alkalosis. In this figure, we see that proton loss (e.g., from vomiting) leads to increases in pH and [HCO_3^-]. These increases in [HCO_3^-] will be accompanied by increases in HCO_3^- filtration and loss in urine. If a maintenance factor (e.g., volume depletion, primary mineralocorticoid excess) is present, however, that raises the tubular transport of HCO_3^- (T_{max}), increased renal losses of HCO_3^- are prevented, and metabolic alkalosis is maintained. Note that the higher pH causes a decrease in alveolar ventilation (V_A, Chapter 9) and the $PaCO_2$ increases.

congestive heart failure, nephrotic syndrome, hepatic cirrhosis) increases the T_{max} and plasma threshold for HCO_3^-. This occurs through both proximal (increased proximal tubule reabsorption of Na and water) and distal (mineralocorticoid effect) mechanisms. Catecholamines and angiotensin II stimulate the Na^+-H^+ exchanger isoform in the luminal membrane of proximal tubule (NHE3). Proton excretion into urine generates intracellular bicarbonate that is transported across the basolateral membrane into blood. Mineralocorticoids act distally to directly stimulate the H^+ ATPase, and indirectly raise the driving force for proton excretion by increasing lumen electronegativity (through stimulation of the epithelial sodium channel).

Chloride Depletion

Sodium and chloride losses result in ECF volume depletion. Studies have shown that chloride is independently (i.e., besides being a marker for extracellular fluid volume) involved in HCO_3^- reabsorption. In fact, even despite ECF expansion, chloride depletion increases the plasma threshold for HCO_3^-, thereby raising ECF $[HCO_3^-]$.

Aldosterone

Mineralocorticoids increase distal sodium reabsorption which, in turn, increases renal HCO_3^- generation and effectively raises the *plasma threshold* and T_{max} for HCO_3^-. These effects can occur in the absence of decreases in effective arterial blood volume. Aldosterone's predominant effect is in the distal nephron. Shown in Figure 8.2 is a model of two of the three major cell types in the collecting duct, the principal cell and the alpha intercalated cell. The principal cell, is responsible for sodium reabsorption and potassium secretion. The alpha intercalated cell mediates acid secretion and, therefore, bicarbonate reabsorption and generation. Potassium secretion is passive and dependent strictly on the electrochemical gradient. Potassium secretion can be increased by raising intracellular

Figure 8.2

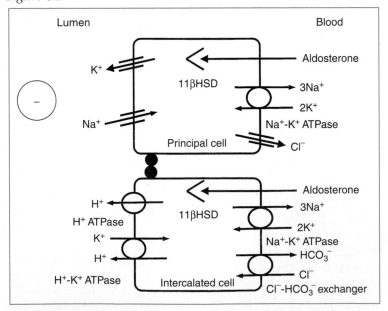

Collecting duct cell model. Proteins involved in sodium, potassium, and acid-base homeostasis are shown in both principal cells and alpha intercalated cells.

potassium, lowering luminal potassium, or making the lumen more electronegative. Indeed the major factors that control distal potassium secretion operate by changing these driving forces. Stimulation of the Na^+-K^+ ATPase by aldosterone increases intracellular potassium. Aldosterone also increases distal sodium reabsorption by causing the insertion of sodium channels, as well as synthesis of new sodium channels. In the long term aldosterone also increases the expression of the Na^+-K^+ ATPase in most epithelial cells, and directly stimulates the H^+ ATPase present in the luminal membrane of the intercalated cell. It also acts indirectly by increasing lumen electronegativity (through sodium reabsorption). Aldosterone binds to its receptor in the cytoplasm; this complex then translocates to the nucleus and stimulates gene transcription.

Surprisingly, it was found that glucocorticoids have similar affinity to that of aldosterone for the mineralocorticoid receptor. In addition glucocorticoids circulate at many times the concentration of aldosterone. So how could aldosterone ever have an effect? The answer to this question lies in the fact that target tissues for aldosterone, such as collecting duct cells, possess the enzyme type II 11β-hydroxysteroid dehydrogenase (HSD) that degrades active cortisol to inactive cortisone. If this enzyme is congenitally absent (apparent mineralocorticoid excess), inhibited (licorice), or overwhelmed (Cushing's syndrome), then glucocorticoids can exert a mineralocorticoid-like effect in the collecting duct.

Potassium Depletion

Potassium depletion also may increase the apparent T_{max} and *plasma threshold* for HCO_3^- and, thus, act as a maintenance factor for metabolic alkalosis. One potential mechanism for this is that potassium depletion may promote a relative intracellular acidosis and that this relative intracellular acidosis makes renal H^+ excretion more favorable; however, there is considerable evidence against this appealing concept. For one, there are orders of magnitude concentration differences involved when we compare protons to potassium ions. The $[H^+]$ in ECF is only about 40 nM (although intracellular concentrations may be slightly higher), whereas potassium concentrations may change by 1.0–2.0 mmol/L. More problematic is the observation that investigators failed to detect a decrease in renal intracellular pH during experimental potassium depletion with ^{31}P NMR spectroscopy. Moreover, in human studies, metabolic alkalosis can be corrected almost completely without correction of potassium depletion. More likely mechanisms for the increased T_{max} for HCO_3^- resulting from K depletion follow. First, potassium depletion results in cellular potassium depletion in proximal tubule. This, in turn, would be expected to hyperpolarize the basolateral membrane and increase the driving force for bicarbonate exit via the Na-$3HCO_3^-$ cotransporter. Second, potassium depletion upregulates H^+-K^+ ATPase in the collecting duct intercalated cell. It is likely that this upregulation results in increased H^+ secretion in this segment. This, in turn, would result in HCO_3^- generation and addition to ECF.

Hypercapnia

The apparent T_{max} and *plasma threshold* for HCO_3^- are raised by increases in $PaCO_2$. This is probably related to the decreases in intracellular pH that occur during acute and chronic hypercapnia. Analogous to our discussion in Chapter 7, increases in $PaCO_2$ that occur during metabolic alkalosis as part of normal respiratory compensation, impair the ability of the kidney to return serum bicarbonate concentration to normal.

KEY POINTS
Maintenance of Metabolic Alkalosis

> 1. Pathogenesis of metabolic alkalosis requires factors, that initiate or generate it and those that maintain it.

2. Several factors increase the apparent T_{max} for HCO_3^- and thus, increase net HCO_3^- reabsorption by the kidney. These include decreases in effective arterial blood volume, chloride depletion, increases in aldosterone, potassium depletion, and hypercapnia.
3. The most important maintenance factor is volume depletion.

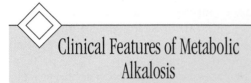

Clinical Features of Metabolic Alkalosis

Signs and symptoms of metabolic alkalosis are nonspecific. Patients who present with muscle cramps, weakness, arrhythmias, or seizures, especially in the setting of diuretic use and vomiting, should prompt consideration of metabolic alkalosis. Most signs and symptoms are due to decreases in ionized calcium that occur as the increased pH causes plasma proteins to bind calcium more avidly. At a pH above 7.6, malignant ventricular arrhythmias and seizures may be seen. It is interesting to note that humans tolerate alkalosis less well than acidosis.

Examination of arterial blood gases will demonstrate an increased pH, increased [HCO_3^-], and increased $PaCO_2$ with the increase in $PaCO_2$ being between 0.6 and 1 times the increase in [HCO_3^-]. Serum electrolytes reveal increased total CO_2 content (TCO_2), which is the sum of the serum [HCO_3^-] and dissolved CO_2, decreased chloride concentration and, typically, decreased potassium concentration. Hypokalemia occurs predominantly from enhanced renal losses. Renal potassium excretion results from maintenance factors involved in the pathogenesis of the metabolic alkalosis. Elevated concentrations of mineralocorticoids (or substances with mineralocorticoid-like activity) are almost always involved as a maintenance factor. Severe metabolic alkalosis may also be associated with an increased serum anion gap (SAG) (increases up to 10–12 meq/L). This is due to small

increases in lactate concentration resulting from enhanced glycolysis secondary to disinhibition of phosphofructokinase. The majority of the increase in SAG, however, is due to the increased electronegativity of albumin with elevated pH.

KEY POINTS
Clinical Features of Metabolic Alkalosis

1. There are no specific signs or symptoms of metabolic alkalosis. Many of the symptoms may be related to associated hypocalcemia.
2. Severe alkalosis (pH >7.6) can cause malignant arrhythmias, as well as seizures.

Differential Diagnosis

The first step in evaluation of the patient with metabolic alkalosis is to subdivide them into those that have ECF chloride depletion as a maintenance factor (chloride responsive) (Table 8.1) from those that do not (chloride resistant) (Table 8.2). This is accomplished by measuring urinary chloride. At first

Table 8.1
Causes of Chloride-Responsive Metabolic Alkalosis

Gastrointestinal causes
Vomiting or gastric drainage
Villous adenoma of the colon
Chloride diarrhea
Renal causes
Diuretic therapy
Posthypercapnia
Poorly reabsorbable anions
Exogenous alkali administration or ingestion
Bicarbonate administration
Milk-alkali syndrome
Massive transfusion of blood products
   (sodium citrate)

Table 8.2

Causes of Chloride-Resistant Metabolic Alkalosis

> **With hypertension**
> Primary aldosteronism
> Renal artery stenosis
> Renin-producing tumor
> Cushing's syndrome
> Licorice or chewing tobacco
> Apparent mineralocorticoid excess
> Congenital adrenal hyperplasia
> Liddle's syndrome
> **Without hypertension**
> Bartter's syndrome and Gitelman's syndrome
> Current diuretic use
> Profound potassium depletion
> Hypercalcemia (nonhyperparathyroid etiology)
> Poststarvation (refeeding alkalosis)

glance this might be surprising since urinary sodium concentration and fractional excretion of sodium are examined most commonly as indicators of volume depletion. These may be misleading in metabolic alkalosis, however, especially if the kidney is excreting bicarbonate that will obligate increased sodium excretion. Urine chloride concentration allows one to classify patients into chloride-responsive and chloride-resistant categories (Figure 8.3). In general, chloride-responsive metabolic alkalosis corrects when volume expansion or improvement of hemodynamics occur. In contrast, chloride-resistant metabolic alkalosis does not correct with these maneuvers. Patients with chloride-responsive metabolic alkalosis typically have urine chloride concentrations less than 20 meq/L, whereas patients with chloride-resistant metabolic alkalosis have urine chloride concentrations exceeding 20 meq/L.

Figure 8.3

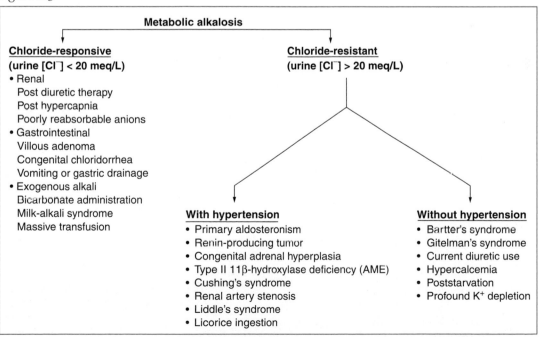

Differential diagnosis of metabolic alkalosis. The differential diagnosis of metabolic alkalosis based on the urine [Cl⁻] is demonstrated. The urine [Cl⁻] is used to separate chloride-responsive causes of metabolic alkalosis (where the urine [Cl⁻] is <20 meq/L) from the chloride resistant causes of metabolic alkalosis where the urine [Cl⁻] is generally >20 meq/L. These chloride-resistant causes can be further separated by whether the patient is hypertensive (volume expanded) or not. Abbreviation: AME, apparent mineralocorticoid excess.

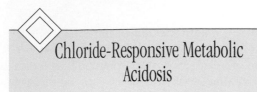

Chloride-Responsive Metabolic Acidosis

Vomiting and Gastric Drainage

Patients with persistent vomiting or nasogastric suctioning may lose up to 2 L/day of fluid containing a proton concentration of 100 mmol/L. Given that for each H^+ secreted a HCO_3^- molecule is generated, gastric parietal cells can excrete up to 200 mmol of HCO_3^- per day. This constitutes a very significant initiation factor; however, it is the sodium, chloride, and potassium losses that allow metabolic alkalosis to be maintained. It is notable that potassium losses are more significant in urine than in vomitus, which generally contains only about 10 meq/L of potassium.

Metabolic alkalosis that develops with vomiting is often mild. Similar to protracted vomiting, gastric drainage, generally via a nasogastric tube, also causes a metabolic alkalosis.

Colonic Villous Adenoma

Rarely, a colonic villous adenoma has significant secretory potential. This type of adenoma may produce profound diarrhea that contains excessive amounts of protein, sodium, potassium, and chloride. These diarrheal losses of sodium, potassium, and chloride and the relatively low HCO_3^- concentration in the fluid may lead to metabolic alkalosis—in contrast to the typical metabolic acidosis that more commonly complicates diarrheal states.

Congenital Chloridorrhea

Congenital chloridorrhea is a rare congenital syndrome arising from a defect in small and large bowel chloride absorption causing chronic diarrhea with a fluid that is rich in chloride leading to metabolic alkalosis. This disorder is the result of a

mutation in the *downregulated in adenoma* (DRA) gene. DRA functions as a Cl-bicabonate and Cl-sulfate exchanger and is expressed in the apical membrane of colonic epithelium.

Diuretic Therapy

Loop diuretics that exert their effects in the thick ascending limb of Henle (e.g., furosemide, bumetanide) and thiazide diuretics that act in the distal tubule (e.g., hydrochlorothiazide and metolazone) may facilitate volume depletion, as well as directly stimulate renin secretion (loop diuretics). These diuretics can, thus, provide both initiation and maintenance factors and produce metabolic alkalosis. If the diuretic is still active urinary chloride concentration is typically elevated. If the diuretic is cleared from the circulation and is no longer active (typically 24–48 hours after a dose) urinary chloride concentration is low, reflecting a normal renal response to volume depletion. Metabolic alkalosis associated with hypokalemia is a common complication of diuretic use, and should suggest the possibility of diuretic abuse. Diuretics are commonly abused in patients with anorexia nervosa.

Posthypercapnia

The kidney responds to chronic elevations in $PaCO_2$ by raising the plasma HCO_3^- concentration. If hypercapnia is subsequently corrected rapidly, as occurs with intubation and mechanical ventilation, the elevated serum HCO_3^- concentration will persist for at least several hours until renal correction is complete. Note that sufficient chloride must be present to allow for this renal correction, and many patients with diseases leading to hypercapnia are also treated with diuretics that may cause chloride depletion.

Poorly Reabsorbable Anions

Large doses of some beta-lactam antibiotics, such as penicillin and carbenicillin, may result in hypokalemic metabolic alkalosis. The initiation and maintenance factor is the delivery of large quantities of poorly reabsorbable anions to the distal nephron with attendant increases in H^+ and potassium excretion.

Cystic Fibrosis

Metabolic alkalosis may develop in children with cystic fibrosis due to chloride losses in sweat that has a low $[HCO_3^-]$. The maintenance factor is the resultant volume depletion caused by these losses.

Alkali Administration

As discussed earlier, the normal kidney rapidly excretes alkali. Ergo, a sustained metabolic alkalosis requires a maintenance factor. In these settings continuous and/or massive administration of alkali may cause metabolic alkalosis. This alkali load may be in the form of HCO_3^- or, more commonly, substances whose metabolism yields HCO_3^- as with citrate or acetate. In particular, it is clear that patients with chronic kidney disease whose ability to excrete a HCO_3^- load is decreased may develop sustained metabolic alkalosis following alkali administration. Baking soda is the richest source of exogenous alkali containing 60 meq of bicarbonate per teaspoon. Many patients ingest baking soda as a "home remedy" to treat dyspepsia and various GI problems.

Milk-Alkali Syndrome

The milk-alkali syndrome is classically noted in patients with GI upset who consume large amounts of antacids containing calcium and absorbable alkali. Calcium carbonate or Tums is the drug most often ingested for this purpose. Volume depletion (or at least the lack of ECF volume expansion) along with hypercalcemia-mediated suppression of parathyroid hormone (PTH)

secretion contribute to the maintenance of metabolic alkalosis. The resulting hypercalcemia also decreases renal blood flow and glomerular filtration, further impairing renal correction of metabolic alkalosis. Nephrocalcinosis may develop with chronic antacid ingestion, a pathologic factor that decreases GFR further, and thus more profoundly reduces the kidney's ability to excrete an alkali load.

Transfusion of Blood Products

Infusion of more than 10 units of blood containing the anticoagulant citrate can produce a moderate metabolic alkalosis, analogous to alkali administration discussed earlier. In many cases, some degree of prerenal azotemia may contribute to the maintenance of metabolic alkalosis. Through an identical mechanism, patients given parenteral hyperalimentation with excessive amounts of acetate or lactate may also develop metabolic alkalosis.

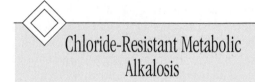

Chloride-Resistant Metabolic Alkalosis

Renal Artery Stenosis

Renal artery stenosis is a frequent clinical problem that develops in the elderly and those with advanced vascular disease. The most common cause of a chloride-resistant metabolic alkalosis with associated hypertension is renovascular disease. This is discussed in more detail in Chapter 21.

Primary Aldosteronism

With primary aldosteronism, excess aldosterone acts as both the initiation and maintenance factor for metabolic alkalosis. Several mechanisms are involved; some are the result of increased sodium reabsorption and potassium secretion, whereas others are independent of sodium or potassium transport. Increased H^+ secretion promotes reclamation of filtered HCO_3^- and generation of new HCO_3^-, which is ultimately retained in the ECF. Interestingly, although the increased ECF volume tends to mitigate the alkalosis by decreasing proximal tubular bicarbonate reabsorption, distal processes aid in maintenance of an elevated plasma HCO_3^- threshold. In primary aldosteronism, the clinical features of a hypokalemic metabolic alkalosis are produced, often in concert with hypertension that results from ECF volume expansion.

Primary aldosteronism may be caused by an adrenal tumor, which selectively synthesizes aldosterone (Conn's syndrome) or hyperplasia (usually bilateral) of the adrenal cortex. The diagnosis of a primary mineralocorticoid excess state depends on the demonstration that ECF volume is expanded (e.g., nonstimulatable plasma renin activity) and nonsuppressible aldosterone secretion is present (e.g., demonstration that exogenous mineralocorticoids and high salt diet or acute volume expansion with saline do not suppress plasma aldosterone concentration). Recent data suggest that primary aldosteronism may occur in as many as 8% of adult hypertensive patients; however, most of these patients do not have a significant metabolic alkalosis. In some families, glucocorticoid remediable aldosteronism (GRA) develops from a gene duplication fusing regulatory sequences of an isoform of the 11β-hydroxylase gene to the coding sequence of the aldosterone synthase gene. The diagnosis of this entity should be entertained in subjects in whom family members also have difficult to control hypertension. Clinical confirmation is generally pursued with the measurement of elevated concentrations of 18-OH-cortisol and 18-oxocortisol in urine prior to genetic analysis. Patients with GRA can often be successfully treated with glucocorticoid supplementation.

Cushing's Syndrome

Cushing's syndrome is characterized by excessive corticosteroid synthesis. Tumors that secrete ectopic adrenocorticotropic hormone (ACTH) are more likely to cause hypokalemia and metabolic alkalosis than pituitary tumors. Most corticosteroids (specifically cortisol, deoxycorticosterone, and corticosterone) also have significant mineralocorticoid effects and produce hypokalemic metabolic alkalosis. Hypertension typically is present. Collecting duct cells contain type II 11β-HSD that degrades cortisol to the inactive metabolite cortisone. Cortisol secretion in response to ectopic ACTH may be so high, however, that it overwhelms the metabolic capacity of the enzyme. In addition, type II 11β-HSD may be inhibited by ACTH.

Bartter's and Gitelman's Syndrome

Bartter's syndrome is characterized by hyperreninemia, hyperaldosteronemia in the absence of hypertension or sodium retention. This rare condition generally presents in childhood. Histologically, hyperplasia of the juxtaglomerular apparatus was observed, but this is not specific. The disorder is caused by an abnormality in thick ascending limb chloride reabsorption (cell model shown in Figure 8.4). This results in high distal nephron sodium and chloride delivery, renin-angiotensin-aldosterone system activation, and development of hypokalemic metabolic alkalosis. The primary disturbance was initially felt to be an abnormality in the prostaglandin system; however, it is now clear that increased renal prostaglandins in these patients is secondary. Recent genetic studies elucidated the molecular basis of the disease. Bartter's syndrome is caused by one of five abnormalities. Specifically, inherited inactivity of the apical Na^+-K^+-$2Cl^-$ transporter, the ROMK potassium channel, the basolateral chloride channel (CLC-K_b), the beta-subunit of the basolateral chloride channel (Barttin) or a gain of function

Figure 8.4

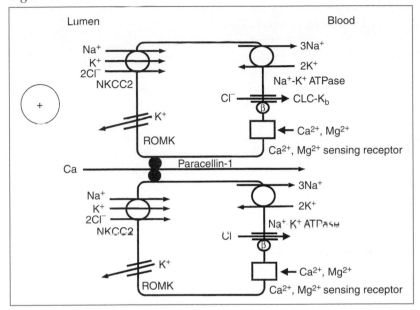

Thick ascending limb cell model. Proteins involved in ion transport in thick ascending limb are shown. Abnormalities of five of these proteins result in Bartter's syndrome and are discussed in the text.

mutation in the calcium-sensing receptor, proteins that are each essential to thick ascending limb of Henle function, can each result in Bartter's syndrome. A closely related condition, Gitelman's syndrome, is caused by mutations in the thiazide-sensitive Na-Cl transporter important in distal tubule function. Gitelman's syndrome may present in adults and is probably more common than Bartter's syndrome.

Both Bartter's and Gitelman's syndromes can closely mimic diuretic abuse. In fact, Bartter's syndrome and Gitelman's syndrome can be functionally imitated by the pharmacologic administration of loop and thiazide diuretics, respectively. Therefore, it is important to consider surreptitious diuretic use as an alternative to these diagnoses, especially if patients present de novo as adolescents or adults with previously normal serum potassium

and bicarbonate concentrations. Measuring diuretic concentrations in urine is often part of the initial workup.

Liddle's Syndrome

Liddle's syndrome is a rare autosomal dominant disorder resulting from a mutation in either the beta- or gamma-subunit of the sodium channel expressed in the apical membrane of the collecting duct. The mutation increases sodium reabsorption by blocking removal of the channel from the membrane. The molecular mechanism was discussed in Chapter 2. Metabolic alkalosis, hypokalemia, and severe hypertension characterize this genetic disorder.

Licorice

Glycyrrhizic and glycyrrhetinic acid, which are found in both licorice and chewing tobacco, may cause a hypokalemic metabolic alkalosis accompanied by hypertension, and thus, simulate primary aldosteronism. Recent studies demonstrate that this chemical inhibits type II 11β-hydroxysteroid dehydrogenase activity and "uncovers" the mineralocorticoid receptor which is normally "protected" by this enzyme from glucocorticoid stimulation. As glucocorticoids circulate at much higher concentrations than mineralocorticoids and produce comparable stimulation of the mineralocorticoid receptor, the result is a clinical syndrome similar to primary aldosteronism without elevated plasma aldosterone concentration.

Profound Potassium Depletion

Severe hypokalemia (serum $[K^+]$ <2 meq/L) may result in metabolic alkalosis. Urine chloride concentration exceeds 20 meq/L in this setting. In some reports, affected individuals did not demonstrate mineralocorticoid excess, and their alkalosis did not correct with sodium repletion until potassium was repleted. This indicates that severe hypokalemia may sometimes convert a chloride responsive to a chloride-resistant metabolic alkalosis. We should stress, however, that correction of metabolic alkalosis without repletion of potassium deficits was shown. Therefore, while hypokalemia contributes to the maintenance of metabolic alkalosis and should be corrected, potassium supplementation does not appear necessary to correct metabolic alkalosis.

Hypercalcemia (Suppressed PTH)

Patients with hypercalcemia from malignancy or sarcoid, and not from hyperparathyroidism, may develop a mild metabolic alkalosis. This is likely to be due to the calcium-mediated suppression of

PTH, which may raise the plasma threshold for HCO_3^-.

Poststarvation (Refeeding Alkalosis)

After a prolonged fast, administration of carbohydrates may produce a metabolic alkalosis that persists for weeks. The initiation factor for this form of metabolic alkalosis is not known, but increased renal sodium reabsorption secondary to ECF volume depletion is responsible for maintenance of the alkalosis.

KEY POINTS
Chloride-Resistant Metabolic Alkalosis

1. Metabolic alkalosis is classified based on urine chloride concentration into chloride responsive and chloride resistant.
2. The most common causes of chloride-responsive metabolic alkalosis are diuretics and vomiting.
3. Chloride-resistant metabolic alkaloses are due to conditions associated with increased aldosterone concentration or an aldosterone-like effect (type II 11β-HSD associated disorders or a sodium channel mutation).

Approach to the Patient with Chloride-Resistant Metabolic Alkalosis

As shown in Figure 8.3 patients are initially subdivided based on the presence or absence of hypertension. Those patients with hypertension can then be further categorized based on their renin

Table 8.3

Renin and Aldosterone Concentrations in Patients With Chloride-Resistant Metabolic Alkalosis and Hypertension

	RENIN CONCENTRATION	ALDOSTERONE CONCENTRATION
Primary aldosteronism	Decreased	Increased
Renal artery stenosis	Increased	Increased
Renin-producing tumor	Increased	Increased
Cushing's syndrome	Decreased	Decreased
Licorice ingestion	Decreased	Decreased
Apparent mineralocorticoid excess	Decreased	Decreased
Liddle's syndrome	Decreased	Decreased

and aldosterone concentrations shown in Table 8.3. Many of these disorders are discussed in more detail in Chapter 21.

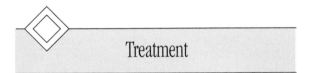

Treatment

Treatment of metabolic alkalosis, as with all acid-base disturbances, hinges on correction of the underlying disease state; however, the severity of the acid-base disturbance itself may be life threatening in some cases, and requires specific therapy. This is especially true in mixed acid-base disturbances where pH changes are in the same direction (such as a respiratory alkalosis from sepsis and a metabolic alkalosis secondary to vomiting). In these circumstances increased pH may become life threatening resulting in seizures or ventricular arrhythmias that require rapid reduction in systemic pH through control of ventilation. In this clinical condition, intubation, sedation, and controlled hypoventilation with a mechanical ventilator (sometimes using inspired CO_2 and/or supplemental oxygen to prevent hypoxia) is often lifesaving.

In the past, administration of either HCl, arginine chloride, or ammonium chloride was used to correct metabolic alkalosis, these agents can result in significant potential complications. Hydrochloric acid may cause intravascular hemolysis and tissue necrosis, while ammonium chloride may result in ammonia toxicity. In addition, their effect is not rapid enough to prevent or treat life-threatening complications. Therefore, in the setting of a clinical emergency, controlled hypoventilation must be employed. Once the situation is no longer critical, partial or complete correction of metabolic alkalosis over the ensuing 6–8 hours with HCl administered as a 0.15 M solution through a central vein is preferred. Generally, the "acid deficit" is calculated assuming a bicarbonate distribution space of 0.5 times body weight in liters, and about half of this amount of HCl is given with frequent monitoring of blood gases and electrolytes.

In less urgent settings, metabolic alkalosis is treated after examining whether it is chloride-responsive or not. Chloride-responsive metabolic alkalosis is responsive to volume repletion. Coexistent hypokalemia should also be corrected. Chloride-resistant metabolic alkaloses are treated by antagonizing the mineralocorticoid (or mineralocorticoid-like substance) that maintains renal H^+ losses. This sometimes can be accomplished with spironolactone, eplerenone, or other distal K-sparing diuretics like amiloride.

It is not unusual that the actual cause of metabolic alkalosis is due to a therapy that is essential in the management of a disease state. The hypokalemic metabolic alkalosis that develops from loop diuretic use in the nephrotic syndrome patient is an example where continued diuretic use is needed to manage the patient's severe edema. A creative approach to such clinical scenarios is the addition of the proximal diuretic acetazolamide, which will decrease the plasma threshold for HCO_3^- by inhibiting proximal tubule HCO_3^- reabsorption. The prescription of a proton pump inhibitor will decrease gastric H^+ losses in the patient who requires prolonged gastric drainage. In those with far advanced chronic kidney disease and severe metabolic alkalosis hemodialysis may be required.

KEY POINTS
Treatment of Metabolic Alkalosis

1. With life threatening pH elevation (e.g., pH >7.6 with seizures and ventricular arrhythmias), rapid pH reduction is accomplished by control of ventilation.
2. HCl or its congeners do not work fast enough to prevent or treat life-threatening complications.
3. Once the situation is no longer critical, partial or complete correction of metabolic alkalosis over 6–8 hours with HCl administered as a 0.15 M solution through a central vein can be carried out.

4. Chloride-responsive metabolic alkalosis corrects with volume replacement and improved hemodynamics.
5. Chloride-resistant metabolic alkalosis may need treatment with mineralocorticoid receptor antagonists or sodium channel blockers.

Additional Reading

Adrogue, H.J., Madias, N.E. Management of life-threatening acid-base disorders. First of two parts. *N Engl J Med* 338:26–34, 1998.

Adrogue, H.J., Madias, N.E. Management of life-threatening acid-base disorders. Second of two parts. *N Engl J Med* 338:107–111, 1998.

Dell, K.M., Guay-Woodford, L.M. Inherited tubular transport disorders. *Semin Nephrol* 19:364–373, 1999.

DuBose, T.D. Jr. Reclamation of filtered bicarbonate. *Kidney Int* 38:584–589, 1990.

Filley, G.F. *Acid-Base and Blood Gas Regulation.* Lea & Febiger, Philadelphia, PA, 1971.

Greenberg, A. Diuretic complications. *Am J Med Sci* 319:10–24, 2000.

Galla, J.H. Metabolic alkalosis. *J Am Soc Nephrol* 11:369–375, 2000.

Hebert, S.C. Bartter syndrome. *Curr Opin Nephrol Hypertens* 12:527–532, 2003.

Monnens, L., Bindels, R., Grunfeld, J.P. Gitelman syndrome comes of age. *Nephrol Dial Transplant* 13:1617–1619, 1998.

Youngsook Yoon and
Joseph I. Shapiro

Chapter 9

Respiratory and Mixed Acid-Base Disturbances

Recommended Time to Complete: 1 day

Guiding Questions

1. How is respiration controlled?
2. What is ventilation?
3. What is respiratory acidosis and how does it occur?
4. What mechanisms are involved in compensation for respiratory acidosis?
5. What is respiratory alkalosis and how does it occur?
6. What mechanisms are involved in the compensation for respiratory alkalosis?
7. What are clues to the presence of a mixed acid-base disturbance?
8. How do we approach the patient with a mixed acid-base disorder?

Respiratory Disturbances

Introduction

Breathing is an automatic, rhythmic, and centrally regulated process by which contraction of the diaphragm and rib cage moves gas in and out of the airways and alveolae of the lungs. Respiration includes breathing, but it also involves the circulation of blood, allowing for O_2 intake and CO_2 excretion.

Two patterns are involved in the control of breathing: automatic and volitional. The automatic component is largely under the control of $PaCO_2$. The control center for automatic breathing resides in the brainstem within the reticular activating system (Figure 9.1). There are two major regions that control automatic ventilation: the medullary respiratory areas and the pontine respiratory group. Interestingly, less is known about volitional control than automatic control of respiration, and we will restrict our further discussion to automatic breathing.

Figure 9.1

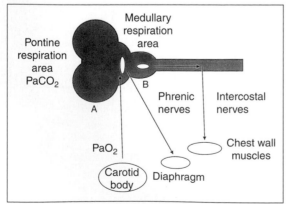

Control of ventilation. Schematic illustrating that central control of ventilation is largely through $PaCO_2$ sensitive chemoreceptors in the pons (A) and medulla (B), whereas peripheral input is largely through PaO_2 sensitive chemoreceptors in the carotid body. Output is to the diaphragm via the phrenic nerves and thoracic muscles largely via intercostal innervations.

Two main types of chemoreceptors, central and peripheral, are involved in the control of automatic breathing. The most important ones are located in the medulla of the central nervous system (CNS). The main peripheral chemoreceptors are within the carotid bodies although less important receptors were identified in the aortic arch. Central chemoreceptors respond to changes in $PaCO_2$ largely through changes in brain pH (interstitial and cytosolic). This is a sensitive system, and $PaCO_2$ control is generally tight. In contrast, respiratory control by oxygen tensions is much less important until PaO_2 falls to below 70 mmHg. This is a reflection of the Hb-O_2 dissociation curve since Hb saturation is generally above 94% until the PaO_2 falls below 70 mmHg. O_2 control of respiration is mediated largely through peripheral chemoreceptors which, in response to low O_2, close adenosine triphosphate (ATP)-sensitive K channels and depolarize glomus cells in the carotid body. The two systems interact, in that, with hypoxia, the central response to $PaCO_2$ is enhanced. As we will discuss later, with chronic hypercapnia, control of respiration by CO_2 is severely blunted leaving some patients' respiration almost entirely under the control of O_2 tensions.

In addition to neural control, the physical machinery of breathing is also extremely important in gas exchange. This physical machinery involves both the lungs, as well as bones and the thorax musculature that interact to move air in and out of the pulmonary air spaces. Just as there may be neural defects that impair respiration, abnormalities of either the skeleton, musculature, or airways, air spaces, and lung blood supply may impair respiration. To some degree, these abnormalities are assessed and characterized by pulmonary function tests. Although it is beyond the scope of this chapter to discuss this topic in detail, it should be clear to the reader that modern pulmonary function tests readily differentiate problems with airway resistance (e.g., asthma or chronic obstructive pulmonary disease) from those of alveolar diffusion (e.g., interstitial fibrosis) or neuromuscular function (e.g., phrenic nerve palsy, Guillian-Barre syndrome). Figure 9.1 shows a simplified schematic of the elements involved in controlling ventilation.

Pulmonary ventilation refers to the amount of gas brought into and/or out of the lung. Pulmonary ventilation is expressed as minute ventilation (i.e., how much air is inspired and expired within 1 minute) or in functional terms as alveolar ventilation (V_A) since the portion of ventilation confined to the conductance airways does not effectively exchange O_2 for CO_2 in alveolae. Since O_2 uptake and CO_2 excretion are so critical, we can reference ventilation with regard to either of these gases, however, since CO_2 excretion is so effective and ambient CO_2 tensions in the atmosphere are so low, pulmonary ventilation generally is synonymous with pulmonary CO_2 excretion. Note that CO_2 is much more soluble than O_2 and exchange across the alveolar capillary for CO_2 is essentially complete under most circumstances, whereas some O_2 gradient from alveolus to the alveolar capillary is always present.

We should also point out that ventilation occurs at the tissue level as well. In this case, rather than inspired air removing CO_2 in its gaseous form, CO_2 produced by cells is largely (about 75%) converted to HCO_3^- and removed from the local cellular environment by blood flow. Although it is an extreme case, when CO_2 tensions in expired gases are monitored during cardiac arrest, the institution of effective circulation is accompanied by a sharp increase in expired CO_2.

KEY POINTS
Respiratory Disturbances

1. CNS respiratory centers receive input from chemoreceptors locally ($PaCO_2$) and peripherally (PaO_2).
2. Ventilation is determined by the integration of neural inputs, neural outputs, muscular responses, flow through airways, and gas exchange between alveolae and pulmonary capillaries.

Respiratory Acidosis

Respiratory acidosis is defined as a primary increase in $PaCO_2$ secondary to decreased effective ventilation with net CO_2 retention. This decrease in effective ventilation can occur from defects in any aspect of ventilation control or implementation. These different causes are summarized in Table 9.1.

Compensation for respiratory acidosis occurs at several levels. Some of these processes are rapid, analogous to what is seen with major compensatory mechanisms for metabolic acidosis or alkalosis, whereas others are slower. This latter fact allows us to clinically distinguish between acute and chronic respiratory acidosis in some cases.

With respiratory acidosis, a rise in $[HCO_3^-]$ is a normal, compensatory response. As is the case for metabolic disorders, a failure of this normal adaptive response is indicative of the presence of metabolic acidosis in the setting of a complex or mixed acid-base disturbance. Conversely, an exaggerated increase in HCO_3^- producing a normal pH indicates the presence of metabolic alkalosis in the setting of a complex or mixed acid-base disturbance.

Mechanisms by which respiratory acidosis increases HCO_3^- concentration are as follows. First and probably foremost, increases in $PaCO_2$ and decreases in O_2 tension stimulate ventilatory drive, in some way antagonizing the process that led to CO_2 retention in the first place. Next, mechanisms by which CO_2 transport occurs from tissues to lungs become operant. In other words, increases in $PaCO_2$ are immediately accompanied by a shift to the right of the reaction

$$H_2CO_3 \leftrightarrow H^+ + HCO_3^-$$

and increases in HCO_3^- concentration result. The amount of this increase in $[HCO_3^-]$ in meq/L is 0.1 times the increase in $PaCO_2$ in mmHg (±2 meq/L). The kidney provides the mechanism for the majority of chronic compensation. Once $PaCO_2$

Table 9.1
Causes of Respiratory Acidosis

Acute	Airway obstruction—aspiration of foreign body or vomitus, laryngospasm, generalized bronchospasm, obstructive sleep apnea
	Respiratory center depression—general anesthesia, sedative overdosage, cerebral trauma or infarction, central sleep apnea
	Circulatory catastrophes—cardiac arrest, severe pulmonary edema
	Neuromuscular defects—high cervical cordotomy, botulism, tetanus, Guillain-Barre syndrome, crisis in myasthenia gravis, familial hypokalemic periodic paralysis, hypokalemic myopathy, toxic drug agents (e.g., curare, succinylcholine, aminoglycosides, organophosphates)
	Restrictive defects—pneumothorax, hemothorax, flail chest, severe pneumonitis, hyaline membrane disease, adult respiratory distress syndrome
	Pulmonary disorders—pneumonia, massive pulmonary embolism, pulmonary edema
	Mechanical underventilation
Chronic	Airway obstruction—chronic obstructive lung disease (bronchitis, emphysema)
	Respiratory center depression—chronic sedative depression, primary alveolar hypoventilation, obesity hypoventilation syndrome, brain tumor, bulbar poliomyelitis
	Neuromuscular defects—poliomyelitis, multiple sclerosis, muscular dystrophy, amyotrophic lateral sclerosis, diaphragmatic paralysis, myxedema, myopathic disease (e.g., polymyositis, acid maltase deficiency)
	Restrictive defects—kyphoscoliosis, spinal arthritis, fibrothorax, hydrothorax, interstitial fibrosis, decreased diaphragmatic movement (e.g., ascites), prolonged pneumonitis, obesity

increases and arterial pH decreases, renal acid excretion and retention of bicarbonate become more avid. Some of this is a direct chemical consequence of elevated $PaCO_2$ and mass action facilitating intracellular bicarbonate formation, whereas other portions involve genomic adaptations of tubular cells involved in renal acid excretion. On this latter topic, enzymes involved in renal ammoniagenesis (e.g., glutamine synthetase), as well as apical and basolateral ion transport proteins (e.g., Na^+-H^+ exchanger, Na^+-K^+ ATPase) are synthesized in increased amounts at key sites within the nephron. In sum, chronic respiratory acidosis present for at least 4–5 days will be accompanied by a $[HCO_3^-]$ increase = 0.4 times the increase in $PaCO_2$ (mmHg) (±3 meq/L). Note that renal correction also never completely returns the arterial pH to the level it was at prior to CO_2 retention.

KEY POINTS
Respiratory Acidosis

1. In respiratory acidosis, the primary disturbance is an increase in $PaCO_2$ secondary to a decrease in effective ventilation with net CO_2 retention.
2. Decreases in effective ventilation can result from defects in any aspect of ventilation control or implementation.
3. In respiratory acidosis, the $[HCO_3^-]$ rises as a normal, compensatory response.
4. A failure of the normal adaptive response indicates the presence of metabolic acidosis in the setting of a complex or mixed acid-base disturbance.
5. The kidney provides the mechanism for the majority of chronic compensation.

Respiratory Alkalosis

Respiratory alkalosis is defined as a primary decrease in $PaCO_2$ secondary to an increase in effective ventilation with net CO_2 removal. This increase in effective ventilation can occur from defects in any aspect of ventilation control or implementation. These different causes are summarized in Table 9.2.

With respiratory alkalosis, a fall in $[HCO_3^-]$ is a normal, compensatory response. As was the case for respiratory acidosis and the metabolic disorders, a failure of this normal adaptive response is indicative of the presence of metabolic alkalosis in the setting of a complex or mixed acid-base

Table 9.2

Causes of Respiratory Alkalosis

Hypoxia
  Decreased inspired oxygen tension
  Ventilation-perfusion inequality
  Hypotension
  Severe anemia
CNS mediated
  Voluntary hyperventilation
  Neurologic disease-cerebrovascular accident
    (infarction, hemorrhage), infection
    (encephalitis, meningitis), trauma, tumor
  Pharmacologic and hormonal stimulation-
    salicylates, ditrophenol, nicotine, xanthines,
    pressor hormones, pregnancy
Hepatic failure
Gram-negative septicemia
Anxiety-hyperventilation syndrome
Heat exposure
Pulmonary disease
  Interstitial lung disease
  Pneumonia
  Pulmonary embolism
  Pulmonary edema
  Mechanical overventilation

Abbreviation: CNS, central nervous system.

disturbance. Conversely, an exaggerated decrease in $[HCO_3^-]$ producing a normal pH indicates the presence of metabolic acidosis in the setting of a complex or mixed acid-base disturbance.

The mechanisms by which respiratory alkalosis decreases $[HCO_3^-]$ are as follows. First and probably foremost, decreases in $PaCO_2$ will inhibit ventilatory drive, in some way antagonizing the process that led to reductions in CO_2 tension in the first place. Decreases in $PaCO_2$ are immediately accompanied by a shift to the left of the reaction

$$H_2CO_3 \leftrightarrow H^+ + HCO_3^-$$

and decreases in $[HCO_3^-]$ result. The amount of this decrease in $[HCO_3^-]$ is (in meq/L) 0.1 times the decrease in $PaCO_2$ in mmHg (with an error range of ±2 meq/L). Again, the kidney provides the mechanism for the majority of chronic compensation. Once $PaCO_2$ decreases and arterial pH increases, renal excretion of acid and retention of bicarbonate are reduced. Some of this is a direct chemical consequence of decreased $PaCO_2$ and mass action antagonizing intracellular bicarbonate formation, whereas other portions involve genomic adaptations of tubular cells involved in renal acid excretion. Essentially, the reverse of what we described for metabolic compensation for respiratory acidosis occurs. In sum, chronic respiratory alkalosis present for at least 4–5 days will be accompanied by a $[HCO_3^-]$ decrease (in meq/L) of 0.4 times the increase in $PaCO_2$ (mmHg) (with an error range of ±3 meq/L). Note that renal correction also never completely returns arterial pH to the level it was at prior to respiratory alkalosis. Moreover, decreases in $[HCO_3^-]$ below 12 meq/L are generally not seen from metabolic compensation for respiratory alkalosis.

KEY POINTS
Respiratory Alkalosis

1. In respiratory alkalosis the primary process is a decrease in $PaCO_2$ secondary to an increase in effective ventilation with net CO_2 removal.

2. With respiratory alkalosis, a fall in $[HCO_3^-]$ is a normal, compensatory response.

3. A failure of this normal adaptive response is indicative of the presence of metabolic alkalosis in the setting of a complex or mixed acid-base disturbance.

4. The kidney provides the mechanism for the majority of chronic compensation.

5. Decreases in $[HCO_3^-]$ below 12 meq/L are generally not seen from metabolic compensation for respiratory alkalosis.

Mixed Disturbances

The first clue to the presence of a mixed acid-base disorder is the degree of compensation. As discussed above, "over compensation" or an absence of compensation are certain indicators that a mixed acid-base disorder is present. For metabolic disorders, the respiratory compensation should be immediate; in these settings, it is relatively easy to determine whether compensation is appropriate (see Chapters 7 and 8). For respiratory disorders, however, it is a bit more complex since metabolic compensation takes days to become complete. Note that mass action will produce about a 0.1 meq/L change in $[HCO_3^-]$ for every 1 mmHg change in $PaCO_2$; ergo, a complete absence of metabolic compensation for respiratory acidosis or alkalosis clearly indicates a second primary problem. For degrees of compensation between 0.1 and 0.4 meq/L/mmHg change in $PaCO_2$, it is difficult if not impossible to distinguish between a failure of compensation (e.g., a primary metabolic disorder) and an acute respiratory disturbance on the blood gas alone. These rules of compensation are illustrated graphically in Figure 9.2. To further address this question, we must return to our description of the anion gap in Chapter 7. Recall that the serum anion gap can be defined as

$$SAG = [Na^+] - [Cl^-] - [HCO_3^-]$$

but this can also be interpreted as

$$SAG = UA - UC$$

To use the SAG in the approach to a complex acid-base disorder, we make the stoichiometric assumption that for a pure organic acidosis

$$\Delta SAG = \Delta[HCO_3^-]$$

Since we don't have "pre" and "post" disorder values, we further assume that the SAG started at 10 meq/L and the $[HCO_3^-]$ started at 24 meq/L. With these assumptions, we can diagnose simultaneous anion gap metabolic acidosis and metabolic alkalosis when the SAG is large and the decrease in $[HCO_3^-]$ is relatively small. A common clinical scenario for this is when vomiting accompanies an anion gap metabolic acidosis such as lactic acidosis in the setting of bowel ischemia. Conversely, we can also diagnose simultaneous non-anion gap metabolic acidosis with anion gap metabolic acidosis if the fall in $[HCO_3^-]$ is much larger than the modestly but significantly increased SAG. Probably the most common example for this would be renal failure where some degree of non-anion gap acidosis and anion gap acidosis coexist. These situations are shown schematically in Figure 9.3. A list of clinical scenarios where complex acid-base disorders often occur is shown in Table 9.3.

It is appropriate at this point to reiterate the reason that one performs analysis of acid-base disorders. Quite simply, it is to gain insight into the clinical problems that the patient is facing. To this end, it is important to realize that the accurate diagnosis of a mixed disorder is more than a matter of semantics. In some cases, it may even be life saving. The following case illustrates this. An 8-year-old boy presents to an emergency room with history of a viral illness followed by progressive obtundation. His arterial blood gas shows a pH of 7.00, $PaCO_2 = 38$ mmHg, $[HCO_3^-] = 9$ meq/L. The serum glucose concentration is elevated, and both urine and blood are positive for ketones. The serum anion gap is calculated at 25 meq/L.

Why is it so important to accurately diagnose that the patient above has a mixed respiratory and

Figure 9.2

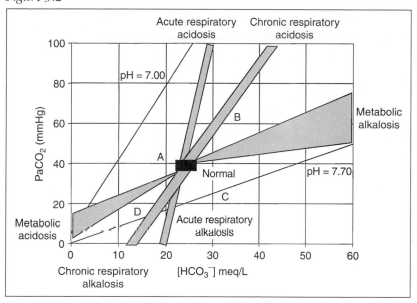

Acid-base nomogram. Acid-base nomogram derived from rules of compensation described in the text. Regions associated with simple acid-base disorders are identified in the shaded regions. A: Mixed respiratory and metabolic acidosis, B: mixed respiratory acidosis and metabolic alkalosis, C: mixed respiratory alkalosis and metabolic alkalosis, and D: mixed respiratory alkalosis and metabolic acidosis. Regions between acute and chronic respiratory acidosis and acute and chronic respiratory alkalosis cannot be uniquely defined (see text). Lines of constant pH 7.00 and 7.70, as well as normal range (black box) shown for reference.

metabolic acidosis (see Figure 9.2) rather than "uncompensated" metabolic acidosis? In the scenario described, it is likely that the child will soon stop breathing. Although the $PaCO_2$ of 38 mmHg is a "normal" value, it is not appropriate compensation and, thus, must be interpreted as another primary disorder. Understanding that this truly represents respiratory acidosis confers appropriate urgency to the clinical situation and also may prompt a search for potential causes of respiratory acidosis. In this case the respiratory acidosis is likely secondary to neuromuscular fatigue, however, in other clinical situations it may prompt a search for causes of central respiratory depression (e.g., sedative administration) or acute airway obstruction.

As was the case for simple acid-base disorders, the key reason for analyzing mixed acid-base

disorders is to create short lists of differential diagnoses to further explore clinically. This is generally accomplished diagnosis by diagnosis. In other words, if a patient were found to have a triple acid-base disorder consisting of respiratory alkalosis, anion gap metabolic acidosis, and metabolic alkalosis, one would examine each of these separately and put them together in the context of the patient.

In Chapters 7 and 8, we stated that the degree of acidosis or alkalosis is rarely life threatening by itself. Although this is true, the exceptional cases generally involve mixed acid-base disorders where both respiratory and metabolic disorders change pH in the same direction. For example, mixed respiratory acidosis and metabolic acidosis that might occur in the setting of cardiac and respiratory arrest may produce low enough pH to

Figure 9.3

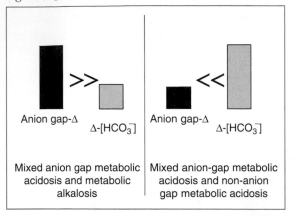

Mixed anion gap metabolic acidosis and metabolic alkalosis	Mixed anion-gap metabolic acidosis and non-anion gap metabolic acidosis

Diagnosis of hidden mixed acid-base disturbances. Schematic illustrating how one can diagnose hidden mixed acid-base disturbances by comparing the change in anion gap to the change in bicarbonate concentration. If the change in anion gap is much larger than the fall in bicarbonate concentration this implies the coexistence of anion gap metabolic acidosis and metabolic alkalosis (left panel). If the change in anion gap is much smaller than the change in the bicarbonate concentration then this implies the presence of an anion gap and non-anion gap metabolic acidosis (right panel).

Table 9.3

Syndromes Commonly Associated with Mixed Acid-Base Disorders

Hemodynamic compromise
Cardiopulmonary arrest
Pulmonary edema
Sepsis
Liver failure
Poisonings
Ethylene glycol intoxication
Methanol intoxication
Aspirin intoxication
Ethanol intoxication
Metabolic disturbances
Severe hypokalemia
Severe hypophosphatemia
Diabetic ketoacidosis
Bowel ischemia
COPD
Renal failure

Abbreviation: COPD, chronic obstructive pulmonary disease.

impair cardiac contractile function and/or vascular tone. Conversely, respiratory alkalosis in combination with metabolic alkalosis (e.g., patient with pulmonary edema treated with potassium wasting diuretics) could develop elevations in pH sufficient to cause seizures and/or cardiac arrhythmias. When these extreme conditions occur, correct therapy is directed at pH control through the control of ventilation. Once the pH is adjusted to one that is not life threatening, the metabolic disturbance(s) are addressed. We reiterate that treatment of the acid-base disorder always involves making the correct clinical diagnosis of the underlying causes and appropriate specific therapy directed at those causes.

KEY POINTS

Mixed Acid-Base Disorders

1. Mixed acid-base disorders may result from the coexistence of primary respiratory and metabolic disorders, the coexistence of metabolic alkalosis with anion gap metabolic acidosis, and/or the coexistence of non-anion gap metabolic acidosis with anion gap metabolic acidosis.

2. To evaluate compensation, one applies the following rules:

   Metabolic acidosis: compensatory change in $PaCO_2$ (mmHg) = 1–1.5 × the fall in $[HCO_3^-]$ (meq/L) or the $PaCO_2$ (mmHg) = 1.5 × $[HCO_3^-]$ + 8 ± 2.

   Metabolic alkalosis: compensatory change in $PaCO_2$ (mmHg) = 0.6–1 × the increase in $[HCO_3^-]$ (meq/L).

   Acute respiratory acidosis or alkalosis: compensatory change in $[HCO_3^-]$ (meq/L) = 0.1 × the change in $PaCO_2$ (mmHg) ± 2 (meq/L).

   Chronic respiratory acidosis or alkalosis: compensatory change in $[HCO_3^-]$ (meq/L) = 0.4 × the change in $PaCO_2$ (mmHg) ± 3 (meq/L).

   Failure to achieve the appropriate degree of compensation implies a second primary disorder.

3. The most dangerous mixed disturbances occur when both metabolic and respiratory alkalosis or metabolic and respiratory acidosis coexist.

4. Stoichiometric equivalence between the change in anion gap and the reduction in [HCO₃⁻] is assumed with anion gap metabolic acidosis. A marked discrepancy between these measurements implies the coexistence of either anion gap metabolic acidosis and metabolic alkalosis or anion gap metabolic acidosis and non-anion gap metabolic acidosis.

5. Triple acid-base disorders are diagnosed when both respiratory and metabolic disturbances are present and either anion gap metabolic acidosis and metabolic alkalosis or anion gap metabolic acidosis and non-anion gap metabolic acidosis coexist.

Adrogue, H.J., Madias, N.E. Management of life-threatening acid-base disorders. Second of two parts. *N Engl J Med* 338:107–111, 1998b.

Constable, P.D. Clinical assessment of acid-base status. Strong ion difference theory. *Vet Clin North Am Food Anim Pract* 15:447–471, 1999.

Epstein, S.K., Singh, N. Respiratory acidosis. *Respir Care* 46:366–383, 2001.

Filley, G.F. *Acid-Base and Blood Gas Regulation.* 1st edition. Lea & Febiger, Philadelphia, PA, 1971.

Kreit, J.W., Eschenbacher, W.L. The physiology of spontaneous and mechanical ventilation. *Clin Chest Med* 9:11–21, 1988.

Mellins, R.B., Haddad, G.G. Respiratory control in early life: an overview. *Prog Clin Biol Res* 136:3–15, 1983.

Orr, W.C. Sleep and breathing: an overview. *Ear Nose Throat J* 63:191–198, 1984.

Stewart, P.A. *How to Understand Acid-Base. A Quantitative Primer for Biology and Medicine.* 1st edition. Elsevier, New York, NY, 1981.

Additional Reading

Adrogue, H.J., Madias, N.E. Management of life-threatening acid-base disorders. First of two parts. *N Engl J Med* 338:26–34, 1998a.

Robert F. Reilly, Jr.

Disorders of Serum Calcium

Recommended Time to Complete: 1 day

Guiding Questions

1. How is extracellular fluid (ECF) ionized calcium regulated?
2. What roles do parathyroid hormone (PTH) and $1,25(OH)_2$ vitamin D_3 (calcitriol) play in this process?
3. What three pathophysiologic processes are involved in hypercalcemia?
4. Which two diseases make up the majority of cases of hypercalcemia and how do their presentations differ?
5. Can you devise a rational treatment plan for the hypercalcemic patient?
6. Why does the hypomagnesemic patient develop hypocalcemia?
7. How does one approach the patient with hypocalcemia?
8. What are the keys to successfully treating hypocalcemia?

Regulation of ECF Ionized Calcium

Despite the fact that only a small percentage of calcium contained in the body resides in ECF, it is ECF ionized calcium that is physiologically regulated. It is regulated by the combined interaction between PTH, the calcium-sensing receptor and calcitriol in the parathyroid gland, bone, intestine, and kidney. Sixty percent of ECF calcium is ultra-filterable and is either ionized and thereby free in solution (50%) or complexed to anions (10%). The other 40% is bound to proteins (mainly albumin). The vast majority of total body calcium exists as hydroxyapatite in bone (99%). The bone calcium reservoir is so large that one cannot become

hypocalcemic without a decrease in bone calcium release due to a defect in either PTH or calcitriol action.

Figure 10.1 illustrates average daily calcium fluxes between ECF and the organ systems involved in its regulation (bone, intestine, and kidney). The average adult takes in 1000 mg and absorbs about 20% in intestine. In the steady state, intestinal absorption is matched by urinary excretion. The kidney excretes approximately 2% (200 mg) of the filtered calcium load.

Another important regulator of calcium homeostasis is the calcium-sensing receptor. The calcium-sensing receptor is expressed in the cell membrane of the parathyroid gland. It is also expressed on the surface of cells in kidney, intestine, lung, and a variety of other organs. In parathyroid gland it couples changes in ECF calcium concentration to the regulation of PTH secretion

Figure 10.1

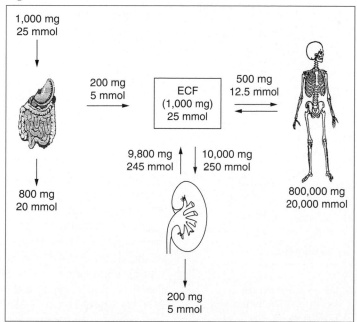

Calcium homeostasis. Daily calcium fluxes between ECF, intestine, kidney, and bone are shown. In the steady state net intestinal absorption and renal excretion of calcium are equal. The majority of calcium in the body is in bone. (With permission from Schrier, R.W. (ed.). *Manual of Nephrology.* Lippincott Williams & Wilkins, Philadelphia, PA, 2000.)

via a complex signaling pathway mediated by phospholipase C and phospholipase A_2. High calcium concentration activates the receptor and inhibits release of PTH. Low calcium concentration stimulates PTH secretion and production, as well as increases parathyroid gland mass. This system responds within minutes to changes in calcium concentration. The parathyroid gland does not contain a large supply of excess storage granules. Basal and stimulated secretion of PTH can only be supported for a few hours in the absence of new hormone synthesis. There is an inverse sigmoidal relationship between calcium concentration and PTH secretion (Figure 10.2). As can be seen in the figure, there is still some basal PTH secretion even at high calcium concentrations. This is important clinically in the patient with secondary hyperparathyroidism and end-stage renal disease. As parathyroid gland mass increases basal PTH secretion increases to the point where it can no longer be suppressed by high dose

Figure 10.2

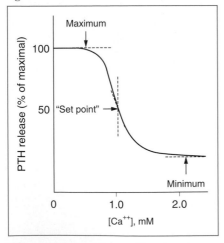

PTH-calcium response curve. There is an inverse sigmoidal relationship between ionized calcium concentration and release of PTH from the parathyroid gland. The set point is that ionized calcium concentration at which PTH release is inhibited by 50%. The minimum arrow illustrates that there is a basal level of PTH release even at high calcium concentrations.

calcitriol therapy and ultimately subtotal parathyroidectomy is required. Calcium-sensing receptor knockout mice demonstrate marked parathyroid hyperplasia suggesting that the receptor also plays a role in parathyroid cell growth and proliferation. The calcium-sensing receptor is expressed in kidney. In the thick ascending limb of Henle it is expressed in the basolateral membrane. Activation of the receptor here by elevated blood calcium concentration results in inhibition of apical sodium entry via the furosemide-sensitive Na-K-2Cl cotransporter. Inhibition of the apical membrane potassium channel by arachidonic acid-derived intermediates reduces the lumen-positive voltage that drives paracellular calcium transport in this segment and increases urinary calcium excretion. The ability of the kidney to concentrate urine is also impaired. In the inner medullary collecting duct the receptor is present in the apical membrane in the very same vesicles that contain water channels. Perfusion of the inner medullary collecting duct with a high calcium solution reduces vasopressin-stimulated water flow by about 40% presumably via activation of the receptor. This may provide a mechanism to inhibit calcium crystallization in states of hypercalciuria. The inhibition of water transport may aid in increasing the solubility of calcium salts.

PTH increases ECF calcium concentration via effects in bone, intestine, and kidney. In the presence of calcitriol, PTH stimulates bone resorption through an increase in osteoclast number and activity. In the intestine PTH acts indirectly through its stimulation of calcitriol formation to increase calcium and phosphorus absorption. Calcitriol increases expression of epithelial calcium channels in the intestine. In the kidney, PTH increases calcium reabsorption in the distal convoluted tubule and connecting tubule, stimulates activity of 1-α-hydroxylase in the proximal convoluted tubule that converts 25(OH) vitamin D_3 to 1,25(OH)$_2$ vitamin D_3, and reduces proximal tubular reabsorption of phosphate and bicarbonate. The end result is an increase in ECF calcium concentration without an increase in phosphorus concentration.

The final step in calcitriol formation is the 1-α-hydroxylation of 25(OH) vitamin D_3 (calcidiol) in proximal tubule. The biosynthetic pathway for calcitriol is shown in Figure 10.3. 7-Dehydrocholesterol in skin is converted to vitamin D_3 by UV light. Vitamin D_3 is then 25 hydroxylated in the liver. This step is poorly regulated and in general 25(OH) vitamin D_3 concentration parallels vitamin D intake. Finally, 1-α-hydroxylation takes place in the inner mitochondrial membrane of proximal tubular cells. Increasing PTH concentration and hypophosphatemia enhance 1-α-hydroxylase activity.

Calcitriol stimulates its own catabolism via activation of 24 hydroxylase. Twenty-four hydroxylase is the major catabolic enzyme in calcitriol target tissues. It is upregulated by calcitriol, hypercalcemia, and hyperphosphatemia.

Calcitriol increases calcium and phosphorus availability for bone formation and prevents hypocalcemia and hypophosphatemia. In intestine and kidney, calcitriol plays an important role in increasing calcium transport via the stimulation of expression of calcium-binding proteins (calbindins). Calbindins bind calcium and move it

Figure 10.3

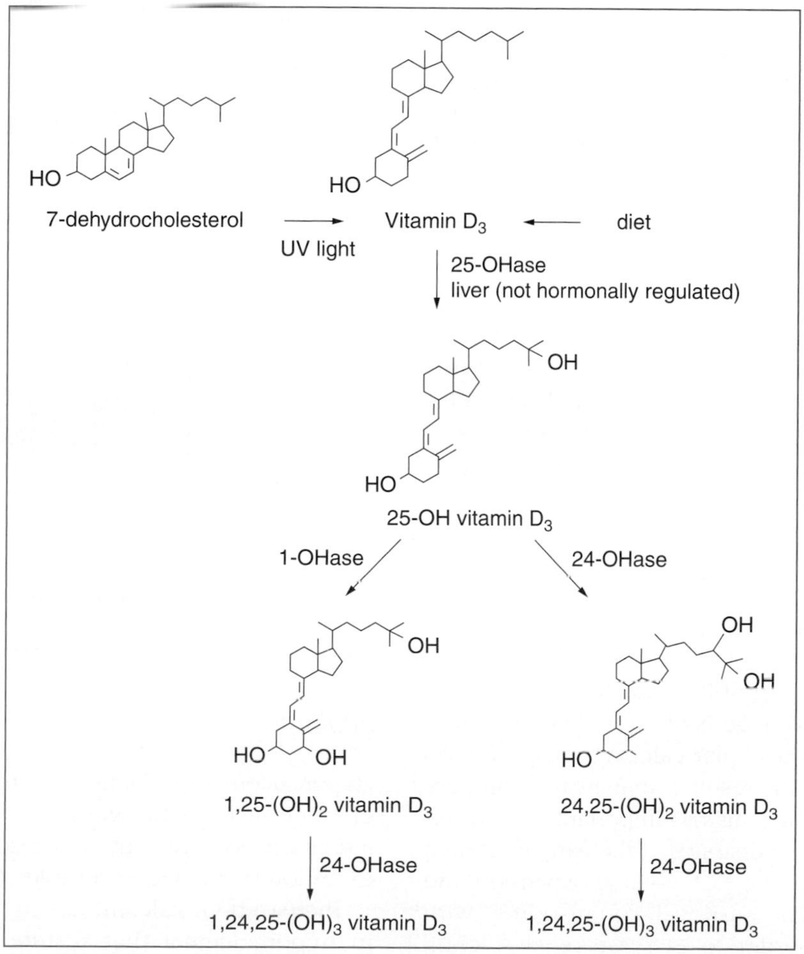

Vitamin D metabolism. The metabolic pathway is illustrated.

from the apical to the basolateral membrane, thereby allowing calcium to move through the cell without an increase in free intracellular calcium. Calcitriol increases expression of the sodium phosphate cotransporter in intestine. In bone, calcitriol has a variety of effects: (1) potentiation of PTH effects; (2) stimulation of osteoclastic reabsorption; and (3) induction of monocyte differentiation into osteoclasts. In parathyroid gland, calcitriol binds its receptor in the cytoplasm and forms a heterodimer with the retinoid X receptor and is translocated to the nucleus. The complex binds to the PTH gene promoter and decreases PTH expression, as well as inhibits parathyroid growth.

Renal calcium excretion plays an important role in calcium homeostasis. Calcium that is not bound to albumin is freely filtered at the glomerulus. The proximal tubule reabsorbs 2/3 of the filtered load. The majority of reabsorption is passive but there is a small active component. Calcium transport in the proximal tubule parallels that of sodium and water. Therefore, calcium reabsorption proximally varies directly with ECF volume. The more expanded the ECF volume, the higher calcium excretion. Calcium excretion is decreased in the setting of volume contraction. The thick ascending limb of Henle reabsorbs 25% of the filtered load. Calcium transport in this segment is passive, paracellular, and dependent on the magnitude of the lumen-positive transepithelial voltage. The lumen-positive voltage is a result of potassium exit across the apical membrane via a potassium channel. Potassium reenters the cell across the apical membrane on the furosemide-sensitive Na-K-2Cl cotransporter. If the Na-K-2Cl cotransporter is inhibited by furosemide, the lumen-positive voltage is dissipated and the driving force for paracellular calcium transport is no longer present. The result is an increase in urinary calcium excretion. This has important clinical relevance in that cornerstones of the early treatment of hypercalcemia are ECF volume expansion and inhibition of the Na-K-2Cl cotransporter with furosemide in order to increase renal calcium excretion. The distal tubule (distal convoluted

tubule and connecting tubule) reabsorbs 10% of the filtered calcium load. This segment is the major regulatory site of calcium excretion under PTH control. Calcium transport is entirely active in this segment. Transport is stimulated by PTH, alkalosis and thiazide diuretics and inhibited by acidosis and hypophosphatemia.

KEY POINTS
Regulation of ECF Ionized Calcium

1. PTH and calcitriol regulate extracellular fluid ionized calcium concentration.
2. Calcium concentration is sensed by the calcium-sensing receptor, which plays an important role in regulating PTH secretion.
3. PTH increases calcium concentration via actions in bone, intestine, and kidney.
4. PTH and hypophosphatemia enhance 1-α hydroxylase activity in the proximal tubule leading to calcitriol formation.
5. Calcitriol increases availability of calcium and phosphorus for bone formation and prevents hypocalcemia and hypophosphatemia.
6. Calcitriol is the most potent suppressor of PTH gene transcription.

Hypercalcemia

Etiology

Hypercalcemia results from increased absorption of calcium from the gastrointestinal (GI) tract, increased bone resorption, or decreased calcium excretion by the kidney (Table 10.1).

Increased GI calcium absorption is important in hypercalcemia that results from the milk-alkali syndrome, vitamin D intoxication, and

Table 10.1

Etiologies of Hypercalcemia

Increased bone resorption
Hyperparathyroidism (primary and secondary)
Malignancy
Thyrotoxicosis
Immobilization
Paget's disease
Addison's disease
Lithium
Vitamin A intoxication
Familial hypocalciuric hypercalcemia
Increased GI absorption
Increased calcium intake
    Milk-alkali syndrome
    Renal failure (calcium and vitamin D
      supplements)
Increased vitamin D concentration
    Vitamin D intoxication
    Granulomatous disease
Decreased renal excretion
Thiazide diuretics

Abbreviation: GI, gastrointestinal.

granulomatous diseases. Milk-alkali syndrome results from excessive intake of calcium and bicarbonate or its equivalent. In addition, alkalosis stimulates calcium reabsorption in the distal tubule of the kidney. Suppression of PTH secretion by hypercalcemia further increases proximal tubular bicarbonate reabsorption. The most common cause of the milk-alkali syndrome in the past was milk and sodium bicarbonate ingestion for therapy of peptic ulcer disease. Today the most common clinical setting is an elderly woman treated with calcium carbonate and vitamin D for osteoporosis. Bulemics taking supplemental calcium or a high calcium diet are also at high risk. The classic triad of milk-alkali syndrome is hypercalcemia, metabolic alkalosis, and elevated serum blood urea nitrogen (BUN) and creatinine concentrations. Treatment of these patients is often complicated by rebound hypocalcemia as a result

of sustained PTH suppression from hypercalcemia. PTH concentrations in these patients are often very low.

Hypercalcemia from increased calcium ingestion alone rarely occurs in the absence of decreases in kidney function or supplementation with vitamin D. Vitamin D intoxication also causes hypercalcemia. Calcitriol stimulates calcium absorption in the small intestine; however, bone release of calcium may also play an important role in these patients. A recent outbreak was reported as the result of over fortification of milk from a home delivery dairy. Other milk-associated outbreaks have resulted from the inadvertent addition of calcitriol to milk. Increased GI calcium absorption and hypercalcemia occur with granulomatous disorders, such as sarcoidosis, mycobacterium tuberculosis, and mycobacterium avium in patients with human immunodeficiency virus (HIV) infection. Macrophages express 1-α-hydroxylase when stimulated and convert calcidiol to calcitriol. Hypercalcemia may be the initial manifestation of extrapulmonary sarcoid. This more commonly results in hypercalciuria than hypercalcemia. Lymphomas can produce hypercalcemia via the same mechanism. The source of calcitriol with lymphomas may be from macrophages adjacent to the tumor and not the malignant cells themselves. Lymphomas may also cause hypercalcemia via cytokine-induced activation of osteoclasts and osteolysis.

Increased bone calcium resorption is the most common pathophysiologic mechanism leading to hypercalcemia. This plays a primary role in the hypercalcemia of hyperparathyroidism, malignancy, hyperthyroidism, immobilization, and Paget's disease. The two most common causes of hypercalcemia are primary hyperparathyroidism and malignancy.

Primary hyperparathyroidism occurs in as many as 1 per 10,000 people in the general population. The pathologic lesion in 80–90% is a solitary adenoma. Of the remaining, as many as 10–20% have diffuse hyperplasia and some of these have the inherited familial syndrome multiple endocrine neoplasia (MEN). MEN type I is associated with pituitary adenomas and islet cell tumors. It has an estimated prevalence of 1 per 50,000. Primary hyperparathyroidism is the initial manifestation occurring in general by age 40–50. The mutation resides in the menin gene. Menin is a tumor suppressor expressed in the nucleus that binds to JunD. Menin mutations occur in approximately 15% of sporadic adenomas. MEN type II is associated with medullary carcinoma of the thyroid and pheochromocytoma. It is subdivided into MEN IIa that is associated with parathyroid hyperplasia and type IIb that is not. MEN type II is caused by mutations in the RET protooncogene that is a tyrosine kinase. In developing tissues including neural crest, kidney, and ureter RET is a receptor for growth and differentiation. Multiple adenomas can occur and parathyroid carcinoma is very rare (<1%).

Hypercalcemia in hyperparathyroidism is the combined result of increased bone calcium resorption, increased calcium absorption from intestine, and increased calcium reabsorption in kidney. In primary hyperparathyroidism hypercalcemia is mild (less than 11.0 mg/dL), and often identified on routine laboratory testing in the asymptomatic patient. Patients present most commonly between the ages of 40 and 60 and women are affected two to three times more often than men. The majority of patients are postmenopausal women.

Secondary hyperparathyroidism may cause hypercalcemia in two clinical settings. In the renal transplant patient although renal function improves, PTH concentration is still elevated as a result of increased parathyroid gland mass. Hypercalcemia generally does not persist more than a year. In the patient with end-stage renal disease and secondary hyperparathyroidism, hypercalcemia can occur with calcium and/or vitamin D supplementation. This occurs primarily in patients with low turnover bone disease (adynamic bone disease).

Malignancy results in hypercalcemia from production of parathyroid hormone-related peptide (PTHrP), local bone resorption in areas of metastasis (cytokine mediated), or calcitriol production (lymphomas). Breast cancer, squamous cell lung cancer, multiple myeloma, and renal cell carcinoma are the most common malignancies associated with hypercalcemia. Hypercalcemia secondary to PTHrP is known as humoral hypercalcemia of malignancy (HHM). A large variety of tumors can produce PTHrP. A partial list includes squamous cell cancers of the head, neck and lung, breast cancer, pancreatic cancer, transitional cell carcinomas, and germ cell tumors. The first 13 amino acids of PTHrP are highly homologous to PTH, and as a result PTHrP binds to the PTH receptor and has similar biologic activity to PTH. PTHrP may be the fetal PTH. PTH is not secreted by the parathyroid gland in utero and does not cross the placenta. Humoral hypercalcemia of malignancy typically presents with severe hypercalcemia (serum calcium concentration >14 mg/dL). At the time of initial presentation the cancer is usually easily identified. An assay for PTHrP is commercially available. PTHrP is immunologically distinct from PTH and as a result is not detected by PTH assays. In patients with HHM PTH concentration will be low. Humor hypercalcemia of malignancy carries a poor prognosis with a median survival of only 3 months. Hypercalcemia from primary hyperparathyroidism and malignancy can be seen in the same patient. Patients with malignancy were reported to have an increased incidence of primary hyperparathyroidism.

Osteolytic metastases produce a variety of cytokines resulting in calcium release from bone. Tumor necrosis factor (TNF) and interleukin-1 (IL-1) stimulate the differentiation of osteoclast precursors into osteoclasts. IL-6 stimulates osteoclast production.

Approximately one-third of patients with multiple myeloma will develop hypercalcemia. Multiple myeloma presents with anemia, hypercalcemia, and localized osteolytic lesions. Release of calcium from bone results from cytokine release (IL-6, IL-1, TNF-β, MIP-1 alpha and MIP-1 beta). Myeloma cells also disturb the ratio of osteoprotegerin and its ligand NF-kappa B ligand (RANKL), which play a critical role in bone remodeling and the regulation of osteoclast to osteoblast activity. By decreasing expression and increasing degradation of osteoprotegerin and increasing RANKL expression in their local environment myeloma cells tip the balance in favor of bone resorption. Lytic bone lesions are characterized by increased osteoclast resorption without new bone formation. This is in contradistinction to bone metastases with breast and prostate cancer where areas of lysis are surrounded by new bone formation. As a result radionuclide bone scans will show uptake at sites of metastasis and not at sites of bone involvement with multiple myeloma.

Increased bone turnover and mild hypercalcemia occur in 5–10% of patients with hyperthyroidism. Hyperthyroid patients may also have an increased incidence of parathyroid adenomas. Immobilization and Paget's disease can cause hypercalcemia; however, this is more common in children. Hypercalciuria is the more common abnormality in adults.

Lithium administration may cause mild hypercalcemia that results from interference with calcium sensing by the calcium-sensing receptor. The calcium-sensing receptor also binds lithium, which acts as an antagonist. Hypercalcemia is generally mild, clinically insignificant, and resolves with discontinuation of the drug. In some cases it persists and may be associated with clinical signs and symptoms. Pheochromocytoma, primary adrenal insufficiency, and the inherited disorder familial hypocalciuric hypercalcemia (FHH) are additional rare causes of hypercalcemia. Pheochromocytoma may produce hypercalcemia via its association with MEN 2a or by the production of PTHrP. Catecholamines are also known to increase bone resorption. Familial hypocalciuric hypercalcemia is inherited in an autosomal dominant fashion. The mutation occurs in the calcium-sensing receptor and results in a receptor that has a decreased affinity for calcium. As a result elevated calcium concentrations are required to suppress PTH. It presents with mild hypercalcemia at a young age, decreased urinary calcium excretion, and a high normal or slightly elevated PTH concentration. Notably signs or symptoms of hypercalcemia are often absent. Familial hypocalciuric hypercalcemia is important because it can be misdiagnosed as primary hyperparathyroidism

and result in unnecessary parathyroid surgery. Patients with FHH often do not have clinical sequelae of excessive PTH activity such as hyperparathyroid bone disease or mental status changes. The presence of hypercalcemia in family members, a lack of previously normal serum calcium measurements, and low urinary calcium suggest familial hypocalciuric hypercalcemia. Some authors advocate using the fractional excretion (FE) of calcium to distinguish FHH from primary hyperparathyroidism with values below 1% suggestive of FHH. This is not recommended, however, given that 25% of patients with primary hyperparathyroidism have a fractional excretion of calcium below 1%.

Increased renal calcium reabsorption contributes to the hypercalcemia of primary hyperparathyroidism and malignancy. Thiazide diuretics cause hypercalcemia due to increased distal tubular calcium reabsorption. Most reported cases, however, have also had associated parathyroid adenomas.

KEY POINTS
Etiology of Hypercalcemia

1. Hypercalcemia results from increased GI calcium absorption, increased bone release of calcium, and/or decreased renal calcium excretion.
2. Of the three pathophysiologic mechanisms increased bone resorption is most common and important.
3. Hypercalcemia from increased GI calcium absorption rarely occurs in the absence of decreased renal function.
4. The most common causes of increased bone calcium release are primary hyperparathyroidism and malignancy.

Signs and Symptoms

As is the case for many electrolyte disorders the severity and rate of rise of the serum calcium concentration determine the extent of clinical signs and symptoms. Patients with primary hyperparathyroidism present with mild asymptomatic hypercalcemia incidentally discovered on routine laboratory examination.

Severe hypercalcemia is associated with prominent neurologic and GI symptoms. Central nervous system symptoms range from confusion to stupor and coma. Seizures can occur as a result of severe vasoconstriction and transient high intensity signals have been documented by magnetic resonance imaging (MRI) that resolve with return of serum calcium concentration to the normal range. Focal neurologic symptoms mimicking a transient ischemic attack although rare were described. Gastrointestinal symptoms are related primarily to decreased gastrointestinal motility that results in nausea, vomiting, constipation, and obstipation. Hypercalcemia-induced pancreatitis can cause epigastric pain. As will be discussed, hypercalcemia decreases expression of renal water channels resulting in polyuria that leads to ECF volume depletion, decreased renal blood flow, and decreased renal function. Hypercalcemia predisposes to digitalis toxicity.

KEY POINTS
Signs and Symptoms of Hypercalcemia

1. Hypercalcemia presents with a wide range of neurologic and GI symptoms.
2. Acute renal failure secondary to prerenal azotemia is commonly associated with hypercalcemia.

Diagnosis

Primary hyperparathyroidism and malignancy are by far the most frequent causes of hypercalcemia making up more than 90% of all cases. Initial evaluation of the hypercalcemic patient includes a careful history and physical examination. Of patients with primary hyperparathyroidism about 20% have signs and symptoms of disease such as kidney stones, neuromuscular weakness, decreased ability to concentrate, depression, or bone disease. One should inquire carefully about use of calcium supplements, antacids, and vitamin preparations. A recent chest radiograph is essential to exclude lung cancers and granulomatous diseases. In patients with primary hyperparathyroidism skeletal radiographs are rarely positive in the present era. Bone densitometry, however, is commonly abnormal. Since primary hyperparathyroidism involves cortical more than cancellous bone, bone density is reduced to the greatest degree in the distal radius. Areas where cancellous bone predominates such as the spine and hip show less of a decrease.

Initial laboratory studies include serum electrolytes, BUN, creatinine, phosphorus, serum and urine protein electrophoresis, and a 24-hour urine collection for calcium and creatinine. A ratio of serum chloride to serum phosphorus concentrations of greater than 33:1 is suggestive of primary hyperparathyroidism. This results from decreased proximal tubular phosphate reabsorption induced by PTH. Laboratory hallmarks of milk-alkali syndrome are a low serum chloride, high serum bicarbonate, and elevated serum BUN and creatinine concentrations. A monoclonal gammopathy on serum or urine protein electrophoresis suggests multiple myeloma. If the diagnosis of multiple myeloma is suspected on clinical grounds, it is important to perform immunofixation electrophoresis (IFE) on both blood and a 24-hour urine sample in order to exclude the diagnosis. In primary hyperparathyroidism and HHM serum phosphorus concentration is often low. In hypercalcemia resulting from milk-alkali syndrome, thiazide diuretics, and FHH 24-hour urinary calcium excretion will be low.

Primary hyperparathyroidism is generally the cause in asymptomatic outpatients with a serum calcium concentration below 11 mg/dL. Malignancy is the most common cause in symptomatic patients with serum calcium concentration above 14 mg/dL. Factors favoring the diagnosis of primary hyperparathyroidism include a prolonged history, development in a postmenopausal woman, a normal physical examination, and evidence of MEN.

After initial evaluation, an intact PTH concentration is obtained. Primary hyperparathyroidism is the most common cause of an elevated PTH. PTH concentration is generally 1.5–2.0 times the upper limit of normal. Some patients may have mildly elevated serum calcium concentration with a PTH concentration that is in the upper range of normal (inappropriately elevated). Others may have a serum calcium concentration in the upper quartile of the normal range and a slightly elevated PTH concentration. Both of these subgroups of patients were demonstrated to have parathyroid adenomas. An elevated PTH concentration may also be seen rarely with lithium and FHH. If the patient is on lithium and it can be safely discontinued PTH concentration should be remeasured in 1–3 months. In all other etiologies of hypercalcemia, PTH is suppressed. PTHrP is immunologically distinct from PTH and specific assays are commercially available. C-terminal fragment PTHrP assays may be increased in pregnancy and in patients with kidney disease.

If malignancy is not obvious and PTH concentration is suppressed, one needs to rule out vitamin D intoxication or granulomatous diseases by measuring calcidiol and calcitriol concentrations. Ingestion of vitamin D or calcidiol will result in an increased calcidiol concentration and often mild to moderately elevated calcitriol concentration. Elevated calcitriol concentrations are observed with ingestion of calcitriol and in those diseases where stimulation of 1-α-hydroxylase occurs including granulomatous diseases, lymphoma, and primary hyperparathyroidism. If hyperthyroidism is suspected, thyroid function tests are obtained.

KEY POINTS
Diagnosis of Hypercalcemia

1. Primary hyperparathyroidism and malignancy comprise 90% of all cases of hypercalcemia.
2. Primary hyperparathyroidism is most often secondary to a parathyroid adenoma.

Hypercalcemia is mild, asymptomatic, and detected on routine laboratory testing.
3. Hypercalcemia of malignancy is severe, symptomatic, and carries a poor prognosis. It is commonly caused by production of PTHrP, a peptide similar but not identical to PTH.
4. After a careful history, physical, and initial laboratory evaluation patients are further characterized based on PTH and PTHrP concentrations.

Treatment

Treatment of hypercalcemia will depend on the degree of elevation of serum calcium concentration and is directed at increasing renal excretion, blocking bone resorption, and reducing intestinal absorption.

The first step to enhance renal calcium excretion is expansion of the ECF volume; subsequently, loop diuretics are added with the goal of maintaining urine flow rate at 200–250 mL/hour. The hypercalcemic patient is invariably volume contracted. Hypercalcemia causes arteriolar vasoconstriction and reduces renal blood flow. Calcium acts directly in the thick ascending limb of Henle to decrease sodium reabsorption and reduce the driving force for calcium reabsorption. Hypercalcemia also antagonizes the effects of antidiuretic hormone in collecting duct. The subsequent volume contraction that results increases proximal sodium and calcium reabsorption and further increases serum calcium concentration. With chronic kidney disease higher doses of loop diuretics are needed. If glomerular filtration rate (GFR) is low and hypercalcemia severe ($\geq$17 mg/dL), hemodialysis may be indicated. Hemodialysis is also helpful in patients with neurologic impairment or in those with concomitant congestive heart failure. Volume expansion and loop diuretics alone may be sufficient in the patient with mild-to-moderate hypercalcemia ($\leq$12.5 mg/dL).

When hypercalcemia is moderate or severe bone calcium resorption must be inhibited. In the short term, calcitonin is used because of its rapid onset (within a few hours). The usual dose is 4 IU/kg subcutaneously every 12 hours. It not only inhibits bone resorption but also increases calcium excretion by the kidney. Its effect, however, is not large and serum calcium concentration is reduced by only 1–2 mg/dL. Another downside is tachyphylaxis that develops with repeated use. Therefore, another agent that decreases bone resorption in addition to calcitonin should be used.

Bisphosphonates are the drug of choice to inhibit bone resorption. Their effects are additive to calcitonin. Bisphosphonates are concentrated in bone where they interfere with osteoclast formation, recruitment, activation, and function. Bisphosphonates have a long duration of action (weeks) but their disadvantage is that they have a slow onset (48–72 hours). Pamidronate is currently the most commonly used bisphosphonate to treat hypercalcemia. Sixty or ninety mg is given intravenously over 4 hours. The dose varies depending on the degree of hypercalcemia (60 mg when calcium concentration <13.5 mg/dL, 90 mg when calcium concentration >13.5 mg/dL). Serum calcium concentration slowly falls over days. A single dose lasts 7–14 days. In general serum calcium concentration will normalize within 7 days. Pamidronate use is not recommended in those with severe decreases in GFR. Renal toxicities of bisphosphonates include focal sclerosis with pamidronate and acute renal failure with zolendronate and pamidronate.

Mithramycin cannot be used in patients with severe liver, kidney, or bone marrow disease. Its onset of action is 12 hours with a peak effect at 48 hours. Due to its severe side-effect profile (hepatotoxicity, proteinuria, thrombocytopenia, and GI upset) mithramycin is rarely used. The dose is 25 μg/kg intravenously over 4 hours daily for 3–4 days. In one study hepatotoxicity was noted in 26% of patients, nausea and vomiting in 23%, as well as bleeding tendencies due to abnormalities in several coagulation factors and platelet dysfunction.

Gallium nitrate also inhibits bone resorption. Gallium accumulates in metabolically active regions of bone. It reduces bone resorption by inhibiting the H^+ ATPase in the ruffled membrane of osteoclasts and blocking osteoclast acid secretion. It has been used to treat hypercalcemia of malignancy. One hundred to two hundred mg/m^2 is given as a continuous infusion for 5 consecutive days. Gallium nitrate is contraindicated if the serum creatinine concentration is above 2.5 mg/dL. It is rarely used.

Agents that decrease intestinal calcium absorption are generally reserved for outpatients with mild hypercalcemia. Corticosteroids were used successfully in patients with vitamin D overdose, granulomatous diseases, and some cancers (lymphomas and multiple myeloma). Ketoconazole and hydroxychloroquine were also employed. Ketoconazole reduces calcitriol concentration by approximately 75% via inhibition of 1-α-hydroxylase. Hydroxychloroquine was used in patients with hypercalcemia and sarcoidosis and works via a similar mechanism. Oral phosphorus can be tried, but is contraindicated in patients with an elevated serum phosphorus concentration or renal dysfunction. Oral phosphorus is often poorly tolerated (diarrhea) and reduces serum calcium concentration only slightly (1 mg/dL).

Finally, whether to surgically remove a solitary parathyroid adenoma remains controversial. Suggested surgical criteria include serum calcium concentration more than 1 mg/dL above the upper limit of normal, an episode of acute symptomatic hypercalcemia, overt bone disease, cortical bone mineral density more than 2 standard deviations below age, sex, and race adjusted means, reduced renal function (more than 30%), a history of nephrolithiasis or nephrocalcinosis, urinary calcium excretion that exceeds 400 mg/day, or young age (<50 years). At least half of affected patients will meet these criteria. In approximately 75% of patients who do not elect surgery, average serum calcium and PTH concentrations generally do not change. In the remaining 25%, however, signs and symptoms worsen with increasing hypercalcemia, hypercalciuria, and decreasing bone mineral density. Patients below the age of 50 and those with nephrolithiasis are at higher risk of progression. If surgery is not performed it is recommended that serum calcium concentration be monitored every 6 months and serum creatinine concentration and bone mineral density measured yearly.

As minimally invasive parathyroid surgery becomes more accepted these criteria will be broadened. With minimally invasive surgery adenomas are first localized with a sestamibi scan and/or ultrasound preoperatively and parathyroidectomy is performed under local anesthesia. PTH assays are performed in the operating room. Given PTH's short half life (4 minutes), after the adenoma is removed PTH concentration is measured within minutes to verify that surgery was successful. If PTH concentration does not decline, the patient is placed under general anesthesia and more extensive neck exploration is performed looking for a second adenoma. Up to 5% of patients may have a previously undetected second adenoma. In patients whose surgery is successful the rate of kidney stone formation declines. Over the next several years bone density often increases in hip and back but not in the distal third of the radius. Patients treated medically with bisphosphonates can have some increase in vertebral bone density but serum PTH concentrations remain elevated. Calcium-sensing receptor agonists can normalize serum calcium concentration but in studies of up to 3 years duration bone density does not increase.

KEY POINTS
Treatment of Hypercalcemia

1. Initial therapy of hypercalcemia is directed at ECF volume expansion.
2. After ECF volume is expanded a loop diuretic is added to increase renal calcium excretion.
3. If hypercalcemia is moderate-to-severe additional measures are required. Drugs that reduce calcium release from bone are added. The drug of choice in the short term is calcitonin and in the long term is the bisphosphonate pamidronate.
4. In special circumstances mithramycin, gallium nitrate, or hemodialysis may be required.

Hypocalcemia

Pathophysiologic Mechanisms

Hypocalcemia results from decreased intestinal calcium absorption or decreased bone resorption. Since there is a large reservoir of calcium in bone, sustained hypocalcemia can only occur if there is an abnormality of PTH or calcitriol effect in bone.

Total serum calcium is comprised of three components: an ionized or free fraction; calcium complexed with anions; and bound to proteins. True hypocalcemia results only when the ionized calcium fraction is decreased (about half of total serum calcium concentration). Normal range for ionized calcium concentration is 4.2–5.0 mg/dL or 1.05–1.25 mmol/L. The first step in evaluation of a low total serum calcium concentration is to attempt to determine whether the ionized fraction is reduced. One way to address this question is to compare the total serum calcium concentration to the serum albumin concentration. As a general rule of thumb for every 1 g/dL decrease in serum albumin concentration from its normal value (4 g/dL), one can expect a 0.8 mg/dL decrement in total serum calcium concentration. For every 1 g/dL fall in serum albumin concentration, 0.8 mg/dL must be added to the total serum calcium concentration to correct it for the degree of hypoalbuminemia. Prediction of ionized calcium from albumin-corrected total calcium concentration should be done with caution. This correction may be unreliable in certain patient populations such as the critically ill trauma patient.

Calcium binding to albumin is also affected by pH. As pH decreases, ionized calcium will increase and vice versa. This effect is fairly minor and ionized serum calcium concentration will only increase 0.2 mg/dL for each 0.1 decrease in pH. If clinical suspicion of true hypocalcemia is high then ionized calcium concentration should be measured directly.

True hypocalcemia is the result of either decreased PTH secretion or vitamin D concentration or end-organ resistance. Less commonly, hypocalcemia results from either extravascular calcium deposition or intravascular calcium binding. Extravascular deposition occurs with pancreatitis, "hungry bone syndrome" postparathyroidectomy, or tumor lysis syndrome. Intravascular calcium binding was reported with foscarnet use (pyrophosphate analogue) and after massive transfusion (citrate) usually in the presence of hepatic or renal failure. The most common etiologies of true hypocalcemia grouped by their pathophysiologic mechanisms are illustrated in Table 10.2.

KEY POINTS
Pathophysiologic Mechanisms of Hypocalcemia

1. True hypocalcemia results from decreased GI calcium absorption, decreased bone resorption or, less commonly, acute shift of calcium out of ECF or calcium binding within the intravascular space.
2. Given the large reservoir of calcium in bone, sustained hypocalcemia cannot occur without an abnormality of PTH or calcitriol action in bone.
3. When interpreting total serum calcium concentration one needs to take into account the serum albumin concentration and systemic pH.

Table 10.2
Etiologies of Hypocalcemia

Decreased PTH action or effect
Hypomagnesemia
Decreased PTH secretion
Postsurgical
Polyglandular autoimmune syndrome (type I)
Familial hypocalcemia
Infiltrative disorders
End-organ resistance to PTH
Pseudohypoparathyroidism (type I and II)
Defects in vitamin D metabolism
Nutritional
Malabsorption
Drugs
Liver disease
Renal disease
Vitamin D-dependent rickets
Shift of calcium out of the ECF
Acute pancreatitis
Hungry bone syndrome
Tumor lysis syndrome
Miscellaneous
Osteoblastic metastases
Toxic shock syndrome
Sepsis
Pseudohypocalcemia

Abbreviations: PTH, parathyroid hormone; ECF, extracellular fluid.

Etiology

Hypoparathyroidism is caused by several acquired and inherited disorders resulting from decreased PTH synthesis or release, or resistance to PTH action. Polyglandular autoimmune syndrome type I is the most common cause of idiopathic hypoparathyroidism. Chronic mucocutaneous candidiasis and primary adrenal insufficiency are also part of the spectrum of this disease. Mucocutaneous candidiasis presents in early childhood and involves skin and mucous membranes without systemic spread. This is subsequently followed by hypoparathyroidism after several years. Adrenal insufficiency generally develops last with an onset in adolescence. Up to half of these patients have antibodies directed against the calcium-sensing receptor. Mutations in the AIRE gene (autoimmune regulator), which is a transcription factor, cause the disease. Affected patients are at risk for developing other autoimmune disorders including pernicious anemia, vitiligo, hypothyroidism, hepatitis, and type I diabetes mellitus.

Familial hypocalcemia is the result of autosomal dominant activating mutations in the calcium-sensing receptor resulting in a receptor that is more sensitive to ECF ionized calcium concentration. Two patients were described with autoantibodies that activate the calcium-sensing receptor. One patient had Graves's disease and the other Addison's disease. In a cell culture system these antibodies bound the receptor, activated second messenger systems, and suppressed PTH secretion. In patients with end-stage renal disease that undergo parathyroidectomy for secondary or tertiary hyperparathyroidism, remineralization of bone (hungry bone syndrome) may result in acute hypocalcemia. With surgical removal of a parathyroid adenoma, transient hypocalcemia may result due to suppression of normal gland function by the adenoma. Hypocalcemia can occur after thyroid surgery and may be either transient (11.9%) or permanent (0.9%). Patients undergoing central lymph node dissection for thyroid cancer are at high risk. Hypocalcemia or hypophosphatemia that persists for 1 week despite calcium replacement are risk factors for permanent hypoparathyroidism. Infiltrative disorders (hemochromatosis and Wilson's disease) and infection with HIV can cause hypoparathyroidism.

The most common etiology of decreased PTH secretion and/or effect is severe hypomagnesemia. Hypomagnesemia decreases PTH secretion, as well as results in end-organ resistance to PTH. End-organ resistance begins to occur at serum magnesium concentration ≤1.0 mg/dL. More severe hypomagnesemia (serum magnesium concentration ≤0.5 mg/dL) is required to decrease PTH secretion. Patients with hypocalcemia secondary to hypomagnesemia will not respond to calcium or vitamin D replacement until the magnesium deficit is replaced. It often takes several days after magnesium is corrected for serum calcium concentration to return to normal.

Rare genetic disorders can cause PTH end-organ resistance (pseudohypoparathyroidism types I and II). Pseudohypoparathyroidism is subdivided based on whether nephrogenous cyclic AMP (cAMP) increases in response to PTH administration (Ellsworth-Howard test). In type II there is a normal response and in type I there is a decreased response. In type I the mutation arises in the $Gs\alpha1$ protein of the adenylate cyclase complex. Parathyroid hormone binds to its receptor but cannot activate adenylate cyclase. The defect in type II is due to resistance to the intracellular effects of cyclic AMP and the mutation has yet to be identified. Some patients with type II disease will respond to theophylline.

Disorders of vitamin D metabolism are important causes of hypocalcemia. A wide variety of disorders can interfere with this complex pathway including decreased vitamin D intake, GI malabsorption, drugs, liver disease, renal disease, and vitamin D-dependent rickets. Despite the fact that milk is supplemented with vitamin D in the United States one study of noninstitutionalized adults showed that 9% had low 25(OH) vitamin D_3 concentration. Patients who are poorly nourished with little sunlight exposure, as well as the institutionalized elderly, are at particular risk. Postmenopausal women and adolescents are also at increased risk. Vitamin D deficiency may result from GI malabsorption given that vitamin D is a fat-soluble vitamin. Anticonvulsant drugs induce the cytochrome P450 system and increase metabolism of vitamin D. It is likely, however, that anticonvulsants cause hypocalcemia via a variety of other mechanisms as well, including direct inhibition of bone resorption, impaired GI calcium absorption, and resistance to PTH. Vitamin D deficiency results from severe parenchymal liver disease since one of the steps involves hydroxylation in the liver. Chronic kidney disease impairs 1-α-hydroxylation, the final step in the formation of calcitriol. Vitamin D-dependent rickets exists in two forms. Type I is caused by impaired 1-α-hydroxylation of calcidiol to calcitriol. Since end-organ response is intact type I patients respond to calcitriol. Type II disease is caused by inactivating mutations in the vitamin D receptor and results in end-organ resistance to calcitriol. Serum calcitriol concentration is elevated in these patients and they respond poorly to supplemental calcitriol.

Other causes of hypocalcemia include tumor lysis syndrome, hyperphosphatemia, acute pancreatitis, and sepsis. Ionized hypocalcemia is common in patients in the intensive care unit (ICU) occurring in up to one-third to two-thirds and many of these are septic. Hypocalcemia is an independent predictor of increased mortality in the ICU. The mechanism of hypocalcemia in sepsis is unknown. Postulated mechanisms include a decrease in PTH concentration, decreased calcitriol concentration, and peripheral resistance to PTH action.

Pseudohypocalcemia was reported after magnetic resonance angiography. Gadolinium, used as a contrast agent in the procedure, interferes with some assays used to measure serum calcium concentration. The effect is short lived but can result in very low spurious calcium determinations (decreases of 3 mg/dL or more). The patients, as expected, exhibit no symptoms.

KEY POINTS
Etiology of Hypocalcemia

1. Hypoparathyroidism results from decreased synthesis, release, or peripheral tissue resistance to PTH.
2. The most common cause of idiopathic hypoparathyroidism is polyglandular autoimmune syndrome type I. It manifests with hypoparathyroidism, adrenal insufficiency, and mucocutaneous candidiasis.

3. Severe hypomagnesemia is the most common cause of hypoparathyroidism.
4. Disorders of vitamin D metabolism such as nutritional deficiency, liver disease, anticonvulsant use, and chronic kidney disease are important causes of hypocalcemia.

Signs and Symptoms

The degree of hypocalcemia and rate of decline of the serum calcium concentration determine whether hypocalcemic symptoms occur. The point at which symptoms occur depends on multiple factors including pH, and whether other electrolyte abnormalities are present (hypomagnesemia and hypokalemia). Symptoms are primarily those of enhanced neuromuscular activation. Circumoral and distal extremity paresthesias are common complaints, as is carpopedal spasm. Altered mental status, irritability, and seizures may also occur. Hypotension, bradycardia, and laryngospasm may be present on physical examination. One should test for the presence of Chvostek's and Trousseau's sign. Chvostek's sign is brought out by gently tapping just below the zygomatic arch over the facial nerve with the mouth slightly open. A positive sign, which is a facial twitch, is occasionally observed in normal patients. To test for Trousseau's sign a blood pressure cuff is inflated to 20 mmHg above systolic pressure for 3 minutes. A positive sign is flexion of the wrist, metacarpophalyngeal joints, and thumb with hyperextension of the fingers.

KEY POINTS
Signs and Symptoms of Hypocalcemia

1. Signs and symptoms depend on the degree and rate of decline of serum calcium concentration.

2. The serum calcium concentration at which symptoms develop varies depending on the presence or absence of other associated electrolyte or acid-base disturbances.
3. Symptoms of neuromuscular excitability predominate.
4. On physical examination one should look for the presence of Chvostek's and Trousseau's signs.

Diagnosis

An algorithm for the differential diagnosis of hypocalcemia is shown in Figure 10.4. Common causes are hypomagnesemia (most common), chronic kidney disease, and vitamin D deficiency. When total serum calcium concentration is low one first evaluates the serum albumin concentration and, if necessary, measures ionized serum calcium concentration. After the presence of true hypocalcemia

Figure 10.4

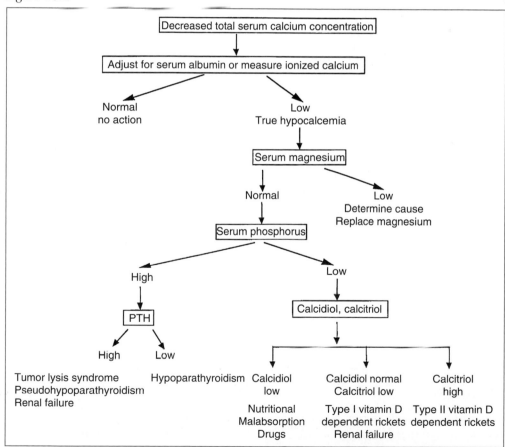

Evaluation of the hypocalcemic patient. After adjusting for serum albumin concentration one evaluates serum magnesium concentration. Patients are further subdivided based on serum phosphorus, PTH, and calcidiol and calcitriol concentrations. (With permission from Schrier, R.W. (ed.). *Manual of Nephrology*. Lippincott Williams & Wilkins, Philadelphia, PA, 2000.)

is established, blood is sent for serum BUN, creatinine, magnesium, and phosphorus concentrations.

Serum magnesium concentration is evaluated next. As stated previously, the most common cause of hypocalcemia is hypomagnesemia. Hypocalcemia will not correct before magnesium losses are replenished.

One then examines serum phosphorus concentrations. If kidney function is normal hyperphosphatemia suggests hypopara-thyroidism or pseudohypoparathyroidism. These disorders can easily be differentiated by measuring PTH concentration. PTH concentration is low in primary hypoparathyroidism due to gland failure, whereas with end-organ resistance as in pseudohypoparathyroidism PTH concentration will be elevated. Pseudohypoparathyroidism is further subdivided by infusing PTH and subsequently measuring urinary phosphate and cAMP concentrations.

Disorders of vitamin D metabolism are characterized by hypophosphatemia. Hypocalcemia stimulates the parathyroid gland to secrete PTH that results in renal phosphate wasting. To determine the defect in vitamin D metabolism serum calcidiol and calcitriol concentrations are measured. If, on the other hand, the kidney is responding appropriately to phosphate depletion the FE will be below 1%. If the FE of phosphate is high, then serum calcidiol and calcitriol concentrations are measured. Calcidiol levels are low with malabsorption, liver disease, phenobarbital, nutritional deficiency, and nephrotic syndrome. Calcitriol levels are low with chronic kidney disease and increased in type II vitamin D-dependent rickets.

KEY POINTS
Diagnosis of Hypocalcemia

1. The most common causes of hypocalcemia are magnesium deficiency, chronic kidney disease, and vitamin D deficiency.
2. If total serum calcium concentration is decreased one evaluates the serum albumin

concentration to attempt to estimate whether ionized calcium concentration is decreased.
3. Hypomagnesemia is the most common cause of hypocalcemia.
4. If hypomagnesemia is not present serum phosphorus concentration and renal phosphate excretion are examined.
5. Hyperphosphatemia in the absence of chronic kidney disease suggests decreased PTH concentration or effect.
6. Decreased serum phosphorus concentration is indicative of a defect in vitamin D metabolism.

Treatment

Treatment will vary depending on the degree and cause of hypocalcemia. In life-threatening circumstances such as with seizures, tetany, hypotension, or cardiac arrhythmias, intravenous calcium at a rate of 100–300 mg over 10–15 minutes is administered. In general, intravenous calcium should be used initially in the symptomatic patient or the patient with severe hypocalcemia (total calcium corrected for albumin ≤7.5 mg/dL). Hypocalcemia that is mild in an outpatient setting is corrected with oral calcium supplementation. A vitamin D preparation may need to be added if the response to oral calcium is insufficient.

If life-threatening symptoms are not present the administration of 15 mg/kg of elemental calcium over 4–6 hours can be expected to increase total serum calcium concentration by 2–3 mg/dL. A variety of intravenous preparations can be used including 10% calcium gluconate—10 mL ampules (94 mg of elemental calcium), (2) 10% calcium glucoptate—5 mL ampule (90 mg elemental calcium), and (3) calcium chloride—10 mL ampule (272 mg elemental calcium). After the first ampule is administered generally over several minutes, an infusion is begun at 0.5–1.0 mg/kg/hour. The infusion rate is subsequently adjusted based on serial serum calcium determinations. Magnesium deficits must first be corrected or treatment will be ineffective. In the patient who also has metabolic acidosis, hypocalcemia should be corrected first. Correction of acidosis before hypocalcemia will result in a further decrease in ionized calcium concentration and exacerbate symptoms.

Patients with hypoparathyroidism are often treated with vitamin D supplements since administration of calcium alone is often ineffective. Serum calcium concentration should be maintained at a level where the patient is symptom free. This is generally at or just below the lower limit of normal. An elemental calcium dose of 1–3 g/day is usually required. Several oral preparations can be used and are shown in Table 10.3. Supplements should be taken between meals to ensure optimal absorption. Calcium citrate is more bioavailable than calcium carbonate especially in patients with increased gastric pH. If higher doses of elemental calcium are required, a vitamin D preparation should be added. In the presence of severe hyperphosphatemia it is advisable to delay calcium supplementation until serum phosphorus concentration is below 6 mg/dL. This may not always be possible and clinical judgment must be used in the severely hypocalcemic patient.

Calcitriol is the most potent vitamin D preparation, has a rapid onset of action, a short duration of action, but is also the most expensive. A dose of 0.5–1.0 µg/day is often required. As one moves from calcidiol to cholecalciferol, and to ergocalciferol, cost decreases and duration of action increases. Some of these agents, however, may be less efficacious in the presence of renal or hepatic disease.

In hypoparathyroidism distal tubular calcium reabsorption is decreased due to a lack of PTH. The increased filtered calcium load resulting from calcium and vitamin D replacement can lead to hypercalciuria, nephrolithiasis, and nephrocalcinosis. Patients with hypoparathyroidism excrete more calcium than normal for any given serum calcium concentration. If urinary calcium excretion exceeds 350 mg/day and serum calcium concentration is acceptable, sodium intake should be restricted and if this is not effective a thiazide diuretic added in order to reduce urinary calcium excretion.

Patients with hypocalcemia postparathyroidectomy require large doses of supplemental calcium. In this setting the serum potassium must be monitored carefully since for unclear reasons these patients are at increased risk of hyperkalemia. Treatment of hypocalcemia in the setting of the tumor lysis syndrome is directed at lowering serum phosphorus concentration.

Table 10.3
Oral Calcium Preparations

PREPARATION	TABLET (MG)	ELEMENTAL CALCIUM/TABLET (MG)
Calcium carbonate	500	200
Calcium citrate	950	200
Calcium lactate	650	85
Calcium gluconate	1000	90

KEY POINTS
Treatment of Hypocalcemia

1. Management of the hypocalcemic patient depends on its severity and cause.
2. Acute symptomatic hypocalcemia is treated with intravenous calcium.
3. Of the available vitamin D preparations calcitriol is the most potent, has a rapid onset of action, a short duration of action, but is also the most expensive.
4. Serum calcium concentration is maintained at the lower limit of normal in patients with hypoparathyroidism to minimize hypercalciuria.
5. If hypercalciuria develops salt restriction or thiazide diuretics can be employed.

Additional Reading

Brown, A.J., Dusso, A., Slatopolsky, E. Vitamin D. *Am J Physiol* 277:F157–F175, 1999.

Bushinsky, D.A. Calcium. *Lancet* 352:306–311, 1998.

Fiorino, A.S. Hypercalcemia and alkalosis due to the milk-alkali syndrome: a case report and review. *Yale J Biol Med* 69:517–523, 1996.

Guise, T.A., Mundy, G. Evaluation of hypocalcemia in children and adults. *J Clin Endocrinol Metab* 80: 1473–1478, 1995.

Mundy, G.R., Guise, T.A. Hypercalcemia of malignancy. *Am J Med* 103:134–145, 1997.

Potts, J.T. Jr., Fradkin, J.E., Aurbach, J.D., Bilezikian, J.P., Raisz, L.G. Proceedings of the NIH consensus development conference on diagnosis and management of asymptomatic primary hyperparathyroidism. *J Bone Miner Res* 6:S1–S165, 1991.

Rankin, W., Grill, V., Martin, T.J. Parathyroid hormone-related protein and hypercalcemia. *Cancer* 80:S1564–S1571, 1997.

Reber, P.M., Heath III, H.H. Hypocalcemic emergencies. *Med Clin North Am* 79:93–106, 1995.

Vetter, T., Lohse, M.J. Magnesium and the parathyroid. *Curr Opin Nephrol Hypertens* 11:403–410, 2002.

Zahrani, A.A., Levine, M.A. Primary hyperparathyroidism. *Lancet* 349:1233–1236, 1997.

Robert F. Reilly, Jr.

Chapter

11

Disorders of Serum Phosphorus

Recommended Time to Complete: 1 day

Guiding Questions

1. Of the regulators of serum phosphorus concentration, which are most important?
2. What is the most common cause of hyperphosphatemia?
3. What are the advantages and disadvantages of various phosphate binders that are available for the treatment of hyperphosphatemia?
4. How does one evaluate the hypophosphatemic patient?
5. How well documented are the clinical consequences of hypophosphatemia?
6. Does the patient with moderate hypophosphatemia require phosphorus replacement?

Regulation

Phosphorus circulates in the bloodstream in two forms, an organic fraction made up primarily of phospholipids and an inorganic fraction. Of these two fractions, it is the inorganic fraction, which makes up approximately one-third of the total serum phosphorus, that is assayed in the clinical laboratory. The normal range in most laboratories is 2.5–4.5 mg/dL (0.8–1.45 mmol/L). The majority (75%) of inorganic phosphorus is free in solution and exists as either divalent ($HPO_4^=$) or monovalent ($H_2PO_4^-$) phosphate. The relative amounts of each ion depend on the systemic pH. At pH 7.4, 80% is in the divalent form. Of the remainder, 15% is protein bound. A small fraction of inorganic phosphorus is complexed with calcium or magnesium. In normal individuals there is a diurnal variation in serum phosphorus concentration. Serum phosphorus concentration is at its lowest in the morning, gradually rises during the day, and peaks in the evening. The change in serum phosphorus concentration may be as much as 1 mg/dL. Whether this diurnal variation persists in disease states characterized by hypophosphatemia is not as clear, although diurnal variation was noted in patients with primary hyperparathyroidism.

The largest reservoir of phosphorus in the body is in the skeleton (80%). The vast majority of the remainder of total body phosphorus is in skeletal muscle and viscera with only 1% in extracellular fluid (ECF). Of the intracellular pool only a very small fraction is inorganic and can be used for synthesis of high-energy phosphate-containing molecules (adenosine triphosphate [ATP]). Phosphorus homeostasis is summarized in Figure 11.1.

Figure 11.1

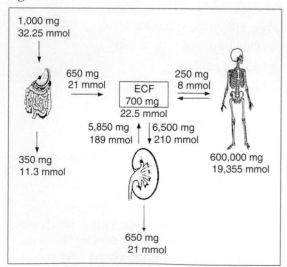

Phosphorus homeostasis. Daily phosphorus fluxes between ECF, intestine, kidney, and bone are shown. In the steady state net intestinal absorption and renal excretion are equal. The majority of phosphorus in the body is in bone. (With permission from Schrier, R.W. (ed.). *Manual of Nephrology.* Lippincott Williams & Wilkins, Philadelphia, PA, 2000.)

On average approximately 800–1400 mg of phosphorus is ingested daily. Of this total 640–1120 mg is absorbed primarily in duodenum and jejunum. The majority of phosphorus absorption in the intestine is passive but there is a small active component regulated by vitamin D.

Parathyroid hormone (PTH) and calcitriol are important regulators of phosphorus homeostasis via their actions in bone, intestine, and kidney. Recently, a newly described molecule fibroblast growth factor-23 (FGF-23) was described that also may play a role in phosphorus homeostasis and will be discussed more fully below. Excretion of phosphate by the kidney, however, is the prime regulator of serum phosphorus concentration. The majority of phosphate is reabsorbed in the proximal tubule (80%). Phosphorus enters this cell via the sodium-phosphate cotransporter, which is regulated directly by PTH and serum phosphorus concentration. The kidney is capable of reducing phosphate excretion to very low levels in states of phosphorus depletion. Exit pathways for phosphate transport across the basolateral membrane of the proximal tubular cell are not well defined.

Three types of sodium-phosphate cotransporters are expressed in the kidney (Npt-I, -II, and -III). Npt-II is further subdivided into three isoforms a, b, and c. Properties of Npt transporter isoforms are illustrated in Table 11.1. Phosphorus concentration and PTH regulate Npt-IIa. Npt-IIa is electrogenic and transports three sodium ions for each $HPO_4^=$) and is expressed in the proximal tubule of the kidney. Both PTH and exposure to high phosphorus concentration result in endocytic retrieval of Npt-IIa from the brush border membrane to small endocytic vesicles. These vesicles are shuttled to lysosomes by a microtubule-mediated process and degraded. There is little to no recycling back to the proximal tubular cell membrane once transporters are endocytosed. New transporters must then be resynthesized and routed to the apical membrane via a subapical compartment. Acute regulation involves changes in endocytic rates. Endocytosis occurs between microvilli at intermicrovillar clefts and involves

Table 11.1

Sodium-Phosphate Cotransporter Isoforms

ISOFORMS	PHOSPHATE TRANSPORTED (%)	CELLULAR LOCALIZATION	TRANSPORT MODE	OTHER TRANSPORT FUNCTIONS
Npt-I	15	Apical	Electrogenic	Cl channel, organic anions
Npt-II	84	Apical		
a			Electrogenic	
b			Electrogenic	
c			Electroneutral	
Npt-III	0.5	Basolateral	Electrogenic	

clathrin. Megalin may also play a role. It is mediated by a variety of protein kinases. This process is summarized in Figure 11.2.

Npt-IIb is expressed in the brush border of enterocytes. It lacks the dibasic amino acid motif (RK) at the C-terminus of the protein that is critical for endocytosis and, therefore, is not regulated in the short term by PTH, as is Npt-IIa. The primary up regulators of Npt-IIb are a low phosphorus diet and calcitriol. Npt-IIb expression is also stimulated by estrogens and inhibited by glucocorticoids and epidermal growth factor.

Figure 11.2

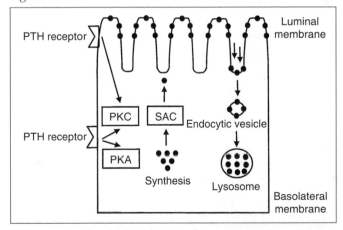

Cellular model of proximal tubular phosphate transport. Sodium-phosphate cotransporters (Npt-IIa) are distributed along the luminal membrane (dark circles). In response to PTH, transporters localize to the intermicrovillar region where they are endocytosed and degraded in lysosomes. This appears to be a unidirectional process. New transporters must be resynthesized and routed to the apical membrane via a subapical compartment (SAC). PTH binds to receptors in both the luminal and basolateral membrane. Parathyroid hormone receptor-mediated signaling pathways (protein kinase A—PKA and protein kinase C—PKC) differ at the basolateral and luminal membranes.

In bone, the end result of PTH action is release of phosphorus into the ECF. In small intestine, PTH acts indirectly via its stimulation of 1α-hydroxylase to produce calcitriol. Calcitriol in turn stimulates phosphorus absorption in the small intestine where the majority of phosphorus is reabsorbed. Importantly, in the large intestine there is a component of unregulated secretion (100–200 mg/day) that can increase with diarrhea and contribute to the pathogenesis of hypophosphatemia. In the kidney, PTH increases phosphate excretion via its actions in proximal tubule. The end result of PTH action is to maintain serum calcium concentration without a concomitant increase in serum phosphorus concentration.

Calcitriol on the other hand ensures that calcium and phosphorus are present in sufficient concentration for bone formation and it acts in concert with PTH to protect against hypocalcemia and hypophosphatemia. This is aided by the fact that PTH and hypophosphatemia are the main stimulators of 1α-hydroxylase and calcitriol production in proximal tubule. In the end, however, the main determinant of serum phosphorus concentration is the ability of the renal proximal tubule to excrete the dietary phosphorus load and conserve phosphorus in the presence of hypophosphatemia.

KEY POINTS

Regulation of Serum Phosphorus Concentration

1. Serum phosphorus consists of an organic and inorganic fraction; of these only the inorganic fraction is assayed in the clinical laboratory.
2. PTH and calcitriol regulate serum phosphorus concentration via effects in bone, intestine, and kidney.
3. PTH has both direct and indirect effects on phosphorus homeostasis. Directly, it increases bone resorption and reduces reabsorption of phosphate in the proximal tubule. It acts indirectly in the intestine via stimulation of 1α-hydroxylase with a resultant increase in calcitriol production.

4. Calcitriol enhances phosphorus transport in the intestine and potentiates PTH effects in bone, which act to increase calcium and phosphorus entry into blood.
5. The main determinant of serum phosphorus concentration is the ability of the proximal tubule to excrete the dietary phosphorus load and to conserve phosphorus in the presence of hypophosphatemia.

Hyperphosphatemia

Etiology

Hyperphosphatemia most commonly results from decreased renal phosphate excretion. This occurs from either a decrease in the filtered load of phosphate due to decreased glomerular filtration rate (GFR) as with acute renal failure or chronic kidney disease (CKD) or increased proximal tubular phosphate reabsorption. An acute phosphorus load from either exogenous or endogenous sources can also cause hyperphosphatemia. Chronic kidney disease is the cause in greater than 90% of cases. Etiologies of hyperphosphatemia grouped by pathophysiologic categories are shown in Table 11.2.

As GFR declines below 60 mL/minute/1.73 m² renal phosphorus excretion increases. Once GFR falls below 30 mL/minute/1.73 m², however, phosphate reabsorption is maximally inhibited and renal excretion cannot increase further. At this point, dietary intake will exceed renal excretion and serum phosphorus concentration must increase. A new steady state is established at a higher serum phosphorus concentration. Approximately 15% of patients with a GFR of 15–30 mL/minute/1.73 m² and 50% of those with a GFR <15 mL/minute/1.73 m² have a serum phosphorus concentration >4.5 mg/dL.

Table 11.2

Etiologies of Hyperphosphatemia

Decreased renal excretion
Decreased glomerular filtration rate
    Acute renal failure
    Chronic kidney disease
Increased renal phosphorus reabsorption
    Hypoparathyroidism
    Acromegaly
    Thyrotoxicosis
    Drugs—bisphosphonates
    Tumoral calcinosis
**Acute phosphorus addition to extracellular
fluid**
Endogenous
    Tumor lysis syndrome
    Rhabdomyolysis
    Severe hemolysis
Exogenous
    Vitamin D intoxication
    Sodium phosphate-containing bowel
      preparation solutions
    High-dose liposomal amphotericin B
    Improperly purified fresh frozen plasma
Pseudohyperphosphatemia

Increased renal phosphate reabsorption is an uncommon pathophysiologic mechanism for the development of hyperphosphatemia. It occurs in hypoparathyroidism as a result of decreased PTH concentration. In acromegaly insulin-like growth factor stimulates phosphate transport. Bisphosphonates directly increase renal phosphate reabsorption but this effect is usually offset by secondary hyperparathyroidism that results from decreases in serum calcium concentration. Tumoral calcinosis is an autosomal recessive disease associated with hyperphosphatemia and soft tissue calcium deposition. The mutated gene GALNT3 encodes a glycosyltransferase that is involved in O-linked glycosylation. The mechanism whereby this mutation increases renal phosphate reabsorption remains unclear.

Serum phosphorus concentration also increases as a result of an acute large phosphorus load. Phosphorus can be released from an endogenous source (within cells), as in tumor lysis syndrome, hemolysis, or rhabdomyolysis. Exogenous sources of phosphorus reported to cause hyperphosphatemia include phosphorus-containing laxatives and enemas, high-dose liposomal amphotericin B (contains phosphatidylcholine and phosphatidylserine), and solvent detergent-treated fresh frozen plasma (contained improper amounts of dihydrogen phosphate used as a buffer in the purification process). Oral sodium phosphate solution is commonly used as a bowel preparation agent for colonoscopy. It can be given in a small volume (45 mL 18 and 6 hours before the procedure) and is less expensive than polyethylene glycol-based solutions. The 90 mL contains 43.2 g of monobasic sodium phosphate and 16.2 g of dibasic sodium phosphate. A variety of rare renal complications occur with its use. Fatal hyperphosphatemia was reported in a renal transplant patient, serum phosphorus concentration 17.8 mg/dL, who received a single oral dose of 90 mL and suffered a cardiorespiratory arrest 6 hours later. The patient presented with nausea, vomiting, abdominal pain, and rectal bleeding. Autopsy showed ischemic colitis. Four other deaths were reported. Two of these four patients had end-stage renal disease and therefore, an impaired ability to excrete a phosphorus load. A group of five patients was reported with acute renal failure (mean serum creatinine concentration 4.9 mg/dL) secondary to acute nephrocalcinosis after oral sodium phosphate bowel cleansing. Their mean age was 69.2 years and mean serum creatinine concentration was 0.9 mg/dL before administration of the bowel preparation. All had calcium phosphate precipitation in distal tubules and collecting ducts and severe tubular damage. Four were prescribed angiotensin converting enzyme inhibitors or angiotensin receptor blockers and two were taking diuretics. At 6 weeks renal function was unchanged in four of the five patients. Another study showed that the rise in serum phosphorus concentration that occurs after ingestion of oral sodium phosphate was directly correlated with patient age. When given to normal volunteers ages 21–41 with normal renal function, oral phosphasoda caused a rise in serum phosphorus concentration to 7.6 mg/dL and a fall in serum calcium concentration to 8.4 mg/dL. There were no adverse clinical effects of these changes. As many as 37% of patients with a creatinine clearance greater than 70 mL/minute have an increase in serum phosphorus concentration to greater than 8.0 mg/dL. Taken together these studies indicate that oral sodium phosphate solution should be used with caution in those above age 55, those with decreased gastrointestinal (GI) motility, patients with decreased glomerular filtration rates, and in the presence of volume depletion.

Tumor lysis syndrome is seen classically with the treatment of Burkitt's lymphoma or acute lymphoblastic leukemia. It is characterized by hyperphosphatemia, hypocalcemia, hyperuricemia, and hyperkalemia following release of intracellular contents of dying malignant cells. Acute renal failure is a common consequence. Hyperphosphatemia classically occurs about 24–48 hours after onset of chemotherapy. Malignant lymphoid cells are reported to contain up to four times as much phosphorus as normal lymphocytes. Precipitation of calcium phosphate in the nephron can result in acute nephrocalcinosis and acute renal failure.

Prevention of acute urate nephropathy is directed at reducing uric acid formation or converting it to a more soluble compound to facilitate its renal excretion. Purines are metabolized to hypoxanthine and xanthine. Xanthine is then converted to uric acid by xanthine oxidase, which can be inhibited by allopurinol. Allopurinol has a half-life of 0.5–2.0 hours. It is metabolized to oxypurinol that also inhibits xanthine oxidase which is renally excreted with a half-life of 18–30 hours. Allopurinol must be used with caution in patients with decreased GFR. Uric acid can be converted to the more soluble sodium urate by increasing urinary pH to greater than 6.5 with administration of sodium bicarbonate. This must be done with caution because calcium phosphate precipitation increases at urinary pH greater than 6.5.

Higher primates do not express urate oxidase that converts uric acid to the more soluble allantoin. Recombinant urate oxidase (rasburicase) was recently approved by the FDA. It cannot be used in patients with glucose-6-phosphate dehydrogenase deficiency since hydrogen peroxide generated during allantoin formation may cause hemolysis. Tumor lysis syndrome can occur in patients with solid tumors when there is a decrease in glomerular filtration rate or tumor burden is large. An increased lactate dehydrogenase (LDH) concentration (>1500 IU), hyperuricemia, large tumor burden, and high tumor sensitivity to treatment are predictive of the development of tumor lysis syndrome.

KEY POINTS
Etiology of Hyperphosphatemia

1. Hyperphosphatemia results from decreased renal phosphate excretion or an acute phosphorus load from either exogenous or endogenous sources.
2. Acute renal failure or CKD is the cause in the vast majority of cases.
3. As GFR declines below 60 mL/minute/1.73 m^2 renal phosphate excretion increases.
4. Once GFR falls below 30 mL/minute/1.73 m^2 phosphate reabsorption is maximally inhibited and renal phosphate excretion cannot increase further.
5. Fifteen percent of patients with a GFR of 15–30 mL/minute/1.73 m^2 and 50% of those with a GFR <15 mL/minute/1.73 m^2 have a serum phosphorus concentration >4.5 mg/dL.

Signs and Symptoms

Signs and symptoms of hyperphosphatemia are primarily the result of hypocalcemia. The most common explanation offered for hypocalcemia is that the calcium-phosphorus product exceeds a certain level and calcium deposits in soft tissues and serum calcium concentration falls. A calcium-phosphate product of >72 mg²/dL² is commonly believed to result in this so-called "metastatic" calcification. It is difficult, however, to find the original studies and data on which this belief is based.

Short-term intravenous infusion of phosphorus is known to depress serum calcium concentration. No evidence of increased soft tissue calcification was documented in these studies. In addition, the hypothesis that hypocalcemia results from soft tissue deposition is inconsistent with the observation that serum calcium concentration continues to decline for up to 5 days after short-term phosphorus infusion is discontinued and long beyond the time period when serum phosphorus concentration normalizes. Short-term infusions of phosphorus increase bone deposition of calcium and reduce bone resorption. Hypocalcemia can also result from decreased calcitriol concentration as a result of suppression of 1α-hydroxylase by increased serum phosphorus. These effects may be more important than physicochemical precipitation.

In patients with end-stage renal disease and high serum phosphorus concentration, it is being increasingly demonstrated that vascular calcification is a highly regulated process and that smooth muscle cells in the blood vessel wall are capable of transforming to an "osteoblast-like" phenotype and expressing what were previously believed to be osteoblast-specific genes. This suggests that hyperphosphatemia plays a direct role in vascular calcification and increased cardiovascular morbidity and mortality that may result.

KEY POINTS

Signs and Symptoms of Hyperphosphatemia

> 1. Symptoms of an acute rise of serum phosphorus concentration are related to hypocalcemia.
> 2. Hypocalcemia may be the result of precipitation of calcium phosphate in tissues and/or the acute effects of hyperphosphatemia on bone deposition and release of calcium.

Diagnosis

Clinically unexplained persistent hyperphosphatemia raises the suspicion of pseudohyperphosphatemia, the most common cause of which is paraproteinemia secondary to multiple myeloma. No consistent relationship of immunoglobulin type or subclass was identified. This is a method-dependent artifact and paraprotein interference may be a general problem in some automated assays. The assay must be rerun with sulfosalicylic acid deproteinized serum in order to eliminate the artifact. Otherwise, the cause is generally acute renal failure or CKD. An algorithm for the differential diagnosis of hyperphosphatemia is shown in Figure 11.3.

KEY POINTS

Diagnosis of Hyperphosphatemia

> 1. Paraproteins may result in a false elevation of serum phosphorus concentration.
> 2. Acute renal failure and CKD remain the most common causes of hyperphosphatemia.

Treatment

The cornerstone of management of the hyperphosphatemic patient with CKD is reduction of intestinal phosphorus absorption. Early in CKD hyperphosphatemia can be controlled with dietary phosphorus restriction. Dietary phosphorus absorption is linear over a wide range of intakes, 4–30 mg/kg/day. Therefore, absorption will depend on the amount of phosphorus in the diet and its bioavailability. The majority of dietary phosphorus is contained in three food groups: (1) milk and related dairy products such as cheese; (2) meat, poultry, and fish; and (3) grains. Processed foods may contain large amounts of phosphorus and in one study an additional 1154 mg/day of phosphorus was ingested secondary to phosphorus-containing additives in fast food with no change

Figure 11.3

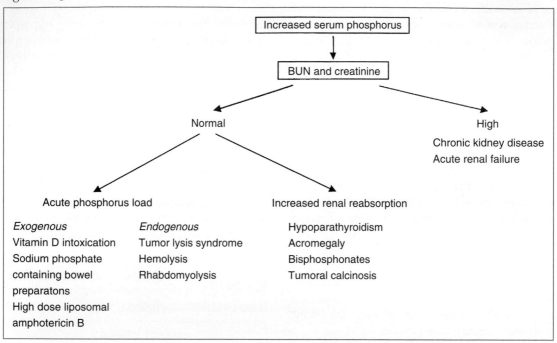

Evaluation of the hyperphosphatemic patient. Serum concentrations of blood urea nitrogen (BUN) and creatinine are evaluated first. Renal failure is the most common cause of hyperphosphatemia. If renal function is normal an acute phosphorus load or increased renal phosphate reabsorption are likely responsible.

in dietary protein intake. Phosphorus contained in plants is largely in the form of phytate and humans do not express the intestinal enzyme phytase that is necessary to degrade phytate and release phosphorus. Phosphorus in meats and dairy products is well absorbed. The inorganic salts of phosphorus contained in processed foods are virtually completely absorbed and patients with hyperphosphatemia should avoid these foods including hot dogs, cheese spreads, colas, processed meats, and instant puddings. Dietary estimates of phosphorus ingestion commonly underestimate phosphorus intake.

As CKD worsens phosphate binders must be added. The optimal choice of a phosphate binder remains controversial. The ideal binder should efficiently bind phosphate, have minimal effects on comorbid conditions, have a favorable side effect profile, and be low in cost. Unfortunately,

none of the currently available phosphate binders fulfill all of these criteria. Calcium-containing binders are low in cost but may contribute to net positive calcium balance and accelerate calcium deposition in vasculature. Aluminum-containing phosphate binders can be employed in the short term but should be avoided chronically in CKD patients because of aluminum toxicity (osteomalacia and dementia). Sevelamer hydrochloride, a synthetic calcium-free polymer, has a favorable side effect profile but is costly. In selecting between a calcium-containing binder and sevelamer hydrochloride one must balance the higher cost of sevelamer hydrochloride against potential benefits of decreased vascular calcification. In the hyperphosphatemic patient with coexistent hypocalcemia it is preferable to first lower the serum phosphorus concentration below 6 mg/dL, if possible, before treating the hypocalcemia.

KEY POINTS
Treatment of Hyperphosphatemia

1. Early in CKD dietary phosphorus restriction alone can normalize serum phosphorus concentration.
2. As GFR continues to fall phosphate binders must be added.
3. The choice of the optimal phosphate binder remains controversial.

Hypophosphatemia

Etiology

Hypophosphatemia results from one or a combination of three basic pathophysiologic processes: redistribution of ECF phosphorus into intracellular fluid (ICF); decreased intestinal phosphorus absorption; or increased renal phosphorus excretion. The differential diagnosis of hypophosphatemia based on pathophysiologic process is shown in Table 11.3.

The two most common causes of a phosphorus shift into cells are respiratory alkalosis and the "refeeding syndrome." The rise in intracellular pH that occurs with respiratory alkalosis stimulates phosphofructokinase, the rate-limiting step in glycolysis and phosphorus is incorporated into ATP. Severe hypophosphatemia with phosphorus concentrations less than 0.5–1.0 mg/dL is common. In 11 normal volunteers hyperventilation to a $PaCO_2$ of 13–20 mmHg caused a fall in serum phosphorus concentration within 90 minutes from a mean of 3.1 mg/dL to 0.8 mg/dL. At the same time phosphate excretion in urine dropped to near zero. Hypophosphatemia was reported with a rise in pH even within the normal range in ventilated chronic obstructive pulmonary disease (COPD) patients. In concert with the pH rise that occurs

Table 11.3
Etiologies of Hypophosphatemia

Decreased net GI absorption
Decreased dietary intake
Phosphate-binding agents
Alcoholism
Shift into intracellular fluid
Respiratory alkalosis
Refeeding
Diabetic ketoacidosis
Hungry bone syndrome
Sepsis
Increased renal excretion
Primary hyperparathyroidism
Secondary hyperparathyroidism from vitamin D deficiency
X-linked hypophophatemic rickets
Autosomal dominant hypophosphatemic rickets
Oncogenic osteomalacia
Fanconi's syndrome
Osmotic diuresis
Partial hepatectomy
Pseudohypophosphatemia

after intubation, serum phosphorus concentration falls over the span of several hours.

With refeeding, the time of onset of hypophosphatemia depends on the degree of malnutrition, caloric load, and amount of phosphorus in the formulation. In undernourished patients it develops in 2–5 days. It was reported with enteral as well as parenteral refeeding. The fall is more marked in patients with liver disease. In adolescents with anorexia nervosa the decline in serum phosphorus concentration was directly proportional to the percent loss of ideal body weight. Serum phosphorus concentration generally does not decline below 0.5 mg/dL with glucose infusion alone. Carbohydrate repletion and insulin release enhance intracellular uptake of phosphorus, glucose, and potassium. The combination of total body phosphorus depletion from decreased intake and increased cellular uptake during refeeding leads to profound hypophosphatemia. Phosphorus also moves into cells with treatment of diabetic ketoacidosis, and in the "hungry bone syndrome" that occurs after subtotal parathyroidectomy for secondary hyperparathyroidism in patients with end-stage renal disease. Renal phosphate loss from osmotic diuresis also contributes to the hypophosphatemia of DKA. In "hungry bone syndrome" serum calcium and phosphorus concentration often fall abruptly in the immediate postoperative period. From a clinical standpoint hypocalcemia is the more important management issue. Catecholamines and cytokines may also cause a phosphorus shift into cells and this may be the mechanism whereby sepsis results in hypophosphatemia.

Decreased GI absorption alone is an uncommon cause of hypophosphatemia since dietary phosphorus intake invariably exceeds GI losses and the kidney is extraordinarily effective at conserving phosphorus. Decreased dietary intake must be combined with phosphate binder use or increased GI losses as with diarrhea. In Bartter's original description of diet-induced hypophosphatemia 75–100 days of a low phosphorus diet and phosphate-binding antacids were required before symptoms developed. The primary symptom was musculoskeletal weakness that resolved with phosphorus replacement. Steatorrhea and malabsorption can result in calcitriol deficiency, secondary hyperparathyroidism, and increased renal excretion of phosphate.

Increased renal phosphate excretion is seen in primary hyperparathyroidism, as well as secondary hyperparathyroidism from disorders of vitamin D metabolism. In primary hyperparathyroidism the serum phosphorus concentration is rarely below 1.5 mg/dL. Although PTH increases renal phosphate excretion, this is partially offset by PTH action to increase calcitriol that in turn increases GI phosphorus absorption. On the other hand, secondary hyperparathyroidism from calcitriol deficiency may be associated with severe hypophosphatemia if the patient has normal renal function.

Three rare diseases associated with isolated renal phosphate wasting deserve further discussion because their pathogenic mechanism was recently elucidated. These include X-linked hypophosphatemia (XLH), autosomal dominant hypophosphatemic rickets (ADHR), and oncogenic hypophosphatemic osteomalacia. XLH is an X-linked dominant disorder with a prevalence of 1:20,000. It is manifested by growth retardation, rickets, hypophosphatemia, renal phosphate wasting, and a low serum calcitriol concentration. XLH is caused by mutations in the PHEX (phosphate regulating gene with homology to endopeptidases) gene. PHEX is a member of the M13 family of metalloproteinases. The gene is expressed in bones, teeth, and the parathyroid gland but not in the kidney. In bone, PHEX is expressed in the cell membrane of osteoblasts and plays a role in osteoblast mineralization. The mutated protein is not expressed in the cell membrane and is degraded in endoplasmic reticulum. How a defect in a membrane protein expressed in osteoblasts results in renal phosphate wasting is unclear. PHEX may play a role in the activation or inactivation of peptide factors involved in skeletal mineralization, renal phosphate transport, and vitamin D metabolism.

Subsequently, the genetic defect responsible for autosomal dominant hypophophatemic rickets (ADHR) was identified. ADHR has a similar phenotype to XLH but is inherited in an autosomal dominant fashion with variable penetrance. Mutations in a novel fibroblast growth factor, FGF-23, cause ADHR. FGF-23, a 251-amino acid protein, is secreted and inactivated at a cleavage site into N- and C-terminal fragments. Mutations in ADHR occur at the proteolytic site and prevent cleavage.

Oncogenic hypophosphatemic osteomalacia (OHO) is caused by overproduction of FGF-23 by mesenchymal tumors. The tumor is often difficult to localize. Overproduction of FGF-23 results in hypophosphatemia, renal phosphate wasting, suppression of 1α-hydroxylase, and osteomalacia. Tumor resection is curative. Immunohistochemical staining of these tumors shows an overabundance of FGF-23.

FGF-23 can be detected in the circulation of healthy individuals suggesting it plays a role in normal phosphorus homeostasis. When administered to animals FGF-23 causes hypophosphatemia, increased renal phosphate excretion, suppression of $1,25(OH)_2$ vitamin D_3, and osteomalacia. Biologic activity of FGF-23 is limited to the full-length molecule and it is degraded by protease cleavage. In ADHR missense mutations in FGF-23 occur at the cleavage site and prevent its proteolysis. The enzyme responsible for FGF-23 cleavage is unknown. One report suggested that it was cleaved by PHEX but this was not confirmed in subsequent studies.

XLH is the result of inactivating mutations of PHEX. PHEX belongs to a family of zinc-dependent proteases that cleave small peptides. The substrate of PHEX is unknown. Some authors have postulated that FGF-23 is the substrate of PHEX; however, its large size (251 amino acids) makes this unlikely. More recent studies indicate that FGF-23 is likely cleaved by subtilisin-like proprotein convertases. It is more likely that other small molecular weight intermediates link PHEX and FGF-23. Renal phosphate wasting also occurs in the immediate postoperative period after partial hepatectomy. The mechanism is unclear. Serum FGF-23 concentrations in these patients are normal.

FGF-23 when injected into experimental animals reduces calcitriol concentration within 3 hours. This occurs as a result of decreased calcitriol synthesis (decreased expression of 1α-hydroxylase) and increased degradation (increased expression of 24-hydroxylase). Serum phosphorus concentration and Npt-IIa fall after 9–13 hours. This effect occurs in parathyroidectomized animals indicating that it is PTH-independent. It is likely that only a part of the phosphaturic effect of FGF-23 is related to decreased calcitriol concentration. Injection of calcitriol into mice results in an increase in FGF-23 concentration and FGF-23 knockout mice have high serum calcitriol concentrations. Taken together these studies indicate that FGF-23 plays a central role in feedback regulation of calcitriol concentration.

Fanconi's syndrome is characterized by renal phosphate wasting, glycosuria in the face of a normal serum glucose, and aminoaciduria. A variety of inherited diseases are associated with Fanconi's syndrome including cystinosis, Wilson's disease, hereditary fructose intolerance, and

Lowe's syndrome. Acquired causes include multiple myeloma, renal transplantation, and drugs. Implicated drugs include ifosfamide, streptozocin, tetracyclines, valproic acid, ddI, cidofovir, adefovir, tenofovir, and ranitidine.

Tenofovir is being increasingly reported as a cause of Fanconi's syndrome in human immunodeficiency virus (HIV)-positive patients. Tenofovir is an acyclic nucleoside phosphonate that is excreted by glomerular filtration and tubular secretion. It enters the proximal tubular cell across the basolateral membrane on the human organic anion transporter 1 (hOAT1) and exits into urine on the multidrug resistance-associated protein 2 (Mrp-2). Since ritonavir inhibits Mrp 2, its use with tenofovir could result in increased toxicity. Renal injury occurs from weeks to months after starting treatment. In addition to Fanconi's syndrome, decreases in creatinine clearance and nephrogenic diabetes insipidus (DI) were also reported. The Chinese herb Boui-ougi-tou, used for treatment of obesity, also causes Fanconi's syndrome. Dent's disease is caused by a mutation in the chloride channel CLCN-5. It results in hypophosphatemia and renal phosphate wasting associated with low molecular weight proteinuria, hypercalciuria, nephrolithiasis, nephrocalcinosis, and chronic kidney disease. A urinalysis for glycosuria should be performed when the diagnosis of Fanconi's syndrome is being considered. The diagnosis is established by measuring serum and urinary amino acids and glucose and calculating the fractional excretion of each.

KEY POINTS
Etiology of Hypophosphatemia

1. The most common pathophysiologic processes that reduce serum phosphorus concentration are decreased GI absorption, shifts of phosphorus from ECF into ICF and increased renal excretion.
2. Intracellular phosphorus shifts are the most common cause of hypophosphatemia in hospitalized patients.

3. Decreased GI absorption alone is a rare cause of hypophosphatemia.
4. The most common causes of increased renal phosphorus excretion are primary and secondary hyperparathyroidism.
5. In primary hyperparathyroidism serum phosphorus concentration is rarely below 1.5 mg/dL.
6. Secondary hyperparathyroidism due to calcitriol deficiency may cause severe hypophosphatemia.

Signs and Symptoms

Hypophosphatemia causes a variety of signs and symptoms. Their severity varies with the degree of severity of hypophosphatemia. With the exception of two studies there is little evidence that moderate hypophosphatemia (serum phosphorus concentration between 1.0 and 2.5 mg/dL) results in any clinically significant morbidity. Moderate hypophosphatemia does not impair myocardial contractility. It increases insulin resistance but the clinical significance of this is unclear. Correction of moderate hypophosphatemia did improve diaphragmatic function in patients with acute respiratory failure. Eight intubated patients were given a short-term infusion of phosphorus (10 mmol [310 mg] over 4 hours). Mean serum phosphorus concentration increased from 1.72 to 4.16 mg/dL. Transdiaphragmatic pressure increased in all patients. One can question the clinical relevance of this finding given the small number of patients and lack of clinically important end points. In the second study a group of 16 patients were evaluated in the early stages of sepsis. Ten of the 16 patients had significant atrial and ventricular arrhythmias. Those patients with arrhythmias had a significantly lower serum phosphorus concentration, 2.8 mg/dL, than those that did not, 3.19 mg/dL. There was no increase in mortality in the hypophosphatemic patients.

On the other hand, severe hypophosphatemia (serum phosphorus concentration <1.0 mg/dL) is associated with morbidity. Failure to wean from mechanical ventilation without correction of severe hypophosphatemia was demonstrated. In one study severe hypophosphatemia increased the length of time patients spent on a ventilator (10.5 versus 7.1 days) and in the hospital (12.1 versus 8.2 days). This was also shown after cardiac surgery where patients with severe hypophosphatemia required more time on the ventilator (2.1 versus 1.1 days), a longer hospital stay (7.8 versus 5.6 days), and cardioactive drugs for a longer period of time.

Although hypophosphatemia causes a leftward shift in the oxygen dissociation curve, the clinical significance of this is unclear. Severe hypophosphatemia produces reversible myocardial dysfunction and an impaired response to pressors. Correction of severe hypophosphatemia increases myocardial contractility by 20%. The effect of short-term correction is variable between patients with some showing minimal to no response and others showing larger responses. Severe hypophosphatemia rarely, if ever, results in clinical congestive heart failure. A variety of neuromuscular symptoms were noted including paresthesias, tremor, and muscle weakness. Hematologic disturbances include increases in red cell fragility that lead to hemolysis. Hemolytic anemia was reported in two patients with serum phosphorus concentrations of 0.1 and 0.2 mg/dL, respectively. Red cell ATP was reduced to very low levels. *In vitro* studies in humans show that a serum phosphorus concentration less than 0.5 mg/dL decreased chemotaxis, phagocytosis, and bacterial killing by white cells. Whether this could predispose to infection is unknown. Severe hypophosphatemia causes rhabdomyolysis in dogs only if there is a preexisting subclinical myopathy. There are very few reports of rhabdomyolysis in man.

KEY POINTS
Signs and Symptoms of Hypophosphatemia

1. Correction of moderate hypophosphatemia improves diaphragmatic function in patients with acute respiratory failure. The clinical importance of this is unclear.

2. Moderate hypophosphatemia does not impair myocardial contractility.

3. Severe hypophosphatemia impairs the ability to wean patients from mechanical ventilation and prolongs hospital stay.

4. Myocardial contractility is decreased in severe hypophosphatemia; however, this rarely, if ever, results in clinical congestive heart failure.

5. Very severe hypophosphatemia increases red cell fragility that can lead to hemolysis.

6. Severe hypophosphatemia causes rhabdomyolysis in dogs only if there is a preexisting subclinical myopathy. There are very few reports of rhabdomyolysis in humans.

Diagnosis

A summary of the diagnostic approach to the patient with hypophosphatemia is illustrated in Figure 11.4. One can use the fractional excretion (FE) of phosphorus, the 24-hour urinary phosphorus excretion, or the calculated renal threshold phosphate concentration (TmPO$_4$/GFR) to distinguish among pathophysiologic mechanisms of hypophosphatemia. The FE of phosphorus is calculated using the formula:

$$\frac{U_P \times S_{Cr}}{U_{Cr} \times S_P} \times 100$$

Urine and serum creatinine (Cr) and phosphorus (P) concentrations are all expressed in mg/dL.

Figure 11.4

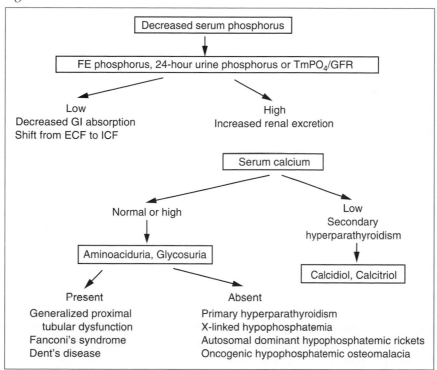

Evaluation of the hypophosphatemic patient. The first step in the evaluation of the hypophosphatemic patient is the evaluation of renal phosphorus excretion. Decreased renal phosphorus excretion suggests a gastrointestinal cause or a shift in phosphate from ECF to ICF. Increased renal phosphorus excretion is further subdivided based on serum calcium concentration. Abbreviations: FE, fractional excretion; TmPO4/GFR, renal tubular maximum reabsorptive capacity for phosphate (expressed as a function of the glomerular filtrate rate)

A FE of phosphorus below 5% or a 24-urine phosphorus less than 100 mg/day indicates that the kidney is responding properly to decreased intestinal absorption or the shift of phosphorus into cells. If renal phosphorus wasting is the pathophysiologic reason for hypophosphatemia, then the FE of phosphorus exceeds 5% and the 24-hour urine phosphorus excretion is greater than 100 mg. Primary and secondary hyperparathyroidism are the most common causes of renal phosphate wasting.

In the patient with increased renal phosphorus excretion one next evaluates the serum calcium concentration. In secondary hyperparathyroidism serum calcium concentration is low provided that renal function is intact. If secondary hyperparathyroidism from vitamin D deficiency is suspected, calcidiol and calcitriol concentrations will help identify the defect. In the patient with a normal or elevated serum calcium concentration one subdivides patients based on whether they have isolated renal phosphate wasting or a generalized proximal tubular disorder. Of the isolated phosphate wasting disorders primary hyperparathyroidism is by far the most common. It is associated with high serum calcium concentration and a low serum phosphorus concentration. The diagnosis is established by measuring PTH concentration. Three rare disorders make up the remainder of patients in this category. These include X-linked hypophosphatemia, autosomal dominant hypophosphatemic rickets, and oncogenic hypophosphatemic osteomalacia.

The generalized proximal tubular disorders are much less common and include Fanconi's syndrome and Dent's disease. If severe hypophosphatemia is noted and the patient is either asymptomatic or serum phosphorus concentration remains low despite repletion then one should consider the possibility of pseudohypophosphatemia. As is the case with pseudohyperphosphatemia paraproteins can also result in a spuriously low serum phosphorus concentration. This artifact is avoided if deproteinized serum is analyzed.

Key Points
Diagnosis of Hypophosphatemia

1. The first step in evaluation of the hypophosphatemic patient is examination of renal phosphorus excretion with a FE, a 24-hour urine, or renal threshold phosphate concentration. This separates patients with renal phosphate wasting from those with decreased intake and intracellular shifting of phosphorus.
2. The most common cause of hypophosphatemia from intracellular shifts of phosphorus in hospitalized patients is respiratory alkalosis.
3. If increased renal phosphate excretion is detected one next examines the serum calcium concentration.
4. Secondary hyperparathyroidism is the most common cause of renal phosphate wasting associated with hypocalcemia.
5. If serum calcium is normal or elevated, primary hyperparathyroidism is the most common cause.

Treatment

There is little evidence that treatment of moderate hypophosphatemia (serum phosphorus concentration 1.0–2.5 mg/dL) is necessary except perhaps in the patient being mechanically ventilated. Severe hypophosphatemia (≤ 1 mg/dL) or symptoms are indications for treatment. One must keep in mind that serum phosphorus concentration may not be a reliable indicator of total body phosphorus stores since the majority of phosphorus is contained within cells. Hypophosphatemia is commonly associated with other electrolyte disturbances (hypokalemia and hypomagnesemia). One must cautiously replete phosphorus in patients who have impaired ability to excrete phosphorus loads (those with decreased GFR). Most hypophosphatemic patients can be corrected

Table 11.4
Phosphate Preparations

PREPARATION	CONTENTS	PHOSPHORUS	SODIUM	POTASSIUM
K-phos-neutral	Dibasic Na phosphate Monobasic Na phosphate Monobasic K phosphate	250 mg/tab	13 meq/tab	1.1 meq/tab
K-phos original	Monobasic K phosphate	114 mg/tab	—	3.7 meq/tab
Fleets phospho-soda	Monobasic Na phosphate Dibasic Na phosphate	129 mg/mL	4.8 meq/mL	—
Neutra-phos-K	Monobasic K phosphate Dibasic K phosphate	250 mg/cap	—	13.6 meq/cap
Neutra-phos	Monobasic and dibasic Na and K phosphates	250 mg/cap	7.1 meq/cap	6.8 meq/cap
IV Na phosphate	Monobasic Na phosphate	93 mg/mL	4.0 meq/mL	—
IV K phosphate	Monobasic K phosphate	93 mg/mL	—	4.4 meq/mL

with up to 1 g of supplemental phosphorus per day orally. Several forms of oral and intravenous phosphorus replacement therapy are listed in Table 11.4. Oral repletion is most commonly limited by the development of diarrhea.

Intravenous phosphorus administration may be complicated by hypocalcemia and hyperphosphatemia and is only justified in those with severe symptomatic phosphorus depletion. Sodium phosphate should be employed except in patients that require concomitant potassium supplementation. During intravenous replacement blood chemistries including serum phosphorus, calcium, magnesium, and potassium concentrations should be monitored closely. Once serum phosphorus concentration has risen above 1 mg/dL, an oral preparation is begun and intravenous phosphorus is discontinued. In the severely malnourished patient, such as an adolescent with anorexia nervosa, refeeding must be accomplished slowly. Serum phosphorus concentration should be monitored closely and the patient placed on telemetry, since sudden death and ventricular arrhythmias were reported with refeeding.

KEY POINTS
Treatment of Hypophosphatemia

1. Treatment of moderate hypophosphatemia should be considered in the ventilated patient.
2. Severe hypophosphatemia (≤ 1 mg/dL) or symptoms are indications for treatment.
3. The safest mode of therapy is oral.
4. Intravenous phosphorus replacement carries the risk of hypocalcemia and is only warranted in patients with severe symptomatic phosphorus depletion.

Additional Reading

Brooks, M.J., Melnik, G. The refeeding syndrome: an approach to understanding its complications and preventing its occurrence. *Pharmacotherapy* 15: 713–726, 1995.

Bugg, N.C., Jones, J.A. Hypophosphatemia. *Anaesthesia* 53:895–902, 1998.

Crook, M. Phosphate: an abnormal anion? *Br J Hosp Med* 52:200–203, 1994.

DiMeglio, L.A., Econs, M.J. Hypophosphatemic rickets. *Rev Endocr Metab Disord* 2:165–173, 2001.

Econs, M.J., Francis, F. Positional cloning of the PEX gene: new insights into the pathophysiology of x-linked hypophosphatemic rickets. *Am J Physiol* 273:F489–F498, 1997.

Kalemkerian, G.P., Darwish, B., Varterasian, M.L. Tumor lysis syndrome in small cell carcinoma and other solid tumors. *Am J Med* 103:363–367, 1997.

Lotz, M., Zisman, E., Bartter, F. Evidence for a phosphate depletion syndrome in man. *N Engl J Med* 278:409–415, 1968.

Murer, H., Tenenhouse, H.S. Disorders of renal tubular phosphate transport. *J Am Soc Nephrol* 14:240–247, 2003.

Nelson, A.E., Robinson, B.G., Mason, R.S. Oncogenic osteomalacia: is there a new phosphate regulating hormone? *Clin Endocrinol* 47:635–642, 1997.

Sabbagh, Y., Tenenhouse H.S. Novel phosphate-regulating genes in the pathogenesis of renal phosphate wasting disorders. *Pflugers Arch- Eur J Physiol* 444:317–326, 2002.

Robert F. Reilly, Jr.

Disorders of Serum Magnesium

Recommended Time to Complete: 1 day

Guiding Questions

1. How is extracellular fluid (ECF) magnesium concentration regulated?
2. What role does the thick ascending limb of Henle play in this process?
3. Which are the most important causes of hypomagnesemia?
4. Why is hypomagnesemia associated with both hypocalcemia and hypokalemia?
5. How does one approach the patient with hypomagnesemia?
6. What are the most common causes of hypermagnesemia?
7. Why are patients with chronic kidney disease (CKD), gastrointestinal (GI) disorders, and the elderly at increased risk for hypermagnesemia?

Regulation

Magnesium is the fourth most abundant cation in the body and second most abundant within cells. It plays a key role in a variety of cellular processes. Magnesium is an important cofactor for ATPases and thereby, in the maintenance of intracellular electrolyte composition. Ion channels involved in nerve conduction and cardiac contractility are regulated by magnesium. Over 300 enzymatic systems depend on magnesium for optimal function including those involved in protein synthesis and deoxyribonucleic acid (DNA) replication. Magnesium deficiency is implicated in the pathogenesis of hypertension, type II diabetes mellitus, atherosclerosis, and asthma.

Normal serum magnesium concentration is between 1.4 and 2.1 mg/dL (0.6–0.86 mmol/L). Only 1% of the 21–28 g of magnesium in the body is contained within the ECF. Of the remainder, 67% is in bone and 20% in muscle. The distribution of magnesium within the body is shown in Figure 12.1. In bone the majority of magnesium is complexed in hydroxyapatite crystals. Approximately 30% of magnesium in bone is exchangeable with the ECF compartment. The rate of exchange is unclear. Magnesium within muscle and red cells is largely complexed to intracellular ligands and has limited ability to move from intracellular fluid (ICF) to ECF in conditions of total body magnesium depletion.

Magnesium is regulated by both the GI tract and the kidney, with kidney playing the more important role. The average North American diet contains approximately 200–350 mg of magnesium. The average daily requirement in men is 220–400 mg and in women is 180–340 mg. The North American diet is only marginally adequate with respect to magnesium. The majority is complexed to chlorophyll in green leafy vegetables. Seafoods, nuts, meats, and grains are high in magnesium.

Magnesium absorption is inversely proportional to intake. Under normal circumstances 30–40% is absorbed. This can vary from a low of 25% with large magnesium intakes to a high of 80% with dietary magnesium restriction. The majority of magnesium absorption occurs in the small intestine via both a paracellular and transcellular pathway. Magnesium absorption is affected by water absorption and prolonged diarrheal states result in significant intestinal magnesium losses. Secretions from the upper GI tract are relatively low in magnesium (1 mg/dL) while those from the colon are relatively high in magnesium (18 mg/dL).

Figure 12.1

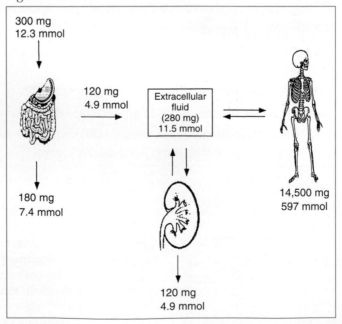

Magnesium homeostasis. Daily magnesium fluxes between ECF, intestine, kidney, and bone are shown. In the steady state net intestinal absorption and renal excretion of magnesium are equal.

Figure 12.2

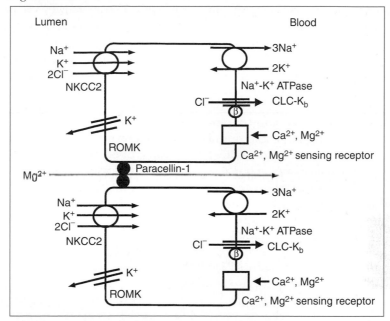

Thick ascending limb magnesium transport model. Five transporters expressed in the thick ascending limb of Henle are associated with a Bartter's-like syndrome: type I—sodium-potassium-chloride cotransporter; NKCC2; type II—the ROMK potassium channel; type III—ClC-Kb, the basolateral chloride channel; type IV—barttin, a β subunit required for the trafficking of ClC-K (both ClC-Ka and ClC-Kb) channels to the plasma membrane; and type V—severe gain-of-function mutations in the calcium-sensing receptor.

The primary regulator of ECF magnesium concentration is the kidney. Renal reabsorption of magnesium varies widely to maintain homeostasis. Reabsorption is reduced to near zero in the presence of hypermagnesemia or CKD. With magnesium depletion secondary to GI causes the fractional excretion of magnesium can be reduced to 0.5%.

Only 30% of magnesium is bound to albumin. The remainder is freely filtered across the glomerulus. Twenty percent of magnesium is reabsorbed in the proximal tubule in adults. Extracellular fluid volume status affects magnesium reabsorption in this segment. Volume contraction increases and volume expansion decreases magnesium reabsorption. The bulk of magnesium reabsorption occurs in the thick ascending limb of Henle (60–70%).

Magnesium is reabsorbed paracellularly with the lumen-positive voltage acting as driving force (Figure 12.2). The voltage is generated by potassium exit across the apical membrane through the ROMK channel. Potassium recycling is essential for Na+-K+-2Cl− function given that the luminal concentration of potassium is much lower than that of sodium or chloride. Magnesium moves across the tight junction through a specific channel, paracellin-1, that transports magnesium and calcium.

Although a variety of peptide hormones increase magnesium reabsorption including parathyroid hormone (PTH), calcitonin, glucagon, and antidiuretic hormone, magnesium concentration at the basolateral surface of the thick ascending limb is the major determinant of magnesium reabsorption. In hypermagnesemic states magnesium reabsorption approaches zero and in hypomagnesemia the loop reabsorbs virtually all of the filtered magnesium reaching it. This effect is presumably mediated via the calcium magnesium-sensing receptor expressed along the thick ascending limb basolateral surface. The receptor senses elevated calcium and magnesium concentration and transduces this signal to the apical membrane resulting in an inhibition of sodium entry via the Na^+-K^+-$2Cl^-$ cotransporter and potassium recycling via ROMK. This dissipates the lumen-positive voltage and decreases the driving force for magnesium reabsorption.

Approximately 5–10% of magnesium is reabsorbed in distal convoluted tubule (Figure 12.3). Magnesium transport here is active and transcellular.

Magnesium enters the cell passively through a channel and exits actively via an unknown mechanism. Despite differences in transport mechanisms compared to thick ascending limb, PTH, calcitonin, glucagon, antidiuretic hormone, and hypomagnesemia increase magnesium reabsorption in this segment. Amiloride increases magnesium reabsorption in distal nephron and is used therapeutically to reduce renal magnesium loss. Thiazide diuretics, on the other hand, cause mild magnesium wasting. Distal magnesium loss is partially offset by increased proximal reabsorption due to mild ECF volume contraction. The collecting duct plays a very limited role in magnesium reabsorption.

KEY POINTS
Magnesium Regulation

1. Magnesium plays a key role in a variety of cellular process.
2. Magnesium is regulated by both the GI tract and the kidney, with the kidney playing the more important role.
3. Twenty percent of magnesium is reabsorbed in the proximal tubule in adults. Volume contraction increases and volume expansion decreases proximal magnesium reabsorption.
4. The majority of magnesium reabsorption occurs in the cortical thick ascending limb. Magnesium is reabsorbed passively across the paracellular space with the lumen-positive voltage acting as the driving force.
5. It is the concentration of magnesium at the basolateral membrane of the cortical thick ascending limb that is the major determinant of magnesium reabsorption.
6. Approximately 5–10% of magnesium is reabsorbed in the distal convoluted tubule. Magnesium transport here is active and transcellular. Amiloride increases magnesium reabsorption in the distal nephron and can be used therapeutically to reduce renal magnesium loss. Thiazide diuretics cause mild magnesium wasting.

Figure 12.3

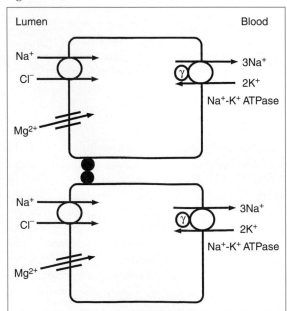

Distal convoluted tubule magnesium transport model. Transporters expressed in distal tubule that are associated with renal magnesium wasting include the thiazide-sensitive Na^+-Cl^- cotransporter (Gitelman's syndrome), the γ subunit of the Na^+-K^+ ATPase (isolated dominant hypomagnesemia), and TRMP6 a magnesium channel (primary intestinal hypomagnesemia).

Hypomagnesemia

Etiology

Hypomagnesemia is caused by decreased oral intake, increased GI losses, increased renal excretion, and shifts of magnesium from ECF to ICF. GI and renal losses are the most common causes of hypomagnesemia.

Magnesium depletion was first appreciated in animals in 1932 with the report of locoism in cattle. Locoism or "grass staggers" closely resembles magnesium depletion in humans and occurs within 1–2 weeks after grazing on early spring grass that is high in ammonium. The ammonium complexes magnesium and phosphate-forming insoluble struvite in the intestinal lumen preventing magnesium absorption. Cattle develop signs and symptoms of neuromuscular excitability, hypomagnesemia, hypocalcemia, and hypokalemia. In 1960, Vallee, Wacker, and Ulmer first reported magnesium deficiency in man. They described five patients with carpopedal spasm, Chvostek's and Trousseau's signs, and seizures.

GI causes of hypomagnesemia include decreased intake, malabsorption, diarrheal states, and primary intestinal hypomagnesemia. Clinically significant magnesium depletion from decreased oral intake alone is rare due to the ubiquitous nature of magnesium in foods and the kidney's ability to conserve magnesium. Hypomagnesemia was described in a number of patients with malabsorption. Serum magnesium concentration in these patients tends to correlate with the degree of steatorrhea. Presumably intestinal free fatty acids bind to magnesium forming insoluble soaps. Magnesium malabsorption is improved with a low-fat diet. Magnesium depletion can occur in any severe diarrheal state. Fecal magnesium increases as stool water increases and colonic secretions are high in magnesium.

Primary intestinal hypomagnesemia is an autosomal recessive disorder characterized by hypomagnesemia and hypocalcemia. Patients present in the first 6 months of life with symptoms of neuromuscular excitability including seizures secondary to hypomagnesemia and hypocalcemia. The hypocalcemia is resistant to therapy with calcium or vitamin D analogues. Passive intestinal magnesium transport is normal and large doses of oral magnesium reverse the hypomagnesemia and hypocalcemia. Mutations in the TRMP6 gene cause this disorder. TRMP6 is a member of the transient receptor potential (TRP) channel family and is expressed in the intestine and distal nephron. TRMP6 is likely the pathway whereby magnesium crosses the apical membrane of epithelial cells in intestine and distal nephron. Renal magnesium wasting was described in these patients consistent with TRMP6 expression in the kidney.

Renal losses of magnesium are due to primary defects in renal tubular reabsorption or secondary to a variety of systemic and local factors to which the kidney is responding normally. Primary renal defects are more likely to cause severe hypomagnesemia than secondary defects. Drug- or toxin-induced injury is the most common cause of primary renal magnesium wasting. Offending drugs include aminoglycosides, cis-platinum, amphotericin B, pentamidine, cyclosporin, and tacrolimus. With cis-platinum hypomagnesemia may persist for years after the drug is discontinued. Cyclosporin-induced hypomagnesemia is often associated with normal or elevated serum potassium and resolves rapidly after discontinuation of the drug. Hypomagnesemia may occur up to 2 weeks after a course of pentamidine. Hypomagnesemia was reported after tubular damage resulting from acute tubular necrosis, urinary tract obstruction, and delayed renal allograft function. This may result from increased flow in the loop of Henle that decreases magnesium reabsorption in this segment.

A variety of uncommon inherited renal magnesium wasting diseases are described. They are subdivided based on whether the genetic defect is in a protein expressed in the loop of Henle or in distal convoluted tubule.

Inherited diseases affecting magnesium reabsorption in the loop of Henle include familial hypomagnesemia with hypercalciuria and nephrocalcinosis (FHHNC), autosomal dominant hypocalcemia (ADH), and Bartter's syndrome. In FHHNC the paracellular channel through which magnesium moves is mutated, while in ADH and Bartter's syndrome the driving force stimulating passive magnesium transport (lumen-positive voltage) is dissipated.

FHHNC is characterized by renal magnesium and calcium wasting. It presents in early childhood with recurrent urinary tract infections, nephrolithiasis, and a urinary concentrating defect. The associated hypercalciuria, incomplete distal renal tubular acidosis, and hypocitraturia result in nephrocalcinosis and a progressive decrease in glomerular filtration rate. One-third develop end-stage renal disease by early adolescence. Mutations in paracellin-1 cause FHHNC. Paracellin-1 is expressed in the tight junction of the thick ascending limb of Henle. It likely functions as a paracellular calcium- and magnesium-selective channel.

Approximately 50% of patients with ADH have associated hypomagnesemia. ADH results from an activating mutation in the calcium magnesium-sensing receptor. Activating mutations shift the set point of the receptor and increase its affinity for calcium and magnesium. This signal is transduced to the apical membrane resulting in an inhibition of apical sodium entry and potassium exit. The resulting reduction in lumen-positive transepithelial voltage reduces the driving force for magnesium and calcium reabsorption in the loop of Henle.

Bartter's syndrome is caused by a variety of genetic defects in the thick ascending limb of the loop of Henle that present with renal salt wasting, hypokalemic metabolic alkalosis, and increased renin and aldosterone concentrations. Mutations in five ion transport proteins were described. All play a key role in transcellular sodium transport and generation of the lumen-positive voltage that is the driving force for magnesium and calcium transport. These include the Na^+-K^+-$2Cl^-$ cotransporter (NKCC2); the apical membrane potassium channel (ROMK); the basolateral membrane chloride channel (ClC-Kb); barttin, the β subunit of the basolateral membrane chloride channel; and

severe gain of function mutations of the calcium-sensing receptor. The phenotype varies depending on the gene mutated. Mutations in NKCC2 and ROMK are associated with severe salt wasting, neonatal presentation, and nephrocalcinosis. For unclear reasons hypomagnesemia is not common. Mutations in ClC-Kb present during adolescence and 50% have hypomagnesemia. Mutations in barttin are associated with sensorineural deafness and hypomagnesemia was not reported.

Genetic disorders resulting in magnesium wasting in the distal tubule include isolated dominant hypomagnesemia (IDH) and Gitelman's syndrome. IDH is an autosomal dominant disorder associated with hypocalciuria and chrondrocalcinosis. It is due to a defect in the FXYD2 gene that encodes the γ subunit of the basolateral Na^+-K^+ ATPase in distal convoluted tubule. Mutations result in subunit retention in the Golgi complex. How a mutation in this subunit results in isolated renal magnesium wasting and increased calcium reabsorption is unclear. Gitelman's syndrome results from loss of function mutations in the thiazide-sensitive sodium chloride cotransporter (NCCT). Mutant NCCT is trapped in the Golgi and not trafficked to the apical membrane. Patients present in adolescence with symptoms of hypomagnesemia and almost always have associated hypocalciuria. Gitelman's syndrome results in more profound hypomagnesemia than is seen with chronic thiazide therapy. The reason for this is unclear.

A variety of systemic and local factors affect magnesium reabsorption in the proximal tubule, thick ascending limb of Henle, and distal convoluted tubule resulting in secondary renal magnesium wasting. In the proximal tubule magnesium reabsorption is decreased by volume expansion as might occur after saline infusion and osmotic diuresis. In the loop of Henle magnesium reabsorption is inhibited by furosemide. This effect is mild due to an associated increase in proximal reabsorption. Hypercalcemia also results in magnesium wasting. Calcium binds to the calcium magnesium-sensing receptor in the basolateral membrane of the loop of Henle decreasing the lumen-positive voltage that drives paracellular magnesium transport. Thiazide diuretics act in distal convoluted tubule to inhibit magnesium transport.

Shifts of magnesium from the ECF to the ICF can occur as with calcium. These are uncommon causes of hypomagnesemia and can result after parathyroidectomy, refeeding, and in patients with hyperthyroidism. Hypomagnesemia develops in patients with burns due to magnesium losses through skin. Magnesium loss is proportional to the skin area burned.

KEY POINTS
Etiology of Hypomagnesemia

1. GI and renal losses are the most common causes of hypomagnesemia.
2. GI causes of hypomagnesemia include decreased oral intake, malabsorption, diarrheal states, and primary intestinal hypomagnesemia.
3. Clinically significant magnesium depletion from decreased oral intake alone is uncommon due to the ubiquitous nature of magnesium in foods.
4. Renal magnesium losses are due to primary defects in renal tubular reabsorption or secondary to systemic and local factors that the kidney is responding to normally.
5. Primary renal defects cause severe hypomagnesemia more often than secondary defects. Drug- and toxin-induced injuries are the most common causes of primary renal magnesium wasting.
6. Common secondary renal causes of hypomagnesemia include volume expansion, osmotic diuresis, furosemide, hypercalcemia, and thiazide diuretics.
7. A variety of inherited renal magnesium wasting diseases were described and can be subdivided based on whether the genetic defect is in the loop of Henle or in distal convoluted tubule.

Signs and Symptoms

It is difficult to attribute specific symptoms to hypomagnesemia due to its common association with metabolic alkalosis, hypocalcemia, and hypokalemia. Symptoms commonly attributed to hypomagnesemia involve the neuromuscular and cardiovascular systems. Increased neuromuscular excitability manifests as weakness, tetany, positive Chvostek's and Trousseau's signs, and seizures. A decreased concentration of either magnesium or calcium can lower the threshold for nerve stimulation.

Magnesium effects a variety of ion channels in the heart. Specifically, it regulates potassium channels that open in the absence of magnesium. It is a critical cofactor for the Na^+-K^+ ATPase and hypomagnesemia decreases pump activity. As a result, intracellular potassium decreases with hypomagnesemia and depolarizes the cardiac myocyte resting membrane potential. The threshold for generation of an action potential is reduced and the potential for arrhythmias increased. Hypomagnesemia is associated with a variety of atrial and ventricular arrhythmias. Decreased intracellular potassium also decreases the speed of potassium efflux resulting in a prolonged repolarization time. Hypomagnesemia aggravates digitalis toxicity since both decrease the activity of the Na^+-K^+ ATPase. Magnesium depletion produces acute changes in the electrocardiogram such as peaked T waves and widening of the QRS complex. In severe magnesium depletion the T wave diminishes in amplitude, the QRS widens further, and the PR interval becomes prolonged. These effects are also seen with hypokalemia and may be secondary to changes in serum potassium concentration.

Hypokalemia is frequently associated with hypomagnesemia. There are at least two possible explanations for this. Magnesium is an inhibitor of ROMK, the apical membrane potassium secretory channel in the loop of Henle and distal nephron. A decrease in intracellular magnesium releases the inhibitory effect and increases potassium secretion. The second is that renal magnesium and potassium losses are unrelated but both occur in patients with specific diseases such as alcoholism, diabetic ketoacidosis, osmotic diuresis, and diuretic use.

Severe magnesium depletion alters calcium homeostasis and results in hypocalcemia. Chronic hypomagnesemia suppresses PTH release from the parathyroid gland and this effect is rapidly reversed by intravenous magnesium infusion. This suggests that magnesium's effect is more likely due to inhibition of PTH release rather than on PTH synthesis. Balance studies show that the hypocalcemia is not associated with a net negative calcium balance indicating that it results from alterations in internal homeostatic mechanisms. Hypomagnesemia-induced hypocalcemia may result from skeletal resistance to the effects of PTH. In vitro studies show that magnesium depletion interferes with PTH-stimulated cyclic adenosine monophosphate (cAMP) generation. End-organ resistance occurs at serum magnesium concentrations ≤ 1.0 mg/dL. Serum magnesium concentrations ≤ 0.5 mg/dL are required to decrease PTH secretion.

KEY POINTS
Signs and Symptoms of Hypomagnesemia

1. Specific symptoms are difficult to attribute to hypomagnesemia due to its common association with metabolic alkalosis, hypocalcemia, and hypokalemia.
2. Hypomagnesemia results in increased neuromuscular excitability manifested by tetany, positive Chvostek's and Trousseau's signs, and seizures.
3. Hypomagnesemia is associated with a variety of atrial and ventricular arrhythmias.
4. Magnesium depletion produces acute changes in the electrocardiogram due to its effects on a variety of ion channels in heart.
5. Hypokalemia is frequently associated with hypomagnesemia.
6. Severe magnesium depletion suppresses PTH release from the parathyroid gland and causes skeletal resistance to PTH resulting in hypocalcemia.

Diagnosis

The two major sources of magnesium loss are GI tract and kidney (Table 12.1). The most common GI causes are malabsorption and diarrheal states. A careful history and physical examination should reveal the presence of these disorders. Hypomagnesemia from decreased oral intake alone and primary intestinal hypomagnesemia are rare.

Renal magnesium wasting is caused by primary defects in renal tubular reabsorption or secondary to systemic and local factors that the kidney is responding to normally. Drug- or toxin-induced injury is the most common cause of primary renal magnesium wasting. A careful drug exposure history is obtained for aminoglycosides, *cis*-platinum, amphotericin B, pentamidine, and cyclosporin. A variety of rare inherited renal magnesium wasting diseases should be considered.

Systemic and local factors can affect magnesium reabsorption in proximal tubule, thick

Table 12.1
Etiologies of Hypomagnesemia

Increased gastrointestinal losses
Decreased oral intake
Malabsorption
Diarrhea
Primary intestinal hypomagnesemia
Increased renal losses
Primary
Drugs
Toxins
Miscellaneous tubular injury
Genetic disorders
Secondary
Osmotic diuresis, saline infusion
Diuretics
Hypercalcemia
Shifts from the extracellular to the intracellular space
Hungry bone syndrome
Refeeding syndrome
Hyperthyroidism

ascending limb of Henle, and distal tubule. Osmotic diuresis reduces proximal tubular reabsorption of magnesium. Loop diuretics such as furosemide cause mild renal magnesium wasting due to an associated increase in proximal tubular magnesium reabsorption secondary to volume contraction. Hypercalcemia results in renal magnesium wasting. Thiazide diuretics act in distal convoluted tubule to block magnesium transport. As with loop diuretics, their effect is mild due to enhanced proximal tubular magnesium reabsorption from ECF volume contraction.

Shifts of magnesium from ECF to ICF are uncommon causes of hypomagnesemia but should be looked for after parathyroidectomy, refeeding, and in patients with hyperthyroidism.

An algorithm for the evaluation of the hypomagnesemic patient is illustrated in Figure 12.4. If the diagnosis is not readily apparent from the

history, either a 24-hour urine for magnesium or a spot urine for calculation of the fractional excretion of magnesium is obtained. The fractional excretion of magnesium is calculated from the equation below:

$$FE_{Mg} = \frac{U_{Mg} \times S_{Cr}}{(0.7 \times S_{Mg}) \times U_{Cr}}$$

The serum magnesium concentration is multiplied by 0.7 since only 70% of magnesium is freely filtered across the glomerulus.

When magnesium losses are extrarenal the kidney will conserve magnesium. The 24-hour urinary magnesium excretion is less than 30 mg and the fractional excretion of magnesium less than 4%. If renal magnesium wasting is the cause of hypomagnesemia renal magnesium excretion is increased. The 24-hour urinary magnesium excretion is greater than 30 mg and the fractional

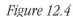

Figure 12.4

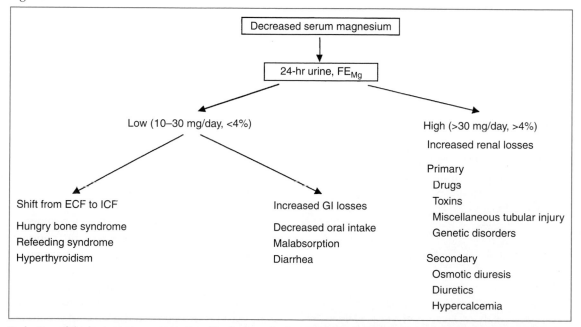

Evaluation of the hypomagnesemic patient. The first step in the evaluation of the hypomagnesemic patient is the evaluation of renal magnesium excretion. Decreased renal magnesium excretion suggests a gastrointestinal cause or a shift in magnesium from the ECF to the ICF. Increased renal magnesium excretion may be primary or secondary. Abbreviations: FE, fractional excretion; ECF, extracellular fluid; ICF, intracellular fluid; GI, gastrointestinal.

excretion of magnesium greater than 4%. In a study of 74 patients with hypomagnesemia the mean fractional excretion of magnesium in patients with renal magnesium wasting was 15% (range 4–48%).

Serum magnesium concentration may not accurately reflect total body magnesium stores. In patients with unexplained hypocalcemia, hypokalemia, or symptoms of neuromuscular excitability, the possibility of normomagnesemic magnesium depletion should be considered. In this setting, especially in patients at high risk for magnesium depletion, a therapeutic trial of magnesium replacement may be warranted. Magnesium replacement carries little risk provided renal function is normal. Some authors advocate performing a magnesium-loading test. A magnesium load is administered (2.4 mg/kg over 4 hours) and its renal excretion monitored over the next 24 hours. If less than 80% of the load is excreted this is considered evidence of total body magnesium depletion. Unfortunately, the test is of limited use. It is often positive in the setting of diarrhea, malnutrition, and diuretic use even in the absence of symptoms and may be falsely negative with renal magnesium wasting.

KEY POINTS
Diagnosis of Hypomagnesemia

1. A careful history and physical examination often reveals the cause of hypomagnesemia.
2. The most common cause of primary renal magnesium wasting is drug- or toxin-induced injury.
3. If the diagnosis is not apparent from the history, a 24-hour urine for magnesium or a fractional excretion of magnesium is obtained.
4. The possibility of normomagnesemic hypomagnesemia should be considered in patients with unexplained hypocalcemia, hypokalemia, and symptoms of neuromuscular excitability.

Treatment

The route of magnesium repletion varies depending on the severity of associated symptoms. The acutely symptomatic patient with seizures, tetany, or ventricular arrhythmias thought to be related to hypomagnesemia should be administered magnesium intravenously. In the life-threatening setting 4 mL (2 ampules) of a 50% solution of magnesium sulfate diluted in 100 mL of normal saline (200 mg) can be administered over 10 minutes. This is followed by 600 mg of magnesium given over the next 12–24 hours. The goal is to increase the serum magnesium concentration above 1.0 mg/dL. Magnesium is administered cautiously in patients with impaired renal function and serum concentration monitored frequently. In the setting of CKD the dose is reduced by 50–75%. Since renal magnesium excretion is regulated by the concentration sensed at the basolateral surface of the thick ascending limb of Henle, an acute infusion results in an abrupt increase in serum concentration and often a dramatic increase in renal magnesium excretion. For this reason much of intravenously administered magnesium is quickly excreted by the kidney.

In the absence of a life-threatening condition magnesium is administered orally. Oral administration is more efficient because it results in less of an acute rise in serum magnesium concentration. Some of the more common oral magnesium preparations are shown in Table 12.2. Slow release preparations of magnesium chloride and magnesium lactate are preferable since they cause less diarrhea. Diarrhea is the major side effect of magnesium repletion that limits therapy. A range of 300–1200 mg/day in divided doses is generally required. Attempts are also made to correct the underlying condition. Drugs that result in renal magnesium wasting should be minimized. Amiloride increases magnesium reabsorption in the distal convoluted tubule and collecting duct and may reduce renal magnesium wasting or decrease the dose of magnesium replacement if diarrhea becomes problematic. Amiloride is not used in patients with impaired renal function because of the risk of hyperkalemia.

Table 12.2

Oral Magnesium Preparations

PREPARATION	MOLECULAR WEIGHT	FORMULA	MG MG/GM	MEQ MG/GM
Mg carbonate	84	$MgCO_3$	289	24
Mg chloride	203.3	$MgCl_2 \cdot 6H_2O$	119	10
Mg gluconate	414.6	$(CH_2OH(CHOH)_4COO)_2Mg$	58	5
Mg lactate	202.4	$Mg(C_3H_5O_3)_2$	120	10
Mg oxide	40.32	MgO	602	50
Mg sulfate	246.5	$MgSO_4 \cdot 7H_2O$	98	8

Certain cardiovascular conditions deserve special comment. Hypomagnesemia was implicated in ventricular and atrial arrhythmias in patients with cardiac disease. Patients with mild hypomagnesemia in the setting of an acute myocardial infarction (MI) have a two-to threefold increased incidence of ventricular arrhythmias in the first 24 hours. This relationship persists for as long as 2–3 weeks after an MI. Magnesium should be maintained in the normal range in this setting.

The American Heart Association Guidelines for Cardiopulmonary Resuscitation recommend the use of intravenous magnesium for the treatment of torsade de pointes and refractory ventricular fibrillation. Torsade de pointes is a ventricular arrhythmia often precipitated by drugs that prolong the QT interval. The exact mechanism of action of magnesium is unknown. Magnesium does not shorten the QT interval and its effect may be mediated via the inhibition of sodium channels.

Hypomagnesemia is common after cardiopulmonary bypass and may result in an increased incidence of atrial and ventricular arrhythmias. Studies on prophylactic magnesium repletion in this setting are conflicting with some showing a reduction in the incidence of atrial fibrillation postcardiac surgery and others no effect.

Studies of magnesium administration in the setting of ischemic heart disease show conflicting results. In animal models magnesium limits ischemia reperfusion injury if given prior to reperfusion. Two large clinical trials examined this issue in the setting of acute MI in humans. In LIMIT-2 a randomized, placebo-controlled, double-blind study in 2316 patients with acute MI, magnesium was given prior to the onset of thrombolysis. There was a 24% reduction in relative risk of mortality in the first month in the treatment group. ISIS-4, however, showed no benefit from magnesium in the setting of acute MI. In this study magnesium was not given until after thrombolysis and an average of 8 hours after the onset of chest pain. Animal models show that the benefit is lost if magnesium is administered after reperfusion.

Epidemiologic studies revealed an association between hypomagnesemia and atherosclerotic cardiovascular disease. The Atherosclerosis Risk in Communities Study (ARIC) followed a cohort of 15,792 subjects over a 4–7-year period. The relative risk of coronary heart disease in men and women increased as serum magnesium concentration decreased. This finding was statistically significant only in women. Men and women that developed coronary heart disease during the study had a lower serum magnesium concentration. Other studies showed that as the magnesium concentration of drinking water increased the incidence of ischemic heart disease decreased. Magnesium deficiency in animal models promotes atherosclerosis. Hypomagnesemia activates macrophages, stimulates the peroxidation of lipoproteins, and increases circulating concentrations of proinflammatory cytokines. Magnesium repletion is associated with improvement in lipid profile, a decrease in insulin resistance, reduction of free radical generation, and inhibition of platelet reactivity. All of these factors play a role in the atherosclerotic process.

KEY POINTS
Treatment of Hypomagnesemia

1. The route of magnesium repletion varies depending on the severity of associated symptoms. The treatment goal is to increase the serum concentration above 1.0 mg/dL.
2. Magnesium is administered cautiously in patients with impaired renal function and serum concentration monitored frequently.
3. Magnesium is administered orally in the absence of a life-threatening condition. Amiloride may reduce renal magnesium wasting but should not be used in patients with impaired renal function.
4. Magnesium should be maintained in the normal range in the setting of ischemic heart disease.
5. Hypomagnesemia is associated with an increased risk of a variety of cardiovascular conditions including atrial and ventricular arrhythmias, torsade de pointes, and atherosclerotic cardiovascular disease.

Hypermagnesemia

Etiology

The kidney is capable of excreting virtually the entire filtered load of magnesium in the presence of an increased serum magnesium concentration

Table 12.3
Etiologies of Hypermagnesemia

Intravenous magnesium load in the absence of chronic kidney disease
Treatment of preterm labor
Treatment of eclampsia
Oral magnesium load in the presence of chronic kidney disease
Laxatives
Antacids
Epsom slats
Miscellaneous
Salt water drowning

or a decrease in the glomerular filtration rate. For this reason hypermagnesemia is relatively uncommon. Some of the more common etiologies are shown in Table 12.3. It most often occurs with magnesium administration in the setting of a severe decrease in glomerular filtration rate. It was recently reported with magnesium-containing cathartics in patients with renal failure, intravenous magnesium for postpartum eclampsia in patients with renal failure, and in patients using Epsom salts (magnesium sulfate) as a mouthwash.

The most common cause of hypermagnesemia is CKD. As glomerular filtration rate falls the fractional excretion of magnesium increases. This allows magnesium balance to be maintained until the glomerular filtration rate falls well below 30 mL/minute. Mild hypermagnesemia resulting from decreased renal excretion of magnesium can occur with lithium intoxication and familial hypocalciuric hypercalcemia. This is due to the interaction of lithium with the basolateral calcium magnesium-sensing receptor in the thick ascending limb of Henle. Antagonism of this receptor causes enhanced magnesium reabsorption.

Intravenous administration of magnesium can result in hypermagnesemia even in the absence of CKD. The typical setting is obstetrical with magnesium infused for the management of preterm labor or eclampsia. Typical protocols often result in serum magnesium concentrations of 4–8 mg/dL. Hypermagnesemia due to oral magnesium ingestion occurs most commonly in the setting of CKD. Cathartics, antacids, and Epsom salts are frequently the source of magnesium. Advanced age, CKD, and GI disturbances that enhance magnesium absorption such as decreased motility, gastritis, and colitis are contributing factors. A rare setting where magnesium concentration may be elevated is salt water drowning. Seawater is high in magnesium (14 mg/dL) with the Dead Sea having the highest recorded concentration (394 mg/dL).

KEY POINTS
Etiology of Hypermagnesemia

1. In the presence of an increased serum magnesium concentration or a decrease in the glomerular filtration rate the kidney is capable of excreting virtually the entire filtered load of magnesium.
2. Hypermagnesemia most commonly occurs with magnesium administration in patients with severe decreases in glomerular filtration rate.
3. Hypermagnesemia with oral magnesium ingestion occurs most commonly in the setting of CKD.

Signs and Symptoms

Hypermagnesemia can result in significant neuromuscular and cardiac toxicity. Magnesium blocks the synaptic transmission of nerve impulses. Initially this results in lethargy and drowsiness. As magnesium concentration increases deep tendon reflexes are diminished (4–8 mg/dL). Deep tendon reflexes are lost and mental status decreases at serum magnesium concentrations of 8–12 mg/dL. If the magnesium rises further (>12 mg/dL) flaccid paralysis and apnea may ensue. Parasympathetic

blockage resulting in fixed and dilated pupils that mimics brainstem herniation was reported. Smooth muscle can be affected resulting in ileus and urinary retention.

In cardiac tissue, magnesium blocks calcium and potassium channels required for repolarization. At serum magnesium concentrations above 7 mg/dL hypotension and ECG changes such as PR prolongation, QRS widening and QT prolongation are noted. At magnesium concentrations greater than 10 mg/dL ventricular fibrillation, complete heart block, and cardiac arrest occur.

KEY POINTS
Signs and Symptoms of Hypermagnesemia

1. At magnesium concentrations between 4 and 8 mg/dL deep tendon reflexes are diminished. Deep tendon reflexes are lost and mental status decreases at serum magnesium concentrations of 8–12 mg/dL. At serum magnesium concentrations greater than 12 mg/dL flaccid paralysis and apnea may ensue.
2. Magnesium blocks calcium and potassium channels required for repolarization in the heart.
3. Hypotension and ECG changes such as PR prolongation, QRS widening, and QT prolongation are noted at serum magnesium concentrations above 7 mg/dL.
4. Fatal complications such as ventricular fibrillation, complete heart block, and cardiac arrest were reported at magnesium concentrations greater than 10 mg/dL.

Diagnosis

Hypermagnesemia is often iatrogenic. A careful medication history is essential to determine the source of the magnesium, whether intravenous, as in the treatment of obstetrical disorders, or oral.

Laxatives, antacids, and Epsom salts are the most common oral sources of magnesium. High doses of intravenous magnesium may result in hypermagnesemia in the absence of kidney disease. Hypermagnesemia from increased gastrointestinal absorption of magnesium often requires some degree of renal impairment. The elderly are at increased risk, often because the degree of decrease in glomerular filtration rate is not adequately appreciated based on the serum creatinine concentration. For example, an 85-year-old Caucasian female weighing 50 kg with a serum creatinine of 1.5 mg/dL may have a creatinine clearance as low as 20 mL/minute. The elderly often have decreased intestinal motility that further increases intestinal magnesium absorption.

KEY POINTS
Diagnosis of Hypermagnesemia

1. Hypermagnesemia is commonly iatrogenic.
2. Hypermagnesemia from intravenous infusion of magnesium can occur in the absence of kidney disease.
3. Some degree of renal impairment is often present in patients developing hypermagnesemia from increased GI absorption of magnesium.
4. The elderly are at increased risk.

Treatment

Since the majority of cases of hypermagnesemia are iatrogenic, caution should be exercised in the use of magnesium salts especially in patients with CKD, those with GI disorders that may increase magnesium absorption, and in the elderly. Patients with CKD should be cautioned to avoid magnesium-containing antacids and laxatives. If the patient has hypotension or respiratory depression calcium (100–200 mg of elemental calcium over 5–10 minutes) is administered intravenously. The source of magnesium should be stopped.

Renal magnesium excretion is increased with a normal saline infusion and/or furosemide administration. In the patient with severe CKD or end-stage renal disease dialysis is often required. Hemodialysis is the modality of choice if the patient's hemodynamics can tolerate it, since it removes more magnesium than continuous venovenous hemofiltration or peritoneal dialysis.

KEY POINTS
Treatment of Hypermagnesemia

1. Caution should be exercised in the use of magnesium salts in high-risk patients.
2. Intravenous calcium can be used if the patient has significant hypotension or respiratory depression.
3. The source of magnesium should be stopped. If renal function is normal, saline infusion and/or furosemide administration are employed if the rate of renal magnesium excretion needs to be increased.
4. In severe hypermagnesemia hemodialysis is often required in those with significant CKD or end-stage renal disease.

Additional Reading

Agus, Z.S. Hypomagnesemia. *J Am Soc Nephrol* 10:1616–1622, 1999.

Agus, M.S, Agus, Z.S. Cardiovascular actions of magnesium. *Crit Care Clin* 17:175–186, 2001.

Al-Ghamdi, S.M., Cameron, E.C., Sutton, R.A. Magnesium deficiency: pathophysiologic and clinical overview. *Am J Kidney Dis* 24:737–752, 1994.

Cole, D.E., Quamme, G.A. Inherited disorders of renal magnesium handling. *J Am Soc Nephrol* 11:1937–1947, 2000.

Elisaf, M., Panteli, K., Theodorou, J., Siamopoulos, K.C. Fractional excretion of magnesium in normal subjects and in patients with hypomagnesemia. *Magnes Res* 10:315–320, 1997.

Fiser, R.T., Torres, A. Jr., Butch, A.W., Valentine, J.L. Ionized magnesium concentrations in critically ill children. *Crit Care Med* 26:2048–2052, 1998.

Konrad, M., Weber, S. Recent advances in molecular genetics of hereditary magnesium-losing disorders. *J Am Soc Nephrol* 14:249–260, 2003.

Simon, D.B., Lu, Y., Choate, K.A., Velazquez, H., Al-Sabban, E., Praga, M., Casari, G., Bettinelli, A., Colussi, G., Rodriguez-Soriano, J., McCredie, D., Milford, D., Sanjad, S., Lifton, RP. Paracellin-1, a renal tight junction protein required for paracellular Mg^{2+} resorption. *Science* 285:103–106, 1999.

Topf, J.M, Murray P.T. Hypomagnesemia and hypermagnesemia. *Rev Endocr Metab Disord* 4:195–206, 2003.

Weisinger, J.R., Bellorin-Font, E. Magnesium and phosphorus. *Lancet* 352:391–396, 1998.

Robert F. Reilly, Jr.

Nephrolithiasis

Recommended Time to Complete: 2 days

Guiding Questions

1. Why do stones form in the urinary tract?
2. How does one evaluate the patient with renal colic and what is the likelihood that a stone will pass spontaneously?
3. What are the important risk factors for the formation of calcium-containing stones?
4. Is there an optimal approach to the patient with a single calcium-containing stone?
5. How does one evaluate and treat the patient with multiple recurrent calcium-containing stones?
6. Which risk factors are most important for the formation of uric acid stones?
7. What role does bacterial infection play in struvite stones?
8. Why is medical therapy difficult in patients with cystine stones?
9. Which prescription and over-the-counter drugs form stones in the urinary tract?

Introduction

Kidney stones are a common problem facing nephrologists, urologists, and general internists in the United States with an annual incidence of 10–20 per 10,000. The frequency of stone formation varies with sex and race. Men are affected 3–4 times more often than women and Caucasians more frequently than African Americans or Asians. By age 70 as many as 20% of all Caucasian men and 7% of all Caucasian women will have formed a kidney stone. The peak incidence for the initial episode of renal colic occurs early in life between the ages 20 and 35. In women there is a second peak at age 55. Nephrolithiasis is a major cause of morbidity due to pain (renal colic), renal parenchymal damage from obstruction of the urinary tract, and infection.

Calcium-containing stones make up approximately 80% of all stones in the United States and contain calcium oxalate either alone or in combination with calcium phosphate. The remainder are composed of uric acid or struvite. Cystine stones are rare in adults. In more arid climates, such as the Middle East, uric acid stones are more common than calcium-containing stones. Studies based on samples received by stone analysis laboratories suggest that 10–20% of all stones are made up of struvite but this is due to an overrepresentation of stones from surgical specimens.

A kidney stone is an organized mass of crystals that grows on the surface of a renal papilla. They result whenever the excretory burden of a poorly soluble salt exceeds the volume of urine available to dissolve it. Supersaturation of urine with respect to a stone-forming salt is necessary but not sufficient for stone formation. Interestingly, in normal patients urine is often supersaturated with respect to calcium oxalate, calcium phosphate, and uric acid yet stone formation does not occur. Other factors such as heterogeneous nucleation and inhibitors of crystallization play an important role in the pathogenesis of stone formation.

Heterogeneous nucleation refers to the principle that crystallization requires less energy when a surface is present on which it can grow, as opposed to in the absence of a surface (homogeneous nucleation). Normal urine contains several inorganic and organic inhibitors of crystallization. Citrate, magnesium, and pyrophosphate are the most important of these.

A recent study of 19 stone formers shed additional light on the pathophysiology of kidney stone formation. Surprisingly, the initial site of crystal formation was on the basolateral surface of the thin limb of the loop of Henle in 15 patients with idiopathic hypercalciuria. Stones consisted of a core of calcium phosphate surrounded by a shell of calcium oxalate. The crystal nidus eroded through the surface of the renal papilla into the renal pelvis. Why calcium phosphate precipitates in this region of the nephron remains unclear. Another four patients formed stones after intestinal bypass surgery. In this subgroup calcium phosphate crystals initially attached to the luminal membrane of inner medullary collecting duct (IMCD) cells. The deposit acted as a nidus for further calcium oxalate precipitation resulting in luminal occlusion and stone growth out into the renal pelvis. Further studies are needed to examine those factors important for calcium salt precipitation in the renal medulla and crystal attachment in the IMCD.

KEY POINTS

Kidney Stones

1. Nephrolithiasis is a common clinical problem whose frequency varies with sex and race.
2. Calcium oxalate stones are the most common stone in the United States.
3. Supersaturation is required but not sufficient for stone formation.
4. Other factors such as heterogeneous nucleation and inhibitors play an important role in the pathogenesis of stone formation.

The Patient with Renal Colic

Stones form on the surface of a renal papilla and if they remain there do not produce symptoms. If the stone dislodges it can impact anywhere between the ureteropelvic and ureterovesicular junction resulting in renal colic. Renal colic presents as severe flank pain that begins suddenly, peaks within 30 minutes, and remains constant and unbearable. It requires narcotics for relief and is associated with nausea and vomiting. The pattern of pain radiation may provide a clue as to where in the urinary tract the stone is lodged. Pain radiating around the flank and into the groin is common for a stone trapped at the ureteropelvic junction. Signs of bladder irritation such as dysuria, frequency, and urgency are associated with stones lodged at the ureterovesicular junction (the narrowest portion of the ureter). Pain may radiate to the testicles or vulva. Struvite stones are often incidentally discovered on plain abdominal radiograph since they are generally too large to move into the ureter. The abdominal, rectal, and pelvic examination are directed at ruling out other potential etiologies of abdominal pain. Physical examination is remarkable for costovertebral angle tenderness and muscle spasm.

A complete blood count, serum chemistries, and urinalysis are required to evaluate patients. The white blood cell (WBC) count may be mildly elevated due to the stress of the acute event. A WBC count greater than 15,000 cells/mm^3 suggests either another intraabdominal cause for the pain or pyelonephritis behind an obstructing calculus. An elevation of the serum blood urea nitrogen (BUN) and creatinine concentrations is not common and if present is usually secondary to prerenal azotemia from volume depletion. Obstruction of a solitary functioning kidney, as is the case after a renal transplant, will result in acute renal failure. Any patient with abdominal pain should have a careful urinalysis performed. Approximately 90% of patients with renal colic will have microscopic hematuria.

If nephrolithiasis is suspected after the initial evaluation, one must next establish a definitive diagnosis. A radiograph of the abdomen can identify radio-opaque stones larger than or equal to 2 mm in size (calcium oxalate and phosphate, struvite, and cystine stones). Radiolucent stones (uric acid) and stones that overlie the bony pelvis are often missed. Unfortunately, two-thirds of kidney stones trapped in the ureter will overlie the bony pelvis. As a result, an abdominal radiograph is most valuable to rule out other intraabdominal processes. It is not sensitive enough to exclude nephrolithiasis with certainty. An ultrasound examination readily identifies stones in the renal pelvis, but is much less accurate for detecting ureteral stones. The intravenous pyelogram (IVP) was formerly the gold standard for the diagnosis of renal colic. It identifies the site of the obstruction, although the stone itself may not be visualized. Structural or anatomic abnormalities and renal or ureteral complications can be detected. Major disadvantages of the IVP include the need for intravenous contrast and the prolonged waiting time required to adequately visualize the collecting system in the presence of obstruction. As a result, spiral computerized tomography (CT) is the test of choice in the majority of emergency departments. Spiral CT is highly sensitive, rapid, and does not require contrast. It may also identify the site of obstruction. An example of a kidney stone detected on spiral CT scanning is shown in Figure 13.1. If the patient does not have a stone the spiral CT may also identify other causes of abdominal pain such as appendicitis and ischemic bowel.

After a stone is identified in the ureter by spiral CT, subsequent management involves an assessment of the likelihood of spontaneous passage, the degree of pain present, and whether there is suspected urinary tract infection (UTI). The probability of spontaneous passage is related to the stone size and its location in the ureter at the time

Figure 13.1

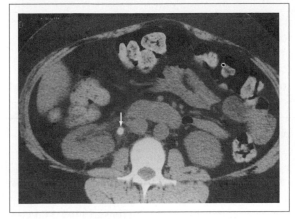

Spiral CT scan of a kidney stone. Shown by the arrow is a kidney stone impacted in the ureter.

of initial presentation (Table 13.1). In general, the smaller the stone and the more distal in the ureter it is located, the higher the likelihood of spontaneous passage. The patient with pain that cannot be managed with oral medication or with evidence of pyelonephritis requires hospital admission for parenteral analgesics and/or antibiotics. Stones unlikely to pass spontaneously require further urologic intervention.

Table 13.1

Likelihood of Spontaneous Kidney Stone Passage

Size
>6 mm—0–25%
4–6 mm—20–60%
<4 mm—50–90%
Location
Upper ureter
  ≥6 mm—<1%
  ≤4 mm—40–80%
Lower ureter
  ≤4 mm—70–95%

KEY POINTS

The Patient with Renal Colic

1. The radiation pattern of renal colic may provide a clue as to where in the ureter the stone is lodged.
2. A WBC count greater than 15,000 cells/mm^3 is indicative of either another intraabdominal cause for pain or pyelonephritis behind an obstructing calculus.
3. Microscopic hematuria is present in 90% of patients.
4. Spiral CT is the diagnostic test of choice in the patient with suspected renal colic.
5. The size of the stone and its location in the ureter at the time of initial presentation determine its likelihood of spontaneous passage.

Risk Factors for Calcium-Containing Stones

Calcium-containing stones make up the majority of stones in the United States and are generally composed of a mixture of calcium oxalate and calcium phosphate. In mixed stones calcium oxalate predominates, and pure calcium oxalate stones are more common than pure calcium phosphate stones. Calcium phosphate precipitates in alkaline urine, whereas calcium oxalate precipitation does not vary with pH. Since urine is acidic in most patients on a standard Western diet, calcium oxalate stones are more common. Hypercalciuria, hypocitraturia, hyperuricosuria, hyperoxaluria, low urine volume, and medullary sponge kidney are the major risk factors for calcium-containing stone formation. Patients may form calcium-containing stones with a single or any combination of risk factors. Some patients form

Table 13.2

Abnormal Values for Calcium Oxalate Stone Risk Factors

	MG/24 HOURS	
SUBSTANCE	MALE	FEMALE
Calcium	>200	>200
Uric acid	>800	>750
Oxalate	>45	>45
Citrate	<320	<320

calcium-containing stones with no risk factors indicating that our knowledge of the stone-forming process is incomplete. The upper limits of normal in a 24-hour urine for some of these risk factors in men and women are shown in Table 13.2.

Hypercalciuria is present in as many as two-thirds of patients with calcium-containing stones. It results from an increased filtered load, decreased proximal tubular reabsorption, or decreased distal tubular reabsorption. Proximal tubular calcium reabsorption is similar to sodium. Whenever proximal sodium reabsorption is decreased there is a parallel decrease in proximal calcium reabsorption and vice versa. Distal nephron calcium reabsorption is stimulated by parathyroid hormone (PTH) and diuretics (thiazides and amiloride) and inhibited by acidosis and phosphate depletion.

The most common cause of hypercalciuria (90%) is idiopathic. In three families the absorptive hypercalciuria phenotype was localized to a region of chromosome 1 (1q23.3-q24). Although the precise mechanism is unknown these patients have increased $1,25(OH)_2$ vitamin D_3 (calcitriol) concentration, low PTH concentration, and reduced bone mineral density. Three potential pathophysiologic mechanisms were proposed: increased intestinal calcium absorption; enhanced bone demineralization; and decreased renal calcium or phosphorus reabsorption. Patients with idiopathic hypercalciuria can be subdivided on the basis of a fast and calcium load study into

absorptive hypercalciuria types I, II, and III and renal leak hypercalciuria. This is based on the assumption that if the physiologic mechanism is identified this information will guide specific therapy. In practice, however, this is often unnecessary. Randomized controlled trials of pharmacologic intervention did not subdivide patients in this fashion.

Other important causes of hypercalciuria include primary hyperparathyroidism, renal tubular acidosis (RTA), sarcoidosis, immobilization, Paget's disease, hyperthyroidism, milk-alkali syndrome, and vitamin D intoxication. Filtered calcium load is increased in primary hyperparathyroidism due to bone calcium release and increased intestinal calcium absorption mediated by calcitriol. In the subset of patients with hypercalciuria increased filtered load overcomes distal PTH action to increase calcium excretion. In RTA, an increased filtered calcium load results from bone calcium release in response to buffering of systemic acidosis. Acidosis also directly inhibits distal tubular calcium reabsorption. In sarcoidosis macrophages produce calcitriol via activation of 1α hydroxylase leading to increased intestinal calcium absorption with a resultant increase in filtered load. Immobilization, Paget's disease, and hyperthyroidism result in calcium release from bone and increase the filtered load.

Citrate is an important inhibitor of calcium oxalate precipitation in urine. It complexes calcium in the tubular lumen and as a result there is less calcium available to associate with oxalate. Citrate also deposits on the surface of calcium oxalate crystals and prevents them from growing and aggregating. This latter effect may be more important. It was estimated that the transit time of a crystal through the nephron is 2–3 minutes. This is too short a period for growth of a single crystal to occlude the tubular lumen or form a stone; however, crystal aggregation is a much more rapid process and may play a role in either the occlusion of the tubular lumen or stone growth on the surface of the renal papilla. Chronic metabolic acidosis as occurs with chronic diarrhea or distal RTA and an acid-loading diet high in protein enhance proximal tubular citrate reabsorption and reduce urinary citrate concentration. Hypokalemia also causes hypocitraturia. Sodium-citrate cotransporter expression in the apical membrane of proximal tubule is upregulated with hypokalemia.

Hyperuricosuria is an important risk factor for calcium-containing stone formation. Uric acid and monosodium urate decrease calcium oxalate and calcium phosphate solubility by several mechanisms. They act as a nidus on which calcium salts can precipitate. As discussed above less energy is required to form a crystal on a surface (heterogeneous nucleation). Uric acid can bind to macromolecular inhibitors and decrease their activity.

Oxalate in urine is derived from two sources. The majority comes from endogenous production in liver. The remainder (10–40%) is derived from dietary oxalate and ascorbic acid. The most common causes of hyperoxaluria include enteric hyperoxaluria from inflammatory bowel disease, small bowel resection, or jejuno-ileal bypass; dietary excess; and the very uncommon inherited disorder primary hyperoxaluria. In enteric hyperoxaluria, intestinal hyperabsorption of oxalate occurs via two mechanisms. Free fatty acids bind calcium and decrease the amount available to complex oxalate increasing free oxalate, which can then be absorbed. In addition, bile salts and fatty acids increase colonic oxalate permeability. Intestinal fluid losses also decrease urine volume, and bicarbonate and potassium losses can lead to hypocitraturia.

Low urine volume is a very common risk factor for calcium-containing stone formation. The risk of stone formation in the United States is largest in areas where temperature is highest and humidity lowest (the stone belt of the Southeast and Southwest).

Studies show that 3–12% of patients with calcium-containing stones have medullary sponge kidney. One should have a high index of suspicion for medullary sponge kidney in women and those that do not have any of the previously discussed risk factors for calcium-containing stone formation. It occurs in 1 in 5000 patients and involves men and women with equal frequency. The medullary and inner papillary collecting ducts are irregularly enlarged resulting in urinary stasis that promotes precipitation and attachment of crystals to the tubular epithelium. An IVP establishes the diagnosis revealing linear papillary striations or collections of contrast media in dilated collecting ducts. Patients present in the fourth or fifth decade with kidney stones or recurrent urinary tract infection that may be associated with a distal RTA.

Nanobacteria were isolated in all 30 calcium-containing stones in one report. Nanobacteria grow in protein- and lipid-free environments. They can nucleate carbonate apatite on their surface at physiologic pH. A subsequent study, however, failed to detect nanobacteria in 10 calcium-containing stones. A recent study called into question the existence of nanobacteria. The development of biomineralization that had been attributed to nanobacteria could not be inhibited by sodium azide (a potent inhibitor of mitochondrial respiration). Amplification of nanobacterial DNA from stone samples appears to have resulted from contamination with DNA from other bacterial species. In addition, biomineralization was shown to reoccur in diluted samples by self-propagation of microcrystalline apatite. The role of these bacteria in calcium-containing stone formation is unclear at present.

KEY POINTS
Risk Factors for Calcium-Containing Stones

1. Important risk factors for calcium-containing stone formation are hypercalciuria, hypocitraturia, hyperuricosuria, hyperoxaluria, low urine volume, and medullary sponge kidney.
2. Hypercalciuria is most commonly idiopathic but other important causes are primary hyperparathyroidism, RTA, and sarcoidosis.

3. Calcium phosphate stones suggest the diagnosis of RTA or primary hyperparathyroidism.
4. Citrate is the most important inhibitor of calcium oxalate precipitation in urine.
5. Uric acid and monosodium urate act as a nidus for the precipitation of calcium oxalate by a variety of mechanisms.
6. Anatomic abnormalities of the urinary tract should be suspected when patients in low-risk groups (women) form stones.

The Patient with a Single Calcium-Containing Stone

The assessment of the patient with an initial calcium-containing stone includes a careful history and physical examination evaluating for a family history of stone disease, skeletal disease, inflammatory bowel disease, and urinary tract infection. Environmental risk factors such as fluid intake, urine volume, immobilization, diet, medications, and vitamin ingestion are examined. Initial laboratory studies include blood chemistries, urinalysis, and either an abdominal radiograph or a spiral CT to assess stone burden. Stone analysis is always performed if the patient saved the stone. One study showed that in 15% of cases analyses of 24-hour urines would not have correctly predicted the chemical composition of the stone. Stone analysis is inexpensive, establishes a specific diagnosis, and can help direct therapy.

Most authors recommend that the patient with a single isolated stone and no associated systemic disease be managed with nonspecific forms of treatment including increased fluid intake and a normal calcium diet. Increasing fluid intake is the cheapest way to reduce urinary supersaturation.

In a prospective randomized trial of 199 first-time stone formers followed for a 5-year period, the risk of recurrent stone formation was reduced 55% by increasing urine volume to greater than 2 L/day with water intake. If the patient will not drink water, lemonade is a sensible, but unproven, alternative. Lemon juice is low in oxalate and high in citrate. One should keep in mind that the likelihood of future stone formation is high, approximately 50% in the subsequent 5–8 years. In high-risk subgroups (Caucasian males), patients with significant morbidity from the initial event (nephrectomy), or patients with a solitary functioning kidney, a more aggressive approach may be warranted (see the section on the patient with multiple or recurrent calcium-containing stones).

In the past, patients with calcium-containing stones were advised to follow a low-calcium diet. Recent studies, however, suggest that a low-calcium diet may increase the risk of stone formation. The postulated mechanism is that ingested calcium complexes dietary oxalate and a reduction in dietary calcium results in a reciprocal increase in intestinal oxalate absorption. This increases urinary supersaturation of calcium oxalate. Confounding factors may also play a role, however, in that high calcium diets are also associated with increased ingestion and excretion of phosphorus, magnesium, and citrate, as well as increased urine pH and volume, factors that also reduce the incidence of stone formation. Recently, a randomized prospective trial compared patients on a low-calcium diet to those on a normal calcium, low-sodium, and low-protein diet. The relative risk of stone formation was reduced 51% in those consuming a normal calcium diet. Based on these findings the safest approach is to recommend a normal calcium diet.

The Atkins diet adversely impacts several risk factors for calcium-containing stone formation. In one study net acid excretion increased 56 meq/day, urinary citrate fell from 763 mg to 449 mg/day, urinary pH declined from 6.09 to 5.67, and urine calcium excretion increased from 160 mg to 248 mg/day. High-protein, low-carbohydrate diets are best avoided in patients with a history of calcium-containing kidney stones.

The question of whether supplemental calcium increases the risk of nephrolithiasis in women is unclear. One report suggested that any use of supplemental calcium raises the relative risk of stone disease 20%. Surprisingly, the risk did not increase with increasing dose. The timing of calcium ingestion (with meals or between meals) was not addressed.

KEY POINTS
Risk Factors for Calcium Containing Stones

1. The majority of first-time calcium-containing stone formers can be managed by increasing fluid intake.
2. Stone analysis is cheap and may help guide future management.
3. Dietary calcium restriction should be avoided.
4. Supplemental calcium may increase the risk of stone formation in some patients.

The Patient with Multiple or Recurrent Calcium-Containing Stones

Complicated calcium-containing stone disease is defined as the presence of multiple stones, new stone formation, enlargement of existing stones, or passage of gravel. This is established based on initial evaluation and these patients require a full metabolic evaluation. Serum calcium concentration is measured and if any value is above 10 mg/dL a PTH concentration must be obtained. Blood chemistries are evaluated for the presence of RTA. At least two 24-hour urine collections are obtained on the patient's usual diet for calcium, citrate, uric acid, oxalate, sodium, creatinine, and pH. Further therapeutic intervention depends on the results of these collections. An IVP may be indicated to evaluate the possibility of structural abnormalities predisposing to stone formation especially if the stone disease is unilateral. If a specific disease is identified such as primary hyperparathyroidism, sarcoidosis, enteric hyperoxaluria, or primary gout, it is treated appropriately.

The patient with complicated disease is managed with both nonspecific and specific treatment. Nonspecific therapies such as increased fluid intake and a normal calcium diet were discussed above. Specific therapies vary depending on risk factor assessment derived from 24-hour urine testing. Treatment is based on therapies shown to be effective in randomized placebo-controlled clinical trials with a follow-up period of at least 1 year, the results of which are shown in Table 13.3. This is critical because of the "stone clinic effect." After a patient develops a symptomatic kidney stone, the next several months are often characterized by a period of decreased risk for new stone formation (*stone clinic effect*). At least two factors play a role in this process: regression to the mean and increased adherence to nonspecific treatments (increased fluid intake). Pharmacologic agents that reduced the risk of stone formation in randomized placebo-controlled trials are thiazides, allopurinol, potassium citrate, and potassium magnesium citrate.

Hypercalciuria is the most common abnormality and is treated with thiazide diuretics. Clinical trials showing benefit used hydrochlorothiazide 25 mg bid, chlorthalidone 50 mg daily, or indapamide 2.5 mg daily. Thiazides directly increase distal tubular calcium reabsorption and indirectly increase calcium reabsorption in the proximal tubule by inducing mild volume contraction. For thiazides to be maximally effective, one must maintain volume contraction and avoid hypokalemia. They usually decrease urine calcium excretion by 50%. If ineffective, the usual reason is a high sodium intake. Proximal reabsorption of sodium and calcium is decreased and urinary calcium excretion increased

Table 13.3
Randomized Placebo-Controlled Trials

TREATMENT	DOSE	PATIENT GROUP
Water	Urine volume >2L	Unselected
HCTZ	25 mg bid	Unselected
Chlorthalidone	50 mg qd	Unselected
Indapamide	2.5 mg qd	Hypercalciuria
Allopurinol	300 mg qd	Hyperuricosuria
K$^+$ citrate	60 meq qd	Hypocitraturia
K$^+$-Mg^{2+} citrate	40 meq qd	Unselected

Abbreviations: HCTZ, hydrochlorothiazide; bid, twice a day; qd, once a day.

with volume expansion. A 24-hour urine for sodium will detect the patient with increased sodium intake. Amiloride acts in a more distal site, collecting duct, than thiazides and is added if needed. Three randomized controlled trials in recurrent stone formers showed a reduced risk for new stone formation with thiazides. Although patients in these trials had calcium-containing stones, the majority were not hypercalciuric, suggesting that thiazides have effects in addition to decreasing urine calcium or that reduction of urine calcium decreases the risk of recurrent stone formation even in the absence of hypercalciuria.

Sodium cellulose phosphate and orthophosphate were used in patients who cannot tolerate thiazides, however, these therapies are often poorly tolerated as well. Slow-release neutral phosphate may be better tolerated from a gastrointestinal standpoint. A randomized controlled trial of potassium acid phosphate showed no effect compared to placebo.

Potassium citrate or potassium magnesium citrate were employed in patients with and without hypocitraturia. Each reduced the relative risk of stone formation in placebo-controlled trials. In patients taking thiazides potassium magnesium citrate has the advantage that it replaces diuretic-induced potassium and magnesium losses. Patients with struvite stones should not receive citrate because it may increase stone growth.

Citrate increases intestinal aluminum absorption in chronic kidney disease patients and should be avoided. The use of citrate preparations is often complicated by diarrhea. Slow release citrate (10–20 meq with meals) is generally well tolerated but is relatively expensive. If urinary citrate excretion is <150 mg/day 60 meq is given in divided doses with meals. A total of 30 meq/day is given if urinary citrate excretion is >150 mg/day.

Hyperuricosuria is best treated with allopurinol. It is unclear whether alkalinization is of benefit since heterogeneous nucleation can be caused by sodium urate, as well as uric acid. Citrate administration might reduce the precipitation of calcium oxalate on the surface of uric acid crystals but this is unproven.

The degree of hyperoxaluria often provides a clue as to its etiology. Dietary hyperoxaluria is generally mild with urinary oxalate excretion between 40 and 60 mg/24 hours and is managed with a low-oxalate diet. Enteric hyperoxaluria is more severe with urinary oxalate excretion between 60 and 100 mg/24 hours. Initially, it is treated with a low-fat, low-oxalate diet. Calcium carbonate and/or cholestyramine can be added if this is unsuccessful. Primary hyperoxaluria is a rare autosomal recessive disorder and urinary oxalate excretion is often in excess of 100 mg/24 hours. It is the result of one of two enzyme defects in glyoxalate metabolism that leads to enhanced conversion of glyoxalate to oxalate. Type I disease is the result of a defect in hepatic peroxisomal alanine:glyoxalate aminotransferase. Pyridoxine is a cofactor of this enzyme. Type II disease is due to a defect in cytosolic glyoxalate reductase/D-glycerate dehydrogenase. Treatment of primary hyperoxaluria is difficult. Pyridoxine supplementation and maintenance of a high urine output can be tried. The disease often recurs in the transplanted kidney. Combined liver-kidney transplant may be the best treatment option for children with progressive type I disease.

If metabolic evaluation fails to detect risk factors for calcium-containing stone formation an IVP is performed to rule out medullary sponge kidney. One also needs to consider whether a trial of citrate alone or citrate plus hydrochlorothiazide is warranted. Both agents are relatively inexpensive and have limited toxicity. In addition, a significant percentage of patients in randomized placebo-controlled trials of thiazides and citrate had no detectable risk factors for stone formation. There is good reason to suspect, therefore, that these therapies would be effective in this subgroup of patients.

If thiazides, allopurinol, or citrate are prescribed, it is important to repeat the 24-hour urine in 6–8 weeks to examine the effect of pharmacologic intervention on urinary supersaturation of calcium oxalate, calcium phosphate, and uric acid. Several commercial laboratories provide this service. Computer programs (EQUIL) and algorithms are also capable of calculating supersaturation from a 24-hour urine collection.

This approach directed at specific and nonspecific risk factor reduction for calcium-containing stone disease decreases the frequency of recurrent stone formation, and reduces the number of cystoscopies, surgeries, and hospitalization.

KEY POINTS
The Patient with Multiple or Recurrent Calcium-Containing Stones

1. Complicated calcium-containing stone disease is present if the patient has multiple stones, evidence of the formation of new stones, enlargement of old stones, or the passage of gravel. This subgroup of patients requires complete metabolic evaluation.
2. Therapy is based on an analysis of risk factors for calcium-containing stones.
3. Treatment is guided by results of randomized placebo-controlled trials.
4. Urinary supersaturation of calcium oxalate, calcium phosphate, and uric acid is monitored with treatment.

Uric Acid Stones

Uric acid stones represent 5–10% of stone disease in the United States. Their highest incidence is reported in the Middle East, where as many as 75% of stones contain uric acid. This is secondary in part to the arid climate and reduced urinary volume. Unlike other mammals, humans do not express uricase that degrades uric acid into the much more soluble allantoin. Therefore, uric acid is the major metabolic end product of purine metabolism. Stones made up of uric acid are by far the most frequent radiolucent stone.

Uric acid has low solubility at acidic pH. It is a weak organic acid with two dissociable protons. Only the dissociation of the first proton, which occurs at a pK_a of 5.5, is of clinical relevance. At a pH of less than 5.5 it remains as an undissociated acid (uric acid), which is much less soluble than the salt (sodium urate). As pH increases, it dissociates into the more soluble salt, sodium urate. At pH 4.5 only 80 mg/L of uric acid is soluble, whereas at pH 6.5 1000 mg/L of sodium urate is dissolved. Because of the dramatic increase in solubility as urinary pH increases, uric acid stones remain the only kidney stones that can be completely dissolved with medical therapy alone. Patients with uric acid stones exhibit a lower urinary pH and ammonium ion excretion than normals. As many as 75% have a defect in renal ammoniagenesis in response to an acid load. Urinary buffers other than ammonia are titrated more fully with a resultant urine pH approximating 4.5. Patients with defects in ammoniagenesis, such as the elderly and those with polycystic kidney disease, are at increased risk for uric acid stones. There is also a high incidence of uric acid stones in patients with type II diabetes mellitus (34%). It has been suggested that a renal manifestation of insulin resistance may be reduced urinary ammonium excretion and decreased urine pH. Given the current epidemic of obesity and diabetes mellitus in the United States population uric acid stones may increase in frequency in the future.

The second most important risk factor for uric acid stone formation is decreased urine volume. Hyperuricosuria is the third and least important risk factor and is seen in less than 25% of patients with recurrent uric acid stones. The importance of urinary pH compared to uric acid excretion is illustrated by the fact that a three-fold increase in uric acid excretion from 500 to 1500 mg would not overcome the effect of a pH change from 5.0 to 6.0 that increases uric acid solubility sixfold.

Another determinant of uric acid solubility is the cations present in urine. Uric acid solubility is decreased by higher sodium concentration, and increased by higher potassium concentration. This may explain calcium phosphate stone formation that can occur during sodium alkali therapy but not with potassium alkali therapy. The sodium load increases urinary calcium excretion and reduces uric acid solubility while potassium does not.

Uric acid stones are more likely to pass spontaneously than calcium oxalate or phosphate stones, because of their smooth contour. Although a definitive diagnosis is established by stone analysis, uric acid stones are suggested by the presence of a radiolucent stone, or the presence of uric acid crystals in unusually acidic urine. Xanthine, hypoxanthine, and 2,8-dihydroxy-adenosine stones are radiolucent but are very rare. When a radiolucent stone fails to dissolve

with standard alkali therapy their presence should be suspected.

Etiologies are subdivided based on the three major risk factors. Low urine volume is important in gastrointestinal disorders such as Crohn's disease, ulcerative colitis, diarrhea, and ileostomies, as well as with dehydration. Acidic urinary pH plays an important role in primary gout and gastrointestinal disorders. Hyperuricosuria is subdivided based on whether hyperuricemia is present (primary gout, enzyme disorders, myeloproliferative diseases, hemolytic anemia, and uricosuric drugs) or absent (dietary excess). Primary gout is an inherited disorder transmitted in an autosomal dominant fashion with variable penetrance. Hyperuricemia, hyperuricosuria, and persistently acid urine are its hallmarks. Uric acid stones are present in 10–20% of patients. In a sizeable group (40%) stones occur before the first attack of gouty arthritis. Since urine is always acidic in patients with primary gout, the risk of uric acid stones will vary directly with serum and urinary uric acid concentration (Tables 13.4 and 13.5).

As might be expected therapy is directed at reversal of the three risk factors. First, urine volume is increased to 2 L/day or greater. Next, potassium citrate is employed to alkalinize the urine to pH 6.5. The starting dose is 10 meq tid with meals and one titrates upward to achieve the desired urine pH. More than 100 meq/day is rarely required.

Table 13.4

Risk of Uric Acid Stones in Patients with Primary Gout as a Function of Serum Urate Concentration

SERUM URATE (MG/DL)	WITH STONES (%)
5.1–7.0	11
7.1–9.0	18
9.1–11.0	25
11.1–13.0	28
>13.1	53

Adapted with permission from Yu, TE and Gutman AB, *Ann Intern Med* 67:1133–1148, 1967.

Table 13.5

Risk of Uric Acid Stones in Patients with Primary Gout as a Function of Urinary Urate Excretion

URINARY URATE EXCRETION (MG/24 HOURS)	WITH STONES (%)
<300	11
300–499	21
500–699	21
700–899	34
900–1,099	38
>1100	50

Adapted with permission from Yu, TE and Gutman AB, *Ann Intern Med* 67:1133–1148, 1967.

Sodium alkali therapy is less preferable since it may cause hypercalciuria. In a study of 12 patients with uric acid stones, alkali therapy resulted in complete stone dissolution in 1 to 5 months. Increases in urine pH above 6.5 are not necessary and should be avoided because of the potential risk of calcium phosphate precipitation. If early morning urine remains acidic acetazolamide (250 mg) is added before bedtime. If hyperuricosuria is present, one should first attempt to decrease purine consumption in the diet. Allopurinol is used in patients whose stones recur despite fluid and alkali, patients with difficulty tolerating this regimen (diarrhea), or when uric acid excretion is greater than 1000 mg/day. If allopurinol is administered in patients with massive uric acid overproduction as in the tumor lysis syndrome, adequate hydration must be ensured to avoid precipitation of xanthine and hypoxanthine.

KEY POINTS

Uric Acid Stones

1. Uric acid stones make up approximately 5–10% of kidney stones in the United States.
2. The three most important risk factors are decreased urine pH, decreased urine volume, and increased urinary uric acid excretion.
3. Of the three risk factors low urine pH is most important.
4. Due to their uniform round shape uric acid stones are more likely to pass spontaneously than calcium-containing stones.
5. Uric acid stones are the most common radiolucent stone.
6. Uric acid stones can be completely dissolved with medical therapy.

Struvite Stones

Struvite stones are composed of a combination of magnesium ammonium phosphate (struvite—$MgNH_4PO_4 \cdot 6H_2O$) and carbonate apatite $(Ca_{10}(PO_4)_6CO_3)$. It is suggested that they comprise 10–15% of all stones, however, this is likely an overestimation. These percentages are based on reports from chemical stone analyses and surgical specimens are overrepresented in these studies. It is likely that their true prevalence is less than 5% of kidney stones. Prior to more recent therapeutic urologic advances, they were the cause of significant morbidity and mortality. Struvite stones are the most common cause of staghorn calculi, although any stone may form a staghorn. Urine is supersaturated with struvite in only one circumstance—infection with urea splitting organisms that secrete urease. Urease-producing bacterial genuses include *Proteus, Morganella, Providencia, Pseudomonas, and Klebsiella. Escherichia coli* and *Citrobacter* do not express urease.

Women with recurrent UTI, patients with spinal cord injury or other forms of neurogenic bladder, and those with ileal ureteral diversions are at high risk for struvite stone formation. Struvite stones can present as fever, hematuria, flank pain, recurrent UTI, and septicemia. They grow and fill the renal pelvis as a staghorn calculus and are radio-opaque due to the carbonate apatite component. Rarely do they pass spontaneously and in many cases they are discovered incidentally. Loss of the affected kidney occurs in 50% of untreated patients.

For struvite stones to form, it is necessary that the urine be alkaline (pH greater than 7.0) and supersaturated with ammonium hydroxide. Urea is hydrolyzed to ammonia and carbon dioxide (Figure 13.2). Ammonia is converted to ammonium hydroxide. Carbon dioxide hydrates to form carbonic acid and then loses protons to form bicarbonate and carbonate. Elevated concentrations of ammonium hydroxide and carbonate at alkaline pH never occurs under physiologic conditions and is seen only with urinary tract infection with a urease-producing organism. The stone behaves like an infected foreign body. A symbiotic relationship develops, whereby bacteria provide conditions suitable for stone growth and the stone acts as a protected environment for the bacteria.

The majority of staghorn calculi are composed of struvite. Struvite stones are larger and less radiodense than calcium oxalate stones. The association of a kidney stone and an infected alkaline urine is highly suggestive of a struvite stone.

Definitive diagnosis, however, can only be established by stone analysis. If a UTI is associated with an acidic urine and a staghorn calculus, it is likely that the two are unrelated. All staghorn calculi should be cultured and sent for stone analysis after percutaneous nephrolithotomy or extracorporeal shock wave lithotripsy (ESWL) treatment. Stone culture is important since urine cultures are not always representative of the organism(s) present in the stone. *Proteus mirabilis* is the most common urease-producing organism isolated. If the culture is negative, one should consider the possibility of infection with *Ureaplasma urealyticum*. Some patients have stones that contain a mixture of struvite and calcium oxalate. A metabolic evaluation should be performed since these patients often have an underlying metabolic abnormality and are at higher risk for stone recurrence.

Open surgical removal is no longer the treatment of choice for staghorn struvite calculi given the high recurrence rate (27% after 6 years), however, and the persistence of UTI (41%). A combination of percutaneous nephrolithotomy and ESWL is currently the treatment of choice and is associated with improved outcomes compared with surgery. Total elimination of the stone is difficult. Small particles containing bacteria that

Figure 13.2

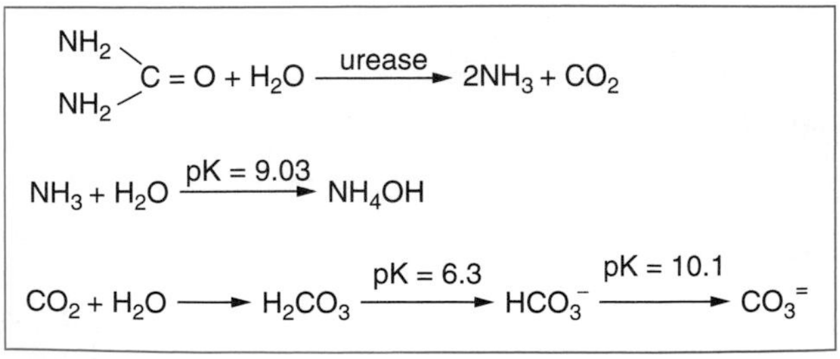

$$\begin{matrix} NH_2 \\ \diagdown \\ C = O + H_2O \xrightarrow{\text{urease}} 2NH_3 + CO_2 \\ \diagup \\ NH_2 \end{matrix}$$

$$NH_3 + H_2O \xrightarrow{pK = 9.03} NH_4OH$$

$$CO_2 + H_2O \longrightarrow H_2CO_3 \xrightarrow{pK = 6.3} HCO_3^- \xrightarrow{pK = 10.1} CO_3^=$$

Pathophysiology of struvite stone formation. Struvite does not form under physiologic conditions. Urease converts urea to ammonia and carbon dioxide. Ammonia hydrates to form ammonium hydroxide. The resultant high pH converts bicarbonate to carbonate. The combination of high pH, ammonium hydroxide, and carbonate provide the conditions for formation of magnesium ammonium phosphate and carbonate apatite (struvite).

can act as a nidus for further stone growth are difficult to remove. Culture-specific antimicrobial agents are employed as prophylaxis against recurrent infection after complete stone removal. If a struvite stone is not completely removed, recurrent UTIs and stone growth will occur. Most patients with residual fragments progress despite treatment with antibiotics. Reducing the bacterial population often slows stone growth but stone resolution with antibiotics alone is unlikely. Urease inhibitors (acetohydroxamic acid) can decrease urinary supersaturation of struvite, reduce stone growth, and can result in dissolution of stones. Acetohydroxamic acid is associated with severe toxicities, however, including hemolytic anemia, thrombophlebitis, and nonspecific neurologic symptoms (disorientation, tremor, and headache). The half-life is prolonged in patients with chronic kidney disease (normal: 3–10 hours; chronic kidney disease: 15–24 hours). Acetohydroxamic acid should not be used if the serum creatinine concentration is greater than 2.0–2.5 mg/dL or the glomerular filtration rate less than 40 ml/minute. It is teratogenic and also should not be administered in patients taking iron supplements.

KEY POINTS
Struvite Stones

1. Struvite stones are the most common cause of staghorn calculi.
2. Women with recurrent UTIs make up the majority of patients and struvite stones.
3. Struvite stones form only when urine is infected with urease-producing bacteria.
4. The stone should always be sent for culture since urine cultures may not be representative of the organisms in the stone.
5. The combination of percutaneous nephrolithotomy and ESWL has replaced open nephrolithotomy as the treatment of choice.
6. In order to cure the patient the stone must be completely removed.

7. Stone growth is suppressed by antimicrobial therapy but a cure is unlikely without urologic intervention.

Cystine Stones

Cystinuria is secondary to an inherited defect (autosomal recessive) in proximal tubular and intestinal reabsorption of dibasic amino acids (cysteine, ornithine, lysine, and arginine). As a consequence increased amounts of these amino acids are excreted by the kidney. Clinical disease results from the poor solubility of cystine (dimer of cyteine) in water. Stones are radiodense due to the sulfhydryl group of cysteine. Cystine stones are less radiodense on radiography than calcium or struvite stones and typically have a homogeneous structure without striation. They are rare in adults, but make up as many as 5–8% of stones in children. The prevalence of cystinuria is approximately 1 per 7000 in the United States. Stones consisting entirely of cystine occur only in homozygotes. Normal adults excrete less than 20 mg of cystine per gram of creatinine per day. Most patients form their first stone before age 20. Men are generally more severely affected than women. Patients present with bilateral large staghorn calculi and elevated serum BUN and creatinine concentrations. Hexagonal cystine crystals are often seen in first morning void urine. Calcium oxalate and calcium phosphate stones can be seen in heterozygotes with cystine acting as a nidus.

Urinary supersaturation occurs at cystine concentrations greater than 250 mg/L. In order to prevent cystine stones urinary concentration should be maintained below 200 mg/L. Given that the pK_a of cysteine is 6.5 its solubility will gradually increase as pH increases from 6.5 to 7.5. Homozygotes excrete an average of 800–1000 mg/day, therefore, 4 L of urine must be produced daily to maintain cystine solubility. Cystine crystals when seen in first morning void urine are diagnostic of cystinuria, but this is an uncommon observation. Acidifying urine to pH 4 with acetic acid and storage overnight may bring out crystals in dilute or alkaline urine. The sodium-nitroprusside test, which can detect cystine at a concentration of 75 mg/L, is a commonly employed screening test. Nitroprusside complexes with sulfide groups and the test may be falsely positive in those taking sulfur-containing drugs. A positive screening test should be followed by 24-hour urine cystine quantitation. Homozygotes excrete greater than 250 mg/g of creatinine.

The hallmark of treatment is water, water, and more water. The amount is based on the patient's cystine excretion. In order to reduce urinary cystine concentration below 250 mg/L a urine output of 4 L/day is often necessary. This requires approximately two 8 oz glasses of water every 4 hours. The patient should also drink two large glasses of water when awakening to void during the night. This is a difficult regimen to comply with and water alone is often ineffective when urinary cystine excretion exceeds 500 mg/day. Alkalinization is a secondary measure used in those who do not respond to water alone. Since the dissociation constant of cysteine is 6.5, a urinary pH of 7.5 must be achieved in order for 90% of cystine to be in the ionized form. The risk of calcium phosphate stone formation is increased at this pH. Potassium citrate is preferable to sodium citrate or bicarbonate since extracellular fluid volume expansion that occurs with sodium salts will increase urinary cystine excretion.

D-penicillamine, alpha-mercaptopropionylglycine, or captopril is used if water and alkali are ineffective. These drugs are thiols that bind to cysteine and form compounds that are more soluble in aqueous solution than cystine. The D-penicillamine-cysteine complex is 50 times more soluble than cystine and the captopril-cysteine complex is 200 times more soluble. Alpha-mercaptopropionylglycine is better tolerated than D-penicillamine.

D-Penicillamine binds pyridoxine and pyridoxine (50 mg/day) should be administered to prevent deficiency. Zinc supplements help prevent the anosmia and loss of taste that can occur with D-penicillamine. Captopril, although it has fewer side effects, may be less efficacious in decreasing urinary cystine concentration.

KEY POINTS
Cystine Stones

1. Cystinuria is secondary to an autosomal recessive defect in proximal tubular and jejunal reabsorption of dibasic amino acids.
2. The amino acid cysteine dimerizes to form cystine that has limited solubility in water (250 mg/L).
3. Homozygotes excrete upward of 1000 mg of cystine daily.
4. Water is the hallmark of treatment but is often of limited use in patients who excrete more than 500 mg of cystine.
5. Ancillary measures include alkalinization of the urine with potassium citrate, and agents that form dimers with cysteine including alpha-mercaptopropionylglycine, D-penicillamine, and captopril.

Drug-Related Stones

A variety of prescription drugs precipitate in urine including sulfonamides, triamterene, acyclovir, and the antiretroviral agent indinavir. Of the sulfa drugs sulfadiazine is more likely to precipitate than sulfamethoxazole. This occurs most commonly after several days of high-dose therapy for *Toxoplasmosis gondii* or *Pneumocystis carinii* infection and often presents as acute renal failure.

The risk is increased with hypoalbuminemia. Treatment involves discontinuation of the drug, alkalinization of the urine to pH >7.15, and maintenance of high urine flow rate.

Triamterene is a weak base that can precipitate and form stones in the urinary tract. Triamterene and parahydroxytriamterene sulfate are the major stone constituents. In one series 22% of reported stones contained only triamterene, 14% had >90% triamterene, and 42% had <20% triamterene mixed with calcium oxalate and uric acid. The annual incidence was estimated at 1 in 1500 patients among those prescribed the drug. Most patients were taking 75 mg for several years but some were taking only 37.5 mg for 3–6 months. Triamterene should be avoided in patients with a previous history of calcium oxalate or uric acid stones. There are rare case reports of crystal-induced acute renal failure.

Acyclovir use can result in crystal-induced acute renal failure, especially if the drug is infused rapidly intravenously or the dose is not adjusted for renal dysfunction. The incidence is reduced by slow infusion over 1–2 hours with vigorous prehydration. There are rare case reports of acute renal failure with oral therapy in those who were dehydrated or received too high a dose.

Indinavir has limited solubility at physiologic pH and 15–20% of the drug is excreted unchanged in urine. Microscopic hematuria occurs in up to 20% of patients. Nephrolithiasis develops in 3%, and 5% will experience either dysuria or flank pain that resolves when the drug is discontinued. Recently, it has been increasingly recognized that indinavir can cause an insidious increase in serum BUN and creatinine concentrations associated with pyuria. Nelfinavir may also crystallize in the urine and cause stones.

As many as 1 in 2000 stones are composed primarily of ephedrine. This results from abuse of over-the-counter cold formulations or the ingestion of Ma-huang. Ma-huang is rich in ephedrine, norephedrine, pseudoephedrine, and norpseudoephedrine. Ephedrine was recently removed from the market in the United States. Guaifenesin and its

metabolites have been detected in kidney stones. Topiramate is an antiepileptic medication that inhibits carbonic anhydrase and causes both type I and type II RTA. Calcium phosphate and calcium oxalate stones were reported with its use.

KEY POINTS
Drug-Related Stones

1. A variety of prescriptions and over-the-counter drugs can precipitate in urine and form stones.
2. A careful medication history should be a part of the evaluation of all patients with nephrolithiasis.

Additional Reading

Asplin, J.R. Uric acid stones. *Semin Nephrol* 16:412–424, 1996.

Coe, F.L., Favus, M.J., Pak, C.Y.C., Parks, J.H., Preminger, G.M. (eds.), *Kidney Stones: Medical and Surgical Management.* Lippincott-Raven, Philadelphia, PA, 1996.

Cohen, T.D., Preminger, G.M. Struvite calculi. *Semin Nephrol* 16:425–434, 1996.

Low, R.K., Stoller, M.L. Uric acid-related nephrolithiasis. *Urol Clin North Am* 24:135–148, 1997.

Moe, O.W., Abate, N., Sakhaee, K. Pathophysiology of uric acid nephrolithiasis. *Encrinol Metab Clin North Am* 31:895–914, 2002.

Pak, C.Y.C. Medical prevention of renal stone disease. *Nephron* 81:S60–S65, 1999.

Parks, J.H., Coe, F.L. Pathogenesis and treatment of calcium stones. *Semin Nephrol* 16:398–411, 1996.

Rodman, J.S. Struvite stones. *Nephron* 81:S50–S59, 1999.

Rutchik, S.D., Resnick, M.I. Cystine calculi: diagnosis and management. *Urol Clin North Am* 24:163–171, 1997.

Sakhaee, K. Pathogenesis and medical management of cystinuria. *Semin Nephrol* 16:435–447, 1996.

Wang, L.P., Wong, H.Y., Griffith, D.P. Treatment options in struvite stones. *Urol Clin North Am* 24:149–162, 1997.

Mark A. Perazella

Urinalysis

Recommended Time to Complete: 1 day

Guiding Questions

1. What information does the urinalysis provide about patients with kidney disease?
2. What are the various components of the urinalysis?
3. Does the dipstick detect all urine proteins?
4. Is the dipstick test for blood specific for red blood cells?
5. Does red blood cell morphology help differentiate the site of kidney bleeding?
6. What information does the presence of cellular casts in the urine sediment provide?
7. Is the presence of uric acid or calcium oxalate crystals always indicative of a renal disease?
8. What factors contribute to the formation of crystals in urine?
9. Is the random spot urine protein:creatinine ratio an accurate estimate of daily protein excretion?
10. Do patterns of urinary findings help differentiate various types of kidney disease?

Introduction

Kidney disease, whether acute or chronic, may present with systemic features of renal injury (hypertension, edema, uremia), renal limited manifestations (flank or loin pain, gross hematuria), or asymptomatically with only abnormalities in blood testing or urinalysis. Kidney disease is fully assessed with complete history and physical examination, directed blood testing, and examination of the urinary sediment. Although the urinary sediment evaluation does not measure level of renal function or shed light on severity of kidney disease, it is extremely important in providing insight into the cause of kidney disease. Thus, in addition to urinalysis, the clinical examination, estimates of glomerular filtration rate (GFR), radiologic testing, and renal biopsy are used in combination to assess the patient with kidney disease. This chapter reviews the components of the urinalysis, as well as their interpretation in patients with kidney disease.

Urinalysis: Role in Kidney Disease

Examination of urine in patients with kidney disease provides invaluable information. It is one of the major noninvasive diagnostic tools available to the clinician. The urinalysis is comprised of several components. These include the appearance of the urine, various parameters measured on dipstick and spot collections, and examination of the urine under the microscope. As will be discussed later, urine microscopy is essential to complete the urinalysis and assess kidney disease. The full urinalysis can provide insight into the cause of kidney injury/disease, some of the functional consequences of renal injury, and the course of kidney disease following various interventions. For example, in a patient suffering from acute glomerulonephritis, the urine sediment can provide information about activity of the inflammatory process. It will not always predict, however, eventual renal outcomes. Thus, normalization of the urine sediment may represent either resolution with full recovery of kidney function or healing of the inflammatory process with residual glomerulosclerosis and nephron loss (chronic kidney disease). In this circumstance, other testing is required to accurately predict the status of kidney disease.

Despite some of the limitations of urinalysis, it should be performed in all patients with kidney disease or suspected kidney problems. The urine specimen is examined within an hour of voiding to provide optimal information and eliminate false-positive or negative results. A midstream specimen is adequate in men. In women, the external genitalia should be cleaned prior to voiding to avoid contamination of the urine with vaginal secretions. Following collection, dipstick testing is performed and the sample centrifuged at 3000 rpm for 3–5 minutes. Urine color and appearance are noted both before and after centrifugation, as this will provide clues to potential causes of the underlying kidney process. The dipstick measures pH, specific gravity, protein (albumin), heme, glucose, leukocyte esterase, bile, and nitrite. The centrifuged specimen is decanted to remove the supernatant and placed in a separate tube. This allows examination of the sediment. A small amount of sediment is placed on a glass slide. A cover slip is applied and both stained and unstained sediment are examined at various powers under the microscope. These aspects of urinalysis are discussed in more detail throughout the chapter.

Urinalysis: Role in Kidney Disease

> 1. Abnormalities in the urinalysis may signal kidney disease in the otherwise asymptomatic patient.
> 2. Findings on the urinalysis provide insight into the cause of acute or chronic kidney disease.
> 3. The evaluation of patients with suspected or known kidney disease should include history, physical examination, directed blood testing, and radiologic studies, as well as complete examination of the urine.

Urinalysis: Components

Appearance

Initial examination of urine consists of assessment of urine color and appearance. Normal urine is typically clear and light yellow in color. It tends to be lighter when more dilute (large water intake or polyuric states) and darker when more concentrated (overnight water restriction, prerenal disease states). The urine may appear cloudy due to infection (white cells, bacteria, proteinaceous material) or crystalluria (uric acid or calcium-containing crystals). The urine can look white from the presence of pyuria or calcium phosphate crystals; green from drugs such as methylene blue, amitriptyline, or propofol; or black due to certain malignancies or ochronosis. Table 14.1 lists some of the substances that can alter urine color. While these urinary colors are unusual, various shades of red or brown are more common. Intermittent excretion of red to brown urine occurs in a variety of clinical settings. Assessment of red/brown urine should proceed through the following steps:

Table 14.1
Substances That May Change the Color of Urine

Substance	Color
Bilirubin	Yellow-amber
Nitrofurantoin	
Chloroquine	
Sulfasalazine	
Serotonin	
Riboflavin	
Phosphate crystals (precipitated)	White
Severe pyuria	
Chyle	
Phenazopyridine	Red-brown
Heme pigments	
Hematuria	
Phenothiazines	
Senna, rhubarb, cascara, aloe	
Phenytoin	
Porphyrins	
Phenolphthalein	
Beets	
Melanin	Brown-black
Homogentisic acid	
Phenol	
Porphobilinogen	
Methyldopa	
Quinine	
Metronidazole	
Ochronosis	
Certain malignancies	
Amitriptyline	Blue-green
Methylene blue	
Biliverdin	
Propofol	
Pseudomonas infection	

1. Centrifuge the urine and examine the sediment and supernatant.
2. Red/brown sediment supports hematuria or acute tubular necrosis (with muddy brown casts).

3. Red/brown supernatant should be examined further with dipstick testing for the presence of heme.

4. Heme negative supernatant may be due to beeturia (beet ingestion in certain hosts), porphyria, or therapy with phenazopyridine (bladder analgesic).

5. Heme positive supernatant may result from either hemoglobinuria or myoglobinuria. These are distinguished by examination of the plasma that will be red with hemoglobinuria and clear with myoglobinuria.

Dipstick Examination of Urine

Urine dipstick allows rapid examination of the urine for several abnormalities. They include specific gravity, pH, protein, blood/heme, glucose, leukocyte esterase, nitrite, and bile. Each of these components of the dipstick, as well as their application to the evaluation of kidney disease will be discussed.

Specific Gravity

The kidney can vary urine osmolality to appropriately maintain plasma osmolality within a very narrow range. Thus, the osmolality of urine varies markedly based on the status of the patient's intravascular volume. To assess whether the kidney's response is appropriate or abnormal for the patient's volume status, measures of concentrating ability are employed. Specific gravity is one such available test. Importantly, the specific gravity and other measures of urine concentrating ability are assessed in correlation with the patient's clinical state. The specific gravity is defined as the weight of a solution compared with that of an equal volume of water. As such, it is a reasonable reflection of concentrating ability. It is most useful in the diagnosis of patients with disorders of water homeostasis (hyponatremia, hypernatremia) and states of polyuria. It can vary

significantly, however, with measured urine osmolality under certain clinical situations. For example, the presence of large molecules in the urine such as glucose and radiocontrast media can produce large changes in specific gravity, while having minimal effects on osmolality. These potential confounders must be accounted for when interpreting the specific gravity.

Urinary pH

Urine pH reflects the degree of acidification of urine; hence it is a measure of the urine hydrogen ion concentration. Urine pH normally ranges from 4.5 to 8.0 based on the prevailing systemic acid-base balance. Examination of urine pH is most useful in the workup of a metabolic acidosis. The appropriate response to metabolic acidosis is an increase in renal acid (buffered hydrogen ion) excretion, with a reduction in urine pH to below 5.5. Urine pH above 5.5 in the setting of metabolic acidosis may signal kidney disease, such as one of the forms of renal tubular acidosis (RTA). Changes in urine pH in response to various provocative tests can help distinguish which type of RTA exists. A urine pH less than 5.5 can also suggest risk for crystal and stone formation from uric acid, as well as medications such as sulfadiazine and methotrexate. Alkaline pH (>7.0) can provide clues to various clinical disorders such as urinary infection with urease-producing organisms (*Proteus mirabilis*) and risk for crystal and stone formation from calcium phosphate and certain drugs (indinavir). Management of these clinical disorders is assessed by measuring urine pH following the appropriate intervention.

Urine Protein

The urine dipstick measures albumin. It does not identify other proteins that may be found in the urine such as immunoglobulins and their light chains, or proteins secreted by tubular cells. Although the dipstick test is highly specific for albumin, it is insensitive in the detection of urinary albumin levels that are less than 300–500 mg/day. This is an important point as this makes the dipstick an unreliable test in the detection of microalbuminuria in certain patient populations. For example, microalbuminuria is an important early manifestation of diabetic nephropathy, one that would prompt changes in disease management. Waiting for dipstick positive proteinuria allows significant amounts of structural damage to occur prior to aggressively managing kidney disease. Similarly, microalbuminuria is associated with cardiovascular disease in nondiabetic patients and its detection would likely alter management in these patients. In addition to the insensitivity of the dipstick protein measurement, the semiquantitative values (trace, 1+, 2+, 3+, 4+) obtained are only rough guides to actual amounts of proteinuria. Furthermore, these values should be interpreted cautiously recognizing that urine concentration, pH, and substances such as iodinated radiocontrast can influence the dipstick reading. For example, dilute urine can underestimate the degree of proteinuria while both concentrated urine and alkaline urine can overestimate proteinuria. Finally, radiocontrast can cause a false-positive dipstick reading for proteinuria. Therefore, the urine should not be tested for at least 24 hours following radiocontrast administration. Other tests to measure proteinuria are discussed later.

Urine Blood/Heme

Dipstick testing of urine for blood/heme is sensitive in detecting both red blood cells and heme pigment (hemoglobin or myoglobin) in urine. As few as one to two red blood cells per high-power field register positive on dipstick, making this test at least as sensitive as urine sediment examination. False-positive results (heme pigments) for hematuria can, however, occur. In contrast, false-negative tests are unusual and a dipstick negative for heme reliably excludes hematuria. Importantly,

the dipstick test for heme is never a substitute for a thorough urine sediment examination. All patients with hematuria on dipstick should have their urine spun down and the sediment examined closely for any abnormalities, especially evidence of glomerular disease (dysmorphic red blood cells, red blood cell casts) or nephrolithiasis (monomorphic red blood cells, crystals).

Urine Glucose

Dipstick testing for glucose is a relatively insensitive measure of hyperglycemia and is not recommended for screening of patients for diabetes mellitus. Significant glycosuria does not occur until the mean plasma glucose concentration is approximately 180 mg/dL. Additionally, it depends on urine volume. Also, glucose detected semiquantitatively on urine dipstick may reflect a kidney abnormality rather than hyperglycemia. Certain disease states may alter the ability of the kidney to reabsorb filtered glucose in the proximal tubule despite normal plasma glucose concentration. This renal glycosuria can manifest as an isolated proximal tubular defect. More commonly, it can develop in association with other defects in proximal tubular reabsorption including hypophosphatemia (phosphaturia), hypouricemia (uricosuria), renal tubular acidosis (bicarbonaturia), and aminoaciduria. This constellation of proximal tubular dysfunction is termed Fanconi's syndrome. This syndrome is hereditary or acquired through diseases (multiple myeloma) or drugs (toxins) that primarily injure proximal tubular cells in kidney. Drugs such as adefovir, cidofovir and tenofovir cause Fanconi's syndrome.

Urine Leukocyte Esterase

Positive dipstick testing for leukocyte esterase represents the presence of white blood cells in urine (pyuria). While the presence of urinary white blood cells most often reflects infection of the urinary tract, it can also be indicative of diseases associated with sterile pyuria. Included are tubulointerstitial nephritis from various causes, crystalluria and nephrolithiasis, and renal mycobacterial infection. As with hematuria, a thorough examination of the urine sediment should be performed in patients with pyuria.

Urine Nitrite

The urine nitrite test is most valuable when used in conjunction with leukocyte esterase to assess a patient for the presence of urinary tract infection. Certain bacteria (*Enterobactericeae*) convert urinary nitrate to nitrite (Figure 14.1). Thus, the combination of leukocyte esterase and nitrite positive tests on dipstick strongly suggests infection with this family of bacteria.

Figure 14.1

INGREDIENTS:
• p-Arsanilic acid
• N-(1-Naphthyl) ethylenediamine dihydrochloride
• Acid buffer

$$\text{Urinary nitrate} \xrightarrow{\text{Bacteria}} \text{Urinary nitrite}$$

Nitrite + p-Arsanilic acid ⟶ Diazonium compound

Diazonium compound + N-(1-Naphthyl) Ethylenediamine → Diazonium complex (pink color)

Laboratory components of the nitrite test used to identify bacteria in the urine. The conversion of nitrate to nitrite results in the production of a pink-colored diazonium complex.

Urine Bile

Bile present on urine dipstick reflects the filtration of serum bilirubin. Normal bile pigment metabolism is shown in Figure 14.2. The finding

Figure 14.2

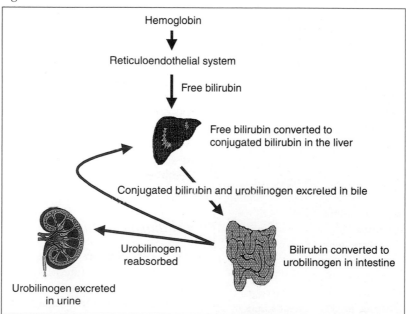

Pathway of normal bile pigment metabolism. Free bilirubin is converted in the liver and intestine to urobilinogen that is subsequently excreted in the urine.

Table 14.2

Conditions Associated with Urine Urobilinogen
and Urine Bilirubin

CONDITION	URINE BILIRUBIN	URINE UROBILINOGEN
Normal	−	+
Hepatitis	+	+
Hepatotoxins	+	+
Biliary obstruction	+	−
Cirrhosis	+	+

of bile pigment is common in patients with various forms of liver disease with associated hyperbilirubinemia. It does not represent a disturbance in kidney function although liver disease may be associated with renal failure (hepatorenal syndrome). Testing for urine bilirubin and urobilinogen separates obstructive jaundice from other forms of liver disease. In this situation, complete biliary obstruction has positive urine bilirubin with negative urobilinogen, while other forms of liver disease are positive for both substances (Table 14.2).

KEY POINTS
Urinalysis: Components

1. Dipstick examination of the urine provides useful information about patients with various forms of kidney disease.
2. A red or brown appearance of urine is appropriately evaluated with dipstick testing and urine sediment examination.
3. Dipstick proteinuria identifies urinary albumin excretion greater than 300–500 mg/day but does not measure nonalbumin proteins.
4. Glycosuria in patients with normal plasma glucose concentration suggests a proximal tubular disturbance in glucose reabsorption. This finding should stimulate investigation

for other defects in proximal tubular function and, if present, evaluation for the cause of Fanconi's syndrome.
5. Urinary tract infection is likely in patients with urine dipstick positive for both leukocyte esterase and nitrite. Isolated positive leukocyte esterase with a negative urine culture result should promote evaluation for causes of sterile pyuria such as tubulointerstitial nephritis.

Urine Sediment Examination

Microscopy of the urine sediment is a very important aspect of the evaluation of patients with known or suspected kidney disease. It is important to also recognize that normal subjects without kidney disease may also have minor amounts of abnormal elements (red blood cells, white blood cells, casts, and crystals) in the urine. For example, a patient without kidney disease may have zero to four white blood cells or zero to two red blood cells in one high-power field and one cast, often hyaline in 10–20 low-powered fields. Additionally, a few crystals made up of uric acid, calcium oxalate, or calcium phosphate may occasionally be observed. A greater number of these elements in the urine is, however, very suggestive of either systemic or renal-related disease states. Various elements found in urine on sediment examination are described below.

Cellular Elements

The most common cell types observed in urine are red blood cells, white blood cells, and epithelial cells. The urine can also contain cells from the bladder, and when contaminated during collection, vaginal squamous cells can be noted. Less commonly, tumor cells from the uroepithelium (bladder and ureteral epithelium), lymphoma, or leukemic cells that have infiltrated the renal parenchyma, and "decoy cells" associated with BK-polyoma virus-induced changes in renal tubular cells or uroepithelial cells are identified in urine sediment. The various cellular elements present in urine are reviewed.

Red Blood Cells

The presence of red blood cells in urine, either microscopic or visible grossly, is called hematuria. Hematuria can be transient and benign, or alternatively, signal a disease of the kidneys or urogenital tract. Microscopic hematuria is defined as two or more red blood cells per high-power field in a spun urine sediment. Red cell morphology is useful to help localize the source of injury or disease within the kidneys or elsewhere in the urinary system. Monomorphic red cells, which appear round and uniform like those seen on a peripheral blood smear, typically suggest extrarenal bleeding (Figure 14.3). In contrast, dysmorphic red cells often indicate a renal lesion, in particular a glomerular process. The morphology of dysmorphic red cells is characterized by blebbing, budding, and partial loss of the cellular membrane. Acanthocytes are one form of dysmorphic red cell that have a ring form with vesicle-shaped protrusions. This process results in altered red cell size (smaller) and shape. Monomorphic and dysmorphic red cells may be difficult to distinguish on routine urine microscopy. Phase contrast microscopy and scanning electron microscopy of urine more accurately identify red cell morphology but are not routinely available in most clinical settings. Persistent hematuria most often signals nephrolithiasis, glomerular pathology, or malignancy of the kidneys or urinary tract.

White Blood Cells

White blood cells in urine, known as pyuria, are larger than red blood cells and have a granular

Figure 14.3

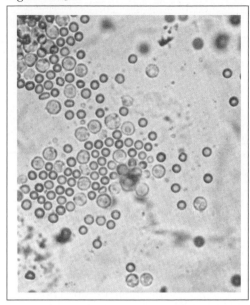

Monomorphic red blood cells in the urine sediment. The red cells are the smaller uniform cells without nuclei. (With permission from Graff, L. (ed.), *A Handbook of Routine Urinalysis.* J.B. Lippincott, Philadelphia, PA, 1983.)

cytoplasm. Neutrophils are the most common white blood cells in urine. They have multilobed nuclei, and often signal infection of the urinary tract or kidney (Figure 14.4). Eosinophils with their bilobed nuclei, may also be observed in urine on Wright's stain or Hansel's stain, which stains the granules bright red. Once thought to indicate the presence of acute interstitial nephritis, urinary eosinophils are seen with various renal processes including cholesterol emboli, glomerulonephritis, urinary tract infection, and prostatitis. Lymphocytes may also be visualized in urine. These cells are observed in urine sediment when lymphocytes, which are present in the renal interstitium, are shed into the urine. Examples are chronic tubulointerstitial diseases such as sarcoidosis and uveitis-tubulointerstitial nephritis syndrome. The nucleus of a lymphocyte is circular and uniform and not divided into lobes.

Figure 14.4

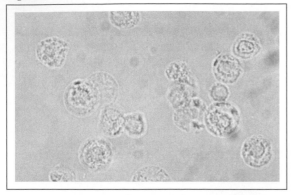

White blood cells in the urine sediment. White cells have a multilobed nucleus and a granular cytoplasm. (With permission from Graff, L. (ed.), *A Handbook of Routine Urinalysis.* J.B. Lippincott, Philadelphia, PA, 1983.)

Epithelial Cells

While epithelial cells can be shed into urine from any part of the genitourinary system, only renal tubular epithelial cells have clinical relevance. In general, renal tubular epithelial cells are several times larger than white blood cells; however, their size varies greatly (Figure 14.5). Also, their nuclei are round and located centrally in the cytoplasm. It is often difficult to distinguish these cells from uroepithelial cells from the lower urinary tract, making the presence of renal tubular epithelial cell casts diagnostically important. Renal tubular epithelial cells and casts are essentially diagnostic of either ischemic or nephrotoxic acute tubular necrosis, but occasionally are seen with glomerular disease. Lipid-filled tubular epithelial cells and free fat droplets (Maltese cross-appearance when polarized) are present in the urine sediment of patients with high-grade proteinuria.

Malignant Cells

Close scrutiny of urine can sometimes discover cancer present in the kidneys or genitourinary tract.

Figure 14.5

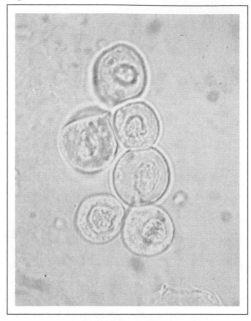

Renal tubular epithelial cells in the urine sediment. Renal tubular epithelial cells have a central uniform nucleus and are larger than white blood cells. (With permission from Graff, L. (ed.), *A Handbook of Routine Urinalysis.* J.B. Lippincott, Philadelphia, PA, 1983)

Atypical lymphocytes or lymphoid cells observed in the urine sediment can represent lymphoma of the kidneys or bladder. Similarly, leukemic cells may be present in urine, signaling leukemic infiltration of the kidneys, or genitourinary tract. Tumor cells of uroepithelial origin are noted in the urine sediment when ureteral or bladder cancer is present.

Decoy Cells

Examination of the urine sediment in renal transplant patients treated with tacrolimus or mycophenylate mofetil can confirm the presence of BK-polyoma virus infection if "decoy cells" are demonstrated. These cells are renal tubular epithelial cells and other uroepithelial cells that manifest changes associated with viral infection. These cells are best visualized employing Papanicolaou-stained urine sediment or phase contrast microscopy of unstained urine sediment. Several cellular findings characterize "decoy cells." They include: (1) ground glass nucleus; (2) chromatin margination; (3) course granules (chromatin patterns); (4) nuclear body inclusions with a peripheral halo; and (5) cytoplasmic vacuoles. Virus particles are seen when scanning electron microscopy is used.

Other Cellular Elements

Bacteria are quite commonly seen in urine sediment during infection of the urinary tract. Rarely, other infectious organisms are seen in the urine sediment. Included are *Candida albicans, Coccidiodes immitis, Mycobacterium tuberculosis, Cryptococcus neoformans, Curvularia* species, and *Schistosoma haematobium*. These organisms are often found associated with white blood cells, red blood cells, abnormal epithelial cells, and cellular casts.

KEY POINTS
Urine Sediment Examination

1. Examination of the urine sediment is crucial to provide insight into the cause of kidney disease.
2. Cellular elements present in the urine sediment include red blood cells, white blood cells, epithelial cells, tumor cells, decoy cells, and various infectious agents.
3. Red blood cell morphology can distinguish glomerular bleeding (dysmorphic cells with blebbing) from nonglomerular bleeding (monomorphic cells).
4. White blood cells in urine are indicative of urinary infection or processes associated with sterile pyuria such as interstitial

nephritis, nephrolithiasis, and renal mycobacterial infection.
5. Tubular epithelial cells are commonly seen when acute tubular necrosis from ischemia or nephrotoxins is present.
6. Rarely, malignant cells are observed in the urine sediment. Examples include renal and bladder lymphoma and uroepithelial tumors of the ureters and bladder.
7. "Decoy cells" represent epithelial cells infected with BK-polyoma virus in renal transplant patients.

Urine Casts

Casts observed in urine are formed within renal tubular lumens and, therefore, conform to the shape of these lumens. They are typically cylindrical with regular margins, but can be fractured during the process of spinning and placing the sediment on the glass slide. All casts have an organic matrix that is composed primarily of Tamm-Horsfall mucoprotein that is synthesized and released at the thick ascending limb of the loop of Henle. Various urinary casts are observed in urine, some in normal subjects. Often, the presence of casts in urine represents significant kidney disease, suggesting an intrarenal origin. The diverse casts that can be viewed in the urine sediment are reviewed below.

Hyaline Casts

These slightly refractile casts (Figure 14.6) are not associated with any particular disease. Hyaline casts may occur in a frequency as high as 5–10 per high-power field. They are found in small volumes of concentrated urine and following diuretic therapy.

Figure 14.6

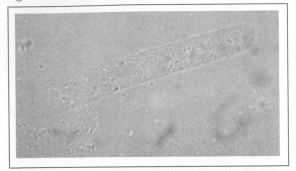

Hyaline cast in the urine sediment. Hyaline casts are acellular and are seen in normal urinary sediment. (With permission from Graff, L. (ed.), *A Handbook of Routine Urinalysis.* J.B. Lippincott, Philadelphia, PA, 1983.)

Figure 14.8

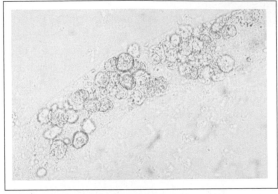

White blood cell cast in the urine sediment. White cell casts are often seen in diseases of the tubulointerstitium. (With permission from Graff, L. (ed.), *A Handbook of Routine Urinalysis.* J.B. Lippincott, Philadelphia, PA, 1983.)

Red Blood Cell Casts

The demonstration of even one red blood cell cast is significant for glomerulonephritis or vasculitis. These casts are difficult to find and require thorough evaluation of the entire sediment on the microscope slide. Red blood cell casts are often found with free dysmorphic red cells (Figure 14.7).

These casts typically contain red cells within a hyaline or granular cast; although sometimes the cast can be tightly packed with red blood cells.

White Blood Cell Casts

Casts containing white blood cells (Figure 14.8) are found most commonly in the urine sediment of patients with acute pyelonephritis or tubulointerstitial disease. Occasionally, these casts are also present with other inflammatory diseases of the kidney such as glomerular disorders, vasculitis, and cholesterol emboli. Like red cell casts, white blood cell casts are often found with free white cells such as neutrophils with pyelonephritis and eosinophils with acute interstitial nephritis.

Figure 14.7

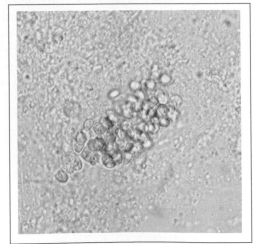

Red blood cell cast in the urine sediment. Red cell casts are the hallmark of glomerulonephritis. (With permission from Graff, L. (ed.), *A Handbook of Routine Urinalysis.* J.B. Lippincott, Philadelphia, PA, 1983.)

Epithelial Cell Casts

Injury to the tubular epithelium with the development of necrosis causes shedding of cells into the lumen. This is the proximate cause of renal tubular epithelial cell casts in urine sediment. The casts contain tubular epithelial cells of varying sizes and shapes admixed with granular material. Free renal tubular epithelial cells are also present in the sediment. While desquamation of these cells is most indicative of tubular injury and necrosis, they are also observed with glomerulonephritis and vasculitis.

Granular Casts

Casts containing granular debris (Figure 14.9) represent degenerating cells of various origins. While most often seen with acute tubular necrosis from degenerating tubular epithelial cells, they can also be degraded red blood cells or white blood cells. Thus, it is important to assess these casts along with other urinalysis findings (protein, other cell types present in urine, and their morphology), as well as the pertinent clinical data.

Waxy Casts

As granular casts continue to degenerate, they form waxy casts. Since this is a relatively slow process, the presence of significant numbers of

waxy casts suggests advanced kidney disease. Once again, the company these casts keep provides useful diagnostic information.

Broad Casts

As their name implies, broad casts are wider than other casts and are thought to form in large (dilated) tubules of nephrons with sluggish urine flow. They often are granular or waxy, and like waxy casts are indicative of advanced kidney disease.

Fatty Casts

Tubular epithelial cells filled with lipid droplets are known as oval fat bodies (Figure 14.10). Those contained in a cast matrix constitute fatty casts. These casts are found in patients with significant levels of proteinuria and lipiduria, and are observed

Figure 14.9

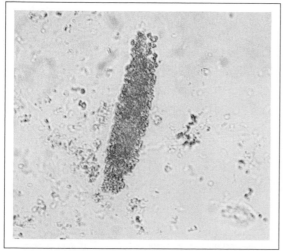

Granular cast in the urine sediment. Granular casts are composed of degenerating cells and reflect tubular injury. They are often seen in acute tubular necrosis. (With permission from Graff, L. (ed.), *A Handbook of Routine Urinalysis*. J.B. Lippincott, Philadelphia, PA, 1983.)

Figure 14.10

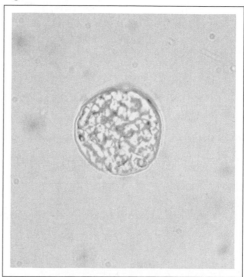

Lipid-filled tubular epithelial cells (oval fat body) in the urine sediment. Oval fat bodies are seen with nephrotic syndrome (With permission from Graff, L. (ed.), *A Handbook of Routine Urinalysis*. J.B. Lippincott, Philadelphia, PA, 1983.)

in the nephrotic syndrome. The droplets are composed of cholesterol and cholesterol esters, both of which can be seen free in the urine.

KEY POINTS
Urine Casts

1. Urinary casts are formed in the tubular space, and as such are cylindrical in shape and composed of an organic matrix consisting of Tamm-Horsfall protein. At times, various cellular elements are contained in the casts.
2. Red blood cell casts are indicative of glomerulonephritis or vasculitis; even one cast is very significant.
3. White blood cell casts are seen in the setting of acute pyelonephritis or interstitial nephritis.
4. Renal tubular epithelial cell casts, along with granular casts and free epithelial cells are commonly seen with acute tubular necrosis.
5. Fatty casts develop in urine in diseases associated with high-grade proteinuria (nephrotic range). They are refractile casts containing tubular epithelial cells filled with cholesterol and cholesterol esters.

Urine Crystals

The formation of crystals in urine depends on a variety of factors. The most important factors include the degree of supersaturation of constituent molecules, urine pH, and the presence or absence of inhibitors of crystallization. These crystals may form in normal subjects, as well as in patients with known disorders associated with crystalluria. Not uncommonly, crystals are admixed with both white and red blood cells. The different crystals seen in urine are reviewed.

Uric Acid Crystals

Acid urine favors the conversion of relatively soluble urate salts into insoluble uric acid. As a result of this milieu, uric acid crystals and amorphous urates form in urine and cause either asymptomatic crystalluria, renal failure from crystal-induced tubular obstruction, or nephrolithiasis. In particular, tumor lysis syndrome can cause severe uric acid crystalluria and acute renal failure. Low urine volumes also contribute to the formation of uric acid crystals and stone formation. These crystals are pleomorphic and can be rhombic or rosette shaped (Figure 14.11). They can be easily identified under polarized light.

Calcium Oxalate Crystals

The formation of calcium oxalate crystals is independent of urine pH. Excess urinary oxalate, as

Figure 14.11

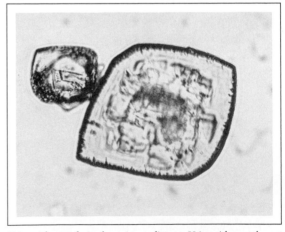

Uric acid crystals in the urine sediment. Uric acid crystals can be rhomboid or needle-shaped and may be a normal finding in an acidic urine. (With permission from Graff, L. (ed.), *A Handbook of Routine Urinalysis*. J.B. Lippincott, Philadelphia, PA, 1983.)

Figure 14.12

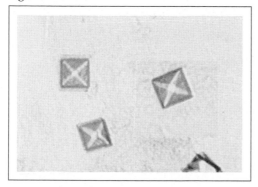

Calcium oxalate crystals in the urine sediment. Calcium oxalate may crystalize in a monohydrate or dihydrate form. The dihydrate form is shown in this figure. (With permission from Graff, L. (ed.), *A Handbook of Routine Urinalysis.* J.B. Lippincott, Philadelphia, PA, 1983.)

seen with ethylene glycol ingestion and short bowel syndrome, is associated with calcium oxalate crystal excretion and nephrolithiasis. Also, hypocitraturia is an important contributor to the formation of calcium oxalate crystals. These crystals are envelope-shaped if calcium oxalate dihydrate (Figure 14.12) or dumbbell or needle-shaped if calcium oxalate monohydrate.

Calcium Phosphate Crystals

In contrast to calcium oxalate crystals, an alkaline pH increases the formation of calcium phosphate crystals. Hypercalciuria also contributes importantly to calcium phosphate crystalluria. These crystals are seen in patients with renal tubular acidosis and can cause cloudy white urine, hematuria, and kidney stones.

Cystine Crystals

Cystine crystals are observed in urine of patients with the hereditary disorder known as cystinuria. The crystals tend to precipitate when their

Figure 14.13

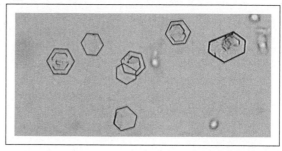

Cystine crystals in the urine sediment. Cystine crystals are hexagon shaped and are the hallmark of cystinuria. (With permission from Graff, L. (ed.), *A Handbook of Routine Urinalysis.* J.B. Lippincott, Philadelphia, PA, 1983.)

concentration exceeds 250 mg/L of urine. Acid urine also increases crystallization. The crystals are hexagonal; their presence in urine is diagnostic of cystinuria (Figure 14.13).

Magnesium Ammonium Phosphate Crystals

Struvite or "infection stones" are made up of two constituents—magnesium ammonium phosphate and calcium carbonate-apatite. Normal urine is never supersaturated with ammonium phosphate, however, infection with certain bacteria increase the ammonia concentration (and hence the pH) through urease production. The alkaline pH (>7.0) decreases the solubility of phosphate and contributes to both crystal and stone formation. Struvite crystals appear as coffin lid covers in the urine sediment (Figure 14.14).

Drug-Associated Crystals

A number of medications can cause crystal formation in urine. Most occur due to supersaturation of a low volume urine with the culprit drug, while others develop due to drug insolubility in either alkaline or acid urine pH. Acyclovir crystals, noted as needle-shaped crystals that polarize, occur when the drug is rapidly infused in volume-depleted

Figure 14.14

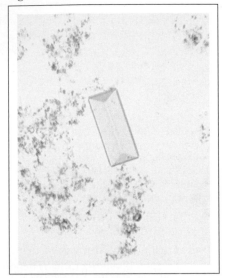

Triple phosphate crystals in the urine sediment. Triple phosphate crystals are shaped like a coffin lid and are only seen in urine infected with urease-producing bacteria. (With permission from Graff, L. (ed.), *A Handbook of Routine Urinalysis.* J.B. Lippincott, Philadelphia, PA, 1983.)

patients. Excess drug dose for the level of renal function also contributes to crystalluria. This can result in acute renal failure. Urine pH is unimportant in the development of acyclovir crystals. Alkaline urine pH contributes importantly to the formation of crystalluria with drugs such as methotrexate, sulfadiazine, and triamterene. Volume depletion with low urinary flow rates also enhances crystalluria with these drugs. All of these medications are associated with acute renal failure, while both sulfadiazine and triamterene also cause renal stone formation. Indinavir, a protease inhibitor, is also associated with crystalluria. Both volume depletion and alkaline urine enhance crystallization and nephrolithiasis from indinavir. Approximately 20% of patients are unable to take indinavir due to symptomatic crystalluria or stone formation. Other therapeutic agents associated with urinary crystals include pyridium, amoxicillin, ampicillin, aspirin, xylitol,

foscarnet, cephalexin, ciprofloxacin, primidone, piridoxylate, and vitamin C.

KEY POINTS
Urine Crystals

1. A variety of crystals can be viewed in urine. Some can occur in normal subjects, as well as patients with defined disease states.
2. Urinary crystals can be asymptomatic, cause hematuria or renal failure, or form kidney stones.
3. Uric acid crystals form in acid urine. Patients may develop acute renal failure and nephrolithiasis from uric acid crystalluria.
4. Calcium oxalate crystals can be envelope-shaped, dumbbell-shaped, or needle-like when viewed in the urine sediment. High urine oxalate and hypocitraturia are common causes of the formation of these crystals.
5. Cystine crystals signal the hereditary disease cystinuria. Crystal formation occurs with excessive cystine concentration in the urine (>250 mg/L), as well as a urine pH <7.0.
6. Medication-induced crystals develop from insoluble drug characteristics, low urine flow rates, and either acid or alkaline pH (depending on the drug). They can be associated with asymptomatic crystalluria, hematuria and pyuria, renal failure, and kidney stone formation.

 Tests of Urinary Protein Excretion

In addition to the aforementioned dipstick tests of urine, other important tests are required in the evaluation of patients with proteinuria and kidney disease. Perhaps one of the most important urinary markers of disease progression is urinary protein excretion. While the dipstick protein measurement is a specific test, it provides only a rough guide to the actual degree of proteinuria. Protein detection on dipstick should stimulate more accurate assessment of proteinuria. High-risk populations like diabetics should have screening with more sensitive measures of albuminuria. The following section will discuss tests that should be employed to more fully evaluate patients with known or suspected kidney disease.

Sulfosalicylic Acid Test

The sulfosalicylic acid (SSA) test, in contrast to the dipstick, detects all proteins in urine. The SSA gained its major usage in the assessment of elderly patients with renal failure, a benign urine sediment, and negative or trace protein on dipstick who were suspected of having myeloma kidney. A strikingly positive SSA test in such a patient is consistent with the presence of nonalbumin proteins, such as immunoglobulin light chains in urine. The SSA is performed by mixing one part urine supernatant with three parts (3%) sulfosalicylic acid. The resultant turbidity is graded as follows with approximate protein concentrations in the parentheses:

0 = no turbidity (0 mg/dL)
trace = slight turbidity (1–10 mg/dL)
1+ = turbidity through which print can be read (15 mg to 30 mg/dL)
2+ = white cloud without precipitate (40 mg to 100 mg/dL)
3+ = white cloud with fine precipitate (150 mg to 350 mg/dL)
4+ = flocculent precipitate (>500 mg/dL)

The rapid availability and accuracy of the random spot urine protein:creatinine ratio has, however, limited the use of the SSA test in clinical medicine.

Spot Protein:Creatinine Ratio

Several studies confirmed the accuracy of the random spot measurement of protein and creatinine in estimating 24-hour urine protein excretion. The protein:creatinine ratio correlates closely with the 24-hour measurement of protein in g/1.73 m^2 of body surface area. The units of measure for the urine protein and creatinine are required to be identical to allow the calculation of the ratio. The following case illustrates the use of spot urinary protein and creatinine in the estimation of daily protein excretion.

A 41-year-old patient with diabetic nephropathy is on therapy with an ACE-inhibitor (lisinopril 40 mg/day). An angiotensin receptor blocker (losartan 100 mg/day) is added in an attempt to reduce proteinuria. Prior to losartan, daily urinary protein excretion was 2.1 g. A random spot urine is sent for protein and creatinine concentration to monitor response to the addition of losartan after 8 weeks of therapy. Urine protein concentration is 110 mg/dL and creatinine concentration is 90 mg/dL (110 mg/dL/90 mg/dL = 1.2); thus the ratio is 1.2. This is equivalent to a urinary protein excretion of 1.2 g/day.

Daily protein excretion above 150 mg/day, when documented on more than one measurement, is considered abnormal and the patient should undergo a thorough investigation to diagnose and treat the underlying kidney disease. The Work Group of the Kidney Disease Outcome Quality Initiative (K-DOQI) of the National Kidney Foundation recommends use of the random spot protein:creatinine ratio to evaluate and monitor proteinuria in patients at risk for or with known kidney disease.

Like the spot protein:creatinine ratio, the random spot albumin:creatinine ratio is invaluable in the diagnosis of microalbuminuria and for monitoring the status of microalbuminuria in patients with diabetes mellitus. This test accurately estimates urine albumin excretion. Albumin concentrations in the 30–300 mg/day range are considered diagnostic of microalbuminuria. Microalbuminuria is confirmed with more than a single urine sample since several factors can increase urinary albumin excretion.

24-Hour Urine Collection

The 24-hour urine collection for protein and creatinine is considered the gold standard measure of urine protein excretion. It is more accurate than the random spot urine protein estimation and allows simultaneous calculation of creatinine clearance. In addition, it detects changes in urine creatinine excretion from vigorous exercise, high meat or vegetarian diet, creatine supplementation, and medications that effect creatinine production. All of these can confound the urine creatinine excretion and render the spot measurement less accurate. Finally, the 24-hour urine collection provides relevant information regarding nutrient and fluid intake by measuring urine volume, urea, sodium, and potassium. The benefits of this test are, however, compromised by its cumbersome nature in the ambulatory setting. Many patients are unwilling to perform these collections on a regular basis, making the random spot protein:creatinine ratio invaluable in monitoring proteinuria.

In patients with diseases associated with the production of monoclonal proteins (immunoglobulins or light chains) and those considered as potentially having these disorders, collection of 24-hour urine is required. Such diseases include multiple myeloma, primary amyloidosis, some lymphomas, and diseases associated with monoclonal light or heavy chain production. This urine collection will allow the measurement of both protein electrophoresis and immunoelectrophoresis, detecting the presence of monoclonal proteins. The 24-hour urine collection is also useful in the evaluation and treatment of patients with certain forms of hypertension (primary aldosteronism and pheochromocytoma) and nephrolithiasis.

KEY POINTS
Tests of Urinary Protein Excretion

1. The SSA test, which measures all urinary proteins, is useful to evaluate patients with negative dipstick protein measurement who are suspected of having a disorder associated with monoclonal immunoglobulin production.

2. The random spot protein:creatinine ratio accurately estimates 24-hour urine protein excretion and is recommended as the test of choice to monitor patients with proteinuric kidney disease.

3. The 24-hour urine collection for protein and creatinine is the most precise measure of proteinuria and provides insight into renal function from the creatinine clearance calculation.

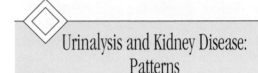

Urinalysis and Kidney Disease: Patterns

As with any test in clinical medicine, urinalysis is most useful diagnostically when different components of the test are combined to allow patterns of urinary findings to associate with different kidney diseases. Often times, the combination of urinary findings will suggest only one or two renal disorders. Below are examples to illustrate the point. Table 14.3 also demonstrates the use of urinalysis and urine sediment examination in the detection of various kidney disease states.

Isolated Hematuria with Monomorphic Red Blood Cells

The differential diagnosis of this combination of findings is limited to crystalluria, nephrolithiasis, or malignancy of the genitourinary system. Rarely, glomerular disorders such as IgA nephropathy or thin basement membrane disease may present in this way. Patients with these glomerulopathies often have, however, dysmorphic red blood cells and red blood cell casts in the urine sediment.

Table 14.3
Urinalysis and Microscopic Examination of the Urine Sediment

TEST	PRERENAL	VASCULITIS	GN	ATN	AIN	POSTRENAL
Specific gravity	High >1.020	Normal/high 1.010–1.020	Normal/high 1.010–1.020	Isosmotic 1.010	Isosmotic 1.010	Isosmotic 1.010
Blood (dip)	Negative	Positive	Positive	±	±	Negative
Protein (dip)	Negative	Positive	Positive	Negative	±	Negative
Sediment examination	Negative, hyaline casts	RBC casts, dysmorphic RBCs	RBC casts, dysmorphic RBCs	Granular casts, RTEs	WBC casts, eosinophils	Negative, sometimes WBCs/RBCs

Abbreviations: GN, glomerulonephritis; ATN, acute tubular necrosis; AIN, acute interstitial nephritis; RBC, red blood cells; WBC, white blood cells; RTE, renal tubular epithelial cells.

Hematuria with Dysmorphic Red Blood Cells, Red Blood Cell Casts, and Proteinuria

Patients with this constellation of findings are likely to have a glomerular disease or renal vasculitis. As discussed in chapter 17, this presentation is termed nephritic syndrome and strongly suggests glomerulonephritis. Importantly, the absence of these findings does not exclude glomerulonephritis. A kidney biopsy may be indicated in this situation.

Hematuria with Dysmorphic Red Blood Cells and Pyuria with White Blood Cells

This combination of urinary findings is seen with various kidney processes. Included are glomerular disease, tubulointerstitial nephritis, vasculitis, urinary obstruction, crystalluria (typically the offending crystal is also present), cholesterol embolization, and renal infarction. All these disease states can injure the kidney and cause an inflammatory lesion within the renal parenchyma.

Free Tubular Epithelial Cells, Epithelial Cell Casts, and Granular Casts

The patient with acute renal failure and this combination of urinary findings is likely to suffer from acute tubular necrosis induced by either an ischemic event or administration of a nephrotoxin, or both. The injured tubular cells are sloughed into the tubular lumen and form a cast in combination with Tamm-Horsfall matrix protein. Marked hyperbilirubinemia can also cause this urinary sediment; usually the serum bilirubin concentration will exceed 10 mg/dL and the dipstick is strongly positive for bile. The cells and casts are also stained with bile.

Free White Blood Cells, White Blood Cell Casts, Granular Casts, and Mild Proteinuria

These urinary findings are seen in patients with tubulointerstitial disease. They include pyelonephritis, drug-induced tubulointerstitial nephritis, and systemic diseases such as sarcoidosis. Rarely, an acute glomerulonephritis or other inflammatory renal disease may have this sediment. Evidence of glomerular disease is, however, also usually present (heme positive dipstick, dysmorphic red blood cells) in these disease processes.

Bland Urine Sediment and High-Grade (4+) Proteinuria

This combination of findings on urinalysis suggests the patient has a glomerular lesion associated with the nephrotic syndrome. A bland urine sediment, defined as the absence of cells or casts, suggests a noninflammatory glomerular lesion. Lipiduria with Maltese crosses and fatty casts may also be present in the urine sediment. Some of the glomerular lesions that cause nephrotic syndrome include membranous glomerulonephritis, focal glomerulosclerosis, minimal change disease, membranoproliferative glomerulonephritis, mesangial proliferative glomerulonephritis, amyloidosis, and diabetic nephropathy.

Additional Reading

Bradley, M., Schulmann, G.B. Examination of the urine. In: Bernard, J.H. (ed.), *Clinical Diagnosis and Management by Laboratory Methods*. W.B. Saunders, Philadelphia, PA, 1984, pp. 380–458.

Faber, M.D., Kupin, W.L., Krishna, G.G., Narins, R.G. The differential diagnosis of acute renal failure. In: *Acute Renal Failure*, 3rd ed., 1993, pp. 133–192.

Fairley, K.F., Birch, D.F. Hematuria: a simple method for identifying glomerular bleeding. *Kidney Int* 21:105–108, 1982.

Fogazzi, G.B., Garigali, G. The clinical art and science of urine microscopy. *Curr Opin Nephrol Hypertens* 12:625–632, 2003.

Haber, M.H., Corwin, H.L. Urinalysis. *Clin Lab Med* 8:415–621, 1988.

Kurtzmann, N.A., Rogers, P.W. *A Handbook of Urinalysis and Urinary Sediment*. Charles C. Thomas, Springfield, IL, 1974.

National Kidney Foundation (NKF) Kidney Disease Outcome Quality Initiative (K/DOQI) Advisory Board. K/DOQI clinical practice guidelines for chronic kidney disease: evaluation. Classification and stratification. Kidney Disease Outcome Quality Initiative. *Am J Kidney Dis* 39(Suppl. 2):S1–S246, 2002.

Perazella, M.A. Crystal-induced acute renal failure. *Am J Med* 106:459–465, 1999.

Pollock, C., Pei-Ling, L., Gyory, A.Z., Grigg, R., Gallery, E.D., Caterson, R., Ibels, L., Mahony, J., Waugh, D. Dysmorphism of urinary red blood cells value in diagnosis. *Kidney Int* 36:1045–1049, 1989.

Schwab, S.J., Christensen, R.L., Dougherty, K., Klahr, S. Quantitation of proteinuria by the use of protein-to-creatinine ratios in single urine samples. *Arch Intern Med* 147:943–944, 1987.

Wesson, M.L., Schrier, R.W. Diagnosis and treatment of acute tubular necrosis. *Ann Intern Med* 137:744–752, 2002.

Wilmer, W.A., Rovin, BH., Hebert, C.J., Rao, S.V., Kumor, K., Hebert, L.A. Management of glomerular proteinuria: a commentary. *J Am Soc Nephrol* 14:3217–3232, 2003.

Mark A. Perazella

Chapter

15

Acute Renal Failure

Recommended Time to Complete: 1 day

Guiding Questions

1. What is acute renal failure (ARF)?
2. What tests are currently used to diagnose ARF?
3. What is the best measure of glomerular filtration rate (GFR)?
4. In what clinical situations are blood urea nitrogen (BUN) and serum creatinine concentrations poor reflections of GFR?
5. Is community-acquired ARF more common than hospital-acquired ARF?
6. What is a simple yet useful classification system for ARF?
7. What are the principal causes of ARF in each category?
8. What are the clinical tools available to diagnose the etiology of ARF?
9. What are the clinical and biochemical consequences of ARF?
10. What are the best available preventive measures and treatments of ARF in the various categories?

Introduction

ARF is broadly defined as a rapid deterioration in kidney function as manifested by a reduction in GFR. It is comprised of a variety of syndromes that are characterized by renal dysfunction that occurs over hours to days. Acute renal failure can occur in the patient with previously normal kidney function or superimposed upon chronic kidney disease. The loss of renal function results in the accumulation of nitrogenous wastes within body fluids that would otherwise be excreted by the kidneys. The most commonly employed markers of ARF are serum creatinine and BUN concentrations, both which rise in this setting. ARF may also cause disturbances in salt and water balance, potassium and phosphorus retention, acid-base homeostasis, and endocrine abnormalities. Descriptive terms in the setting of ARF include the following:

1. **Azotemia.** A buildup of nitrogenous wastes in blood.
2. **Uremia.** A constellation of symptoms and signs of multiple organ dysfunction caused by retention of "uremic toxins" in the setting of renal failure.

Urine output is highly variable in the setting of ARF. It is often oliguric (<400 mL/day), but may be nonoliguric with urine volumes actually exceeding 3 L/day (polyuric). In certain clinical states, urine output will be less than 100 mL/day, defined as oligoanuric or anuric (no urine output). Therefore, it is important to recognize that the presence of urine output does not exclude the possibility of ARF. In general, the level of renal impairment in ARF includes a spectrum ranging from mild and rapidly reversible to very severe with a prolonged course and often a poor outcome. As will be discussed later, the etiology of ARF, as well as the population of patients it occurs in will determine the ultimate clinical course of ARF.

KEY POINTS
Acute Renal Failure

1. Acute renal failure is defined as an abrupt reduction in GFR.
2. Accumulation of nitrogenous wastes, disturbed electrolyte and acid-base balance, and abnormal volume status may result from ARF.
3. Acute renal failure may be polyuric, nonoliguric, oliguric, or anuric based on measured levels of urine output for the 24-hour period.

Measures of Renal Function

Although serum creatinine concentration is the most commonly employed clinical laboratory measure of renal function, it actually is a poor reflection of true GFR in many patients. This problem exists because changes in serum creatinine concentration do not precisely correlate with changes in GFR. The concentration of serum creatinine is influenced by a number of factors.

1. In the setting of kidney disease, creatinine is cleared from the body by the kidney through both glomerular filtration and tubular secretion.
2. Certain drugs compete with tubular secretion of creatinine (trimethoprim, cimetidine) and may increase serum creatinine concentration in the absence of any change in GFR.
3. The reported serum creatinine concentration can be falsely elevated by interference with the laboratory technique used to measure creatinine (certain cephalosporins, endogenous chromophores).
4. The gender and muscle mass of the patient influence the serum creatinine concentration and can mask changes in GFR. This results because muscle is the primary source of creatine, which is nonenzymatically converted to creatinine. Female gender and severe muscle wasting will reduce the production of creatine and limit the rise in serum creatinine concentration that would normally accompany a reduction in GFR.

The relationship between BUN and GFR is even more confounded. First, renal handling of urea includes glomerular filtration, as well as tubular secretion and reabsorption. Thus, any disease state associated with reduced tubular flow rates will increase urea reabsorption in the kidney and increase serum BUN concentration. Second, multiple factors increase serum BUN concentration in the absence of changes in GFR. They include protein loading (total parenteral nutrition, high protein supplements), hypercatabolic states (infection, steroids), gastrointestinal (GI) bleeding (reabsorbed blood converted to urea), and tetracycline antibiotics (increase urea generation). Alternatively, serum BUN concentration may remain very low despite significant renal dysfunction in states such as cirrhosis (reduced urea generation), poor protein intake, and protein malnutrition, all which are associated with decreased urea generation.

In spite of the problems associated with serum creatinine and BUN concentrations as accurate estimates of GFR, they are the most commonly employed laboratory tests to identify ARF. Clinicians use these less than optimal markers of renal function because they are readily available, are familiar to all physicians, and there are no good alternative tests. Better measures of GFR, such as technetium-labeled iothalamate, are not practical in the acute clinical situation and not widely available. Inulin clearance, the gold standard measure of GFR, is strictly a research tool. Estimates of GFR or creatinine clearance, such as those based on the MDRD formulas and Cockcroft-Gault formula, were only tested in patients with stable chronic kidney disease and would probably be inaccurate in the setting of ARF with a rapidly changing GFR. To complicate the diagnosis of ARF further, there is no consensus on a universal definition of ARF. Several studies of this entity employ widely varying definitions. For example, an absolute change in serum creatinine concentration (increase by 0.5–1.0 mg/dL) is used by some investigators. Also, a relative increase in serum creatinine concentration (increase of 25–100%) is employed by others. At times, both definitions of ARF are used. The time interval of increase in serum creatinine concentration to define ARF also varies from study to study, ranging from 24 to 72 hours. Other serum (cystatin C) and urinary markers (kidney injury molecule-1) of renal function are being investigated, but at this time appear no better and are not widely available. Thus, the clinician assesses the patient with suspected ARF using all of the clinical tools currently available while recognizing their limitations.

KEY POINTS
Measures of Renal Function

1. Serum creatinine and BUN concentrations are the most common tests used to identify ARF.
2. An abrupt increase in serum creatinine concentration usually reflects a decline in GFR and signals the development of ARF.
3. Unfortunately, the two commonly used laboratory tests suffer from a number of limitations that reduce their accuracy in the estimation of GFR.
4. Factors besides GFR that influence serum creatinine concentration include gender, muscle mass, and certain drugs.
5. In addition to the level of underlying renal function, serum BUN concentration is influenced by the urea avidity of the kidney (slow urine flow rates), presence of gastrointestinal bleeding, protein intake, catabolic states, protein malnutrition, and cirrhosis.

Epidemiology of Acute Renal Failure

Acute renal failure is a frequent problem in hospitalized patients, whereas it is less common in the community setting. Clearly, the actual incidence and outcomes of ARF are dependent on the definition used, as well as the patient population evaluated. A few studies were published to evaluate the incidence and etiology of community-acquired renal failure, as well as ARF that develops in hospitalized patients.

In a study designed to examine community-acquired ARF, renal failure was defined as an increase in serum creatinine concentration of 0.5 mg/dL in patients with a baseline <2.0 mg/dL, a rise of 1.0 mg/dL in patients with a baseline between 2.0 and 4.9 mg/dL, or a rise of 1.5 mg/dL in patients with a baseline >5.0 mg/dL. The incidence of ARF on admission to the hospital was 0.9%. Approximately half of the patients had ARF superimposed on chronic kidney disease. Prerenal azotemia accounted for 70% of the cases, while obstructive uropathy caused 17%. Intrinsic renal failure from various etiologies resulted in only 11% of the ARF cases. Overall mortality was 15% in patients with ARF. Mortality was highest in patients with intrinsic renal failure (55%) and lowest in patients with prerenal azotemia (7%). As will be seen in the discussion of hospital-acquired ARF, the mortality of community-acquired ARF is much less compared with that seen in the hospital.

Two studies evaluated the incidence of ARF in the hospital. It is worth noting that the incidence of hospital-acquired ARF is higher than community-acquired ARF. In a study performed in 1979, the incidence of ARF was 4.9% of all hospital admissions when a definition of ARF similar to the one employed above was used. Once again, prerenal azotemia was the most common cause of ARF (42%), whereas postoperative ARF resulted in 18%, radiocontrast material in 12%, and aminoglycosides in 7% of episodes. Overall mortality associated with ARF was 29% and mortality was highest in patients with a serum creatinine concentration >3.0 mg/dL (64% versus 3.8% in patients with serum creatinine concentration <2.0 mg/dL). As noted, this study represents trends in ARF that occurred in the late 1970s. In 1996, the same group of investigators performed a similar study to determine if the incidence of and mortality associated with hospital-acquired ARF changed. They postulated that the population of patients studied in this time period were older, possessed higher comorbidities, and received more nephrotoxic medications, placing them at higher risk for ARF. When compared with the study 20 years earlier, the incidence of hospital-acquired ARF increased slightly to 7.2%. Once again, prerenal azotemia remained the most common cause of ARF (39%). This was followed by nephrotoxic drugs (aminoglycosides and non-steroidal anti-inflammatory drugs [NSAIDs])

causing 16%, radiocontrast material causing 11%, and postoperative renal impairment causing 9% of the episodes of ARF. Chronic kidney disease was a common underlying risk factor for ARF as compared with patients with previously normal kidney function. Remarkably, the overall mortality was 19.4%, lower than the mortality noted 20 years prior. This may reflect improved supportive care and advances in several lifesaving technologies. Mortality, however, remained high in patients with serious illnesses, such as sepsis (76%), when ARF developed. As seen previously, the correlation between severity of ARF and mortality was again observed.

The mortality associated with hospitalized ARF depends on the severity of illness and burden of organ system dysfunction. For example, whether quantifying disease severity by number of failed organ systems or Acute Physiology and Chronic Health Evaluation (APACHE) II or III score, the mortality increases as the severity of patient illness increases. As the number of organs failed increased from 0 to 4, the mortality associated with ARF increased from less than 40% to above 90%. Similarly, the mortality associated with ARF progressively increased from less than 10% with an APACHE III score <50, to 52% with a score of 51–70, to 58% with a score of 71–90, to 86% with a score of 91–110, and to 100% with a score >110. As one might suspect when examining these data, the mortality associated with ARF that develops in the medical or surgical intensive care unit is extremely high.

KEY POINTS

Epidemiology of Acute Renal Failure

1. The incidence of ARF varies depending on whether it occurs in the hospital (5–7%) or community setting (0.9%).
2. Prerenal azotemia is the most common cause of ARF in patients with either community- or hospital-acquired ARF.

3. Obstructive uropathy is the second leading cause of ARF in community-acquired renal failure, whereas drug nephrotoxicity and postoperative renal failure are the next most common causes in hospitalized patients.

4. The overall mortality associated with ARF is higher with hospital-acquired ARF (19–29%) than community-acquired ARF (15%).

5. The mortality associated with ARF increases as the severity of patient illness increases (up to 100%).

Classification of Acute Renal Failure

Table 15.1 provides a list of the etiologies of acute renal failure classified as prerenal, intrinsic renal, or postrenal. Figure 15.1 is a schematic representation of the various causes of ARF. A logical approach to ARF is achieved by broadly classifying the clinical causes into the following categories:

1. **Prerenal azotemia.** A decrease in GFR that occurs as a consequence of reduced renal blood (plasma) flow and/or reduced renal perfusion pressure.

Table 15.1

Etiologies of Acute Renal Failure

Prerenal
"True" volume depletion
Extrarenal losses
Nausea/vomiting
Diarrhea, external fistulae
Renal losses
Overdiuresis

Renal salt wasting
Diabetes insipidus
"Effective" volume depletion
Sepsis
Cardiomyopathy
Cirrhosis/hepatic insufficiency
Nephrotic syndrome
Structural renal artery/arteriolar disease
Renal artery stenosis, arteriolo-
nephrosclerosis
Altered intrarenal hemodynamics
NSAIDs, calcineurin inhibitors, ACE
inhibitors, ARBs
Intrarenal
Vascular disease
Arterial, arteriolar, venous
Glomerular disease
Acute glomerulonephritis (immune complex,
vasculitis, anti-GBM)
Thrombotic microangiopathy (TTP/HUS)
Monoclonal immunoglobulin deposition
disease
Acute tubular necrosis
Nephrotoxic
Ischemic
Pigment-related
Crystal-associated nephropathy
Osmotic nephropathy
Acute interstitial nephritis
Medication-induced
Infection (viral, fungal, bacterial)
Systemic diseases
Postrenal
Pelvic/ureteral obstruction
Retroperitoneal disease
Nephrolithiasis
Fungus balls, blood clots
Bladder obstruction
Structural (stones, benign prostatic hyper-
plasia, blood clots)
Functional (neuropathic, drugs)
Urethral obstruction

Abbreviations: NSAIDs, nonsteroidal anti-inflammatory drugs; ACE, angiotensin-converting enzyme; ARB, angiotensin receptor blocker; GBM, glomerular basement membrane; TTP, thrombotic thrombocytopenic purpura; HUS, hemolytic uremic syndrome.

2. **Intrinsic renal azotemia.** A decrease in GFR due to direct parenchymal injury in the kidney, often subdivided by the various anatomical compartments involved (vascular, glomerular, interstitial, tubular).

3. **Postrenal azotemia.** A decrease in GFR due to an obstruction to urine flow anywhere from the pelvis and calyces to the urethra.

Prerenal Azotemia

Acute renal failure is classified as prerenal azotemia when a patient exhibits rising serum BUN and creatinine concentrations due to inadequate blood flow to the kidneys. To provide a framework to understand the concept of prerenal azotemia, the following description of renal

blood flow is provided. The kidneys receive up to 25% of the cardiac output, which results in more than a liter of renal blood flow per minute. This high rate is necessary to not only maintain GFR, but also to preserve renal oxygen delivery (to sustain ion transport and other energy requiring processes). Thus, normal kidney function is dependent on adequate perfusion. It is intuitive that a significant reduction in renal perfusion may be sufficient to diminish filtration pressure and lower GFR. Broad examples of prerenal azotemia include the following causes of renal circulatory insufficiency:

1. Renal circulatory insufficiency from "true" intravascular volume depletion.
   a. Hypovolemia from hemorrhage, renal losses (diuretics), gastrointestinal losses

Figure 15.1

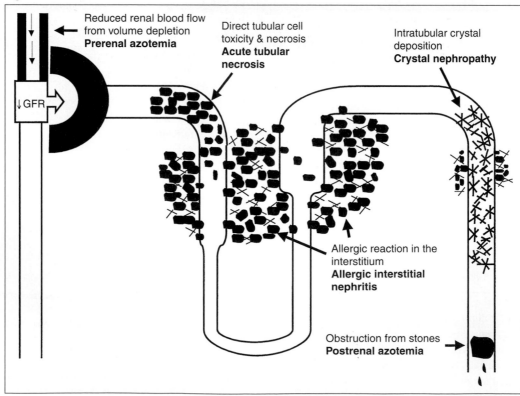

Etiologies of acute renal failure. Common causes of acute renal failure are noted in this schematic representation.

(vomiting, diarrhea), third spacing, and severe sweating.

2. Renal circulatory insufficiency from "effective" intravascular volume depletion.
   a. Impaired cardiac function from cardiomyopathy, hypertensive heart disease, valvular heart disease, pericardial disease, and severe pulmonary hypertension.
   b. Impaired liver function from acute hepatic failure and severe cirrhosis with hepatorenal physiology.
   c. Impaired systemic vascular tone (inappropriate vasodilatation) due to sepsis, medications, and autonomic failure.
3. Renal circulatory insufficiency due to renal artery disease.
   a. Main renal artery disease (renal artery stenosis).
   b. Small renal vessel narrowing (hypertensive arteriolonephrosclerosis).
4. Renal circulatory insufficiency due to altered intrarenal hemodynamics.
   a. Afferent arteriolar vasoconstriction (NSAIDs, calcineurin inhibitors, and hypercalcemia).
   b. Efferent arteriolar vasodilatation (angiotensin-converting enzyme [ACE] inhibitors, angiotensin receptor blockers [ARBs]).

Both "true" and "effective" intravascular volume depletion activate several neurohormonal vasoconstrictor systems as mechanisms to protect circulatory stability. These include catecholamines from the sympathetic nervous system, endothelin from the vasculature, angiotensin II (AII) from the renin angiotensin system (RAS), and vasopressin from the neurohypophysis. All these substances raise blood pressure through arterial and venous constriction. They also possess, however, the ability to constrict the afferent arteriole and reduce GFR, especially when systemic blood pressure is inadequate to maintain renal perfusion pressure. Structural lesions in the renal arterial and arteriolar tree can also reduce perfusion and promote prerenal azotemia. In response to these hemodynamic challenges, renal adaptive responses are stimulated to counterbalance diminished renal perfusion, whether due to

functional or structural causes. Myogenic influences and the production of vasodilator substances constitute these adaptive processes. The myogenic reflex is activated by low distending pressures sensed in the renal baroreceptors, thereby causing afferent arteriolar vasodilatation. Prostaglandins (PGE_2, PGI_2), nitric oxide, and products from the kallikrein-kinin system modify the effects of above-noted vasoconstrictors on the afferent arteriole.

Hepatorenal syndrome (HRS) is a classic example of "effective" intravascular volume depletion as a cause of prerenal azotemia. It is characterized clinically by low blood pressure, oliguria and progressive renal failure in patients with advanced liver disease. Urine findings consistent with HRS include a urine Na^+ concentration <10meq/L, urine osmolality at least 100 mOsm greater than plasma osmolality, and an unremarkable urine sediment. HRS requires careful evaluation of volume status to help distinguish it from prerenal azotemia from "true" intravascular volume depletion. A trial of intravascular volume expansion and/or measurement of central filling pressure are required to differentiate HRS from prerenal azotemia. HRS is a diagnosis of exclusion that carries a poor prognosis. Orthotopic liver transplant is the best treatment while the transjugular intrahepatic portosystemic shunt (TIPS) procedure is beneficial in some patients. Medications such as midodrine, octreotide and vasopressin analogues (terlipressin, and ornipressin) when used in conjunction with intravenous albumin may provide some benefit.

Disturbance of the balance between afferent vasodilatation and efferent vasoconstriction can disrupt intrarenal hemodynamics and precipitate ARF. Medications such as NSAIDs and selective cyclooxygenase-2 (COX-2) inhibitors act to cause prerenal azotemia through inhibition of vasodilatory prostaglandins in patients who require prostaglandin effects to maintain renal perfusion. Despite its vasoconstrictor properties, AII actually acutely preserves glomerular filtration pressure and GFR in states of reduced renal perfusion by constricting the efferent arteriole. This effect in part explains the reduction in GFR that occurs when an ACE inhibitor or an ARB is administered to a patient who is dependent on AII to constrict the efferent arteriole.

In general, prompt correction of the underlying hemodynamic insult causing the reduction in renal perfusion will result in rapid correction of renal blood flow and GFR. This ultimately prevents structural kidney damage in the form of ischemic renal tubular necrosis and preserves tubular function. Recognizing that renal tubular function remains intact is important. In prerenal azotemia, the tubules will reabsorb sodium avidly and maximally concentrate the urine. This protective mechanism preserves intravascular volume, sometimes appropriately as with "true" volume depletion and at other times inappropriately with congestive heart failure. This tubular effect on renal sodium and water reabsorption is useful to identify prerenal azotemia as a cause or contributor to ARF. The urine sodium concentration is usually less than 20 meq/L and the urine osmolarity is very high (greater than plasma). The ratio of the clearance of sodium to creatinine concentrations (fractional excretion of sodium or FENa) is calculated as follows:

$$FENa = \frac{(U_{Na} \times S_{Cr})}{(S_{Na}/U_{Cr})} \times 100 \text{ (expressed in percent)}$$

The FENa is generally useful to separate prerenal azotemia from other causes of ARF. A FENa less than 1% supports a diagnosis of prerenal azotemia and a FENa greater than 2% suggests other causes of ARF. The fractional excretion of urea (FEUrea) is employed to separate prerenal azotemia from acute tubular necrosis (ATN) in patients who have received diuretics. It is calculated from the formula

$$FEUrea = \frac{(U_{Urea} \times S_{Cr})}{(S_{Urea} \times U_{Cr})} \times 100 \text{ (expressed in percent)}$$

A FEUrea greater than 50% suggests ATN, whereas a level less than 35% supports prerenal azotemia. The renal failure index (RFI) is another equation used to separate prerenal azotemia (<1%) from

ARF due to other causes (>2%). Its formula is RFI = $U_{Na} \times (P_{Cr}/U_{Cr}) \times 100$. The urinalysis is unrevealing and the urine sediment is typically bland without cells, protein, or casts in prerenal azotemia.

As will be discussed later, prolonged prerenal azotemia can sometimes result in ATN from ischemic-induced injury. Ischemic ATN will change the clinical picture of ARF. The course of ARF will likely be protracted as compared with prerenal azotemia. In addition, injured renal tubules will no longer have the capacity to reabsorb sodium and water, resulting in a FENa >2% and a urine osmolality fixed around 300 mOsm. This entity will be more fully discussed in the intrinsic renal azotemia section.

KEY POINTS
Prerenal Azotemia

1. Prerenal azotemia occurs when renal blood flow is reduced and causes a reduction in GFR and associated ARF.
2. Prerenal azotemia is broadly classified on the basis of intravascular volume depletion (true versus effective), the presence of structural lesions in the renal arterial/arteriolar system, and altered intrarenal hemodynamics.
3. The urine sodium and osmolality, the FENa, and the RFI are useful to help distinguish prerenal azotemia from other causes of ARF. The FENa and the RFI are both less than 1% with prerenal azotemia.
4. Rapid identification and prompt correction of the prerenal disturbance often improves kidney function quickly.

Intrinsic Renal Azotemia

Acute renal failure that arises from a process that damages one of the compartments of the renal parenchyma is called intrinsic renal azotemia. For ease of organization and simplicity, the renal compartments are divided into the following anatomic sites of injury:

1. Vasculature
   a. Artery (thrombosis superimposed on stenotic renal arterial lesion, thromboembolism with renal artery occlusion, renal artery dissection, large and medium vessel vasculitis)
   b. Arteriole (atheroemboli, vasculitis, scleroderma kidney, fibrinoid necrosis from malignant hypertension, septic emboli)
   c. Venous (renal vein thrombosis)
2. Glomerulus
   a. Acute proliferative glomerulonephritis (immune complex, vasculitis, antiglomerular basement membrane antibody)
   b. Thrombotic microangiopathy (hemolytic uremic syndrome [HUS]/thrombotic thrombocytopenic purpura [TTP])
   c. Monoclonal immunoglobulin deposition disease (light/heavy chain, amyloid, fibrillary/immunotactoid)
3. Tubules
   a. Acute tubular necrosis (ischemic, nephrotoxic)
   b. Pigment nephropathy (hemoglobin, myoglobin)
   c. Crystal deposition (medications, uric acid)
   d. Osmotic nephropathy (sucrose, intravenous immune globulin [IVIG], hydroxyethylstarch, dextran, mannitol)
   e. Cast nephropathy (multiple myeloma)
4. Interstitium
   a. Allergic interstitial nephritis (drugs)
   b. Infection-induced interstitial nephritis (viral, bacterial, tuberculosis, rickettsial)
   c. Systemic diseases associated with interstitial nephritis (sarcoid, systemic lupus erythematosus [SLE], Sjögren's syndrome)
   d. Malignant interstitial infiltration
   e. Idiopathic interstitial nephritis

VASCULATURE

Disease of the blood vessels leading to the kidneys (large- and medium-sized arteries), within the renal parenchyma (small arteries and arterioles), and draining the kidneys (veins) may cause ARF. Large vessel arterial disease that causes ARF consists of the following: (1) thrombosis superimposed on high-grade renal artery stenosis (unilateral in a single functioning kidney or bilateral disease), (2) significant thromboembolism from the heart or an aortic aneurysm causing occlusion of the renal arteries, or (3) dissection of the renal arteries from trauma or a collagen vascular disorder. Patients with these renal disorders often present with flank or abdominal pain, fever, hematuria if urine is still formed, and oligoanuria or anuria. Laboratory testing reveals elevations in serum and urine lactate dehydrogenase (LDH) concentration, urinalysis dipstick positive for blood, and many red blood cells present in the urine sediment. If discovered early enough, treatment of thrombosis and thromboembolism is administration of thrombolytic agents to dissolve clot and restore renal blood flow. Long-term anticoagulation may be required to prevent further renal embolization from the heart. Surgical repair of an aortic aneurysm may be indicated, while percutaneous angioplasty with or without stent placement is a relatively noninvasive procedure to correct significant renal artery stenosis. In certain centers, surgical revascularization of the kidney may be more appropriate. A renal artery dissection clearly is an indication for surgical repair. Vasculitis may affect the large renal blood vessels in Takayasu's arteritis and Giant Cell arteritis. More commonly, the small arterial vessels and arterioles are injured by vasculitis as discussed below.

Embolization of atheromatous material to the interlobar, arcuate, and interlobular arteries in the kidneys induces ischemic injury in downstream tissue while also eliciting a giant cell reaction in the interstitium surrounding the occluded vessel

Figure 15.2

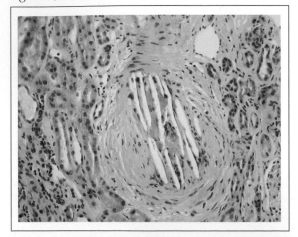

Atheroembolic renal disease. Clefts of atheromatous material occlude the vessel lumen and cause acute renal failure in the setting of cholesterol emboli.

(Figure 15.2). Debris from ulcerated plaques in the aorta and renal arteries are composed primarily of cholesterol crystals. Embolization of the crystals occurs most commonly from invasive procedures (percutaneous arterial interventions and vascular surgery) that disrupt the fibrous cap on the ulcerated plaque; however, thrombolytic therapy and therapeutic anticoagulation can also precipitate embolization. Rarely, this process occurs spontaneously in patients with significant burden of renal artery or aortic plaque. The clinical manifestations of atheroembolic disease include abrupt onset of severe hypertension, acute or subacute renal failure, livedo reticularis, digital/limb ischemia, abdominal pain (pancreatitis or bowel ischemia), GI bleeding, muscle pain, central nervous system (CNS) symptoms (focal neurologic deficits, confusion, amaurosis fugax), and retinal ischemic symptoms. The presenting symptoms depend on the extent and distribution of the cholesterol embolization. Peripheral eosinophilia, hypocomplementemia, elevated sedimentation rate, and eosinophiluria variably accompany the syndrome, while urinary findings range from bland to varying levels of cylinduria and proteinuria

(occasionally nephrotic proteinuria). Diagnosis of this syndrome can be confused by intravenous contrast administration at the time of the invasive procedure. The time course of contrast nephropathy, however, is different from cholesterol emboli. Contrast-associated renal failure develops within 48 hours, peaks within approximately a week, and then recovers over the next several days. In contrast, cholesterol emboli-induced renal failure follows a more delayed onset and protracted course of renal failure with infrequent recovery, development of chronic kidney disease, and sometimes progression to end-stage renal disease. In addition to the clinical and laboratory findings noted, cholesterol embolization syndrome is diagnosed with biopsy of involved organs including kidney and skin. Treatment is based primarily on prevention by avoiding the factors known to precipitate atheroembolization, especially in patients with severe vascular disease. Supportive care with blood pressure control, amputation of necrotic limbs, aggressive nutrition, avoidance of anticoagulation (reduce risk for further embolization), and dialytic support for severe renal failure improves the dismal prognosis associated with this syndrome. Steroids have been used to treat the inflammatory lesion that accompanies renal atheroembolism. A small number of reports describe benefit with steroids, as well as iloprost.

Macroscopic polyarteritis nodosa (PAN) causes arterial injury in medium and small vessels. It is typically idiopathic or may be associated with hepatitis B antigenemia. This type of PAN presents with severe hypertension and renal failure. Diagnosis is confirmed by renal arteriogram demonstrating beading in the arterial tree of the kidney. Disease can also occur in other arterial beds, causing symptoms attributable to disease specific to the affected organ. Scleroderma is a systemic disorder characterized by narrowing of the arteries from the deposition of mucinous material. Multiple organs may be involved including the lungs, heart, GI tract, and skin. Scleroderma renal crisis manifests as ARF and severe hypertension in a patient with a flaring of their disease. ACE inhibitors are an effective therapy to control blood pressure and improve renal function. Poorly controlled or untreated hypertension can cause ARF from severe renal injury related to malignant hypertension. Fibrinoid necrosis with ischemic injury occurs in the kidney. Initial blood pressure control is associated with worsening renal function because the autoregulatory capability of the kidney is impaired and renal perfusion is solely dependent on systemic pressure. Over time, renal function improves.

Renal vein thrombosis is a complication of nephrotic syndrome, especially when the underlying glomerular lesion is membranous nephropathy. Loss of anticoagulant substances in the urine (antithrombin 3, plasminogen activator inhibitor) and increased production of procoagulants (tissue plasminogen activator, fibrinogen) underlies the development of a hypercoagulable state. Thrombosis of the renal vein is thought to cause ARF through raised intrarenal pressures and reduced renal perfusion. Treatment of renal vein thrombosis is thrombolysis and anticoagulation, as well as remission of the underlying glomerular lesion and reduction in proteinuria.

KEY POINTS
Vasculature

1. Intrinsic renal disease is categorized by anatomic compartments that were acutely injured. They include the vasculature, glomerulus, tubules, and interstitium.
2. Acute renal failure from large vessel arterial disease occurs most commonly from thrombosis of preexisting renal artery stenosis or thromboembolism from a cardiac thrombus.
3. Atheroembolic disease causes systemic disease from occlusion of small arteries and arterioles, inducing end-organ

ischemia. Renal atheroemboli is associated with ARF, hypertension, and variable findings in the urine sediment ranging from minor cylinduria to eosinophiluria and proteinuria.
4. Macroscopic PAN presents with severe hypertension and ARF. Arteriogram of the renal arteries reveals a characteristic beading pattern.
5. Scleroderma renal crisis also presents with severe hypertension and ARF. ACE inhibitors are the treatment of choice for this disease.
6. Renal vein thrombosis complicates heavy proteinuria, especially with membranous nephropathy. Acute renal failure likely results from reduced renal perfusion.

GLOMERULUS

Glomerular diseases occur through various mechanisms. Acute proliferative glomerulonephritis may be classified as immune complex, pauci-immune, or anti-glomerular basement membrane (GBM)-related disease. This group of diseases is characterized by glomerular cell proliferation and necrosis, polymorphonuclear cell infiltration, and with severe injury, epithelial crescent formation. TTP and HUS are two of the more common causes of thrombotic microangiopathy. Platelet deposition and endothelial injury with thrombosis of arterioles and glomerular capillaries underlie the renal injury associated with thrombotic microangiopathies. Glomerular damage can be severe with profound ischemia and necrosis (Figure 15.3). Treatment is usually plasmapheresis, plasma exchange, blood pressure control, dialysis when required, and avoidance of platelet transfusions.

Deposition of monoclonal immunoglobulin light and/or heavy chains may also promote glomerular lesions. The type of immunoglobulin, as well as the metabolism and packaging of the

Figure 15.3

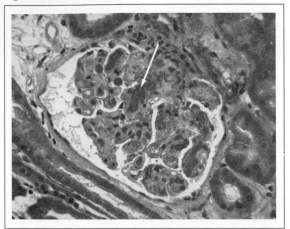

Histopatholgy of thrombotic microangiopathy. As seen in this glomerulus, capillary loops are occluded with microthrombi associated with thrombotic microangiopathy. An occluded capillary loop is shown by the arrow.

immunoglobulin determine which type of glomerular lesion develops. Light chain deposition disease, heavy chain deposition disease, and light/heavy chain deposition disease were all described to cause nodular glomerular lesions. Similarly, amyloidosis forms glomerular nodules. These diseases are separated by appearance on electron microscopy. Light and heavy chain diseases have granular deposits whereas, amyloidosis appears as haphazard fibrils in the 8–12-nm size range. The fibrillary glomerulonephritides (fibrillary and immunotactoid) are sometimes associated with mesangial expansion or glomerular nodules. They more commonly appear as a mesangial proliferative, mesangiocapillary, or membranous lesion. At times, crescents are also present. They are also distinguished from amyloidosis by a larger fibril size (fibrillary: 20 nm; immunotactoid: 30–50 nm) and organized microtubular fibrils (immunotactoid only) seen on electron microscopy.

Acute proliferative glomerulonephritis presents with hematuria and proteinuria, described as a nephritic sediment. Examination of the urine sediment under the microscope classically reveals dysmorphic red blood cells and red blood cell casts. ARF is typically present as are hypertension and edema formation. The thrombotic microangiopathies may also present with a nephritic sediment. Acute renal failure may be severe, as seen with HUS or may be mild, as noted with TTP. A microangiopathic hemolytic anemia and thrombocytopenia are key features of this disease complex. The immunoglobulin deposition diseases more often manifest with nephrotic proteinuria and renal failure. On very rare occasions, these diseases will have hematuria. The glomerular diseases will be covered more fully in chapter 17.

KEY POINTS
Glomerulus

1. Acute proliferative glomerulonephritis may result from an immune complex-disease, pauci-immune vasculitis, or anti-glomerular basement membrane-related disease.
2. The clinical presentation of this renal lesion is hypertension, azotemia, and a nephritic urinary sediment.
3. Other glomerular lesions associated with ARF include the thrombotic microangiopathies and monoclonal immunoglobulin deposition diseases.

TUBULES

ATN is the most common form of intrinsic renal azotemia (Figure 15.4). It probably accounts for greater than 80% of the episodes of intrinsic renal disease. It is classically divided into ischemic, which makes up 50% of ATN, and nephrotoxic ATN, which constitutes the remainder

Figure 15.4

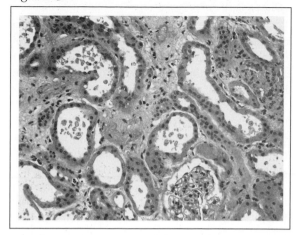

Histopathology of acute tubular necrosis. Acute tubular necrosis is characterized by tubular injury with cellular blebbing, necrosis, and sloughing of cells into the tubular lumen.

of cases. In many instances, ATN results from multiple insults acting together to induce multifactorial renal injury. The end result of either ischemic or toxic insult is tubular cell necrosis and death. Table 15.2 outlines the important factors underlying the pathogenesis of acute tubular necrosis.

Ischemic ATN is an extension of severe and uncorrected prerenal azotemia. Prolonged renal hypoperfusion causes tubular cell injury, which persists even after the underlying hemodynamic insult resolves. Various etiologies precipitate ischemic ATN. Surgical causes include intraoperative and postoperative hypotension with impaired renal perfusion. This occurs relatively frequently following cardiac and vascular surgical procedures. Obstructive jaundice also appears to increase the risk of ischemic ATN. In the medical intensive care unit and on the medical wards, ischemic and multifactorial ATN are common. This relates to the severe comorbidities these patients manifest. Superimposition of sepsis with or without shock, severe intravascular volume depletion from hemorrhage or gastrointestinal/renal fluid losses, or cardiogenic shock can induce severe ischemic ATN. Employment of vasopressors to restore blood

Table 15.2

Pathogenesis of Acute Tubular Necrosis

INTRARENAL HEMODYNAMICS AND VASOCONSTRICTION	TUBULAR CELL INJURY AND NECROSIS	REPERFUSION INJURY FROM INFILTRATING LEUKOCYTES AND T CELLS	ROLE OF GROWTH FACTORS IN RENAL INJURY
Elevated endothelin, increased sympathetic discharge, reduced nitric oxide, loss of renal autoregulation	Disruption of actin cytoskeleton with loss of cell polarity	Recruitment of neutrophils and adhesion of cells, release of ROS, proteases, elastases, other enzymes	Growth factors participate in regenerative process after ischemic injury
Reduction in cortical and medullary blood flow	Generation of reactive oxygen species	Infiltration of T lymphocytes → unknown mechanism of injury	Growth factors may also promote renal injury
Ischemic tubular injury with apoptosis and cell necrosis	Tubular shedding: Backleak of filtrate Cast formation with tubular obstruction	Tubular cell death, interstitial inflammatory infiltrate with fibrosis	Augmentation of tubulointerstitial injury and fibrosis

Abbreviations: ROS, reactive oxygen species.

pressure further reduces renal perfusion. In some cases, ischemic ATN is so profound that cortical necrosis (ischemic atrophy of the renal cortex) develops.

Nephrotoxic ATN occurs when either endogenous or exogenous substances injure the tubules. Tubular toxicity occurs through direct toxic effects of the offending substance, changes in intrarenal hemodynamics, or a combination of these effects. Organic solvents and heavy metals (mercury, cadmium, lead) were a frequent cause of ATN in the past. Over time, many drugs were noted to cause tubular injury by multiple mechanisms. Aminoglycoside antibiotics cause proximal tubular injury. These drugs are reabsorbed into the cell by pinocytosis. Once intracellular, they promote cell injury and death, leading to clinical ATN and ARF. It is notable that acute tubular necrosis from aminoglycosides rarely develops within the first week of therapy. The antifungal agent amphotericin B destroys cellular membranes through sterol interactions. A component of tubular ischemia also contributes via acute afferent arteriolar constriction. ATN develops in a dose-dependent fashion. Newer formulations (liposomal, lipid complex) are less nephrotoxic, but can also precipitate ARF in high-risk patients. Radiocontrast material is a common cause of ARF because it is so widely employed with imaging procedures. Radiocontrast nephropathy develops in patients with underlying risk factors such as kidney disease, especially diabetic nephropathy, and "true" and "effective" intravascular volume depletion. Radiocontrast causes ATN through both ischemic tubular injury (prolonged decrease in RBF) and direct toxicity (reactive oxygen species and osmotic cellular injury). Large volumes of contrast clearly increase risk while low osmolar and isoosmolar radiocontrast reduce the incidence of dye-induced ARF. Drugs such as the antiviral agents cidofovir, adefovir, and tenofovir cause ARF through disruption of mitochondrial and other cellular functions following their uptake from the peritubular blood into the cell via the human organic anion transporter-1 on the basolateral membrane.

Pigment nephropathy represents the renal tubular effects of overproduction of heme moieties in plasma that are filtered at the glomerulus and excreted in urine. Heme pigment, from either hemoglobinuria (massive intravascular hemolysis) or myoglobinuria (severe rhabdomyolysis), induces tubular injury by promoting the formation of reactive oxygen species, as well as by reducing renal perfusion through inhibition of nitric oxide synthesis.

Crystal deposition in distal tubular lumens causes a well-recognized syndrome of ARF following massive rises in uric acid and therapy with certain medications. Keys to developing ARF from crystal deposition are underlying renal disease and intravascular volume depletion. Uric acid nephropathy with tubular obstruction from urate crystals develops in patients suffering from tumor lysis syndrome. Sulfadiazine promotes intratubular deposition of sulfa crystals in an acid urine, acyclovir crystal deposition occurs with large intravenous doses of the drug, while indinavir crystal deposition (Figure 15.5)

Figure 15.5

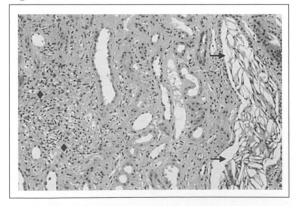

Indinavir nephropathy. Indinavir crystal deposition (shown by the arrows) noted in the tubule of an HIV-infected patient with acute renal failure. (From Reilly R, Tray K, Perazella MA: *Am. J. Kidney Dis.* Vol 38: E23, with permission.)

develops in the setting of volume contraction and urine pH above 5.5. Methotrexate, foscarnet, and large doses of intravenous vitamin C also promote intratubular crystal deposition. Vitamin C, which is metabolized to oxalate, causes deposition of calcium oxalate crystals within tubules.

Acute renal failure can occur in patients with multiple myeloma secondary to either prerenal azotemia or cast nephropathy. Hypercalcemia causes prerenal azotemia by multiple mechanisms including: (1) reduction of renal blood flow by direct renal vasoconstriction; (2) activation of the calcium sensing receptor in the basolateral membrane of the thick ascending limb resulting in inhibition of sodium transport by the Na^+-K^+-$2Cl^-$ cotransporter; and (3) reduced AQP2 expression leading to an acquired nephrogenic diabetes insipidus. In cast nephropathy monoclonal light chains precipitate in the tubular lumen resulting in both obstruction and tubular injury. Light chains have variable nephrotoxicity that may be related to their ability to bind Tamm-Horsfall protein (THP), their ability to self-associate, or their isoelectric point (pI). A higher pI may promote interaction with negatively charged THP. Treatment consists of adequate hydration, management of hypercalcemia, chemotherapy to decrease light chain production, and plasmapheresis to remove circulating light chains.

Finally, the interesting and poorly recognized entity of osmotic nephrosis can promote ARF through the induction of tubular swelling, cell disruption, and occlusion of tubular lumens. The hyperosmolar nature of substances such as sucrose, dextran, mannitol, IVIG (sucrose), and hydroxyethylstarch underlies the pathophysiology of this renal lesion. All of these substances are freely filtered at the glomerulus where they are then reabsorbed by the proximal tubule through pinocytosis. Once inside the cell, they cannot be metabolized further, thereby promoting cellular uptake of water driven by the high osmolality within the cell. Cells then develop severe swelling, disturbing cellular integrity,

and occluding tubular lumens. Acute renal failure results from this abnormal tubular process when patients with underlying kidney disease or other risk factors for ARF (intravascular volume depletion, older age) receive these hyperosmolar substances.

KEY POINTS
Tubules

1. Acute tubular necrosis is the most common cause of intrinsic renal azotemia. Ischemic insults and various nephrotoxins are the major causes.
2. Tubular injury leading to ATN also results from endogenous toxins such as heme pigment. Both massive intravascular hemolysis and rhabdomyolysis are associated with pigmenturia.
3. Crystal deposition in distal tubular lumens is another cause of ARF. Acute tumor lysis syndrome and certain medications underlie crystal nephropathy.
4. Acute renal failure in multiple myeloma may be secondary to hypercalcemia or cast nephropathy.
5. Hyperosmolar substances such as sucrose, IVIG, mannitol, dextran, and hydroxyethylstarch induce tubular cell swelling and ARF. This entity is called osmotic nephropathy.

INTERSTITIUM

Disease of the renal interstitium can result from drugs, certain infectious agents, systemic diseases, and infiltrative malignancies. The syndrome of acute interstitial nephritis (AIN) is characterized by ARF and a myriad of clinical findings. What is constant in AIN is the presence of a cellular infiltrate (lymphocytes, monocytes, eosinophils, plasma cells) and edema (or fibrosis) in the

Figure 15.6

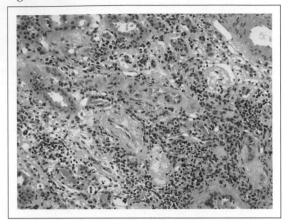

Acute interstitial nephritis. The renal interstitium is infiltrated with lymphocytes, plasma cells, and eosinophils in acute interstitial nephritis.

interstitium of the kidney (Figure 15.6). Tubulitis or invasion of lymphocytes into the tubular cells may also occur. Typically, the glomeruli and vasculature are spared by this process. The clinical presentation varies based on the offending agent and the host response. For example, beta-lactams often cause the classic triad of fever, maculopapular skin rash, and eosinophilia. Other clinical findings include arthralgias, myalgias, and flank pain. In contrast, patients with AIN secondary to NSAIDs rarely develop any extrarenal manifestations. Aside from ARF, patients receiving NSAIDs do not develop a fever, rash, or eosinophilia. Other drugs such as the sulfa-containing agents, rifampin, phenytoin, allopurinol, H_2-blockers, and fluoroquinolones may or may not cause extrarenal manifestations. At times, there might be a slight increase in liver transaminases, representing an associated drug-induced hepatitis. The urinalysis may reveal mild proteinuria, hematuria, and leukocyturia. The urine sediment examination may be bland or demonstrate white blood cells (sometimes eosinophils), red blood cells, and white blood cell casts. The Wright stain or Hansel stain may reveal eosinophils in the urine, but unfortunately neither of these tests are

sensitive or specific for AIN. For example, the most common cause of eosinophiluria is urinary tract infection. In general, renal disease occurs 2–3 weeks following drug exposure, however, it may occur more quickly in patients previously exposed to the inciting agent. Diagnosis is best made by renal biopsy. Characteristic findings are as described above—a cellular infiltrate and either edema or fibrosis in the interstitium. When biopsy is not possible, gallium scan of the kidneys may provide help in ruling out the diagnosis, as it is a sensitive but not specific test. Treatment is most successful when AIN is identified early, allowing withdrawal of the offending agent prior to the development of advanced tubulointerstitial fibrosis. Therapy with steroids is controversial, but may reduce the duration of ARF and perhaps improve functional recovery in patients with severe renal impairment. There are no convincing data, however, to support widespread steroid use.

Infection in the renal interstitium was described as a cause of interstitial nephritis prior to the AIN reported with the drugs noted above. Infection with bacteria such as Staphylococci, Streptococci, Mycoplasma, Diptheroids, and Legionella promotes acute interstitial nephritis. Several viral agents including cytomegalovirus, Epstein-Barr virus, human immunodeficiency virus (HIV), Hantaan virus, parvovirus, and rubeola also cause acute interstitial nephritis. Finally, acute interstitial nephritis may result from other infectious agents such as rickettsia, leptospirosis, and tuberculosis.

A number of systemic illnesses cause disease in the renal interstitium. Sarcoidosis promotes a lymphocytic interstitial nephritis, at times associated with noncaseating granulomas. This leads to renal injury and chronic kidney disease. Steroids reduce the severity of interstitial nephritis with sarcoidosis. Systemic lupus erythematosis (SLE) is an immune complex disease more commonly associated with a proliferative glomerulonephritis. An underrecognized histopathologic finding that occurs with SLE is acute interstitial nephritis. The interstitial inflammatory lesion is due to immune complex deposition in the tubulointerstitium.

This lesion responds to usual therapy given for lupus nephritis. Interstitial nephritis also occurs in Sjögren's syndrome. This also appears to be an immune complex-mediated disease of the renal interstitium.

Malignant infiltration of the kidney is an uncommon cause of clinical renal disease. The malignancies most often associated with interstitial infiltration are the leukemias and lymphomas. Leukemic infiltration causes nephromegaly, acute renal failure, and sometimes urinary K^+ wasting (due to either tubulointerstitial damage or lysozyme production). Renal involvement from lymphomatous infiltration can be in the form of discrete nodules or diffuse interstitial infiltration. Lymphoma may also cause massive kidney enlargement and ARF. Successful treatment of the underlying malignancy typically improves the infiltrative lesion; however, irradiation of the kidneys may also provide additional benefit.

A more complete discussion of all of the diseases that affect the tubulointerstitium will be undertaken in chapter 18. This will include chronic interstitial nephritis and tubulointerstitial disease secondary to glomerular disease. The pathogenesis of tubulointerstitial disease will also be examined.

KEY POINTS
Interstitium

1. Acute interstitial nephritis results from a variety of medications. Beta-lactams such as the penicillins produce the classic syndrome of fever, skin rash, and eosinophilia along with ARF more often than other drugs. In contrast, NSAIDs lack most of the extrarenal manifestations of AIN.
2. Infectious agents such as bacteria, viruses, mycobacteria, rickettsial organisms, and leptospira cause AIN.
3. Acute interstitial nephritis is also a consequence of systemic diseases. Included are sarcoidosis, SLE, and Sjögren's syndrome.

Altered immunity associated with these diseases promotes interstitial disease in such patients.
4. Infiltration of the interstitium with malignant cells occurs most commonly with the leukemias and lymphomas. Massive nephromegaly often accompanies ARF, while tubular damage may manifest as hypokalemia.

Postrenal Azotemia

Anatomic obstruction of urine flow anywhere along the genitourinary system can result in ARF. The process causing postrenal azotemia is called obstructive uropathy. The radiographic (ultrasound, intravenous or retrograde pyelogram, computed tomography [CT] scan) demonstration of a dilated urinary collecting system is termed hydronephrosis. Abnormal kidney function (ARF, tubular defects) that occurs with urinary obstruction is called obstructive nephropathy. For ARF to develop, obstruction must be bilateral (both ureters or below the bladder) or unilateral in a single functioning kidney. It is important to recognize that obstruction may be complete and associated with anuria, or partial (incomplete) and associated with urine volumes varying (and fluctuating) from low to normal to polyuric levels. Either complete or partial obstruction may cause ARF; however, obstructive uropathy that is complete is typically associated with more severe renal failure and clinical manifestations (hypertension, intravascular volume overload, hyperkalemia, and hyponatremia).

The pathogenesis of ARF from urinary obstruction is briefly discussed in this section. A more thorough description will be presented in chapter 19. Following acute obstruction, a triphasic response occurs in the renal plasma flow. An initial and short-lived (2–4 hours) increase in plasma flow develops as vasodilatory prostaglandins are produced in response to the rise in intratubular pressure. This represents an attempt to maintain GFR by overcoming the elevated intratubular pressure. Blood flow begins to decline after 2–5 hours, an effect due to increased ureteral and tubular pressure transmitted to the renal interstitium. Intratubular pressure also returns to normal at 24 hours, after increasing acutely with obstruction. A further decline in renal plasma flow at 24 hours (30–50% of baseline) occurs despite normalization of ureteral and tubular pressures. This fall is due to production of angiotensin II and thromboxane A_2, both vasoconstrictors. These substances also reduce GFR not only by reducing renal plasma flow but by inducing mesangial contraction and reducing the glomerular ultrafiltration coefficient. Despite all these effects, GFR declines progressively but never reaches zero. The explanation for maintained GFR is the continued reabsorption of sodium and water (urine) along the nephron and in lymphatics.

Obstruction of the urinary system can occur anywhere starting at the renal calyces and extending to the urethra. A wide variety of disorders cause ARF from urinary obstruction. They can be classified according to the site or level of obstruction (Table 15.3). In general, the most common causes of obstructive uropathy in the upper urinary tract (above the bladder) include stones and retroperitoneal disease, whereas in the lower tract, prostatic hyperplasia and bladder dysfunction most often obstructs urine flow at this level. The diagnosis of obstructive uropathy should be considered in most patients with ARF since it is highly reversible when identified and treated early on. History may point to upper tract (history of nephrolithiasis or certain cancers, flank pain) or lower tract (prostatism, neuropathic bladder). Physical examination should include assessment of flank tenderness, prostatic enlargement, or palpable bladder. Straight catheterization of the bladder helps evaluate for lower tract obstruction (large residual urine in the bladder). Imaging of the kidneys with ultrasound is the most appropriate initial test to evaluate the patient with ARF and

Table 15.3

Etiologies of Postrenal Azotemia

Ureterocalyceal obstruction
Retroperitoneal disease
    Tumor
    Lymph nodes
    Fibrosis
Papillary necrosis
Nephrolithiasis
Fungus balls
Blood clots
Strictures
    Infection
    Granulomatous disease
    Prior instrumentation
Bladder obstruction
Structural
Stones
Blood clots
Tumor
Benign prostatic hyperplasia
Functional
    Cerebrovascular accident
    Diabetes mellitus
    Spinal cord injuries
    Drugs
    Other neuropathic conditions
Urethral obstruction
Urethritis
Urethral stricture
Blood clots

possible urinary tract obstruction. In general, the sensitivity and specificity of renal ultrasonography for the detection of urinary obstruction (hydronephrosis) are high; however, several clinical situations can reduce its accuracy. Acute obstruction (<48 hours) does not allow the urinary system time to fully dilate, causing a negative ultrasound study for hydronephrosis. In patients with superimposed severe intravascular volume depletion, GFR and urine formation are reduced, limiting dilatation of the urinary system and the ability of ultrasound to detect obstruction. Retroperitoneal disease involving the kidneys and ureters (cancer, fibrosis, and enlarged nodes) encases the collecting system and blunts dilatation. In addition, obese patients and overlying bowel gas reduce visualization of the kidneys and urinary system, potentially confounding ultrasound results. In cases such as these, where the ultrasound findings are equivocal or negative yet the suspicion for urinary obstruction is high, a CT scan may provide more information. CT scan's use stems from its ability to detect the etiology of obstruction (stones, tumor, enlarged lymph nodes) despite the absence of hydronephrosis. If these studies are negative but obstruction is still considered likely, retrograde pyelography can diagnose many forms of upper tract obstruction.

Adequate treatment of obstructive uropathy hinges on early recognition. As time passes with obstruction, especially if complete, reversibility of renal impairment is compromised. Upper urinary tract obstruction is relieved by retrograde ureteral stent placement. When severe retroperitoneal disease and ureteral or bladder cancer limit ureteral stent placement, nephrostomy tube insertion is often required. Relief of lower tract obstruction with a bladder catheter or suprapubic tube (when indicated), like the procedures for upper tract obstruction noted above, is the first step in treatment. Management of electrolyte and fluid balance is the next step in patients with obstructive uropathy. Postobstructive diuresis is a phenomenon that occurs most commonly in patients with bilateral, complete obstruction. Large urine volumes can attend the diuresis that accompanies relief of obstruction. The diuresis is, in part, physiologic in that excess sodium and water are being excreted. Disturbed tubular function, however, may contribute to the excessive diuresis. Tubular abnormalities in sodium and water reabsorption can develop and persist for days (or permanently). Also, elevated levels of atrial natriuretic peptide may also induce diuresis while urea may cause an osmotic diuresis. Judicious fluid repletion is required in this circumstance, avoiding both iatrogenic contribution of postobstructive diuresis, as well as underresuscitation and hypotension.

KEY POINTS
Postrenal Azotemia

1. Anatomic obstruction of urine flow results in an entity called obstructive uropathy. When renal defects develop in this situation, it is termed obstructive nephropathy.
2. Obstruction of the urinary system can be partial or complete, and either unilateral or bilateral. Acute renal failure most often complicates bilateral, complete obstruction.
3. Urine output can fluctuate between polyuria and oliguria in patients with partial obstruction. Bilateral, complete obstruction is characterized by anuria.
4. The pathogenesis of obstructive uropathy includes a reduction in GFR from both elevated intratubular pressure (resisting filtration pressure) and production of vasoconstrictor substances that reduce renal plasma flow.
5. Obstruction of the urinary system is classified as either upper tract (renal pelvis and ureters) or lower tract (bladder and urethra) according to the site of obstruction.
6. Diagnosis of obstructive uropathy entails a complete history (anuria, prostatism, history of bladder, prostate, or cervical cancer) and physical examination (suprapubic fullness, flank tenderness), as well as imaging with renal ultrasound. This imaging test is both sensitive and specific, but can be negative (no hydronephrosis) in the presence of obstruction in a few clinical situations.
7. Treatment of obstruction focuses on rapid identification to preserve renal function. Upper tract obstruction is usually managed with ureteral stent placement or percutaneous nephrostomy tube insertion.

Lower tract disease is managed with a bladder catheter or suprapubic tube.

8. Postobstructive diuresis may develop following relief of complete, bilateral obstruction for several reasons. Excess sodium and water are excreted while obstruction-related tubular defects may occur and cause inappropriate sodium and water wasting. Elevated serum BUN concentrations may also contribute through an osmotic diuresis.

Approach to the Patient with Acute Renal Failure

Evaluation of the patient with ARF should be methodical to ensure that potentially reversible causes are rapidly diagnosed and treated to preserve kidney function and limit chronic kidney disease. A thorough history to identify causes of and risk factors for prerenal azotemia (vomiting, diuretics, diarrhea, heart failure, cirrhosis), potential nephrotoxic drugs (either prescribed or over-the-counter), and risk factors for (prostate disease, cervical cancer) or symptoms of urinary obstruction (prostatism, overflow incontinence, anuria) is required. Physical examination should focus on extracellular fluid volume status to allow initial classification into one of the broad categories of ARF. These include hypotension, an orthostatic fall in blood pressure or flat neck veins (volume depletion), as well as edema, pulmonary rales, or an S3 gallop (cardiac dysfunction). In situations where intravascular volume status is uncertain, measurement of cardiac filling pressures with a Swan-Ganz catheter is useful. Examination for evidence of systemic disease should also be sought. For example, this includes signs of pulmonary hemorrhage (vasculitis, Goodpasture's disease), skin rash (SLE, atheroemboli, vasculitis, cryoglobulins, AIN), and joint disease (SLE, rheumatoid arthritis) to name a few.

Laboratory tests are directed by the differential diagnosis postulated following a complete history and physical examination. Basic tests include a complete blood count to assess for anemia (microangiopathic or immune-mediated) and thrombocytopenia (TTP, HUS, disseminated intravascular coagulation [DIC]). The urinalysis is a key component of the ARF work-up. Table 15.4 outlines the various urine findings in some of the

Table 15.4

Urinalysis and Microscopic Examination of the Urine Sediment

TEST	PRERENAL	VASCULITIS	GN	ATN	AIN	POSTRENAL
Specific gravity	High	Normal/high	Normal/high	Isosmotic	Isosmotic	Isosmotic
Blood (dip)	Negative	Positive	Positive	±	±	Negative
Protein (dip)	Negative	Positive	Positive	Negative	±	Negative
Sediment examination	Negative, hyaline casts	RBC casts, dysmorphic RBCs	RBC casts, dysmorphic RBCs	Granular casts, RTEs	WBC casts, eosinophils	Negative, sometimes WBCs/RBCs

Abbreviations: GN, glomerulonephritis; ATN, acute tubular necrosis; AIN, acute interstitial nephritis; RBC, red blood cell; WBC, white blood cell; RTEs, renal tubular epithelial cells.

different causes of ARF. It is essential to evaluate urine specific gravity, as well as the presence of blood (or heme), protein, or leukocyte esterase on urinary dipstick. A very high urine specific gravity typically suggests a prerenal process while isosthenuria (SG = 1.010) indicates intrinsic renal disease such as ATN. A bland urine with no blood or protein favors a diagnosis of prerenal azotemia. Vascular causes of ARF have a variable urine specific gravity and sometimes hematuria and granular casts. Glomerulonephritis will have variable urine specific gravity, blood and protein (usually), and red blood cells and red blood cell casts. Acute tubular necrosis has isosthenuria, variable heme (positive with rhabdomyolysis and hemolysis) and protein, renal tubular epithelial cells, and pigmented coarsely granular casts. The urine in patients with postrenal azotemia is typically isosthenuric and bland unless there is associated infection (pyuria) or nephrolithiasis (hematuria). Urine chemistries sometimes help distinguish the type of pathology in the kidney. As stated earlier, a low urine sodium and a FENa and RFI (both <1%) support prerenal azotemia. In contrast, urine sodium greater than 20 meq/L and a FENa and RFI both greater than 2% suggest ATN (Table 15.5). Evidence of systemic disease should prompt directed testing using anti-nuclear antibodies (ANA-SLE), anti-nuclear

cytoplasmic antiboby (ANCA-vasculitis), hepatitis serology, serum cryoglobulins (cryoglobulinemia), complement levels, serum and urine immunoelectrophoresis (monoclonal immunoglobulin diseases), and blood cultures (endovascular infection)

Diagnostic imaging tests play an important role in the evaluation of patients with ARF. The modality most often employed is retroperitoneal ultrasonography of the kidneys, ureters, and bladder. This test provides information about kidney size (large or small) and parenchyma (echogenicity), status of the pelvis and urinary collecting system (hydronephrosis), and the presence of structural abnormalities (stones, masses, and enlarged lymph nodes). In the setting of ARF, renal ultrasound's biggest use is in rapidly confirming or excluding the presence of hydronephrosis and a diagnosis of obstructive uropathy. Doppler interrogation of the renal arteries provides important information about renal blood flow and renal artery stenosis; however, this test is highly operator dependent. CT scan of the retroperitoneum also provides important information about the etiology of postrenal azotemia when ultrasound is negative or inconclusive. Magnetic resonance imaging with gadolinium angiography also safely provides important information about renal artery stenosis/ thrombosis.

Percutaneous renal biopsy is sometimes required to determine the etiology of ARF, as well as to direct appropriate therapy. Reasonable criteria to support use of renal biopsy are the following: no obvious cause of ARF (no evidence of hypotension, nephrotoxins); prolonged oliguria (>2–3 weeks); assess for multiple myeloma in the elderly with unexplained renal failure; extrarenal manifestations of systemic disease (SLE, vasculitis); and to determine if AIN is present in patients receiving a potentially culprit drug. Examination of kidney tissue using light microscopy, immunofluorescence staining, and electron microscopy will facilitate an accurate diagnosis in virtually all cases of ARF. Renal biopsy, however, should be employed judiciously

Table 15.5

Urine Chemistries

Lab Test	Prerenal	ATN
Urine Na⁺ (meq/L)	<20	>20
UOsm (mOsm/kg)	>500	<400
RFI (%)	<1	>2
FENa (%)	<1	>2
FEUrea (%)	<35	>50

Abbreviations: ATN, acute tubular necrosis; Na⁺, sodium; U, urine; Osm, osmolality; RFI, renal failure index; FENa, fractional excretion of sodium; FEUrea, fractional excretion of urea.

to avoid complications such as traumatic arteri-ovenous malformation within the kidney, severe bleeding requiring transfusion, other organ injury (liver, spleen, bowel), and kidney loss (severe bleeding requiring embolization or nephrectomy).

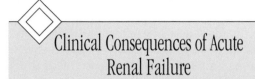

Clinical Consequences of Acute Renal Failure

Failure of kidney function precipitates clinical problems related to toxin excretion, fluid balance, acid/base homeostasis, and electrolyte/mineral regulation. Disturbance of the homeostatic renal processes result in the following:

Retention of nitrogen wastes ⇒ azotemia and uremia

Retention of sodium ⇒ volume overload, hypertension

Retention of water ⇒ hyponatremia

Retention of metabolic acids ⇒ metabolic acidosis

Retention of potassium ⇒ hyperkalemia

Retention of phosphate ⇒ hyperphosphatemia, hypocalcemia

Clinical manifestations of ARF vary based on the severity of renal dysfunction. Uremic symptoms include anorexia, nausea/vomiting, weakness, difficulty mentating, lethargy, and pruritus. Physical examination findings supporting uremia include asterixis, pericardial friction rub, sensory and/or motor neuropathy, and hyper- or hypotension depending on the cause of ARF. Other associated findings of severe uremia include GI ulcerations, bleeding from platelet dysfunction, infection from abnormal WBC function, impaired wound healing, and malnutrition from the catabolic state.

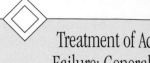

Treatment of Acute Renal Failure: General Principles

Therapy of ARF first requires identification of the etiology and pathogenesis of the inciting process (prerenal, intrarenal, postrenal). Hence, treatment is based on diagnosis directed therapy. Also, the consequences of ARF need to be identified and rapidly managed to avoid serious adverse events (hyperkalemia, pericarditis, and acidosis). Prerenal azotemia is best treated by optimizing renal perfusion. Repletion of intravascular volume and correction of heart failure, liver failure, and other "effective" causes of reduced intravascular volume constitute treatment for this form of ARF. Intrarenal azotemia is managed through directed therapy for the disturbed kidney compartment (vasculature, glomerulus, tubules, interstitium). In certain situations, preventive therapy reduces renal injury. Examples include volume repletion prior to any nephrotoxic or ischemic exposure. Fluid therapy (isotonic saline or sodium bicarbonate), acetylcysteine, and fenoldopam may reduce the renal damage associated with radiocontrast exposure in high-risk subjects. As discussed previously, management of postrenal azotemia mandates rapid identification of the obstruction process and early intervention to relieve obstruction and preserve renal function.

Conservative therapy of many of the consequences of ARF is initially employed. These include correction of volume overload/hypertension, hyponatremia, hyperkalemia, and acidosis. The actual therapies for these clinical situations will be covered in other chapters. Conversion of patients from oliguric to nonoliguric ARF makes management easier, but probably does not improve morbidity or mortality. Azotemia and uremia, as well as the other consequences previously noted may require renal replacement therapy to allow appropriate management when conservative measures are unsuccessful.

Initiation of acute hemodialysis or continuous renal replacement therapies is required in certain patients with ARF. Continuous therapies, which can only be employed in critical care units, include continuous venovenous hemofiltration/hemodialysis/hemodiafiltration (CVVH, CVVHD, CVVHDF) and extended daily dialysis (EDD). Emergent indications include severe hyperkalemia, uremic end-organ damage (pericarditis, seizure), refractory metabolic acidosis, and severe volume overload (pulmonary edema). Other clinical situations that mandate the commencement of renal replacement therapy are uremic symptoms such as anorexia, nausea/vomiting, somnolence, restless legs, and neuropathy. Bleeding from platelet dysfunction and extreme hyperphosphatemia are other reasons to consider initiation of dialysis. Acute hemodialysis is the modality most commonly employed to treat the consequences of ARF. In patients who are critically ill and hemodynamically unstable, continuous therapies are preferred. The continuous modalities allow more precise control of volume, uremia, acid-base disturbances, and electrolyte disorders with less hemodynamic instability (hypotension). They also allow aggressive nutritional support without associated volume overload. Peritoneal dialysis is another gentle therapy for ARF, but it is less commonly used.

Additional Reading

Abuclo, J.G. Diagnosing vascular causes of renal failure. *Ann Intern Med* 123:601–614, 1995.

Bellomo, R., Kellum, J.A., Ronco, C. Acute renal failure: time for consensus. *Intensive Care Med* 27:1685–1688, 2001.

Block, C.A., Manning, H.L. Prevention of acute renal failure in the critically ill. *Am J Respir Crit Care Med* 165:320–324, 2002.

Cockcroft, D.W., Gault, M.H. Prediction of creatinine clearance from serum creatinine. *Nephron* 16:31–41, 1976.

Davda, R.K., Guzman, N.J. Acute renal failure. Prompt diagnosis is key to effective management. *Postgrad Med* 96:89–92, 1994.

Faber, M.D., Kupin, W.L., Krishna, G.G., Narins, R.G. The differential diagnosis of acute renal failure. In: *Acute Renal Failure*, 3rd ed., 1993, pp. 133–192.

Han, W.K., Bailly, N., Abichandani, R., Thadhani, R., Bonventre, J.V. Kidney injury molecule-1 (KIM-1): a novel biomarker for human renal proximal tubule injury. *Kidney Int* 62:237–244, 2002.

Kaufman, J., Dhakel, M., Patel, B., Hamburger, R. Community-acquired acute renal failure. *Am J Kidney Dis* 17:191–198, 1991.

Kellum, J.A., Angus, D.C., Johnson, J.P., Leblanc, M., Griffin M., Ramakrishnan, N., Linde-Zwirble, W.T. Continuous versus intermittent renal replacement therapy: a meta-analysis. *Intensive Care Med* 28:29–37, 2002.

Kellum, J.A., Levin, N., Bouman, C., Lamiere, N. Developing a consensus classification system for acute renal failure. *Curr Opin Crit Care* 8:509–514, 2002.

Klahr, S. Pathophysiology of obstructive uropathy: a 1991 update. *Semin Nephrol* 11:156–168, 1991.

Kramer, L., Horl, W.H. Hepatorenal syndrome. *Semin Nephrol* 22:290–301, 2002.

Lamiere, N., Vanholder, R. Pathophysiologic features and prevention of human and experimental acute tubular necrosis. *J Am Soc Nephrol* 12:S20–S32, 2001.

Levey, A.S., Bosch, J.P., Lewis, J.B., Greene, T., Rogers, N., Roth, D. A more accurate method to estimate glomerular filtration rate from serum creatinine: a new prediction equation. Modification of Diet in Renal Disease Study Group. *Ann Intern Med* 130:461–70, 1999.

Liano, F., Pascual, J., The Madrid Acute Renal Failure Study Group. Epidemiology of acute renal failure: a prospective, multicenter, community-based study. *Kidney Int* 50:811–818, 1996.

May, R.C., Stivelman, J.C., Maroni, B.J. Metabolic and electrolyte disturbances in acute renal failure. In: *Acute Renal Failure*, 3rd ed., 1993, pp. 107–132.

Nash, K., Hafeez, A., Hou, S. Hospital-acquired renal insufficiency. *Am J Kidney Dis* 39:930–936, 2002.

Pascual, J., Liano, F., Ortuno, J. The elderly patient with acute renal failure. *J Am Soc Nephrol* 6:144–153, 1995.

Perazella, M.A. Acute renal failure in HIV-infected patients: a brief review of some common causes. *Am J Med Sci* 319:385–391, 2000.

Perazella, M.A. COX-2 selective inhibitors: analysis of the renal effects. *Expert Opin Drug Saf* 1:53–64, 2002.

Schoolwerth, A.C., Sicca, D.A., Ballerman, B.J., Wilcox, C.S. Renal complications in angiotensin converting enzyme inhibitor therapy. *Circulation* 104:1985–1991, 2001.

Shokeir, A.A., Shoma, A.M., Mosbah, A., Mansour, O., Abol-Ghar, M., Eassa, W., El-Asmy, A. Noncontrast computed tomography in obstructive anuria: a prospective study. *Urology* 59:861–864, 2002.

Thadhani, R., Pascual, M., Bonventre, J.V. Acute renal failure. *N Engl J Med* 334:1448–1460, 1996.

Wesson, M.L., Schrier, R.W. Diagnosis and treatment of acute tubular necrosis. *Ann Intern Med* 137:744–752, 2002.

Mark A. Perazella

Chronic Kidney Disease

Recommended Time to Complete: 2 days

Guiding Questions

1. Why is the rapid growth of the chronic kidney disease (CKD) population a concern?

2. Why are estimation equations of glomerular filtration rate (GFR) used to measure kidney function?

3. Why is a staging system beneficial to appropriately care for CKD patients?

4. What are the major mechanisms of progression of kidney disease?

5. What are the most effective treatments to slow progression of CKD to end-stage renal disease (ESRD)?

6. Is cardiovascular disease (CVD) common in CKD patients?

7. What are the various categories of risk factors for the development of cardiovascular disease in CKD patients?

8. What are the most common causes of anemia in CKD patients?

9. What are the options available to treat anemia in CKD patients?

10. What metabolic mineral disturbances occur in CKD patients?

11. What types of bone disease constitute the spectrum of renal osteo-dystrophy?

12. Why is early referral of CKD patients to nephrologists important?

13. What are the important aspects of preparation of CKD patients for initiation of renal replacement therapy (RRT)?

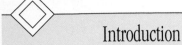

Introduction

CKD is a worldwide health problem. Comprehensive data on CKD provided by the Third National Health and Nutrition Examination Survey (NHANES III) noted, that approximately 800,000 Americans have CKD as manifested by a serum creatinine concentration of 2.0 mg/dL or greater. More than 6.2 million are estimated to have a serum creatinine concentration of 1.5 mg/dL or greater. Data extrapolated from the Framingham study suggest that approximately 20 million people in the United States are at risk for CKD.

The rapid growth in both the incidence and prevalence of CKD will result in a huge influx of patients into the ESRD system. Based on data from the United States Renal Data System (USRDS), the incidence of ESRD has increased steadily for the past 15 years, rising from 142 cases per million population in 1987 to 308 cases per million population in the year 2000. Expansion of the ESRD population will have a significant economic impact on the already overextended Medicare system. For example, Medicare expenditures for the ESRD program in 1996 increased 12.5% over the previous year, costing an estimated $10.96 billion. The increase in both CKD and ESRD populations may also overwhelm the ability of nephrologists and other health care providers to fully provide interventions that will improve the length and quality of patients' lives.

Defining and Staging CKD

Several terms are used to describe the period of kidney disease that precedes the institution of renal replacement therapy such as *pre-ESRD, chronic renal insufficiency, chronic renal failure, and chronic renal disease*. Unfortunately, none of these terms is particularly accurate and may be confusing to nonnephrology physicians. The term *pre-ESRD* gives the impression that dialysis is an inevitable outcome of all kidney diseases. The terms *renal insufficiency, chronic renal failure, chronic renal disease,* and *pre-ESRD* have negative connotations.

These terms also include the word *renal*, which is not easily understood by patients. For these reasons, *chronic kidney disease* is chosen as the defining term.

The definition and classification of CKD are based on measurement of GFR, the best overall measure of kidney function. Factors that influence GFR include structural or functional kidney disease, as well as patient age. In general, the annual decline of GFR with age is approximately 1 mL/minute/1.73 m^2 of body surface area, beginning after the patient reaches approximately 20–30 years of age. Although a chronic decline in GFR to a level of <60 mL/minute/1.73 m^2 is evidence of CKD, substantial kidney damage can exist without a decrease in GFR. In this circumstance, kidney damage is defined as a structural or functional abnormality of the kidney that persists for more than 3 months. Manifestations of kidney damage can include pathologic changes or abnormalities revealed by blood, imaging, or urine tests. Using this definition, CKD is present if the GFR is <60 mL/minute/1.73 m^2. CKD is also present if the GFR is ≥60 mL/minute/1.73 m^2 if other evidence of kidney damage also exists. A classification and staging system based on the level of GFR is noted in Table 16.1. This staging system provides a common language for communication between the various health care providers. It allows more reliable estimates of the prevalence of earlier stages and of populations at increased risk for CKD. In addition, evaluation of factors associated with a high risk of progression can be recognized. Treatments can be more effectively examined and the development of adverse outcomes in this population is more easily determined.

GFR as an Index of Kidney Function

Serum creatinine concentration is commonly employed as an index of kidney function. It is not an accurate measure of GFR, however, and it is especially inaccurate when the serum creatinine concentration is between 1 and 2 mg/dL. This is because creatinine, unlike inulin, is secreted by the renal tubules. As renal function declines, the amount of creatinine secreted by the tubules increases and

Table 16.1

Staging System and Action Plan for CKD

STAGE	DESCRIPTION	GFR (mL/minute/1.73 m²)	ACTION*
0	At increased risk of CKD	≥90 with risk factors†	Screening CKD risk reduction
1	Kidney damage with normal or increased GFR‡	≥90	Diagnosis and treatment Slow progression of CKD Treat comorbidities Cardiovascular disease risk reduction
2	Mild decrease in GFR	60–89	Estimate progression
3	Moderate decrease in GFR	30–59	Evaluate and treat complications
4	Severe decrease in GFR	15–29	Prepare for renal replacement therapy
5	Kidney failure	<15 or dialysis	Renal replacement if uremic

*Includes actions from preceding stages.
†Risk factors: hypertension, dyslipidemia, diabetes mellitus, anemia, systemic lupus erythematosus, and chronic analgesic ingestion.
‡Kidney damage as manifested by abnormalities noted on renal pathology, blood, urine, or imaging tests.
Abbreviations: CKD, chronic kidney disease; GFR, glomerular filtration rate.
Source: Adapted from Kidney Foundation (NKF) Kidney Disease Outcome Quality Initiative (K/DOQI) Advisory Board. *Am J Kidney Dis* 39(2 Suppl. 2): S1–S246, 2002 with permission.

raises the amount of creatinine in the urine. This acts to falsely increase the creatinine clearance (CrCl), resulting in an overestimation of GFR. Serum creatinine concentration is also influenced by body mass, muscle mass, diet, drugs, and laboratory analytical methods. "Normal" ranges of serum creatinine concentrations quoted by laboratories are misleading because they do not take into account the age, race, sex, or body size of the individual.

Inulin clearance is the gold standard test for measuring GFR. Unfortunately, this test is cumbersome, expensive, and not widely available for clinical use. Iothalamate (^{125}I-iothalamate) clearance estimates GFR and is a reasonably accurate substitute for the inulin clearance method. It is also expensive and somewhat cumbersome to perform as a routine clinical test. A 24-hour urine collection for creatinine clearance is the accepted alternative measure of GFR because it is widely available and is familiar to most clinicians. It is often difficult, however, for patients to perform correctly and is less accurate than either

inulin or iothalamate clearance. The adequacy of the 24-hour urine collection is assessed by calculating the urinary creatinine excretion per kg of body weight. Males excrete 20–25 mg creatinine/kg and females excrete 15–20 mg creatinine/kg in the steady state. In addition, this test often overestimates GFR in patients with advanced kidney disease.

To simplify measurement of renal function, GFR estimates from prediction equations are often used. These formulas take into account serum creatinine concentration, age, gender, race, and body size, and are better estimates of GFR than serum creatinine concentration alone. The formulas used are sufficiently accurate. The two most widely used are the Cockcroft-Gault and the Modification of Diet in Renal Disease Study (MDRD) equations. The Cockcroft-Gault equation noted below estimates creatinine clearance:

$$\frac{[140 - \text{age (years)}] \times \text{weight (kg)}}{72 \times \text{serum [creatinine] (mg/dL)}} \times 0.85 \text{ for females}$$

Although it provides an adequate estimate of GFR, the MDRD equations are more accurate. MDRD equation 7 is the preferred formula but it requires serum blood urea nitrogen (BUN) and albumin concentrations. The MDRD formula is as follows:

$$170 \times [\text{serum creatinine (mg/dL)}]^{-0.999}$$
$$\times [\text{age (years)}]^{-0.176} \times [0.762 \text{ if female}]$$
$$\times [1.18 \text{ if African American}]$$
$$\times [\text{BUN (mg/dL)}]^{-0.170}$$
$$\times [\text{albumin (g/dL)}]^{+0.318}$$

An abbreviated form of the MDRD equation that does not require serum BUN or albumin concentrations was also developed and is as follows:

$$186 \times [\text{serum creatinine (mg/dL)}]^{-1.154}$$
$$\times [\text{age (years)}]^{-0.203} \times [0.742 \text{ if female}]$$
$$\times [1.21 \text{ if African American}]$$

The abbreviated form is reasonably accurate. The MDRD equation was tested in over 500 patients with a range of kidney diseases and ethnicities (European Americans and African Americans). GFR values were validated in the sample group using ^{125}I-iothalamate as the gold standard, however, certain patient groups were not well represented in the MDRD study sample. Therefore, clearance measurements are still required in groups who were underrepresented in the MDRD sample to fully validate the formula for all patients. These include: patients at extremes of age and body size; the severely malnourished or obese; patients with skeletal muscle diseases, paraplegia, or quadriplegia; vegetarians; and those with rapidly changing kidney function. The MDRD equation underestimates GFR in patients with relatively normal kidney function.

Prevalence of CKD Stages

Prevalence estimates for each CKD stage were obtained by using a reference group comprised of patients evaluated in NHANES III. In this sample of patients, the MDRD equation was used to estimate GFR. In addition to abnormal GFR levels, the presence of micro- or macroalbuminuria on spot urine specimens was considered sufficient evidence of kidney damage. The level of albuminuria, based on the ratio of albumin (and protein) to creatinine on spot urine samples, was used to estimate the prevalence of the first two stages. The prevalence of each GFR category is noted in Table 16.2.

Table 16.2

U.S. Prevalence of CKD by Stage

STAGE	DESCRIPTION	GFR (mL/minute/1.73 m²)	PREVALENCE* N (1000s)	PERCENT
1	Kidney damage with normal or increased GFR†	≥90	5900	3.3
2	Mild decrease in GFR	60–89	5300	3.0
3	Moderate decrease in GFR	30–59	7600	4.3
4	Severe decrease in GFR	15–29	400	0.2
5	Kidney failure	<15 or dialysis	300	0.1

*Prevalence based on population of 177 million adults age ≥20 years.
†Kidney damage as manifested by abnormalities noted on renal pathology, blood, urine, or imaging tests.
Abbreviation: GFR, glomerular filtration rate.
Source: Adapted from National Kidney Foundation (NKF) Kidney Disease Outcome Quality Initiative (K/DOQI) Advisory Board. *Am J Kidney Dis* 39(2 Suppl. 2):S1–S246, 2002 with permission.

Approach to CKD Patients

The approach to the patient involves establishing the presence of CKD, determining the stage of disease, and enacting an action plan based on the stage. The management of CKD patients requires a multidisciplinary approach involving primary care physicians, nephrologists, endocrinologists, cardiologists, vascular surgeons, physician assistants, nurse practitioners, dietitians, and social workers. The goals of this interdisciplinary approach are to identify patients either with or at increased risk for CKD, to slow the progression of CKD to ESRD, to identify and treat comorbid conditions, to identify and prevent complications of CKD, and to prepare patients mentally and physically for renal replacement therapy. As seen in Table 16.1, the action taken increases from simple screening maneuvers and risk reduction to more complex disease management.

Patients with established CKD are assessed for comorbid conditions. Medications are adjusted for the level of renal function. Blood pressure (BP) monitoring is essential to diagnose hypertension and facilitate optimal blood pressure control. Serum creatinine concentration is measured to allow estimation of GFR. Protein- or albumin-to-creatinine ratios on spot urine samples and urinalysis are performed. Finally, imaging of the kidney by ultrasound is warranted in most CKD patients.

The approach is implemented in a step-wise fashion and individualized for each patient based on the level of kidney function. In a patient with a normal GFR ($\geq$90 mL/minute/1.73 m^2) or a mildly impaired GFR (>60 mL/minute/1.73 m^2) the focus will be on delaying progression and treating comorbid conditions. Progression is best predicted by plotting the reciprocal of the serum creatinine concentration over time. This plot predicts a date when the GFR will reach target levels for the initiation of renal replacement therapy. In general, the cut-off values are 15 mL/minute/1.73 m^2 for diabetic patients and 10 mL/minute/1.73 m^2 for nondiabetic patients.

KEY POINTS
Approach to CKD Patients

1. The incidence and prevalence of CKD are growing rapidly.
2. Equation estimates of GFR as well as other laboratory, pathologic, and radiographic abnormalities allow classification and staging of CKD.
3. The most useful equation to estimate GFR is the MDRD formula.
4. Patients with CKD should be staged and then evaluated and managed using their CKD stage.
5. Management of CKD patients will focus on disease prevention, management of comorbidities, and preparation for renal replacement therapy.

Progression of CKD

Mechanisms of CKD Progression

The initiating event in the development of kidney disease is a pathologic process that produces nephron injury and loss of functioning units. Following a reduction in the number of functioning nephrons, remaining nephrons experience hyperfiltration and glomerular capillary hypertension. Although these changes are initially adaptive to maintain GFR, over time they are deleterious to renal function because of pressure-induced capillary stretch and glomerular injury. The damage caused by glomerular hyperfiltration is important in the pathophysiology that underlies diabetic nephropathy. The hyperfiltering state induced by hyperglycemia upregulates local expression of the renin-angiotensin-aldosterone system (RAAS) and contributes to progressive kidney damage. In this instance, stimulation of the RAAS causes glomerular injury by further raising glomerular capillary pressure through angiotensin II (AII)-driven efferent arteriolar vaso-constriction and facilitating pressure and stretch injury in the capillaries. Taken together, these effects lead to endothelial injury, stimulation of profibrotic cytokines by the mesangium, and detachment of glomerular epithelial cells. Other maladaptive consequences include glomerular hypertrophy with elevated capillary wall stress and increased ammoniagenesis per remnant nephron. This latter effect promotes complement activation and enhanced tubulointerstitial disease.

Another consequence of renal injury and activation of the RAAS is proteinuria. Glomerular capillary hypertension, caused by hyperfiltration and AII effect on efferent arterioles, leads to an increase in glomerular permeability and excessive protein filtration. Pore size is altered by AII, increasing protein leak across the glomerular basement membrane. An activated RAAS may also cause proteinuria through novel effects on nephrin expression in kidney. Nephrin, a transmembrane protein located in the slit diaphragm of the glomerular podocyte, is thought to play a key role in the function of the glomerular filtration barrier. By maintaining slit diaphragm integrity, nephrin limits protein loss across the glomerular basement membrane. When its expression is disrupted, proteinuria and its consequences may result. Data in rat models of proteinuric kidney disease suggest an important interaction between the RAAS and nephrin in modifying glomerular protein permeability. Although proteinuria is a marker for renal disease risk, it is also likely that excess protein in urine contributes to progressive kidney damage. Proteins present in the urine are toxic to the tubules, and can result in tubular injury, tubulointerstitial inflammation, and scarring. Tubular damage is due to protein overloading of intracellular lysosomes, stimulation of inflammatory cytokine expression, and extracellular matrix protein production. These processes induce renal tubulointerstitial fibrosis and glomerular scarring. It was clearly demonstrated that a remission or reduction in proteinuria is associated with nephroprotection.

While it is known that elevated glomerular capillary pressure and capillary stretch lead to scar formation in the glomerulus, an activated RAAS and other inflammatory mediators directly cause irreversible damage in the kidney through other mechanisms. Proinflammatory and profibrotic effects of AII and aldosterone underlie the injury that develops in the renal parenchyma. Advanced glycation end-products also cause renal injury. These various mediators promote fibrosis and scarring in the kidney through multiple untoward effects such as toxic radical formation, enhanced cellular proliferation, and collagen deposition in the glomerulus and tubulointerstitium. Ultimately, glomerulosclerosis and tubulointerstitial fibrosis occur and promote chronic kidney disease.

Risk Factors for Progression of CKD

HYPERTENSION AND THE RAAS

Hypertension is clearly associated with progression of CKD and is the second most common cause of ESRD. Importantly, hypertension is present in the majority of CKD patients, making it a key risk factor for progression. Most studies, with a few exceptions, confirm that hypertension hastens the course of CKD to ESRD in both diabetic and non-diabetic patients. The MDRD study demonstrated that proteinuric patients, when randomized to a lower blood pressure, manifested a slower decline in GFR. Also, a significant correlation between the achieved blood pressure and the rate of decline in renal function, especially in patients with greater than 1 g/day of proteinuria was noted. The Joint National Committee (JNC VII) recommends the following blood pressure target goals:

1. CKD with <1 g/day of proteinuria: 130/85.
2. CKD with >1 g/day of proteinuria: 125/75 to 130/80.

Proteinuria is a powerful risk factor for progression of CKD, especially as levels exceed both 1 and 3 g/day, respectively. Patients with high-grade proteinuria and hypertension are at highest risk to progress to ESRD. Both experimental and clinical data suggest that inhibition of the RAAS is very effective in lowering blood pressure, reducing proteinuria, and slowing progression of kidney disease in both diabetic and nondiabetic patients. This is of particular interest since the leading cause of ESRD in the United States is diabetic nephropathy. Treatment of disease states resulting from or associated with excessive RAAS activity is best achieved by therapies that suppress AII and aldosterone production or inhibit the renal effects of these substances (Figure 16.1).

Inhibition of angiotensin-converting enzyme (ACE) activity decreases AII and aldosterone formation and potentiates the vasodilatory effects of the kallikrein-kinin system by increasing bradykinin formation (Figure 16.1). The ACE inhibitors reduce proteinuria and delay progression of kidney disease in both diabetic nephropathy and other forms of proteinuric kidney disease. In a landmark study, the effect of captopril versus conventional therapy on the occurrence of multiple renal endpoints (time to doubling of serum creatinine concentration, progression to ESRD, or death) was studied in 409 type 1 diabetic patients with proteinuria and CKD. A 50% reduction in the development of these renal endpoints was demonstrated in patients treated with captopril compared with conventional therapy, despite little difference in blood pressure control. The beneficial

Figure 16.1

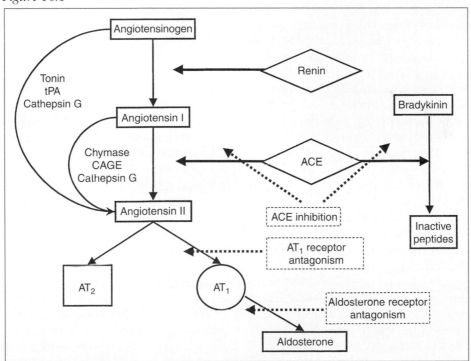

The renin-angiotensin-aldosterone system. Angiotensin II and aldosterone are formed by classical pathways (renin, ACE) and alternate pathways (tonin, tPA, cathepsin G, chymase, CAGE). The pathway is interrupted at various levels by ACE inhibitors, AT_1 receptor antagonists, and aldosterone receptor antagonists. Abbreviations: tPA, tissue plasminogen activator; AT_1, angiotensin type 1; AT_2, angiotensin type 2; CAGE, chymostatin-sensitive angiotensin II-generating enzyme; ACE, angiotensin converting enzyme.

effects of RAAS inhibition also extend to nondiabetic kidney diseases complicated by proteinuria. The ACE Inhibition in Progressive Renal Insufficiency (AIPRI) Study compared the ACE-inhibitor benazepril with placebo in 583 nondiabetic patients with CKD. Benazepril was associated with an overall risk reduction of 53% in the development of the primary renal endpoint (doubling of serum creatinine concentration and need for dialysis) as compared with conventional antihypertensive therapy. In this trial, the absolute benefit of ACE inhibition was most marked in patients with the highest level of proteinuria. The REIN study (stratum 2) confirmed these positive results in a similar group of nondiabetic patients. A 52% risk reduction in progression to kidney disease endpoints was seen with ramipril as compared with placebo. Renoprotection was most impressive in patients with greater than 3 g of proteinuria. A metaanalysis of data obtained from 1860 nondiabetic patients from 11 randomized clinical trials demonstrated significant renal protection with ACE inhibitors. ACE-inhibitor therapy was associated with a reduction in relative risk for the development of ESRD (0.69) and for the doubling of serum creatinine concentration (0.70). Thus, the benefit of ACE inhibition is most pronounced in patients with heavy proteinuria and a reduction in proteinuria correlates with slower declines in GFR.

Angiotensin II type 1 receptor blockers (ARBs) lower blood pressure, reduce proteinuria, and slow progression of kidney disease. Antagonism of the AT_1 receptor (Figure 16.1) and binding of AII to the AT_2 receptor probably underlies their mechanism of action. Recently completed clinical trials suggest that ARBs reduce microalbuminuria and proteinuria and retard the progression of diabetic chronic kidney disease in a fashion similar to the ACE inhibitors. The RENAAL study compared the ARB losartan with conventional therapy in 1513 type 2 diabetics with hypertension and nephropathy. A 16% risk reduction was noted in predetermined primary composite endpoints (time to doubling of serum creatinine concentration,

progression to ESRD, or death) in the losartan group over a mean follow-up of 3.4 years. This study demonstrated a 28% risk reduction in progression to ESRD and 25% reduction in doubling of serum creatinine concentration in patients treated with losartan. An average reduction in the level of proteinuria of 35%, despite similar blood pressure control between the groups, was also noted. Similar findings were described in the IDNT study, which employed irbesartan in patients with type 2 diabetes mellitus and nephropathy. Like ACE inhibitors, interruption of the RAAS with ARBs in diabetics is a logical albeit incomplete strategy to provide renoprotection.

Dual blockade of the RAAS with ACE inhibitors and angiotensin receptor blockers may provide kidney benefit beyond therapy with either drug alone. The CALM study combined lisinopril and candesartan to treat hypertension and reduce microalbuminuria in patients with type 2 diabetes mellitus. Over 24 weeks, dual blockade safely reduced blood pressure and reduced microalbuminuria (50%) as compared with candesartan (24%) and lisinopril (39%) monotherapy. Similarly, a randomized double-blind crossover study in 18 type 2 diabetic patients with proteinuria demonstrated positive renal effects with combination therapy. In patients with IgA nephropathy, the combination of losartan and enalapril were additive in decreasing urinary protein excretion, whereas doubling the dose of either form of monotherapy had no effect on proteinuria. Over 6 months, the combination of lisinopril plus candesartan reduced proteinuria by 70% compared to monotherapy with lisinopril (50% reduction) or candesartan (48% reduction). The COOPERATE study examined the effect of combination therapy on progression of renal disease (time to doubling of serum creatinine concentration or ESRD) in patients with proteinuric kidney disease. In this 3-year study, patients were randomly assigned to trandolapril (3 mg/day), losartan (100 mg/day), or a combination of the 2 drugs. Only 11% of patients on combination therapy reached the renal endpoint, whereas 23% of patients in the two monotherapy arms did so. Not all studies demonstrate that combination therapy is better than maximal dose ACE-inhibitor therapy in decreasing proteinuria. These studies suffer from small patient numbers, surrogate markers of renal protection (proteinuria), and short-term follow-up. Thus, titration of the single agent to maximal dose to control blood pressure and proteinuria is recommended. If proteinuria remains greater than 1 g/day, a second agent to further block the RAAS should be considered.

Aldosterone is associated with renal injury through both hemodynamic and profibrotic effects. Aldosterone antagonism in animals is renoprotective when used alone or in combination with ACE inhibition. Preliminary human data suggest that the combination of an aldosterone receptor antagonist like spironolactone or eplerenone with an ACE inhibitor or ARB significantly reduce proteinuria. This therapy, however, is associated with higher risk of hyperkalemia.

Finally, it is important to recognize that inhibitors of the RAAS can be used safely in most patients with mild-to-moderate CKD. The two major concerns associated with these drugs are the development of hyperkalemia and/or further worsening of kidney function. In regards to hyperkalemia, careful dose titration, dietary changes, avoidance of potassium altering medications (NSAIDs, COX-2 selective inhibitors, and potassium sparing diuretics), and use of loop diuretics allow safe therapy in most patients. Increases in serum creatinine concentration should be tolerated as long as the concentration rises no higher than 30% above baseline and stabilizes within 2 months of therapy. Continued increases should promote drug discontinuation and a search for volume contraction, critical renal artery stenosis, and other potentially correctable problems.

DIABETES MELLITUS

As the prevalence of diabetes mellitus grows in the United States, patients with this disease continue to contribute a significant number of patients to the CKD population. In fact, diabetic kidney disease is the most common cause of ESRD. Thus, it is important to identify and adequately manage these patients to reduce progression of their underlying kidney disease. As shown in the Diabetes Control and Complications Trial (DCCT), intensive insulin therapy to establish tight glucose control prevented de novo kidney disease (microalbuminuria) by 34% and reduced progression of established nephropathy (albuminuria) by 56% in type 1 diabetics. Progression of CKD in type 2 diabetics is an even bigger problem as this group makes up the majority of patients who develop ESRD. Several studies reveal that intensive insulin therapy to maintain the HbA1c level in the 7.0–7.6% range reduces progression of kidney disease (albuminuria/proteinuria) as compared with conventional insulin therapy. Thus, patients with diabetic nephropathy should achieve tight glucose control, defined by a HbA1c concentration of 7.0–7.5%, in addition to BP control with RAAS inhibitors.

DIETARY PROTEIN RESTRICTION

Restriction of dietary protein reduces renal injury in the experimental setting by decreasing glomerular capillary hypertension and reducing production of profibrotic cytokines and growth factors. In humans, it is less clear that a low protein diet is beneficial. The results of various studies are mixed. In the largest study, two levels of protein restriction (low and very low) failed to show a difference in GFR decline between groups after a mean follow-up of 2.2 years. Posthoc analysis identified some benefit of protein restriction when examined by achieved level of protein intake. Patients with very low protein intake had a 1.15 mL/minute/year slower decline in GFR. Two metaanalyses also suggest a benefit with protein restriction. In one, the risk of ESRD or death was reduced by 33% while another noted a small benefit in GFR change (0.53 mL/minute/year) with a low protein diet. Enthusiasm for this approach is tempered by the real risk of malnutrition in

CKD patients. Thus, in the highly motivated patient, a moderately low protein diet (0.6–0.8 g/kg/day) can be employed along with close monitoring of nutritional state.

SERUM LIPID REDUCTION

Experimental work demonstrates that low density lipoprotein (LDL) lipids are toxic to human mesangial cells, an effect that is reversed by 3-hydroxy-3-methylglutaryl-coenzyme A (HMG-CoA) reductase inhibitors (statins). Observational studies in humans suggest that reducing serum lipid levels is associated with preservation of kidney function. Unfortunately, these studies are plagued by small patient numbers and, as a result, are underpowered to allow any conclusions. To address this problem, a metaanalysis of 13 studies revealed a trend toward reduction in proteinuria and a small decrease in the rate of GFR loss with lipid lowering. Despite the absence of conclusive data, it is logical that lipid reduction should be employed in CKD patients to reduce cardiovascular risks and potentially slow progression of kidney disease.

SMOKING CESSATION

Tobacco smoking may injure the kidney through various pathways. Hypertension complicates smoking, a well-known factor associated with kidney disease. Smoking also increases single nephron GFR and may promote progression of kidney disease through hyperfiltration and glomerular capillary hypertension. Finally, smoking raises aldosterone levels. As discussed previously, aldosterone may enhance kidney disease by increasing BP and direct profibrotic effects. In humans, smoking similarly injures the kidney and increases the risk of developing albuminuria in diabetics. Smoking cessation slows progression of kidney disease in patients with diabetic nephropathy and some nondiabetic forms of kidney disease. Given the overall negative health consequences associated with smoking, patients with CKD should be aggressively counseled to quit.

KEY POINTS
Progression of CKD

1. Adaptive changes to nephron injury promote various effects that ultimately contribute to progression of CKD.
2. Hypertension, hyperfiltration, hyperglycemia, high-grade proteinuria, and overactivation of the RAAS cause renal injury and progression of kidney disease to ESRD.
3. CKD patients with high levels of proteinuria are at highest risk to progress to ESRD.
4. Therapies that reduce blood pressure to appropriate goals, reduce proteinuria, and inhibit the RAAS provide the most benefit to slow loss of renal function in diabetic and nondiabetic patients with proteinuric kidney disease.
5. ACE inhibitors and ARBs provide renoprotection in CKD patients; combination therapy with these drugs and aldosterone antagonists may provide further kidney protection but need further validation.
6. Tight glucose control in diabetics reduces progression of micro- and macroalbuminuria.
7. Dietary protein restriction, serum lipid lowering with statins, and smoking cessation may also reduce progression of kidney disease in subgroups of patients.

Cardiovascular Consequences of CKD

CVD is the leading cause of death in CKD patients. There is an increase in the overall prevalence of CVD in these patients. Left ventricular hypertrophy (LVH) and ischemic heart disease (IHD) are the most common manifestations of CVD in this population. This is not surprising given the shared risk factors (hypertension and diabetes mellitus) for both disease entities. Analysis of the Framingham study demonstrates that moderate CKD was associated with twice the prevalence of CVD and higher relative risks for both IHD and cerebrovascular accident (CVA) compared with individuals with normal kidney function. In a recent large cross-sectional study of 5888 elderly Medicare patients, the odds ratio for the presence of CVD was almost 2.5 times higher in CKD patients. In the Heart Outcome Prevention Evaluation (HOPE) trial, myocardial infarctions were more common in the subset of patients with CKD. A similar finding was noted in CKD patients compared with subjects from the general population in France.

The prevalence of left ventricular hypertrophy (LVH) approaches 40% in the early stages of CKD, higher rates occur in patients with lower GFR values. Left ventricular hypertrophy is present in nearly three-quarters of CKD patients initiating dialysis. Indirect evidence suggests that LVH develops progressively in these patients over the years preceding dialysis initiation. In addition, eccentric rather than concentric LVH is found to be twice as prevalent, suggesting a prominent role for anemia in the genesis of hypertrophied left ventricles in CKD patients. In Canada, the prevalence of IHD approaches 39–46% in patients with CKD. Coronary artery disease is also more severe with advanced renal dysfunction. Finally, PVD is prevalent in CKD patients, reaching 20% in one study. It is thus well established that CVD is prevalent in CKD patients.

Chronic kidney disease patients with CVD have worse outcomes than the general population. In ESRD patients commencing dialysis, the presence of LVH is independently associated with increased mortality. The risk of death over the first year following a myocardial infarction in this group is almost twice that of the general population. Similar findings are seen in CKD patients. The presence of mild-to-moderate kidney disease is associated with an increased risk of overall cardiovascular mortality. A number of studies documented a worse outcome after a myocardial

infarction in CKD patients. This may be due in part to undertreatment of these patients with state-of-the-art therapies for cardiovascular disease. Fear of exacerbating underlying kidney function with inhibitors of the renin-angiotensin system, contrast material, and aspirin explain this therapeutic approach. Risk of bleeding complications from thrombolytics employed for acute coronary syndromes in CKD patients with dysfunctional platelets further reduces use of this potentially life-saving therapy. There is also an increased risk for death after cardiac surgery. In the Studies of Left Ventricular Dysfunction (SOLVD) trial, kidney disease confers a higher risk of death among patients with ventricular dysfunction. Similarly, a higher risk of death and other cardiovascular events in CKD patients were noted in the HOPE trial. In summary, CKD patients appear to possess a higher risk of death from CVD.

Many factors increase risk for cardiovascular disease in CKD patients. The pathogenesis of cardiovascular damage in this group is far more complex than in the general population. Risk factors for CVD include those identified in the general population and additional ones associated with kidney disease (Table 16.3). Traditional coronary risk factors are highly prevalent in CKD patients. Diabetes mellitus is the most common cause of kidney disease in the United States and is present in more than 35% of patients with ESRD. Similarly, hypertension and dyslipidemia are rampant. A cross-sectional analysis involving patients enrolled in the Modification of Diet in Renal Disease trial noted that 64% were hypertensive despite therapy and more than half had elevated LDL cholesterol concentrations. "CKD-related" risk factors include the hemodynamic and metabolic abnormalities associated with kidney disease. Risk factors for CVD can be divided into "factors modified by CKD" such as hypertension, dyslipidemia, and hyperhomocysteinemia, and "CKD state-related risk factors" including anemia, hyperparathyroidism, malnutrition, and oxidative stress. Risk factor reduction is likely to be effective in reducing

Table 16.3

Cardiovascular Risk Factors in CKD

TRADITIONAL RISK FACTORS	RISK FACTORS ALTERED BY CKD	CKD-RELATED RISK FACTORS
Hypertension	Dyslipidemia	Hemodynamic overload
Hyperlipidemia	High lipoprotein (a)	Anemia
Diabetes mellitus	Prothrombotic factors	Increased oxidant stress
Tobacco use	Hyperhomocysteinemia	Malnutrition
Physical inactivity	Hypertension	Hyperparathyroidism
	Sleep apnea	Elevated ADMA levels

Abbreviation: ADMA, asymmetric dimethyl arginine.

morbidity and mortality due to cardiovascular disease in patients with CKD as they are in the general population. An approach to risk reduction should target both the traditional coronary risk factors and specific risk factors related to CKD (Table 16.3).

Traditional Risk Factors

HYPERTENSION

Hypertension is a common problem in CKD and is associated with untoward vascular events. From a cardiovascular disease perspective, the treatment of hypertension in CKD is incompletely studied. In stages 3–4, antihypertensive therapy improves LVH, and a recent study of patients with polycystic kidney disease revealed better results in reduction of left ventricular mass (35% versus 21%) in the group of patients whose target BP was 120/80 mmHg versus the conventional <140/90 mmHg. Patients with diabetic nephropathy have a reduction in hospitalization for first heart failure episode with AII receptor blockade. Large cohort studies reveal a protective effect associated with antihypertensive drug therapy. Exposure to calcium channel blockers or beta-blockers was associated with

decreased cardiovascular death in hemodialysis patients. ACE inhibitor effects are inconsistent across studies, but they are probably cardioprotective and reduce heart failure. Thus, hypertension is important in CKD due to its impact on both kidney disease progression and cardiovascular events. Lower BP targets lead to better control of LVH and likely cardiovascular outcomes.

DIABETES MELLITUS

Patients with diabetes mellitus constitute a large portion of the CKD population. This comorbid condition increases their risk of cardiovascular disease. In patients without significant degrees of renal dysfunction, several studies demonstrate the importance of markers of diabetic nephropathy on cardiovascular outcomes. The WHO Multinational Study of Vascular Disease in Diabetes, which included both type 1 and type 2 patients, demonstrated an almost twofold increase in the standardized mortality ratio of diabetic patients who had microalbuminuria. The addition of CKD increased this ratio to two-to threefold depending on sex. It appears that diabetes mellitus is an independent risk factor for the development of de novo ischemic heart disease and de novo heart failure in both CKD and ESRD patients.

SMOKING

Smoking aggravates the excessive cardiovascular risk in CKD patients. A random sample of new ESRD patients in the United States noted that smokers had a 22% greater risk of developing coronary artery disease. Like hypercholesterolemia and older age, smoking strongly predicted the presence of carotid atherosclerosis in ESRD patients. Since smoking has a clear association with cardiovascular disease in CKD patients, attempts at modifying its use are warranted. There are no published studies on the efficacy of different strategies for smoking cessation in patients with CKD or ESRD. Despite this, smoking cessation is an important preventive intervention.

Factors Modified by CKD

DYSLIPIDEMIA

The prevalence of hyperlipidemia in CKD is higher than in the general population but varies depending on the lipid, target population, course of kidney disease, and level of kidney function. Total or LDL cholesterol elevations are common in patients with CKD and nephrotic syndrome and ESRD patients on peritoneal dialysis (PD). Uremic dyslipidemia is characterized by increased plasma triglyceride with normal total cholesterol concentration. Very low density lipoprotein (VLDL) and intermediate density lipoprotein (IDL) concentrations are elevated, whereas LDL and high density lipoprotein (HDL) concentrations are decreased. Increased triglyceride and decreased HDL cholesterol concentrations are more severe in individuals with advanced CKD. Limited data suggest that lipid abnormalities increase cardiovascular disease in CKD patients. For example, the incidence of myocardial infarctions in 147 CKD patients (creatinine clearance of 20–50 mL/minute/1.73 m^2) was approximately 2.5 times higher than in the general population. Patients with myocardial infarctions had lower HDL cholesterol concentrations and higher triglyceride, LDL cholesterol, apolipoprotein B and lipoprotein (a) concentrations. Patients with CKD

should be considered in the highest risk group as defined by the National Cholesterol Education Program guidelines. LDL cholesterol concentrations >100 and >130 mg/dL are treatment initiation thresholds for diet and drug therapy, respectively. Target LDL cholesterol concentrations are <70 mg/dL in CKD patients. Statins are the most effective therapy to reduce total and LDL cholesterol concentrations. They are associated with decreased mortality in ESRD patients. Pharmacologic treatment of hypertriglyceridemia and of low HDL is not recommended unless LDL is also increased. Statins in combination with ezetimibe may further improve LDL cholesterol concentrations. Fibric acid analogs are the most effective in reducing triglycerides in CKD patients.

HYPERHOMOCYSTEINEMIA

Hyperhomocysteinemia, an independent risk factor for atherosclerosis in the general population, is highly prevalent in CKD patients. It may also increase atherosclerosis in this group. Approximately 90% of ESRD patients have elevated plasma homocysteine concentrations, the result of impaired homocysteine metabolism. The clinical impact of lowering homocysteine concentrations by employing folate, vitamin B6 and vitamin B12 supplementation needs to be confirmed, since conventional doses seldom correct the abnormal concentrations observed in patients with stage 4 or 5 CKD.

CKD-Related Risk Factors

ANEMIA

Anemia in ESRD dialysis patients is associated with adverse cardiovascular outcomes. Under uremic conditions, the hemodynamic changes associated with anemia are maladaptive, resulting in cardiac hypertrophy and arteriosclerosis. A decrease in hemoglobin (Hb) level of 1 g/dL incrementally increases the risk of mortality by 18–25% and of left ventricular hypertrophy by approximately 50%. Anemia is also a cardiac risk factor in CKD patients. As an example, CKD patients with a 0.5 g/dL decrease in hemoglobin concentration have a 32% increased risk of left ventricular growth. Correction of anemia may improve cardiovascular outcomes through multiple effects. Regression of LVH occurs in CKD patients after 12 months of erythropoietin treatment aimed at normalizing hematocrit (Hct), in the absence of better blood pressure control. Target hemoglobin is 12 g/dL. This level is safe for most CKD patients, provided that a rapid increase is avoided and blood pressure is controlled.

HYPERPARATHYROIDISM

Disturbances of calcium and phosphate metabolism may increase cardiovascular disease in CKD patients. Elevated serum calcium and phosphate concentrations, secondary hyperparathyroidism, administration of calcium-containing phosphate-binding agents, and vitamin D supplementation were implicated as risk factors for increased cardiovascular complications, possibly through end-organ calcification. Calcifications of the coronary arteries, valves, and myocardial tissue, as well as diffuse myocardial fibrosis are common pathologic findings in uremic hearts. Hyperphosphatemia is strongly associated with mortality in ESRD patients. The adjusted relative risk of death is greater at serum phosphorus concentration >6.5 mg/dL and when the calcium-phosphorus product is >72 mg^2/dL^2. Increased mortality is due to an increase in cardiac deaths, suggesting that correction of hyperphosphatemia is important to reduce cardiac morbidity and mortality, especially in the early stages of CKD. Efforts should be made to reduce hyperphosphatemia and hyperparathyroidism through strict phosphorus control and judicious use of vitamin D derivatives. Non-calcium-containing binders may have additional benefits to reduce cardiovascular complications. Calcimimetics may also play an important role in CVD reduction by improving PTH concentration and calcium-phosphorus product in CKD patients.

KEY POINTS
Risk Factors

1. CVD is common in CKD patients and is associated with increased risk of mortality.
2. Several risk factors are present in CKD patients that increase the prevalence of CVD, including traditional factors, factors modified by CKD, and factors related to the CKD state.
3. Hypertension and diabetes mellitus are the major factors contributing to the large CVD burden in CKD.
4. Anemia increases the development of LVH, a prominent risk factor for untoward cardiovascular events.
5. Calcification of the vasculature from hyperphosphatemia, a high calcium-phosphorus product, and perhaps excessive calcium intake also contribute to CVD.

Anemia of CKD

Anemia is a common and early complication of CKD. It is characterized by normochromic normocytic red blood cells (RBCs). In 5222 prevalent patients with CKD, mild anemia, as defined by Hb level <12 g/dL, was found in 47% of the cohort. The degree of anemia was most marked in patients with the lowest GFRs. Anemia, however, can develop in patients with GFR levels as high as 60 mL/min/1.73 m^2. Anemia guidelines for CKD patients recommend anemia workup and treatment for all stage 3 or 4 CKD patients. Patients with GFRs <60 mL/minute/1.73 m^2 and Hb <11 g/dL (premenopausal females and prepubertal patients) and Hb <12 g/dL (adult males and postmenopausal females) should be evaluated. Hemoglobin is the recommended parameter for the evaluation and management of anemia, given the wider variations seen in hematocrit values and instability of samples.

Anemia evolves in patients with CKD for a variety of reasons. Decreased RBC production, decreased RBC survival, and blood loss all contribute to anemia. The primary cause of anemia in patients with CKD is insufficient production of erythropoietin by the diseased kidneys. This is supported by a state of "relative" erythropoietin deficiency in CKD patients, since levels are inappropriately low for the degree of anemia compared with normal individuals. Finally, an improvement in the RBC count is seen almost uniformly following therapy with exogenous erythropoietin.

A common secondary cause of anemia is iron deficiency. This is defined in CKD as transferrin saturation (TSAT) <20% or ferritin <100 ng/mL according to the NKF-K/DOQI guidelines. Blood loss from phlebotomies associated with laboratory testing, occult gastrointestinal bleeding, decreased iron absorption, dietary restriction, and iron usage by exogenously stimulated erythropoiesis all contribute to the development and maintenance of iron deficiency. In an analysis of data from the NHANES III, 38.3% of 3453 anemic subjects with GFRs between 20 and 60 mL/minute/1.73 m^2 had TSAT values below 20%. Thus, all potential causes of iron deficiency must be fully evaluated in CKD patients. Other secondary causes of anemia in CKD include hypothyroidism, severe hyperparathyroidism, acute and chronic inflammatory conditions, aluminum toxicity, folate and B$_{12}$ deficiencies, shortened red blood cell survival, and hemoglobinopathies.

Evaluation of anemia in CKD patients should include the following tests:

- Hb and/or Hct
- RBC indices
- Reticulocyte count
- A test for occult blood in stool
- Iron parameters: serum iron concentration, total iron-binding capacity (TIBC), percent transferrin saturation, and serum ferritin concentration

Diagnosis of iron deficiency is not always straightforward in CKD patients. Functional iron deficiency, which refers to the imbalance between iron needed to support erythropoiesis and the amount released from storage sites, is often present. A ferritin concentration below 100 ng/mL is usually diagnostic of iron deficiency, however, the ferritin concentration may be elevated secondary to chronic inflammation or infection. Thus it is not always a reliable index of iron deficiency in CKD patients. TSAT is considered the best routinely available test of iron deficiency. A TSAT <20% usually indicates functional iron deficiency. Other tests such as the proportion of hypochromic red blood cells (>10% with mean corpuscular hemoglobin <28 g/dL) and reticulocyte hemoglobin content may improve the diagnosis of functional iron deficiency in CKD patients.

Effects of Anemia in CKD Patients

Anemia plays a major role in the quality of life in CKD patients and has pronounced effects on patient well-being. It may ultimately determine prognosis both prior to and after starting RRT. For these reasons, it is imperative that anemia is addressed and corrected in CKD patients. The relationship between anemia and morbidity and mortality in dialysis patients is well established. There is a growing body of evidence similarly associating anemia and cardiovascular disease in CKD patients. The effect of anemia on CVD appears to start many years prior to the development of ESRD.

Role of Anemia in Cardiovascular Disease and Mortality

Evidence supports a link between anemia and CVD. Anemia is independently associated with the presence of LVH in CKD patients and plays a significant role in its evolution. Evidence in favor of the connection of anemia and LVH includes data generated from a cross-sectional study of 175 patients with mean creatinine clearance of 25.5 mL/minute. A decline in hemoglobin of 1 g/dL was associated with a 6% independent increased risk for LVH. More severe LVH is seen with lower hemoglobin levels. Anemia may also increase oxidative stress. Other factors peculiar to CKD such as the uremic milieu, calcification, hypertension, and volume overload contribute to the maladaptive cardiac response to anemia. Cardiac fibrosis and potentially irreversible LVH may result from these factors.

Correction of anemia in ESRD patients was shown to reduce left ventricular mass index (LVMI), improve ejection fraction (EF), and mitigate ischemic changes that develop during cardiac stress tests. Similar limited data are available in CKD patients, although small numbers of patients with severe LVH and advanced kidney disease were studied. Prospective studies are underway to further elucidate the long-term benefits of anemia correction in earlier stages of CKD and less severe LVH. These earlier interventions raise the interesting role of primary prevention of anemia in CKD patients, which may be important in modulating the development of irreversible cardiac changes.

Other Benefits of Anemia Correction

Correction of anemia in CKD patients maintains benefits beyond solely improving cardiac status. A reduction in mortality during the first 24 months after initiating hemodialysis occurs in patients treated with erythropoietin in the predialysis phase of care. Additional benefits include the following:

1. Improved sense of well-being, quality of life, neurocognitive function, and work capacity.
2. Reduced need for packed red blood cell transfusion.
3. Reduced allosensitization pretransplantation.
4. Reduced hospitalization.

Effect of Anemia Correction on Renal Function

Worsening of renal function with anemia correction by recombinant human erythropoietin (rHuEpo) was an initial concern based on data from an animal model of kidney disease. Uncontrolled hypertension rather than correction of anemia was the probable cause of worsening kidney function. Studies in humans uniformly show no effect of exogenous erythropoietin therapy on renal function in CKD patients. Of interest, a beneficial effect of anemia correction on renal function was noted. Several studies suggest that correction of anemia slows the progression of CKD. The potential mechanisms for such a desirable benefit may relate to the effect of anemia and hypoxia on interstitial fibrosis and the anti-apoptotic effect of erythropoietin. Several in vitro and in vivo studies support a nephroprotective effect of erythropoietin.

Effect of Anemia Correction on BP Control

Anemia correction with rHuEpo may increase BP in CKD patients. Concerns for severe hypertensive crisis and seizures were prominent following initial experience with rHuEpo. The increase in BP that develops with rHuEpo is due to an increase in systemic vascular resistance, as well as direct and indirect pressor effects of rHuEpo. These initial concerns, however, were almost entirely alleviated when the rate of Hb correction was slowed to an average of 1 g/dL/month. Since hypertension may still develop with slower rates of anemia correction, BP monitoring should be a standard part of rHuEpo therapy. Blood pressure control is easily achieved with adjustments in antihypertensive regimens.

Therapy of Anemia in CKD

Recombinant human erythropoietin and darbepoetin both successfully correct anemia in patients with CKD. Optimal target hemoglobin concentrations are unknown but current recommendations suggest Hb concentrations between 11 and 12 g/dL (Hct 33 and 36%). In CKD patients with heart disease and chronic obstructive lung disease, it is medically justifiable to maintain the Hb concentration >12 g/dL. Presently, full correction of anemia cannot be recommended given the absence of scientific evidence supporting either beneficial effects or safety.

Subcutaneous injection is the preferred route of rHuEpo administration. Self-administration is simple and well tolerated by most patients. Some patients experience minor pain at the site of injection. Recombinant human erythropoietin is usually given on a weekly or twice-weekly basis. More frequent dosing may be required at initiation, depending on the degree of anemia. After attaining target Hb concentration, many patients may be subsequently maintained on weekly injections. The recommended starting dose of rHuEpo is 50–100 U/kg/wk. Dosing changes for rHuEpo should not be done more frequently than every week, while the frequency for darbepoetin should be less. Hemoglobin is measured on a weekly basis during the initiation phase of therapy and until the target Hb concentration is attained. Thereafter, biweekly or monthly determinations are usually sufficient.

Darbepoetin is a newer erythropoietic agent with a longer serum half-life than rHuEpo. It differs structurally from rHuEpo by virtue of its higher sialic acid-containing carbohydrate content, an important determinant of the half-life of these molecules. It is generally given no more frequently than once a week; bi- or triweekly use may be sufficient to correct anemia. The starting dose for darbepoetin is 0.45 µg/kg. Most patients will require either a dose of 25 or 40 µg every other week. The safety profile of this long-acting erythropoietic agent is similar to that of rHuEpo.

As erythropoiesis is stimulated and the marrow produces RBCs, iron stores are rapidly used. Many patients will require iron supplementation to maintain erythropoietic responsiveness. Oral supplementation is usually effective but intravenous iron preparations may be required. Iron indices such as TSAT and ferritin are followed on a regular basis to guide iron administration. Suboptimal response to rHuEpo therapy may be the result of gastrointestinal blood loss and primary hematologic disorders. These should be fully investigated as clinically indicated.

KEY POINTS
Anemia of CKD

1. Anemia commonly occurs when GFR reaches 30–40 mL/minute/1.73 m^2 in CKD patients, but may occur earlier.
2. Decreased red cell production (erythropoietin deficiency), reduced red cell survival, and enhanced blood loss (with iron deficiency) contribute to the anemia of CKD.
3. Iron deficiency is the most common cause of exogenous erythropoietin resistance in CKD patients.
4. Correction of anemia is associated with reductions in adverse cardiovascular disease events and hospitalizations, improvements in well being and neurocognitive function, and reductions in red blood cell transfusions and allosensitization pretransplant.
5. Anemia is corrected in CKD patients with either subcutaneous recombinant erythropoietin or darbepoietin.
6. CKD patients receiving exogenous erythropoietin should have their hemoglobin corrected approximately 1 g/dL/month until target is reached to avoid severe hypertension and seizure.

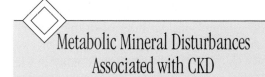

Metabolic Mineral Disturbances Associated with CKD

In CKD patients, the incidence of hyperphosphatemia, hypocalcemia, and secondary hyperparathyroidism increase as GFR declines. Identification and treatment of mineral metabolism disturbances at an early stage in CKD may reduce many of their adverse consequences. These metabolic disturbances ultimately lead to a group of bone disorders collectively known as renal osteodystrophy.

Serum phosphorus concentration increases as GFR declines below 60 mL/minute/1.73 m^2. Approximately 15% of patients with a GFR from 15 to 30 mL/minute and 50% of those with a GFR <15 mL/minute have a serum phosphorus concentration >4.5 mg/dL. Parathyroid hormone (PTH) increases the renal excretion of phosphorus. In the short term, this serves to maintain phosphorus homeostasis. As GFR falls below 30 mL/minute/1.73 m^2 renal phosphate excretion reaches a maximum. Hyperphosphatemia directly increases PTH secretion and stimulates parathyroid cell proliferation and hyperplasia. Hyperphosphatemia also decreases expression of the calcium-sensing receptor. The calcium-sensing receptor is expressed on parathyroid cells and senses the extracellular fluid (ECF) calcium concentration. There is an inverse sigmoidal relationship between serum calcium and PTH concentrations with a nonsuppressible component of PTH secretion even at high serum calcium concentrations. The PTH-calcium response curve is shifted to the right in CKD patients with secondary hyperparathyroidism. Decreased calcium sensing may be due to reduced expression of the calcium-sensing receptor in parathyroid gland.

Concentrations of 1,25(OH)$_2$ vitamin D$_3$ decline early in the course of CKD (GFR ≤ 60 mL/minute/1.73 m^2). 1,25(OH)$_2$ vitamin D$_3$ is a potent suppressor of PTH gene transcription, and parathyroid growth and cell proliferation. The vitamin D receptor and calcium-sensing receptor in the parathyroid are downregulated in CKD. Calcium-sensing receptor expression is also regulated by 1,25(OH)$_2$ vitamin D$_3$. A decrease in calcium-sensing receptor expression decreases the responsiveness of the parathyroid gland to inhibition by calcium.

Hypocalcemia occurs late in the course of kidney disease, typically after changes in serum phosphorus, 1,25(OH)$_2$ vitamin D$_3$, and PTH concentrations. Seven percent of patients with a GFR of 15–30 mL/minute and 25% of patients with a GFR <15 mL/minute are hypocalcemic. This divalent disorder increases PTH concentration by prolonging the half-life of the mRNA and exacerbates secondary hyperparathyroidism.

Secondary hyperparathyroidism is a near universal complication of CKD that develops early in the course of the disease. PTH concentration begins to rise as the GFR falls below 40 mL/minute/1.73 m^2. PTH production and secretion are regulated by phosphorus, 1,25(OH)$_2$ vitamin D$_3$, and calcium. Alterations in these parameters, as noted above, increase the development of secondary hyperparathyroidism.

Renal Osteodystrophy

Renal osteodystrophy is a group of metabolic bone disorders that develop as a consequence of kidney disease. They include osteitis fibrosa, osteomalacia, mixed uremic osteodystrophy, and adynamic bone disease. Osteitis fibrosa develops as a result of increased PTH concentration, which increases osteoblast and osteoclast number and activity (high bone turnover). Osteomalacia is due to 1,25(OH)$_2$ vitamin D$_3$ deficiency. It is characterized by low bone turnover with wide unmineralized osteoid seams and the absence of osteoclasts and erosive surfaces. Mixed uremic osteodystrophy has features of both osteitis fibrosa and osteomalacia. Adynamic bone disease is distinguished by a reduction in bone formation and resorption and is manifested histologically by thin osteoid seams with little or no evidence of cellular activity. It is associated with peritoneal dialysis, higher doses of calcium carbonate as a phosphate binder, the presence of diabetes mellitus, 1,25(OH)$_2$ vitamin D$_3$ treatment, and older age.

In patients with advanced CKD, the spectrum of renal osteodystrophy is similar to that observed in ESRD patients. Osteitis fibrosa is seen in 40–56%, osteomalacia in 2–11%, and adynamic bone disease in 27–48%. Few patients have normal bone histology. In patients with milder kidney disease, osteitis fibrosa and mixed uremic osteodystrophy are the most common histologic lesions found in 40 and 29% of patients, respectively. Osteomalacia is the least common abnormality (4.5% of patients). Normal bone histology is found in approximately 20% of those with less severe kidney disease. Adynamic bone disease is noted in only 6% of those with milder CKD. The largest study examining 176 CKD patients with bone biopsy found osteitis fibrosa in 56%, mixed uremic osteodystrophy in 14%, and adynamic bone disease in 5%. Normal histology was seen in 25% and osteomalacia was observed in only one patient. Patients with normal histology had a significantly higher GFR than those with an abnormal bone biopsy.

PTH is the most common biomarker used for the assessment of bone turnover and classification of renal osteodystrophy. Using second generation intact PTH assays a PTH concentration <65 pg/mL has a sensitivity of 88% and a specificity of 91% for adynamic bone disease. A PTH concentration >400 pg/mL has a sensitivity of 83% and a specificity of 88% for osteitis fibrosa. Although bone biopsy is the gold standard, biomarkers such as PTH are followed longitudinally in patients at high risk to develop renal osteodystrophy and those with bone disease that is likely to become more severe as kidney function deteriorates. Target PTH concentrations in advanced CKD were proposed (Table 16.4) but are extrapolated from the ESRD population. Optimal target PTH concentrations are not established for patients with mild-to-moderate CKD.

One consequence of renal osteodystrophy in ESRD patients is increased risk of hip and vertebral fractures. Those with adynamic bone disease appear to be at highest risk. Analysis of the USRDS database of Caucasians starting dialysis between 1989 and 1996 showed the risk of hip fracture in women was 13.63 per 1000 patient years and in men was 7.45 per 1000 patient years. The relative risk for hip fracture in men and women was 4.44 and 4.40 times higher, respectively, in dialysis patients compared to age and sex-matched

Table 16.4

Suggested Ranges for PTH in Relation to GFR

GFR	PTH
>50 mL/minute/1.73 m^2	Upper limit of normal
20–50 mL/minute/1.73 m^2	1.0–1.5 times the upper limit of normal
<20 mL/minute/1.73 m^2	1.5–2.0 times the upper limit of normal
On dialysis	2.0–3.0 times the upper limit of normal

Abbreviations: GFR, glomerular filtration rate; PTH, parathyroid hormone.

controls. Although the age-specific relative risk was highest in the youngest age groups, the added risk of fracture associated with dialysis increased steadily with advancing age. Risk factors for hip fracture include age, Caucasian race, female sex, low body mass index (BMI), peripheral vascular disease, inability to ambulate, low albumin, and smoking. Data in CKD patients are not available, but their fracture risk is likely higher than the general population.

Treatment of Renal Osteodystrophy

Treatment of renal osteodystrophy in CKD patients includes several targets. Hyperphosphatemia is initially controlled with dietary restriction. Ingestion of foods high in phosphorus should be minimized. As CKD worsens, oral phosphate binders are frequently required. The previous goal of therapy in ESRD patients was to maintain the calcium-phosphorus product below 72 mg^2/dL^2 and the serum phosphorus concentration below 6.5 mg/dL. Concentrations above these increase the relative risk of mortality in ESRD patients. The serum phosphorus goal was recently lowered to ≤5.5 mg/dL and the calcium-phosphorus product to ≤55 mg^2/dL^2. Although no studies on this issue exist in CKD, the recommended goals are similar.

The use of calcium-containing phosphate binders results in net positive calcium balance in ESRD patients. This calcium may deposit in the vasculature and contribute to increased morbidity and mortality from ischemic coronary disease. Calcium-containing binders, although efficient and low in cost, may contribute to excess total body calcium burden. Sevelamer hydrochloride, a synthetic calcium-free polymer has a favorable side effect profile but is costly. Aluminum is the most efficient binder and is relatively inexpensive, however, it has significant long-term toxicity (aluminum-related osteomalacia and dementia). Aluminum-containing phosphate binders should only be used in the short-term management of severe hyperphosphatemia (serum phosphorus concentration ≤8.5 mg/dL). Lanthanum carbonate, another noncalcium containing phosphate binder may also provide safe and effective control of hyperphosphatemia and was recently FDA approved for clinical practice.

Since hypocalcemia is a potent stimulator of PTH secretion, serum calcium concentration should be corrected into the low normal range. This can be achieved with oral calcium, however, it should be employed cautiously as it may increase risk for vascular calcification and the development of adynamic bone disease.

Acidosis is common in CKD patients. This disturbance increases bone loss, potentiates the effect of PTH and decreases 1,25(OH)$_2$ vitamin D$_3$ production. Correction slows the progression of secondary hyperparathyroidism. A serum bicarbonate concentration goal of ≥22 meq/L can be achieved with 1–4 g of sodium bicarbonate daily with close monitoring for hypertension and fluid overload. Addition of a loop diuretic often allows continued sodium bicarbonate therapy in patients with hypertension and edema.

The optimal PTH concentration in CKD patients is not established. If PTH is more than two to four times the upper limit of normal, hyperphosphatemia and hypocalcemia should be corrected. If PTH remains elevated or these conditions are absent then vitamin D therapy will likely be required. Small doses of oral calcitriol (0.25–0.50 g/day) stabilize and decrease PTH concentration. Decreases are primarily seen in patients with a PTH concentration <200 pg/mL. Pulse calcitriol oral therapy (2 g/week dosed once per week) may be more effective and is associated with a lower risk of hypercalcemia.

KEY POINTS
Metabolic Mineral Disturbances Associated with CKD

1. Disturbances in mineral metabolism develop early in CKD and include hyperphosphatemia, hypocalcemia, and low vitamin D concentration and secondary hyperparathyroidism.
2. Renal osteodystrophy consists of a spectrum of bone diseases in CKD patients. They include osteitis fibrosa, osteomalacia, adynamic bone disease, and mixed uremic osteodystrophy.
3. Hip and vertebral fractions are a complication of renal osteodystrophy in CKD patients.
4. Although bone biopsy is the gold standard, PTH concentration is employed to guide management of renal osteodystrophy and use of vitamin D.

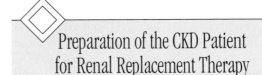

Preparation of the CKD Patient for Renal Replacement Therapy

A critical part of CKD care consists of the emotional and physical preparation of patients for the initiation of RRT. Evaluation and management of the patient with advanced CKD focuses on preparation for RRT. Importantly, improved predialysis care reduces the mortality rate for this high-risk group. To address this issue, the appropriate timing of nephrology referral, ESRD preparatory care, critical components of patient education and those resources available to patients, and the optimal time of RRT initiation is reviewed.

Nephrology Referral of CKD Patients

The population of patients with CKD is not uniformly monitored in the United States. As a result, most CKD patients are not prepared for entry into the world of ESRD. Less than half of new ESRD patients have permanent vascular access in place at the initiation of hemodialysis. Given the well-known advantages of permanent vascular access, there is room for improvement in the preparatory phase of CKD patients.

A major reason for this problem is late referral (1–4 months prior to RRT) of CKD patients to nephrologists. Only about half of incident ESRD patients are seen by a nephrologist 1 year prior to initiation of ESRD care, and 30% are seen less than 4 months before RRT is begun. Late referral is associated with increased morbidity and a graded risk reduction for patient mortality is noted with early referral (>12 months). Multiple factors cause late referral of CKD patients to nephrology specialty care teams. Economic barriers (i.e., lack of insurance), as well as patient factors that include denial, fear, and procrastination. Provider factors, such as underappreciation of severity of kidney disease, fear of alarming the patient, lack of a multidisciplinary care team, and inadequate frequency of patient follow-up may contribute. Lack of training about both the appropriate timing and indications for referral of CKD patients to nephrologists also contribute. Finally, poor communication and feedback from nephrologists following CKD patients promotes late referral.

Late referral to the nephrologist is associated with diminished patient choice, as well as adverse outcomes (Table 16.5). Patients referred late select peritoneal dialysis (PD) as a dialysis modality less often. It also promotes delayed referral for renal transplantation evaluation and eliminates any possibility for preemptive renal transplantation. Resource usage is significantly higher when referral occurs late in the course of CKD, including

Table 16.5
Consequences of Late Referral

Severe metabolic acidosis
Severe hyperphosphatemia
Marked anemia
Hypoalbuminemia
Severe hypertension and volume overload
Low prevalence of permanent dialysis access
Delayed referral for renal transplantation
Higher initial hospitalization rate
Higher costs of initiation of dialysis
Increased 1-year mortality rate
Decreased patient choice in RRT modality selection

Abbreviation: RRT, renal replacement therapy.

higher initial hospitalization rates and cost of initiation of dialysis. Most importantly, overall patient mortality is greater. In contrast, early referral permits multidisciplinary predialysis education and improves vocational outcomes. It also delays progression of CKD, reduces requirements for urgent dialysis, and decreases hospital length of stay. Importantly, it increases native arteriovenous fistula (AVF) creation (Table 16.6). The NIH

Table 16.6
Benefits of Early Referral to Nephrologist

Improved vocational outcomes
Delay in need to initiate RRT
Increased proportion of patients with permanent vascular access, particularly AVF
Patient modality selection differences—greater peritoneal dialysis usage
Reduced need for urgent dialysis
Reduced hospital length of stay and health care costs
Better metabolic parameters at dialysis initiation
Better patient survival

Abbreviations: RRT, renal replacement therapy; AVF, arteriovenous fistula.

Consensus Development Conference Panel published a consensus statement recommending nephrology referral of all CKD patients with a serum creatinine concentration >2 mg/dL in men or >1.5 mg/dL in women. The National Kidney Foundation (NKF) also recommends early referral to the nephrology team.

Components of ESRD Care Preparation

A multidisciplinary clinic approach, consisting of physicians, social workers, nutritionists, and nurse coordinators, enhances the preparation of CKD patients for entry into ESRD care and initiation of RRT. The use of a multidisciplinary predialysis program to reduce urgent dialysis was studied. The proactive CKD care program reduced the number of urgent dialysis starts from 35 to 13%. It also decreased the number of hospital days during the first month of RRT from 13.5 to 6.5 days and resulted in net dollar savings of $4000 per patient. Hence, a multidisciplinary team approach to CKD care improved preparedness for entry into the ESRD system and reduced health care resource usage. Education about the various dialysis options allows patients to make informed choices about the appropriate modality of RRT. Since development of ESRD is emotionally traumatic news for most patients, early nephrology referral allows adequate time for the dialysis care team to assist in this aspect of CKD patient care.

The nephrologist should discuss modality options for RRT including the specifics of hemodialysis, peritoneal dialysis, and preemptive renal transplantation. If PD is the patient's preferred choice of RRT, the patient and/or the family can initiate PD training prior to the actual initiation of dialysis. If hemodialysis is selected, vascular access, preferably an AVF, should be placed. Patients should be counseled to protect their nondominant arm to protect veins for future AVF creation. K/DOQI guidelines strongly encourage placement of permanent vascular access when serum creatinine concentration is greater than

4 mg/dL, the creatinine clearance is <25 cc/minute/1.73 m², or the development of ESRD is anticipated within 1 year. Preemptive renal transplantation requires a significant amount of time for planning and completion of medical testing. In some instances, the patient may elect not to initiate RRT. In this difficult situation, explicit counseling that outlines the serious consequences of this choice is mandatory and should include one or more members of the patient's family. In addition, an evaluation for major depression is required. The presence of depression precludes informed consent and requires further intervention by the family and judicial system (conservatorship). If this decision is ultimately chosen by the patient and is supported by the family, then end-of-life care should be pursued.

As renal disease progresses to ESRD, dietary modifications are necessary to avoid life-threatening volume overload, hyperkalemia, protein and caloric malnutrition, exacerbation of metabolic acidosis, and divalent ion derangements. Consultation with a renal dietician is essential to avoid or reduce the development of these complications. Medication adjustments by the nephrologist will also reduce these complications. Nutritional state should be assessed regularly and dietary counseling undertaken to optimize protein intake without inducing hyperphosphatemia, hyperkalemia, or metabolic acidosis.

To avoid information overload and patient confusion, the introduction of small amounts of new information at successive visits will reduce patient stress and improve understanding of their disease process and ultimate ESRD care plan. It is helpful for the primary provider to assess the patient's understanding of the aforementioned at follow-up visits. Reinforcement of correctly understood information and clarification of erroneous aspects of the patient's education are essential since cognitive deficits may exist in advanced uremia. Early education improves understanding by reducing anxiety and fear through preparation, allowing for choices, assuring informed consent, encouraging independence, and promoting a sense of patient self-control.

Initiation of RRT

Timely initiation of RRT is the final aspect of adequate preparation of the CKD patient. Absolute indications for dialysis include uremic scrositis (especially pericarditis), uremic encephalopathy, refractory metabolic acidosis, hyperkalemia, or uncontrollable volume overload. It is appropriate to commence RRT in patients who are in the presymptomatic stage, when CrCl is <10 cc/minute/ 1.73 m^2 in nondiabetics and <15 cc/minute/ 1.73 m^2 in diabetics. Ultimately, initiation of RRT is based on the combination of kidney function as assessed by estimated GFR (or CrCl), the presence of signs and symptoms of uremia, and patient preference. At the time of initiation of RRT, emotional and physical preparation of patients is key. This approach will allow a smooth transition and more stable entry into ESRD care or preemptive transplantation.

KEY POINTS

Preparation of the CKD Patient for Renal Replacement Therapy

1. The patient with advanced CKD requires emotional and physical preparation for the initiation of RRT.
2. Late referral to the nephrology care team is associated with increased morbidity and mortality in CKD patients.
3. A multidisciplinary clinic approach (physicians, social workers, nutritionists, and nurse coordinators) enhances the preparation of CKD patients for entry into ESRD care.
4. In patients with advanced CKD, dietary modifications are required to avoid life-threatening volume overload, hyperkalemia, acidosis, protein and caloric malnutrition, and disturbances in mineral metabolism.
5. Initiation of RRT is based primarily on the presence of signs of symptoms of uremia, and the level of kidney function.

Additional Reading

Alem, A.M., Sherrard, D.J., Gillen, D.L., Weiss, N.S, Beresford, S.A., Heckbert, S.R., Wong, C., Stehman-Breen, C. Increased risk of hip fracture among patients with end-stage renal disease. *Kidney Int* 58:396–399, 2000.

Astor, B.C., Muntner, P., Levin, A., Eustace, J.A., Coresh, J. Association of kidney function with anemia: the Third National Health and Nutrition Examination Survey (1988–1994). *Arch Intern Med* 162:1401–1408, 2002.

Bakris, G.L., Weir, M.R. Angiotensin-converting enzyme inhibitor-associated elevations in serum creatinine. Is this a cause for concern? *Arch Intern Med* 160:685–693, 2000.

Block, G.A., Port, F.K. Re-evaluation of risks associated with hyperphosphatemia and hyperparathyroidism in dialysis patients: recommendations for a change in management. *Am J Kidney Dis* 35:1226–1237, 2000.

Consensus Development Conference Panel. Morbidity and mortality of renal dialysis: an NIH consensus conference statement. *Ann Intern Med* 121:62–70, 1994.

Garg, A.X., Clark, W.F., Haynes, R.B., House, A.A. Moderate renal insufficiency and the risk of cardiovascular mortality: results from the NHANES I. *Kidney Int* 61:1486–1494, 2002.

Golper, T. The impact of pre-ESRD education on dialysis modality selection. *J Am Soc Nephrol* 11:A1223, 2000.

Healthy People 2010: Chronic Kidney Disease. National Institutes of Health, National Institute of Diabetes and Digestive and Kidney Diseases, Bethesda, MD, 2000.

Hsu, C.Y., McCulloch, C.E., Curhan, G.C. Epidemiology of anemia associated with chronic renal insufficiency among adults in the United States: results from the Third National Health and Nutrition Examination Survey. *J Am Soc Nephrol* 13:504–510, 2001.

Jafar, T., Schmid, C., Landa, M., Giatras, I., Toto, R., Remuzzi, G., Maschio, G., Brenner, B.M., Kamper, A., Zucchelli, P., Becker, G., Himmelmann, A., Bannister, K., Landais, P., Shahinfar, S., de Jong, P.E., de Zeeuw, D., Lau, J., Levey, A.S. Angiotensin converting enzyme inhibitors and progression on non-diabetic renal disease. *Ann Intern Med* 135:73–87, 2001.

Jungers, P., Massy, Z.A., Khoa, T.N., Fumeron, C., Labrunie, M., Lacour, B., Descamps-Latscha, B.,

Man, N.K. Incidence and risk factors of atherosclerotic cardiovascular accidents in predialysis chronic renal failure patients: a prospective study. *Nephrol Dial Transplant* 12:2597–2602, 1997.

Kinchen, K.S., Sadler, J., Fink, N., Brookmeyer, R., Klag, M.J., Levey, A.S., Powe, N.R. The timing of specialist evaluation in chronic kidney disease and mortality. *Ann Int Med* 137:479–486, 2002.

Levey, A.S., Bosch, J.P., Lewis, J.B., Greene, T., Rogers, N., Roth, D. A more accurate method to estimate glomerular filtration rate from serum creatinine: a new prediction equation. Modification of Diet in Renal Disease Study Group. *Ann Intern Med* 130:461–470, 1999.

Levey, A., Eknoyan, G. Cardiovascular disease in chronic renal disease. *Nephrol Dial Transplant* 14:828–833, 1999.

Levin, A. Consequences of late referral on patient outcomes. *Nephrol Dial Transplant* 15(Suppl. 3):8–13, 2000.

Lewis, E.J., Hunsicker, L.G., Bain, R.P., Rhode, R.D. The effect of angiotensin-converting enzyme inhibition on diabetic nephropathy. *N Engl J Med* 329:1456–1462, 1993.

Llach, F., Velasquez Forero, F. Secondary hyperparathyroidism in chronic renal failure: pathogenic and clinical aspects. *Am J Kidney Dis* 38(Suppl. 5):S20–S33, 2001.

Locatelli, F., Bommer, J., London, G.M. Cardiovascular disease determinants in chronic renal failure: clinical approach and treatment. *Nephrol Dial Transplant* 16:459–468, 2001.

Mann, J.F., Gerstein, H.C., Pogue, J., Bosch, J., Yusuf, S. Renal insufficiency as a predictor of cardiovascular outcomes and the impact of ramipril: the HOPE randomized trial. *Ann Intern Med* 134:629–636, 2001.

Maschio, G., Alberti, D., Janin, G., Locatelli, F., Mann, J.F., Motolese, M., Ponticelli, C., Ritz, E., Zucchelli, P. Effect of the angiotensin-converting-enzyme inhibitor benazepril on the progression of chronic renal insufficiency. The angiotensin-converting enzyme inhibition in progressive renal insufficiency study group. *N Engl J Med* 334:939–945, 1996.

National Kidney Foundation (NKF) Kidney Disease Outcome Quality Initiative (K/DOQI) Advisory Board. K/DOQI clinical practice guidelines for chronic kidney disease: evaluation, classification, and stratification. Kidney Disease Outcome Quality Initiative. *Am J Kidney Dis* 39(2 Suppl. 2):S1–S246, 2002.

Rostand, S.G., Drueke, T.B. Parathyroid hormone, vitamin D, and cardiovascular disease in chronic renal failure. *Kidney Int* 56:383–392, 1999.

Shlipak, M.G., Heidenreich, P.A., Noguchi, H., Chertow, G.M, Browner, W.S, McClellan, M.B. Association of renal insufficiency with treatment and outcomes after myocardial infarction in elderly patients. *Ann Intern Med* 137:555–562, 2002.

Silver, J., Kilav, R., Naveh-Many, T. Mechanisms of secondary hyperparathyroidism. *Am J Physiol Renal Physiol* 283:F367–F376, 2002.

Suranyi, M.G., Lindberg, J.S., Navarro, J., Elias, C., Brenner, R.M., Walker, R. Treatment of anemia with Darbepoetin Alfa administered de novo once every other week in chronic kidney disease. *Am J Nephrol* 23:106–111, 2003.

The GISEN group. Randomized placebo-controlled trial of effect of ramipril on decline in glomerular filtration rate and risk of terminal renal failure in proteinuric, non-diabetic nephropathy. *Lancet* 349: 1857–1863, 1997.

UK Prospective Diabetes Study. Efficacy of atenolol and captopril in reducing risk of macrovascular and microvascular complications in type 2 diabetes: UKPDS. *BMJ* 317:713–720, 1998.

Robert F. Reilly, Jr. and
Mark A. Perazella

Chapter 17

Glomerular Diseases

Recommended Time to Complete: 2 days

Guiding Questions

1. What are the clinical presentations of glomerular disease?
2. Which primary renal diseases present as the nephrotic syndrome?
3. What are the five clinical stages of diabetic nephropathy?
4. Can you describe the characteristic findings on urinalysis of the patient with nephritis?
5. How does rapidly progressive glomerulonephritis (RPGN) present and what are its most-common causes?
6. What is the serum anti-neutrophil cytoplasmic antibody test and how is it interpreted?
7. Which glomerular diseases commonly present with isolated abnormalities on urinalysis?

Presentation of Glomerular Diseases

Diseases that adversely affect the structure and function of the glomerulus present to the clinician in a limited number of ways. Glomerular diseases can be grouped into four clinical syndromes. These include the nephrotic syndrome, the nephritic syndrome, rapidly progressive glomerulonephritis (a variant of the nephritic syndrome), and asymptomatic abnormalities on urinalysis. The differential diagnosis varies depending on the clinical syndrome.

The nephrotic syndrome is manifested by severe proteinuria (>3.0–3.5 g/1.73 m^2/day) and hypoalbuminemia. Associated features include to a variable degree: edema; hyperlipidemia; and lipiduria. Nephrotic syndrome results from an increase in glomerular permeability to macromolecules. Etiologies are divided into two broad categories: primary renal diseases; and secondary forms (infection, malignancy, medications, and multisystem diseases). The pathogenesis is not well understood. Abnormalities of the immune system appear to be the predominant mechanism in man. Circulating immune complexes may deposit in glomeruli, or the antigen may be deposited or originate in the glomerular capillary wall and immune complexes (antigen-antibody) form in situ. Less commonly inherited diseases of the podocyte cause congenital nephrotic syndrome. Mutations in genes that produce proteins critical to the maintenance of the normal structure and function of the podocyte foot processes and slit diaphragm result in proteinuria.

The nephritic syndrome is characterized by the presence of hematuria with red blood cell casts, increased serum blood urea nitrogen (BUN) and creatinine concentrations, varying degrees of hypertension, and proteinuria. Nephritic syndrome is secondary to an inflammatory disease of the glomerulus that is manifested by an increase in cellularity on light microscopy. The increased cellularity is secondary to proliferation of endothelial, epithelial, and/or mesangial cells or to glomerular infiltration with inflammatory cells.

RPGN is a variant of the nephritic syndrome. The serum BUN and creatinine concentrations rise rapidly over days to weeks. The hallmark of RPGN on renal biopsy is the cellular or fibrous crescent and this disorder is also referred to as "crescentic" glomerulonephritis. A crescent is a histologic marker of severe injury. It develops when a rent or hole forms in either the glomerular capillary basement membrane or in the basement membrane of Bowman's capsule. When such a disruption occurs, macrophages, inflammatory mediators, and plasma proteins gain access to Bowman's space. A crescent develops from the proliferation of macrophages, fibroblasts, and parietal glomerular epithelial cells. Crescents are often associated with visible areas of necrosis within the glomerular capillary. Rapidly progressive glomerulonephritis is important to recognize because irreversible glomerular damage occurs quickly in the absence of therapy.

Asymptomatic abnormalities on urinalysis include the discovery of hematuria or proteinuria on routine dipstick analysis of urine. This chapter is subdivided into four sections based on the clinical syndromes described above. Individual glomerular diseases are discussed further based on their most common clinical presentation.

KEY POINTS
Presentation of Glomerular Diseases

1. Glomerular diseases present as four clinical syndromes: nephrotic syndrome; nephritic syndrome; RPGN (a variant of the nephritic syndrome); and asymptomatic abnormalities on urinalysis.
2. The nephrotic syndrome is manifested by severe proteinuria (>3.0–3.5 g/1.73 m^2/day) and hypoalbuminemia.
3. Hematuria with red blood cell casts, increased serum BUN and creatinine concentrations, varying degrees of hypertension, and proteinuria are present in the nephritic syndrome.
4. Rapidly progressive glomerulonephritis is a variant of the nephritic syndrome in which the serum BUN and creatinine concentrations rise rapidly over days to weeks. The hallmark of RPGN on renal biopsy is the cellular or fibrous crescent.
5. Glomerular disease may also present as asymptomatic abnormalities on urinalysis.

Nephrotic Syndrome

Under normal circumstances only 30–45 mg of protein is excreted in urine, about one-third of that total is albumin. The upper limit of normal for urinary protein excretion is 150 mg/day and this can increase to 300 mg/day with exercise. The glomerular capillary acts as a barrier to the filtration of serum proteins. This barrier consists of three layers: an endothelial cell; the basement membrane itself; and an epithelial cell. There is both a size barrier [(small proteins are freely filtered (MW 5000 Da), and large ones are restricted (MW 100,000 Da)], as well as a charge barrier (the capillary membrane is negatively charged and repels negatively charged proteins). Disorders of the filtration barrier result in proteinuria and if severe enough the nephrotic syndrome.

The nephrotic syndrome is manifested by severe proteinuria (>3.0–3.5 g/1.73 m^2/day) and hypoalbuminemia. Peripheral edema, an elevated serum cholesterol concentration and lipiduria are often present. Edema results from a change in Starling's forces across the capillary wall. As serum albumin concentration falls plasma oncotic pressure decreases. There may also be an intrarenal defect resulting in increased sodium reabsorption as well. Albumin in the tubular lumen increases activity of the Na$^+$-H$^+$ exchanger in proximal tubule resulting in increased sodium reabsorption. Edema should first be treated with sodium restriction. If this is ineffective then diuretics are added. Milder diuretics that block sodium reabsorption in the distal convoluted tubule or collecting duct (thiazides, triamterene, amiloride, spironolactone, and eplerenone) are often used before more potent loop diuretics.

Hypercholesterolemia is thought to result from an increase in synthesis of hepatic proteins in response to hypoalbuminemia. This is supported by animal studies showing that the degree of cholesterol elevation is inversely related to the fall in plasma oncotic pressure. Animal studies also show that raising oncotic pressure with albumin infusion results in a fall in serum cholesterol concentration toward normal. If serum cholesterol concentration is elevated and the patient does not have hypoalbuminemia, the increase is probably not due to the nephrotic syndrome. There is also a decrease in lipoprotein catabolism. Lipoprotein lipase is decreased as is lecithin-cholesterol acyltransferase (esterifies cholesterol to high density lipoprotein [HDL]). Down regulation of lipoprotein lipase and the very low density lipoprotein (VLDL) receptor results in elevated triglycerides and VLDL.

A variety of coagulation abnormalities are often present in the nephrotic syndrome. Levels of factors V, VIII, and fibrinogen are increased while X, XI, and XII and antithrombin III are decreased. The platelet count tends to be increased, as is platelet aggregation. The end result is that patients are hypercoagulable, and have an increased incidence of both arterial and venous thrombi. Renal vein thrombosis occurs in 5–35% and is more commonly associated with membranous glomerulonephritis. The presentation can be acute or chronic. Acute renal vein thrombosis is manifested by flank pain, hematuria, and a decrease in glomerular filtration rate (GFR). Chronic renal vein thrombosis is often silent and can present as a pulmonary embolus. Since antithrombin III concentration is low, these patients may be relatively heparin resistant and require more heparin than usual to raise the PTT into the therapeutic range.

The risk of infection with encapsulated organisms is increased possibly due to the loss of complement factor B (alternate pathway) and gamma globulin in urine. Patients should be immunized with pneumococcal vaccine.

KEY POINTS
Nephrotic Syndrome

1. The glomerular capillary acts as both a charge and size barrier to the filtration of serum proteins.
2. The nephrotic syndrome is manifested by severe proteinuria (>3.0–3.5 g/1.73 m^2/day) and hypoalbuminemia.
3. Patients with the nephrotic syndrome are hypercoagulable and have an increased incidence of both arterial and venous thrombi.

Primary Renal Diseases That Present as the Nephrotic Syndrome

Minimal Change Disease

Minimal change disease also known as nil disease or lipoid nephrosis derives its name from the fact that the light microscopic (LM) appearance of the glomerulus is normal (Figure 17.1). Immunofluorescence (IF) studies are also negative. On electron microscopy (EM) podocyte epithelial foot processes are fused (Figure 17.2). Some patients have mesangial deposits of IgM and C3. Heavy deposition of IgM (IgM nephropathy) associated with mesangial hypercellularity may carry a worse prognosis. This is thought to represent an intermediate lesion along a path of progression toward focal and segmental glomerulosclerosis (see below).

The pathogenesis may be secondary to a defect in cell-mediated immunity, since in vitro T-cell

Figure 17.2

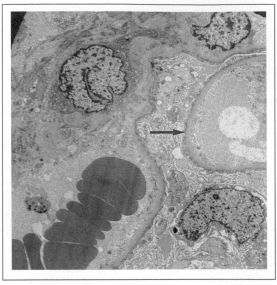

Minimal change disease (electron microscopy). Shown by the arrow is fusion of the foot processes of podocytes. This is the only abnormality seen on the renal biopsy of a patient with minimal change disease.

Figure 17.1

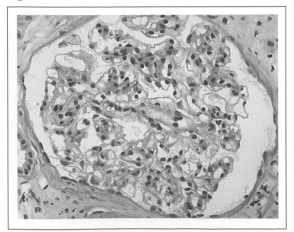

Minimal change disease (light microscopy). The glomerulus on light microscopy in minimal change disease is normal.

function abnormalities are described and minimal change disease can occur in association with Hodgkin's disease, nonsteroidal anti-inflammatory drugs (NSAIDs) and treatment of malignant melanoma with interferon-β. T-cell cultures derived from patients with minimal change disease release a vascular permeability factor. Minimal change disease may result from the production of a lymphokine that is toxic to the glomerular epithelial cell. The toxin reduces the anionic charge barrier of the membrane and leads to albuminuria. In adults minimal change disease is the cause of 10–15% of cases of nephrotic syndrome. In children it is the most common cause of nephrotic syndrome with a peak incidence between ages 2 and 3. It accounts for greater than 90% of cases of nephrotic syndrome in the pediatric population. The urine sediment is generally unremarkable although microscopic hematuria may be present in 20% of patients. Proteinuria is "selective" consisting almost entirely of albumin suggesting that the abnormality in glomerular basement membrane (GBM) is an alteration in the charge barrier. Hypertension is generally absent. Minimal change disease responds well to corticosteroids (within 4 weeks), although relapses are the rule. Relapses may be provoked by an upper respiratory infection. Patients with frequent relapses or those who are steroid-dependent may be treated with cyclophosphamide, chlorambucil, cyclosporin, or levamisol. Oral cyclosporin carries the risk of nephrotoxicity, especially in those treated for longer periods of time. The long-term prognosis with respect to the maintenance of renal function is good.

Focal Segmental Glomerulosclerosis (Focal Sclerosis)

Focal segmental glomerulosclerosis (FSGS) is characterized by sclerosing lesions associated with hyaline deposits involving parts (segmental) of some glomeruli (focal). The sclerosis results from glomerular capillary collapse with an increase in mesangial matrix (Figure 17.3). Mild-to-moderate mesangial hypercellularity may be seen. On EM subendothelial deposits and foot process fusion are present in involved glomeruli. Capillary collapse and folding and thickening of the basement membrane are present in sclerotic glomeruli. Immunofluorescence reveals nonspecific trapping of IgM and C3 in the sclerotic mesangium. As the disease progresses tubular atrophy, interstitial fibrosis, and global glomerular sclerosis occur. Increasing degrees of interstitial fibrosis (>20% of biopsy surface area) is associated with a poorer prognosis. Juxtamedullary nephrons are affected initially.

The etiology of primary FSGS is unknown but humoral factors, glomerular hypertrophy and hyperfiltration, and injury to glomerular cells are postulated. Inherited forms of FSGS are caused by mutations in genes that encode podocyte proteins α-actinin 4, podocin, and nephrin. Focal sclerosis can also be secondary to vesicoureteral reflux, morbid obesity, urinary tract obstruction, analgesic

Figure 17.3

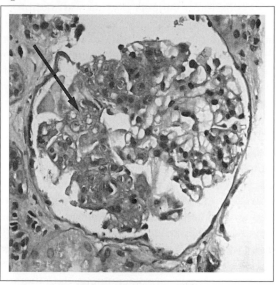

Focal and segmental glomerulosclerosis (FSGS). The left half of this glomerulus is sclerotic (arrow) and the right half is normal, hence the term segmental in FSGS. In the sclerotic region there is glomerular capillary collapse and an increase in mesangial matrix.

nephropathy, chronic renal transplant rejection, heroin nephropathy, human immunodeficiency virus (HIV) infection, and substantial loss of nephron mass. Focal sclerosis is the most common primary renal disease resulting in nephrotic syndrome in African Americans. The urinary sediment is usually remarkable for hematuria and pyuria, and up to 30% of adults may present with asymptomatic proteinuria. Blood pressure is generally elevated, GFR decreased, and the development of slowly progressive renal failure is the usual course. Approximately 50–60% of patients reach end-stage renal disease (ESRD) within 10 years of initial diagnosis. Patients with nonnephrotic range proteinuria have a better prognosis. The clinical course is much more rapid in patients with heroin nephropathy or HIV infection (renal failure often is present within 2 years from the time of initial diagnosis).

HIV-associated nephropathy (HIVAN) is much more common in African Americans than Caucasians. It generally occurs late in the course of HIV infection in patients with a CD4 count of <250 cells/mm³. Patients present with nephrotic syndrome and elevated serum BUN and creatinine concentrations. The kidneys are enlarged on renal ultrasound with increased echogenicity of the renal cortex. On LM there is glomerular collapse, extensive lymphocytic infiltration, and cystic dilation of tubules that are filled with proteinacious material (microcysts). Tubuloreticular inclusion bodies are found within glomerular and nonglomerular endothelial cells. Immune complex-related diseases such as membranoproliferative glomerulonephritis (MPGN), membranous glomerulonephritis, and IgA nephropathy are more common in Caucasians with HIV infection and the nephrotic syndrome. HIV viral proteins induce podocyte injury and apotosis. Studies in HIVAN show that the decrease in GFR was slowed by highly active antiretroviral therapy (HAART), angiotensin-converting enzyme (ACE) inhibitors, and prednisone. Prednisone should be reserved for those patients at low risk of infection since serious infectious complications may arise during its use. A collapsing FSGS was recently reported as a complication of pamidronate therapy.

Focal sclerosis is less responsive to corticosteroids. High-dose corticosteroids often must be employed for 6–9 months before a response is seen. If corticosteroids fail, the second line agent of choice is cyclosporin; cyclophosphamide, and mycophenolate mofetil (MMF) can also be used. Factors associated with a poorer prognosis include persistent high-grade proteinuria, extent of tubulointerstitial fibrosis and degree of glomerulosclerosis on renal biopsy, and a higher serum creatinine concentration. African American race and a lack of response to corticosteroids are also predictors of poor outcome. As many as 30% of patients may develop a recurrence in the transplanted kidney. Those with a rapid progression and with high degrees of proteinuria are at increased risk of recurrence. Treatment of secondary causes of FSGS are directed at the underlying cause such as repair of reflux, weight reduction (obesity), control of hyperfiltration (nephron loss), and HAART (HIVAN).

Mesangial Proliferative Glomerulonephritis

Mesangial proliferative glomerulonephritis generally presents with isolated microscopic hematuria or proteinuria although nephrotic syndrome is also seen. On LM there is an increase in mesangial cell number. Mesangial deposits of immunoglobulin and complement are present on EM. Treatment is often supportive focusing on blood pressure control and proteinuria reduction with drugs that modulate the renin-angiotensin-aldosterone system (RAAS) such as ACE inhibitors and angiotensin receptor blockers (ARBs). Initial treatment is generally with corticosteroids. Nonresponders or partial responders often do not respond to cyclosporin. Deposition of IgM in the mesangium and lack of response to corticosteroids are associated with a poor prognosis.

Membranous Glomerulonephritis

Membranous glomerulonephritis is characterized by uniform, diffuse thickening of the glomerular capillary wall without cellular proliferation (Figure 17.4). The most characteristic

Figure 17.4

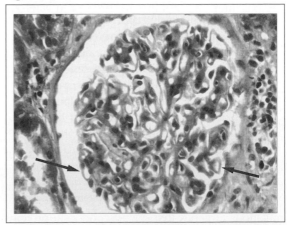

Membranous glomerulonephritis (light microscopy). Shown by the arrows are the diffusely thickened glomerular capillary loops characteristic of this lesion. There is no increase in cellularity.

Figure 17.5

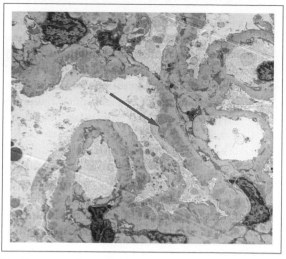

Membranous glomerulonephritis (electron microscopy). Immune deposits in the glomerular basement membrane are shown by the arrow. They are found in the subepithelial space.

Figure 17.6

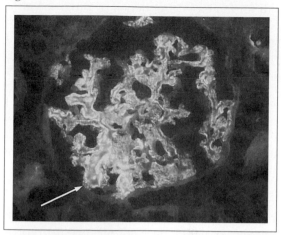

Membranous glomerulonephritis (immunofluorescence microscopy). The staining pattern is granular and corresponds to the punctate accumulation of immune deposits in the glomerular basement membrane and mesangium.

feature is the presence of subepithelial immune deposits on electron microscopy (Figure 17.5). The electron-dense deposits are formed in situ in the glomerular basement membrane. The development of glomerular injury is complement-dependent and is related to the formation of the membrane attack complex (C5b-C9). The membrane attack complex induces matrix production, release of oxidants, and podocyte injury. Glomerular basement membrane accumulates between the deposits, which creates the appearance of spikes. With time the basement membrane extends over the deposits forming domes. Immunofluorescence microscopy shows a granular pattern (Figure 17.6). In the idiopathic lesion mesangial deposits are usually absent. In membranous glomerulonephritis due to secondary causes mesangial deposits are generally present. Subendothelial deposits, tubulointerstitial deposits, the presence of all immunoglobulins in deposits, and mesangial or endocapillary proliferation are suggestive of a secondary cause. Many of these patients have evidence of circulating immune complexes.

Histologic changes associated with a poor prognosis include interstitial fibrosis and segmental glomerulosclerosis.

Membranous glomerulonephritis is the most common primary renal disease that causes nephrotic syndrome in Caucasian adults. Nephrotic syndrome is present in 80% of cases. Hypertension is usually absent and the urinary sediment may show hematuria in approximately half of patients. This lesion is also seen in collagen vascular diseases (systemic lupus erythematosis [SLE], mixed connective tissue disease, and rheumatoid arthritis), infections (hepatitis B, malaria, secondary and congenital syphilis, leprosy, schistosomiasis, and filariasis), drugs (NSAIDs, gold, penicillamine, mercury, probenecid, captopril, and bucillamine), neoplasia (lung, colon, stomach, breast, cervix, and ovary), and miscellaneous disorders (sickle cell disease, thyroiditis, and sarcoid).

Therapy remains controversial due to the high spontaneous remission rate. Without treatment generally one-third of patients spontaneously remit, one-third progress to renal failure, and one-third remain unchanged. Factors associated with an increased frequency of progression to renal failure include male sex, age >50, high-grade persistent proteinuria, hypertension, and an elevated serum creatinine concentration. Excretion of IgG and α_1-microglobulin is a predictor of a poor response to therapy, and progression to renal failure, as is the extent of tubulointerstitial damage on renal biopsy. An initial study suggested that corticosteroids alone decreased the rate of decline in renal function but this was not borne out by subsequent trials. The combination of alternating monthly courses of either corticosteroids and chlorambucil or corticosteroids and oral cyclophosphamide increase the rate of remission of nephrotic syndrome and the probability of survival without renal failure. The majority of therapeutic trials were conducted, however, in patients with a serum creatinine concentration ≤1.7 mg/dL. Uncontrolled trials were carried out in patients with serum creatinine concentrations between 2.0 and 3.0 mg/dL. The combination of prednisone and cyclophosphamide lowered serum creatinine concentration in the short term. It is unclear whether patients with serum creatinine concentrations ≥3.0 mg/dL benefit from therapy. Cyclosporin was used in patients who failed steroid therapy. The rate of remission of nephrotic range proteinuria is increased but conflicting data exist as to whether one can slow progression of disease. Mycophenylate mofetil was employed successfully in small numbers of patients.

Because of the high spontaneous remission rate some authors recommend treating only patients with elevated serum creatinine concentration, a progressive decline in GFR, symptomatic nephrotic syndrome, those at high risk for progression, and patients with thromboembolic disease. Because of the association with renal vein thrombosis and thromboembolic events some recommend treating patients with profound hypoalbuminemia with anticoagulants. Patients who experience a thromboembolic event should be anticoagulated as long as they remain nephrotic.

Membranoproliferative Glomerulonephritis

MPGN is characterized by diffuse proliferation of mesangial cells with the extension of mesangial matrix or cytoplasm into the peripheral capillary wall, giving rise to a thickened and reduplicated appearance. This gives rise to the double contour or "tram-track" appearance of the GBM. There is mixed mesangial and endothelial cell proliferation that results in a lobular distortion of the glomerulus (lobular accentuation) (Figure 17.7). Membranoproliferative glomerulonephritis is divided into several types based on EM.

Type I MPGN, which is the most common form of the disease, is associated with subendothelial electron-dense deposits and marked peripheral capillary interposition of mesangial cell cytoplasm and matrix. Immunofluorescence microscopy reveals glomerular deposition of immunoglobulin, C3, and C4. Patients may present with the nephrotic syndrome, nephritic syndrome, an overlap of these two syndromes, RPGN, or with asymptomatic hematuria and proteinuria. Episodic macroscopic

Figure 17.7

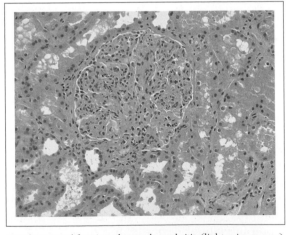

Membranoproliferative glomerulonephritis (light microscopy). There is an increase in both cellularity (proliferation of endothelial and mesangial cells) and mesangial matrix. Open capillary loops are difficult to visualize as a result of endothelial proliferation. The lobules of the glomerulus are distorted (lobular accentuation).

hematuria may also occur. Blood pressure is generally increased, GFR reduced, and anemia present out of proportion to the degree of azotemia. Complement concentrations are low especially in type II MPGN. The classical complement pathway is activated in type I MPGN resulting in a decrease in C4 concentration. Glomerular crescents, hypertension, decreased GFR, and heavy proteinuria are poor prognostic signs. Infection (shunt nephritis, malaria, endocarditis, hepatitis B and C, and HIV), B-cell lymphomas, SLE, mixed connective tissue disease, sickle cell disease, and alpha-1-antitrypsin deficiency are also associated with MPGN type I. Infection with hepatitis C is the most common cause.

Type II MPGN is characterized by intramembranous electron-dense deposits and is often called dense deposit disease. There are dense ribbon-like confluent deposits in the basement membranes of the glomeruli, tubules, and vasculature. In type II MPGN the alternative complement pathway is activated decreasing C3 concentration. Peripheral catabolism of C3 is increased by a circulating IgG known as C3 nephritic factor. This results in an increase in C3 degradation products especially C3c. C3c has an affinity for the lamina densa of the GBM and is deposited there. The depressed complement concentrations do not correlate with disease activity. These patients are generally resistant to therapy.

Subendothelial and subepithelial immune deposits and marked fragmentation of the GBM are found in type III MPGN. It is associated with IgA nephropathy and Henoch-Schönlein purpura (HSP) and is rarely a result of hepatitis C infection. This lesion is not corticosteroid responsive.

KEY POINTS
Primary Renal Diseases that Present as the Nephrotic Syndrome

1. Minimal change disease is the most common cause of nephrotic syndrome in children. Proteinuria is selective and the response rate to prednisone is high.

2. Focal segmental glomerulosclerosis is characterized by sclerosis in a portion (segmental) of some (focal) glomeruli. It is the most common primary renal disease causing nephrotic syndrome in African Americans.

3. Membranous glomerulonephritis is characterized by thickened glomerular capillary walls, the absence of cellular proliferation, and the presence of subepithelial immune deposits. Therapy remains controversial due to the high spontaneous remission rate.

4. Membranoproliferative glomerulonephritis may present with the nephrotic syndrome, nephritic syndrome, an overlap of these two syndromes, or with asymptomatic hematuria and proteinuria. Complement concentrations are low.

Secondary Renal Diseases Commonly Associated with Nephrotic Syndrome in Adults

Diabetes Mellitus

Diabetic nephropathy is the single most common cause of the nephrotic syndrome and ESRD in the United States. Type I diabetics with nephropathy have a 50-fold increase in mortality compared to those without nephropathy. Nephropathy in type I diabetes mellitus rarely develops before 10 years disease duration, and approximately 40% of type I diabetics have proteinuria within 40 years after the onset of disease. The annual incidence of diabetic nephropathy peaks just before 20 years of disease duration and declines thereafter. Those patients who survive 30 years of type I diabetes mellitus without developing nephropathy are at low risk of doing so in the future.

Figure 17.8

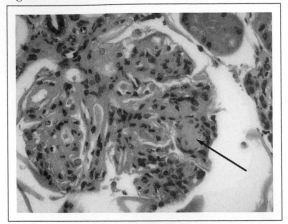

Diabetic glomerulosclerosis (light microscopy). Shown by the arrow is an area of nodular glomerulosclerosis (Kimmelstiel-Wilson's disease). Note also the diffuse increase in mesangial matrix throughout the glomerulus (diffuse glomerulosclerosis).

The glomeruli in patients with diabetic nephropathy may exhibit a form of nodular glomerulosclerosis known as Kimmelstiel-Wilson's disease (Figure 17.8). The nodules form in the peripheral regions of the mesangium and can be single or multiple. They may result from accumulation of basement membrane or injury from micro-aneurysmal dilation of the glomerular capillary. Nodular glomerulosclerosis can occur in association with diffuse glomerulosclerosis. Diffuse glomerulosclerosis results from widening of the mesangial space by an increase in matrix production. Glomerular injury in diabetes mellitus is related to the severity and duration of hyperglycemia and may be related to advanced glycation end products (AGEs). Elevation of serum glucose concentration leads to glycosylation of serum and tissue proteins resulting in AGE formation that can cross-link with collagen. In animal models administration of AGEs induces glomerular hypertrophy and stimulates mesangial matrix production. Upregulation of TGF-β_1 and its receptor likely play an important role in renal cell hypertrophy and stimulation of mesangial matrix production. In addition to glomerular changes,

there is diffuse accumulation of hyaline material in the subendothelial layers of the afferent and efferent arterioles.

The natural history of type I diabetic nephropathy is divided into five stages: (1) time of initial diagnosis; (2) the first decade (characterized by renal hypertrophy and hyperfiltration); (3) the third stage is manifested by glomerulopathy (microalbuminuria) in the absence of clinical disease; (4) clinically detectable disease (the hallmarks of this stage are dipstick positive proteinuria, hypertension, and a progressive decline in renal function); and (5) ESRD.

Stage I. At the onset of diabetes mellitus virtually all patients experience functional changes such as increased kidney size, microalbuminuria that reverses with the control of blood glucose concentration, and an increased GFR that decreases with initiation of insulin therapy in most patients.

Stage II. In stage II GFR may be increased, and it is postulated that this finding predicts the later development of nephropathy but this remains controversial. The pathogenesis of the hyperfiltration is unclear but may be due in part to hyperglycemia and activation of the RAAS. At the onset of diabetes mellitus the renal biopsy is usually normal. Within 1.5–2.5 years GBM thickening begins in nearly all patients. No correlation exists between GBM thickening and clinical renal function. Mesangial expansion begins about 5 years after the onset of disease.

Stage III. Stage III is manifested by microalbuminuria. Microalbuminuria is an albumin excretion rate between 30 and 300 mg/day (20 to 200 µg/min). This amount of albumin excretion is below the level of sensitivity of a urine dipstick. A mid morning albumin to creatinine ratio greater than 30 mg/g is abnormal and correlates well with 24-hour or timed urine collections. Several groups reported the predictive value of a slightly elevated urinary albumin excretion occurring in the first or second decade of diabetes mellitus as a harbinger of the later development of clinical diabetic nephropathy. These studies used thresholds ranging from 15 to 70 µg/minute to classify patients. Microalbuminuria best predicts diabetic nephropathy when it is progressive over time and is associated with hypertension.

Stage IV. Stage IV is defined by the presence of dipstick positive proteinuria and is associated with a slow gradual decline in GFR that may result in ESRD. Classically the rate of decline of GFR was stated to be 1 mL/minute/month, but this number is probably now closer to 0.5 mL/minute/month or less. The rate of progression can be slowed by antihypertensive therapy. It may decline further with combined treatment with ACE inhibitors and ARBs.

Stage V. As the GFR continues to decline ESRD may develop. Diabetic nephropathy is the most common cause of ESRD in the United States. Because of associated autonomic neuropathy and cardiac disease, diabetics often experience uremic symptoms at higher GFRs (15 mL/minute/1.73 m²) than nondiabetics.

Although the five clinical stages of diabetic nephropathy are best characterized in patients with type I diabetes mellitus, they are similar in patients with type II disease with the following exceptions. The ability to date the time of onset of type II diabetes mellitus is more difficult than in patients with type I disease. Therefore, one needs to be more flexible in interpreting the first decade. It may be shorter than 10 years. In virtually 100% of patients with type I diabetes mellitus and diabetic nephropathy, retinopathy is present, while retinopathy is present in two-thirds of those with type II disease and diabetic nephropathy. Therefore, the absence of retinopathy in a patient with type II diabetes mellitus should not dissuade one from the diagnosis in the appropriate clinical setting. On the other hand, the absence of retinopathy in a patient with type I disease would argue strongly against diabetes mellitus as a potential cause of renal disease.

The urinalysis in diabetic nephropathy is generally remarkable for proteinuria with little in the way of cellular elements present. On occasion microscopic hematuria is seen. This should prompt a workup for other causes of hematuria such as transitional cell carcinoma in the patient greater than age 40 (cystoscopy). The most common cause of microscopic hematuria in the patient with diabetic nephropathy is, however, diabetic nephropathy. Macroscopic hematuria or the presence of red cell casts is suggestive of another diagnosis. The presence of nephrotic range proteinuria in the diabetic patient with a preserved GFR should also raise concern that another glomerular lesion is the cause of the nephrotic syndrome. In general, proteinuria is initially mild and progresses to the nephrotic syndrome as the GFR declines in patients with diabetic nephropathy. Treatment of diabetic nephropathy requires a multidrug regimen including tight glucose control, BP control with medications that modulate the RAAS, and statin therapy to reduce lipids. This was reviewed in more detail in Chapter 16.

Systemic Amyloidosis

More than 90% of patients with primary and secondary amyloidosis have renal involvement, approximately 60% have nephrotic syndrome. In patients over the age of 60 with nephrotic syndrome 10% have amyloidosis. On LM diffuse amorphous hyaline material is deposited in glomeruli (Figure 17.9). Amyloid deposits may also be

Figure 17.9

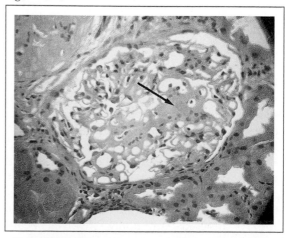

Amyloid (light microscopy). Illustrated by the arrow is a diffuse increase in amorphous hyaline material (amyloid) deposited in the glomerulus.

Figure 17.10

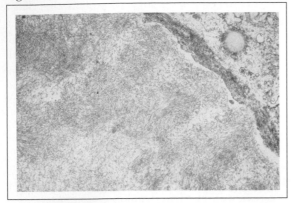

Amyloid (electron microscopy). Shown in the glomerulus is the deposition of nonbranching 8–12 nm fibers that are characteristic of amyloid.

present in tubular basement membranes, arterioles, and small arteries. In more advanced cases nodule formation occurs and the LM picture can resemble advanced diabetic nephropathy. The diagnosis is confirmed by special stains (Congo red, thioflavin-T) and electron microscopy. Amyloid deposits have a characteristic applegreen birefringence under polarized light with Congo red staining. The demonstration of 8–12 nm nonbranching fibrils on EM is diagnostic (Figure 17.10). Patients present with nephrotic syndrome, decreased GFR, and an unremarkable urinary sediment. Clinically apparent extrarenal involvement is often absent. A monoclonal light chain is present in urine in approximately 90% of patients with primary amyloidosis. The diagnosis can be established on biopsy of the rectum, gingiva, abdominal fat pad and skin, as well as on renal biopsy.

In primary amyloidosis (AL amyloid) fibrils consist of the N-terminal amino acid residues of the variable portion of monoclonal light chains. Lambda light chains more commonly form amyloid fibrils (75%) than kappa light chains (25%). Primary amyloid commonly involves heart, kidney, and peripheral nerves. The vast majority of patients have a paraprotein detected in serum or urine (90%). Prognosis is poor with a mean survival of less than 2 years and only a 20% 5-year

survival. Cardiac disease, renal dysfunction, and interstitial fibrosis on kidney biopsy are associated with a worse prognosis. The goal of therapy is to reduce light chain production with chemotherapy. The combination of melphalan and prednisone is most commonly employed with stabilization of renal function and improvement in organ system involvement in some patients. The best results are found with high-dose melphalan followed by bone marrow or stem cell transplant. Toxicity of this regimen is considerable and only a small subset of patients are candidates.

In one study of 350 patients who carried a clinical diagnosis of AL amyloid, 10% had mutations resulting in the formation of amyloidogenic proteins that were responsible for the syndrome. Mutated genes included transthyretin, fibrinogen A alpha-chain, lysozyme, and apolipoprotein A-I. None of these patients had a positive family history. A genetic cause should be suspected in those whose fluorescence staining is negative for light chains and serum amyloid-associated protein A.

In secondary amyloidosis (AA amyloid) fibrils are made up of the N-terminus of serum amyloid-associated protein A. Chronic inflammation (rheumatoid arthritis, inflammatory bowel disease, bronchiectasis, heroin addicts who inject subcutaneously), some malignancies (Hodgkin's disease and renal cell carcinoma), and familial Mediterranean fever stimulate hepatic production of serum amyloid-associated protein A, an acute phase reactant. Monocytes and macrophages take up the protein and cleave it into smaller fragments called AA protein (the major component of secondary amyloid fibrils). Treatment is directed at the underlying process. Correction of the inflammatory or infectious process may improve proteinuria in patients with secondary amyloidosis. Colchicine in high doses is effective in patients with familial Mediterranean fever. Those with preserved renal function are more likely to respond with decreases in proteinuria.

Nonamyloid fibrillar deposits can also cause glomerular disease. They occur most commonly in elderly Caucasians. These diseases, fibrillary glomerulonephritis and immunotactoid glomerulonephritis, are only diagnosed by renal biopsy.

A variety of LM patterns are described including diffuse proliferative glomerulonephritis, mesangial proliferation, membranous glomerulonephritis, and membranoproliferative glomerulonephritis. The diagnosis is established based on EM. In fibrillary glomerulonephritis, fibrils average 20 nm in diameter and are randomly arranged. Immunofluorescence microscopy is positive for IgG, C3, and kappa and lambda light chains. Fibrillary glomerulonephritis is responsible for >90% of nonamyloid fibrillary diseases.

Immunotactoid glomerulonephritis is characterized by fibrils that are 30–50 nm in size. On LM an MPGN type I or diffuse proliferative pattern are most common. Immunofluorescence microscopy is positive for IgG. IgM, IgA, C3, and C1q may also be seen. Some patients have a circulating paraprotein and hypocomplementemia is often present. An association with chronic lymphoproliferative disease was described.

Patients with nonamyloid fibrillar deposits commonly present with nephrotic syndrome, microscopic hematuria, hypertension, and a progressive decline in GFR. There is no proven effective therapy although corticosteroids, cyclophosphamide, and cyclosporin were employed. Some advocate tailoring therapy based on the LM pattern. There is a high rate of recurrence after renal transplantation.

Monoclonal Immunoglobulin Deposition Diseases

Monoclonal immunoglobulin deposition diseases result from the deposition of light chains, heavy chains, or the combination of both in a variety of organs including kidney. In light chain deposition disease (LCDD) immunoglobulin light chains deposit in the glomerulus and do not form fibrils. The deposits in most cases are derived from the constant region of kappa light chains. A paraprotein is detected in the urine or serum by immunofixation electrophoresis in 85% of patients. The most common presentation is nephrotic syndrome associated with hypertension and a decreased GFR. Other organs such as heart, liver, and peripheral nerves may be affected. Light microscopy reveals eosinophilic mesangial nodules. Immunofluorescence microscopy is positive for monoclonal light chains in a linear pattern in the glomerular and tubular basement membrane. Mesangial nodules also stain positive. A subset of patients have associated myeloma cast nephropathy. The prognosis of patients with LCDD is poor and renal dysfunction predicts a poor prognosis. Some patients respond to the combination of melphalan and prednisone.

Heavy chains may also deposit in the glomerulus with a similar clinical presentation and result in heavy chain deposition disease (HCDD). The diagnosis is established by immunofluorescence with antiheavy chain antibodies. Patients with HCDD secrete an abnormal heavy chain with a deletion in the CH1 domain. If the patient produces a heavy chain that fixes complement (IgG 1 or 3) hypocomplementemia may be present.

Systemic Lupus Erythematosis

Renal involvement is common in SLE with half of patients having an abnormal urinalysis or a decreased GFR at the time of initial diagnosis, and 75% eventually manifesting kidney disease. Renal involvement includes mild mesangial proliferation, focal or diffuse proliferative glomerulonephritis, membranous glomerulonephritis, and chronic glomerulonephritis. Although SLE may present as nephrotic syndrome (membranous glomerulonephritis), it more commonly presents as nephritis and is discussed in the following section. Patients may change from one form of renal involvement to another.

KEY POINTS

Secondary Renal Diseases Commonly Associated with Nephrotic Syndrome in Adults

1. Diabetic nephropathy is the most common cause of the nephrotic syndrome and ESRD in the United States. The natural history of diabetic nephropathy is divided into

five stages. The rate of progression can be
slowed by antihypertensive therapy.

2. Nephrotic syndrome may occur in up to
60% of patients with primary and secondary
amyloid. The demonstration of amyloid fibrils on EM is diagnostic.

3. Monoclonal immunoglobulins (light chains
and heavy chains) can deposit in the
glomerulus and cause nephrotic syndrome.
IF staining with the appropriate anti-sera
will be positive.

Nephritic Syndrome (Glomerulonephritis)

Acute nephritic syndrome or glomerulonephritis
is characterized by the abrupt onset of hematuria,
proteinuria, and a rise in serum BUN and creatinine
concentrations. Patients are often hypertensive and
may have peripheral edema. In glomerulonephritis
there is an inflammatory lesion of the glomerular
capillary bed that is often immune-mediated. This is
manifested clinically by red cell casts, hematuria,
and proteinuria. The hallmark of glomerulonephritis on urinalysis is the presence of red cell casts.
Decreased glomerular capillary perfusion decreases
GFR and results secondarily in increased reabsorption of sodium and water. Hypertension, oliguria,
edema formation, and rising serum BUN and creatinine concentrations are the clinical sequellae.

Postinfectious Glomerulonephritis

Acute postinfectious glomerulonephritis occurs
most often in children but can be seen in adults. It
generally occurs 2 weeks after pharyngeal infection with specific nephritogenic strains of group A
β-hemolytic streptococcal infection. The clinical
presentation can vary from microscopic hematuria
and proteinuria on urinalysis to the nephritic syndrome with the abrupt onset of periorbital and
lower extremity edema, mild-to-moderate hypertension, microscopic hematuria, red cell casts,
gross hematuria, and oliguria. The latent interval
from the time of infection to the onset of symptoms is not less than 5 days and not more than
28 days (average 10–21 days). Documentation of a
preceding streptococcal infection may be by throat
or skin culture or serologic changes in streptococcal antigen titers. Antistreptolysin O (ASO)
titers are not as sensitive in patients with skin infection and anti-DNAse B is often used in this setting.
Laboratory evaluation reveals an elevated serum
BUN and creatinine concentration, and low
serum complement concentration (C3). The vast
majority of children recover spontaneously. The
recovery rate is lower in adults. In the rare patient
RPGN may develop. The serum creatinine concentration usually returns to baseline within 4 weeks,
C3 concentration returns to normal in 6–12 weeks,
hematuria generally resolves within 6 months,
however, proteinuria may persist for years. There
is no evidence that immunosuppressive therapy
with corticosteroids is of benefit.

In kidney there is endothelial and mesangial cell
proliferation with leukocytic infiltration resulting in
a picture of diffuse proliferative glomerulonephritis. Electron microscopy reveals large immune
deposits in the subepithelial space. Subendothelial
deposits can occur early in the course of the disease. Immunofluorescence demonstrates complement and IgG. The disease is secondary to an
immunologic process. Many patients have circulating immune complexes while others may develop
in situ immune complexes in the GBM due to
planted bacterial antigens. Treatment includes
antimicrobial agents, blood pressure control, and
supportive therapy.

Systemic Lupus Erythematosis

Renal disease in patients with SLE is associated
with a number of different lesions that involve the

Table 17.1

WHO Classification of Lupus Nephritis

TYPE	NAME	LIGHT MICROSCOPY	IF	EM
I	Normal	Normal	Mild mesangial staining	Few mesangial deposits
II	Mesangial proliferative	Mesangial proliferation with increased mesangial matrix	Mesangial staining	Mesangial deposits
III	Focal proliferative	Focal and segmental mesangial and endothelial proliferation, few areas of necrosis	Mesangial and capillary loop staining	Mesangial deposits, some deposits in subendothelial and subepithelial space
IV	Diffuse proliferative	Diffuse proliferative and necrotizing lesion, wire loops and crescents	Mesangial and capillary loop staining	Deposits in all sites, deposits are larger and more numerous
V	Membranous	Diffuse basement membrane thickening	Capillary loop staining	Subepithelial and often mesangial deposits
VI	Sclerosing	Diffuse sclerosis of glomeruli	—	—

Abbreviations: WHO, World Health Organization; IF, immunofluorescence microscopy; EM, electron microscopy.

glomerulus, blood vessels, and tubulointerstitium. This section focuses on glomerular disease. Immune complex formation underlies the pathogenesis of SLE nephritis. The World Health Organization (WHO) classification divides the lesions associated with SLE into six different patterns or types (Table 17.1). Type I is normal LM with evidence of mesangial deposits on EM and mesangial immunoglobulin staining on IF microscopy. Type II is characterized by mesangial proliferation, defined as increased mesangial matrix and hypercellularity (LM), mesangial immunoglobulin staining (IF), and dense deposits (EM) within the mesangium. Focal proliferative glomerulonephritis constitutes type III WHO SLE nephritis. On LM, "focal" represents disease in some but not all glomeruli, whereas "segmental" means that less than 50% of glomeruli have evident

disease. As such, focal and segmental mesangial and endothelial proliferation is seen; necrosis (cell death) may also be present in these areas. Immune staining is seen in the mesangium and capillary loops on IF. Deposits in the mesangium, subendothelial, and subepithelial areas are often visualized on EM. Type IV lupus nephritis is a diffuse proliferative glomerulonephritis. Light microscopy demonstrates proliferative changes and necrosis diffusely throughout the glomerulus. Crescents and thickening of capillary loops (wire loops) may also be seen (Figure 17.11). Immune staining is noted in the mesangium and capillary loops on IF, while EM shows deposits in all sites. The EM deposits are typically more numerous and larger with type IV disease. Type V nephritis is a membranous lesion. It is characterized by diffuse thickening of the GBM without cellular

Figure 17.11

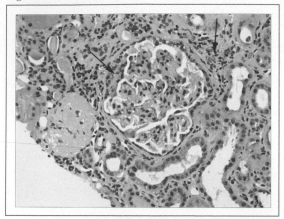

Lupus nephritis (light microscopy). There is an increase in cellularity due to mesangial and endothelial proliferation, as well as an accumulation of mesangial matrix. An early crescent is seen at the arrow on the left. The arrow on the right shows an infiltration of mononuclear cells in the interstitium. The association of interstitial nephritis with glomerulonephritis is suggestive of the diagnosis of vasculitis.

proliferation. A granular pattern of staining is noted on IF. Subepithelial immune deposits are present on EM, although mesangial deposits are often found as well. A sclerosing glomerular lesion is seen with type VI lupus nephritis. This represents an end-stage kidney lesion.

An abnormal urinalysis (hematuria and proteinuria) is typically seen at the time of diagnosis of SLE. Approximately 50% of patients with newly diagnosed SLE will have an abnormal urinalysis with or without renal dysfunction. In this setting, proteinuria is the most common urinary abnormality, noted in 80% of patients. Hematuria and/or pyuria develop in nearly 40% of patients at sometime during the course of disease. In general, lupus nephritis develops early following diagnosis, although decreased kidney function (increased serum creatinine concentration) is relatively uncommon within the first few years of diagnosis. Younger patients appear to develop renal disease earlier. While SLE is associated more commonly with certain HLA genotypes (HLA-B8, DR2, DR3, and DQW1) and complement

component deficiencies (C2 and C4 deficiencies), nephritis tends to be more severe in African Americans, children, and in those patients with genetic abnormalities of Fc receptors. The course of renal disease is typically benign for types I and II SLE nephritis. Often there are no obvious signs of renal disease, although hematuria and/or proteinuria with preserved kidney function is seen. In type III, proteinuria and hematuria are commonly present, rarely patients may develop nephrotic range proteinuria. Mild renal dysfunction and hypertension can occur. Diffuse proliferative nephritis (type IV) is universally complicated by hematuria and proteinuria. Renal failure, which can be severe, hypertension, and nephrotic range proteinuria are common. Type III and, in particular, type IV nephritis are both associated with severe and rapid loss of kidney function when left untreated. In addition to type III and type IV lesions, poor renal prognosis is associated with high activity index and chronicity index, presence of cellular crescents and interstitial fibrosis, and severe vascular lesions. The activity index is based on six histologic categories of active lesions that may be reversible (cellular proliferation, leukocyte infiltration, fibrinoid necrosis, cellular crescents, hyaline thrombi or wire loops, and mononuclear cell interstitial infiltration), whereas chronicity index measures four histologic components of irreversible damage (glomerular sclerosis, fibrous crescents, interstitial fibrosis, and tubular atrophy). Membranous nephropathy, which has a variable course of disease, is associated with high-grade proteinuria, and 90% develop nephrotic syndrome at some point in the disease course. Hematuria, hypertension, and renal failure may be seen.

As an immune complex disease, the pattern of SLE-associated glomerular injury that develops is related to the site of formation of the immune deposits. Loss of self-tolerance and generation of an autoimmune response are associated with alterations in cytotoxic, suppressor, and helper T cells numbers. Altered T cell signaling, cytokine production, and polyclonal activation of B cells results in the production of idiotypic autoantibodies against nuclear antigens, DNA, Sm, RNA, Ro, La, and other nuclear antigens. Thus, the complexes are composed of nuclear antigens and complement fixing IgG1 antibodies. Immune complex deposition in kidney results from either complexes formed in the circulation (mesangial and proliferative) or binding of circulating antibodies to antigens previously planted in the subepithelial space (membranous). Location of deposits determines the type of inflammatory response. Deposits in the mesangium or subendothelial space are close to the vascular space, and, as a result activate complement. This generates the chemoattractants C3a and C5a, stimulating influx of neutrophils and mononuclear cells. A proliferative glomerular lesion, including mesangial, focal, and diffuse proliferative nephritis, is created. In contrast, deposits on the subepithelial space activate complement but do not attract inflammatory cells due to their separation from the vascular space. A nonproliferative lesion complicated by proteinuria (membranous) with disease limited to the glomerular epithelial cell develops.

Diagnosis of SLE nephritis most often occurs following identification of extrarenal disease. Occasionally, renal manifestations and renal histology precede systemic disease, or recognition of atypical symptoms of SLE. In addition to urinary findings such as hematuria (with or without red blood cell casts) and proteinuria (both low and high grade), blood testing, such as serum creatinine concentration, antinuclear antibody titer, antidouble stranded DNA, and serum complement concentration are also useful. Renal biopsy is the gold standard test to diagnose and direct therapy in lupus nephritis. In addition, biopsy allows for prediction of prognosis. Histologic features such as WHO class, activity and chronicity indices, and other findings when employed with clinical features can help guide therapy. For example, aggressive cytotoxic treatment is employed for lesions that are potentially reversible and less aggressive approaches, employing supportive therapy in those with advanced, irreversible histopathology.

Therapy of lupus nephritis is based primarily on WHO classification, with types III and IV undergoing treatment. A combination of intravenous "pulse" cyclophosphamide and intravenous methylprednisolone are more effective than either alone. Cyclophosphamide is infused monthly ($0.5-1.0$ g/m^2, titrated to maintain white blood cell count above 3000 cells/mm^3) for 6 months followed by every 3 months for an additional 24 months. Prolonged maintenance therapy is associated with the best outcome. Due to toxicity, a shorter maintenance course is recommended for patients with diffuse proliferative lupus nephritis with mild clinical disease. Corticosteroids are often tapered over a period of months to doses optimal to control extrarenal manifestations of SLE. Oral azathioprine (0.5–4 mg/kg/day) and mycophenolate mofetil (500–3000 mg/day) were employed successfully as maintenance therapies for lupus nephritis. Plasmapheresis appears to add little benefit to routine immunosuppressive therapy, although some patients with resistant disease garner some benefit. Patients should be monitored for both remission (during therapy) and relapse of lupus nephritis (following therapy) with the same clinical tools used to diagnose renal disease.

When routine treatment of lupus nephritis is unsuccessful, other modalities were employed for both initial and maintenance therapy. African-American race is associated with resistance to routine immunosuppressive regimens for diffuse proliferative glomerulonephritis. Limited evidence supports use of mycophenolate mofetil (versus cyclophosphamide) as an initial therapy for diffuse proliferative lupus nephritis. Mycophenolate mofetil reduced both serum creatinine concentration and proteinuria at 1 year in a small number of patients who failed cyclophosphamide. At this time, it might be best to reserve this drug for female patients who are concerned about fertility. Cyclosporin stabilized renal function and reduced proteinuria in a small number of patients with type IV lupus nephritis that were resistant to cyclophosphamide. Intravenous immunoglobulin promoted histologic, immunologic, and clinical improvement in nine patients resistant to routine therapy. The efficacy of this therapy needs further evaluation in controlled studies. High-dose chemotherapy with stem cell transplantation was examined in patients with active diffuse proliferative nephritis and other severe extrarenal manifestations of SLE refractory to aggressive immunosuppressive treatment. Seven patients with this type of disease underwent this regimen. At 25 months of follow-up, all patients had no clinical or serologic evidence of SLE. Other experimental therapies for lupus nephritis on the horizon include immunoadsorption, anti-CD 40 ligand (to block costimulatory pathways between T and B cells), and LJP-394, a small molecule that blocks production of anti-DNA antibodies. Large, randomized studies are required to fully test these interventions.

Treatment of lupus-associated membranous nephropathy is unclear as the renal prognosis and natural history of this lesion are uncertain. Treatment is probably indicated if renal function declines or nephrotic syndrome is severe and associated with complications. Prednisone alone or in combination with other immunosuppressive regimens (cyclophosphamide, cyclosporin, or chlorambucil) was employed. Cyclophosphamide and cyclosporin appeared superior to prednisone alone in small studies of patients with this lesion. Combination therapy with corticosteroids plus chlorambucil was better than corticosteroids alone for inducing either complete or partial remission.

Thrombotic Microangiopathies

The thrombotic microangiopathies consist of a spectrum of diseases that are characterized by the formation of platelet microthrombi within vessels, thrombocytopenia, and microangiopathic hemolytic anemia. Formation of microthrombi in the microcirculation leads to multisystem end-organ ischemia and one of two clinical presentations (Table 17.2), consistent with either hemolytic uremic syndrome (HUS) or thrombotic thrombocytopenic purpura (TTP). There is, however,

Table 17.2

Clinical Features of the Thrombotic Microangiopathies

	D+ HUS	TTP
CNS symptoms	+	+++
Fever	+	+++
Colitis	+++	+
Multiorgan disease	+	+++
Hematuria/proteinuria	+++	++
Renal failure	+++	+
Death despite treatment	5%	15%
Recurrences	1%	20%

Abbreviations: +, rare; +++, common; D+HUS, hemolytic uremic syndrome associated with diarrhea; TTP, thrombotic thrombocytopenic purpura; CNS, central nervous system.

overlap between the two with regard to the clinical manifestations of the thrombotic microangiopathy. Hemolytic uremic syndrome and TTP can also be separated based on pathogenesis of the coagulation disorder. Thrombotic thrombocytopenic purpura is most often associated with either a congenital or acquired defect in a metalloproteinase-converting enzyme (ADAMTS13) for von Willebrand's factor (vWF). Absence of or reduced activity of this enzyme leads to abnormally large vWF in the circulation, which promotes aggregation of platelets and formation of microthrombi. In contrast, with HUS endothelial cell damage in the vasculature is thought to be the primary event that precipitates coagulation and microthrombi formation. It is not associated with a defect in the vWF-cleaving protease, but can have abnormal vWF in the circulation during acute illness.

Renal histology in the thrombotic microangiopathies is characterized by microthrombi within small vessels, including small arteries, arterioles (including afferent arterioles), and glomerular capillary loops. Ischemic retraction of glomeruli and ischemic injury in the tubulointerstitium is present. Over time, glomerulosclerosis and tubulointerstitial fibrosis are seen. Electron microscopy demonstrates small vessel microthrombi consisting of platelets and fibrin. No immune deposits are seen.

Immunofluorescence staining is also negative except for fibrin deposition in vessel walls.

HEMOLYTIC UREMIC SYNDROME

Hemolytic uremic syndrome develops from various disease processes. The sporadic or endemic variety associated with diarrhea (D+HUS) is linked to Shiga toxin exposure. The classic example is *Escherichia coli* strain O-157:H7. This bacterium produces the culprit toxin, which is associated with acute endothelial inflammation and injury, as well as accelerated thrombogenesis, resulting in bloody diarrhea and HUS. Other organisms produce neuraminidase, a promoter of diffuse endothelial injury, and may also cause HUS. Atypical, non-diarrhea-associated HUS (D–HUS) is more heterogeneous. It consists of familial forms, including both autosomal dominant and recessive disorders that can frequently relapse. Non-diarrhea-associated HUS can also occur following exposure to various drugs and therapeutic agents. Included are cyclosporin, tacrolimus, mitomycin-C, gemcitabine, methotrexate, oral contraceptives, ticlodipine, irradiation, quinine, and anti-T-cell antibodies. Pregnancy (HELLP—hemolysis-elevated liver enzymes-low platelets syndrome), certain malignancies, systemic diseases (scleroderma, SLE, antiphospholipid antibody syndrome), malignant hypertension, HIV infection, and bone marrow transplantation are associated with D–HUS. Hereditary complement deficiency (Factor H deficiency) was also described to cause this form of HUS. Finally, an idiopathic form of D–HUS can occur.

The majority of HUS in children is associated with diarrhea (D+HUS), whereas less than 50% of adult cases are D+HUS. Vectors for toxin-producing bacteria are beef, fermented salami, as well as contaminated water, fruit, and vegetables. Unpasteurized apple cider, apple juice, and dairy products are also sources. Numerous outbreaks are due to person-to-person contact. Development of HUS occurs during the warmer months. In children, bloody diarrhea from colitis is common and abdominal pain, which can be associated with intussception, bowel necrosis,

and rectal prolapse can occur. The onset of HUS occurs approximately 1 week after diarrhea, presenting as pallor, lethargy, irritability, severe hypertension, and decreased urine output. Clinical or chemical pancreatitis, seizures, and other end-organ disturbances occur less commonly.

Treatment is supportive as most interventions are too risky and often with marginal or no benefit. In particular, the benefit of plasma exchange is unclear; however, anecdotal reports suggest some modest benefit in those with D–HUS. Blood pressure control and optimal management of renal failure, often using dialysis, are key to improved outcomes. Children with HUS have a good prognosis. Approximately 90% experience functional recovery whereas 5% die in the acute phase of illness. In those who recover, 10% are left with some form of chronic kidney disease. In contrast, adults have worse outcomes. Overall mortality is up to 30%, and chronic kidney disease occurs in approximately 20–30% of survivors, many requiring renal replacement therapy for end-stage renal disease. Mortality is highest (greater than 50%) in those with postpartum, cancer, or mitomycin-C-associated HUS. Recurrence develops in 25% of cases. The poor outcome is likely explained by the much higher incidence of D–HUS in adults.

THROMBOTIC THROMBOCYTOPENIC PURPURA

Thrombotic thrombocytopenic purpura occurs most often from either congenital or acquired abnormalities in the vWF-cleaving protease (ADAMST13). The primary defect is abnormal (enhanced) platelet aggregation due to large, circulating vWFs present due to reduced protease activity, resulting in microthrombi formation. Congenital forms may be acute and nonrelapsing or, more commonly, chronic and relapsing. The chronic, relapsing form of TTP may be familial (autosomal recessive) or sporadic, both associated with a deficiency of vWF-cleaving protease. Acquired forms occur following exposure to various drugs such as ticlopidine, mitomycin-C, oral contraceptives, quinine, cyclosporin, and cocaine. Scleroderma, pregnancy, HIV infection, and SLE are also associated with TTP. Acute, nonrelapsing forms of TTP are more commonly acquired. An autoantibody directed against the vWF-cleaving protease, that is able to inactivate the enzyme, occurs with most acquired forms of TTP.

In contrast to HUS, TTP occurs predominantly in women (70%) and is not seasonal. Peak incidence is in the third and fourth decades and TTP is rare in infants and the elderly. This is probably due to the more common association with acquired causes of TTP, which outnumber congenital forms. Fever and bleeding are common presenting features of TTP. Central nervous system (CNS) manifestations occur initially in approximately 50% of patients, but eventually develop in nearly 90% of those with TTP, and are the most prominent feature of the syndrome. Headache, visual symptoms, somnolence, and focal neurologic findings occur commonly. Seizures develop in 30% of patients. The CNS changes can fluctuate and be fleeting. Purpura is common, while gastrointestinal bleeding occurs from severe thrombocytopenia. Renal manifestations include hematuria, proteinuria, and azotemia. Severe renal failure, in contrast to HUS, is much less common but can occur. Heart and lung may also suffer thrombotic complications of TTP.

The rationale of plasma infusion and plasma exchange in TTP is based on targeting the vWF-cleaving protease abnormality. Treatment with fresh frozen plasma infusion is very effective for TTP-associated with a deficiency of the vWF protease. Alternatively, intensive plasmapheresis with plasma infusion is appropriate for disorders associated with an autoantibody to the vWF protease. Plasma exchange is associated with a response in 70–90% of patients with TTP. Treatment should be continued until remission is achieved. In general, at least seven consecutive daily treatments followed by alternate day exchanges for those improving are recommended. Therapies for those who fail plasma exchange are vincristine, corticosteroids, intravenous immunoglobulin, and antiplatelet agents. Except for vincristine, the efficacy of these treatments for TTP is unclear. Splenectomy is risky and its benefit is marginal. Platelet transfusions are generally felt to be contraindicated because they may worsen clinical signs and symptoms.

KEY POINTS
Nephritic Syndrome (Glomerulonephritis)

1. Nephritis or the nephritic syndrome is characterized by the abrupt onset of hematuria, proteinuria and acute renal failure. Patients often have associated hypertension and peripheral edema. The hallmark of glomerulonephritis on urinalysis is the presence of red cell casts.

2. Acute postinfectious glomerulonephritis occurs most often in children after pharyngeal infection with specific nephritogenic strains of group A β-hemolytic streptococcal infection.

3. Immune complex formation underlies the pathogenesis of SLE nephritis. Location of deposits determines the type of inflammatory response.

4. The WHO classification divides the lesions associated with SLE into six different types. Type III (focal proliferative glomerulonephritis) and, in particular, type IV nephritis (diffuse proliferative glomerulonephritis) are both associated with severe and rapid loss of kidney function when left untreated.

5. Therapy of lupus nephritis is based primarily on WHO classification.

6. The thrombotic microangiopathies consist of a spectrum of diseases that are characterized by the formation of platelet microthrombi within vessels, thrombocytopenia and microangiopathic hemolytic anemia.

7. Hemolytic uremic syndrome develops from various disease processes. The sporadic or endemic variety associated with diarrhea is linked to Shiga toxin exposure. The onset occurs approximately 1 week after diarrhea, presenting with severe hypertension and decreased urine output.

8. Thrombotic thrombocytopenic purpura is associated with either a congenital or acquired defect in a metalloproteinase-converting enzyme for von Willebrand factor. Central nervous system manifestations are the most prominent feature. Purpura is common, while gastrointestinal bleeding occurs from severe thrombocytopenia. Renal manifestations include hematuria, proteinuria, and azotemia.

Rapidly Progressive Glomerulonephritis

RPGN is characterized by crescent formation and a rapid decline in renal function. A crescent is made up of proliferating epithelial cells that line Bowman's capsule and infiltrating macrophages (Figure 17.12). Crescents result when the GBM is severely damaged with breaks observed on EM. This allows fibrin, plasma proteins, macrophages, monocytes, plasma cells, and platelets to gain access to Bowman's space. Patients present with rising serum BUN and creatinine concentrations and may have oliguria. Without adequate treatment irreversible renal failure may develop in weeks. Rapidly progressive glomerulonephritis is subdivided into three types based on immunofluorescence microscopy: (1) anti-GBM antibody disease; (2) pauci-immune glomerulonephritis; and (3) immune complex disease.

Type 1–Anti-GBM Antibody Disease (Goodpasture Syndrome)

Goodpasture syndrome is characterized by circulating antibodies to the GBM in association with glomerulonephritis and pulmonary hemorrhage. Rarely, clinical evidence of an anti-neutrophil cytoplasmic antibody (ANCA)-associated vasculitis may be seen concurrently with anti-GBM disease. Hemoptysis, pulmonary infiltrates, and pulmonary hemorrhage result from cross-reactivity of anti-GBM antibody to the alveolar capillary basement membrane. The autoantibodies recognize an epitope in the alpha-3 chain of type IV collagen. The binding of antibody to antigen induces an inflammatory response that results in glomerular injury. The initial injury is a focal and segmental necrosis followed by extensive crescent formation. Immunofluorescence microscopy shows linear deposition of IgG in the GBM (Figure 17.13). Electron microscopy does not reveal dense deposits, excluding immune complex disease.

Anti-GBM disease is uncommon; the annual incidence is one to two cases per million population/year. It makes up less than 10% of all cases of crescentic glomerulonephritis seen on renal biopsy. The disease incidence has two peaks, the first is in the third decade in men, and the second in the sixth and seventh decades with men and women equally affected. Young males more often present with the pulmonary renal syndrome while elderly females more commonly develop renal-limited disease. Smoking predisposes to the development of pulmonary hemorrhage. Dyspnea,

Figure 17.12

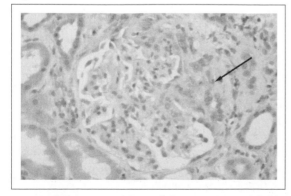

Crescent (light microscopy). A cellular crescent is seen by the arrow.

Figure 17.13

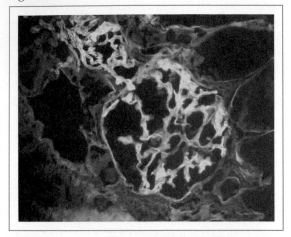

Goodpasture syndrome (immunofluorescence microscopy). Immunofluorescence staining in this patient with Goodpasture syndrome shows the classic linear IgG staining pattern. Note that there is no granularity as in Figure 17.5.

either intermittent or continuous, cough, and hemoptysis are the major symptomatic features of Goodpasture syndrome. Hemoptysis can be massive, minor, or absent. Lack of hemoptysis does not exclude pulmonary disease or hemorrhage. Pulmonary symptoms may develop over hours or slowly over weeks. Tachypnea, cyanosis, and inspiratory rales are signs of pulmonary disease. Arterial blood gas may demonstrate hypoxemia from alveolar hemorrhage. Occasionally, subclinical bleeding in the lungs results in iron deficiency anemia. Nephritis from anti-GBM disease is associated with hematuria, dysmorphic red cells, and red blood cell casts on urine sediment. Proteinuria and an elevated serum creatinine concentration are often present at the time of diagnosis. Renal function can deteriorate rapidly in the absence of therapy. Some patients, especially the elderly, present with renal manifestations and no pulmonary symptoms. In the absence of pulmonary hemorrhage, patients are considered to have renal-limited anti-GBM disease.

The diagnosis is suspected based on clinical and laboratory findings. The chest radiograph demonstrates patchy or diffuse infiltrates in the central lung fields. The changes are most often symmetric, but rarely can occur asymmetrically. Renal ultrasound typically appears normal. Anti-GBM antibodies may be detected in serum, but this is not a sensitive test (excessive number of false-negative results). Circulating anti-GBM antibodies are detected in serum using a specific enzyme-linked immunosorbent assay (ELISA) or radioimmunoassay. The test is based on the principle that purified GBM components are coated on plastic microtiter plates, diluted serum is applied, and anti-GBM antibodies bind the GBM components. Antibody binding is detected by using a secondary antibody that binds to human IgG. In general, the ANCA test is negative, but may be positive when a vasculitis occurs concurrently with anti-GBM disease. Although rarely performed, lung biopsy is diagnostic when it reveals linear IgG staining along the pulmonary basement membrane. Alveoli are often filled with red blood cells and hemosiderin-laden macrophages. Renal histology is typically obtained in these cases and, as described above, is diagnostic.

Anti-GBM disease is a true autoimmune disease of the kidney and lung. The pathogenesis is thought to be due to both the presence of anti-GBM antibodies and T-cell-mediated immunity to GBM antigens. Glomerular basement membrane antigens are expressed in thymus, and autoreactive CD4[+] T cells are increased. These T cells provide help to autoreactive B cells in the production of anti-GBM antibodies. These autoantibodies are directed against the noncollagenous 1 domain of the alpha-3 chain of type IV collagen in kidney and lung. Antibody binding leads to inflammation with complement deposition, leukocyte recruitment, and tissue injury and destruction. Genetic factors may play a role, as HLA-DR2 is associated with the development of anti-GBM disease. Environmental influences such as smoking, infection, certain geographical locations, and organic solvents or hydrocarbons are associated with Goodpasture syndrome.

Treatment is directed at removing culprit autoantibodies and suppressing their production. To this end, intensive plasma exchange, glucocorticoids, and immunosuppressive agents such as cyclophosphamide and azathioprine are employed. Most therapeutic protocols use a combination regimen consisting of prednisolone, cyclophosphamide, and plasma exchange. Prednisolone is employed at 1 mg/kg/day (maximum 80 mg/day) with a weekly dose reduction to 20 mg/day, followed by a slow taper over the next 1–2 years. Oral cyclophosphamide at 2.5 mg/kg/day (maximum 150 mg/day) is given for 4 months (dose adjusted based on white blood cell count) and converted to azathioprine for the next 1–2 years. Daily 4 L exchanges with 4.5% albumin for 2 weeks (or until no detectable anti-GBM antibodies) is the plasma exchange regimen. Key to success is initiation of therapy prior to the serum creatinine concentration reaching 5.7 mg/dL. The probability of achieving a 5-year survival without dialysis was 94% in these patients, where it decreased to 50% in patients with higher serum creatinine concentrations not yet requiring dialysis. Dialysis dependence at the time of therapy was associated with a dismal 13% chance of dialysis-free survival. Interestingly, there was no influence of anti-GBM titer on outcome, although 100% glomerular crescents on biopsy portended a poor renal prognosis.

Type 2–Pauci-Immune Glomerulonephritis

Pauci-immune glomerulonephritis is characterized by no or very little immunoglobulin deposition on immunofluorescence. This group of diseases is associated with ANCA. Most patients have evidence of a systemic vasculitis such as Wegener's granulomatosis, microscopic polyarteritis, or Churg-Strauss syndrome.

WEGENER'S GRANULOMATOSIS

Wegener's granulomatosis is a necrotizing vasculitis involving small-sized vessels. Although Wegener's granulomatosis can affect any organ system, it classically involves the kidney, as well as the upper and lower respiratory tract. Pathologic examination of lesions in the nasopharynx and lung reveals a necrotizing granulomatous vasculitis. In kidney the vasculitis manifests as a necrotizing glomerulonephritis with crescent formation. Granulomas are rarely seen on renal biopsy.

The disease most commonly develops in middle aged or elderly adults but can occur at any age. The initial presentation is often nonspecific with a variety of prominent constitutional symptoms including fever, night sweats, anorexia, weight loss, and fatigue. Upper respiratory and pulmonary symptoms are prominent early on such as rhinorrhea, sinusitis, otitis media, epistaxis, cough, and hemoptysis. A "limited" form of Wegener's is described that affects the upper and lower respiratory tract and not the kidneys. Renal involvement generally, but not always, follows the development of extrarenal involvement. Microscopic hematuria, red blood cell casts, proteinuria, and an elevated serum creatinine concentration are often present at the time of diagnosis. Some patients present with the renal lesion and nondiagnostic systemic symptoms. In the absence of upper and lower respiratory involvement these patients are often considered to have microscopic polyarteritis. It is likely that Wegener's granulomatosis, "limited" Wegener's, and microscopic polyarteritis are all part of a spectrum of the same disease since patients with "limited" Wegener's often develop renal involvement, patients with microscopic polyarteritis often subsequently develop pulmonary involvement, and the ANCA test is typically positive in all three syndromes. A variety of other organ systems may also be involved including the musculoskeletal system (myalgias, arthralgias), peripheral and central nervous system (mononeuritis multiplex, cranial nerve abnormalities), cardiovascular (pericarditis, myocarditis), skin (palpable purpura, ulcerative lesions), and eyes (conjunctivitis, episcleritis, uveitis, proptosis).

The diagnosis is suspected based on clinical and laboratory findings. The chest radiograph shows solitary or multiple nodules in the middle or lower lung fields. The nodules are poorly defined and often undergo central necrosis.

The ANCA test is frequently positive in a cytoplasmic pattern (cANCA) and has a high sensitivity and specificity in the presence of active classic Wegener's granulomatosis (>90%) but is not sufficient to either rule in or rule out the diagnosis. In "limited" Wegener's the ANCA may be negative in as many as 40% of patients.

The ANCA test is performed by incubating the patient's serum with ethanol-fixed human neutrophils. Indirect immunofluorescence is carried out and two patterns are observed. A diffuse cytoplasmic pattern is caused by antibodies directed against proteinase 3 and a perinuclear pattern is caused by antibodies directed against myeloperoxidase. A positive immunofluoresence should be followed by an ELISA for proteinase 3 and myeloperoxidase. Approximately 70% of patients with microscopic polyarteritis will have a positive pANCA. The pANCA pattern is, however, nonspecific and is seen in a wide variety of inflammatory diseases. It can also be caused by antibodies against a host of azurophilic granule proteins including catalase, lysozyme, lactoferrin, and elastase. The pANCA can also be falsely positive in patients with positive antinuclear antibodies (ANA).

Wegener's granulomatosis is an immune-mediated disorder. It likely results from an inciting inflammatory stimulus and a pathologic immune reaction to shielded antigens on neutrophil granule proteins. These anti-neutrophil cytoplasmic antibodies interact with activated neutrophils and endothelial cells and cause tissue damage. The inciting inflammatory event remains unclear. Given that the initial symptoms often involve the respiratory tract, research has focused on infectious and noninfectious inhaled agents without identifying a causal agent. It is possible that an inflammatory event exposes neoepitopes on granule proteins that generate an immune response that then undergoes epitope spreading. Activated neutrophils have increased surface expression of proteinase 3, are more likely to degranulate and release reactive oxygen species, and have increased binding to endothelial cells resulting in tissue damage.

Confirmation of the diagnosis requires histologic examination of tissue. If lesions are present in the nasopharynx these should be biopsied because of the low morbidity. Granulomatous inflammation is often observed but granulomatous vasculitis is seen in only one-third of patients. If there are no nasopharyngeal lesions the kidney is often biopsied since it is less invasive than an open lung biopsy (transbronchial biopsy often does not provide sufficient tissue to exclude the diagnosis). A kidney biopsy will not differentiate between Wegener's granulomatosis and microscopic polyarteritis since granulomas are rarely seen on renal biopsy. The characteristic finding in both disorders is a focal necrotizing glomerulonephritis with or without crescent formation. Immunofluorescence studies are negative. Serum complement concentrations are normal. This distinction is often not important clinically given that the treatment of both conditions is the same.

The mortality rate in untreated Wegener's granulomatosis is high, 80% within 1 year and 90% within 2 years. Mean survival in untreated patients is only 5 months. Although corticosteroids alone may yield transient improvement, this is generally only temporary. One-year survival with corticosteroids alone is 33%. Long-term remissions are obtained in those treated with cyclophosphamide. One-year survival with cyclophosphamide is 80–95%. Early institution of therapy is paramount. The presence of severe dialysis requiring acute renal failure during the acute phase of illness does not preclude aggressive therapy. Enough renal function can return to allow the discontinuation of dialysis. Patients with respiratory involvement or fulminant disease are begun on 4 mg/kg/day of oral cyclophosphamide for the first 3 or 4 days. When disease is active but relatively stable one can use 2 mg/kg/day orally. Intermittent IV pulse cyclophosphamide given at monthly intervals ($0.5–1$ g/m^2) was also employed. Oral prednisone (1 mg/kg/day in divided doses) is given and is especially helpful in reducing acute inflammation in the pericardium, eye, and skin. Intravenous pulse methylprednisolone (1 g for 3 days) is used in patients with rapidly progressive renal failure or respiratory disease. Corticosteroids are continued until the disease is controlled and then tapered to an alternate-day schedule. Cyclophosphamide is continued until there is no evidence of disease activity. Patients in remission after 3 or 4 months can be switched to oral azathiaprine or methotrexate to reduce the incidence of complications providing the ANCA is negative. Approximately 80–90% of patients can be placed into remission. Maintenance therapy is generally continued for 12–24 months after complete remission is induced. Systemic symptoms often improve quickly. The pulmonary and renal abnormalities require 3–6 months after cyclophosphamide begins to remit. Late relapses can occur. Given the toxicity of oral cyclophosphamide, monthly pulse intravenous dosing was evaluated with mixed results. Some studies showed equal and others reduced efficacy. Plasmapheresis is of limited benefit but may be of value in those with pulmonary hemorrhage, patients who require dialysis during the initial phase, and those with anti-GBM antibodies.

CLASSIC POLYARTERITIS NODOSA

Classic polyarteritis nodosa (PAN) involves small and medium-sized muscular arteries. Lesions tend to be segmental and commonly occur at arterial bifurcations with distal spread occasionally involving arterioles. There is prominent neutrophilic infiltration with destruction of the vascular wall. Fibrinoid necrosis occurs with disruption of the internal elastic lamina, ischemia, and infarction. Aneurysm formation develops in the weakened vessel wall, and scarring during the healing process leads to further obliteration of the vascular lumen. The arcuate and interlobular arteries are primarily involved in the kidney. The glomerular lesion is a focal, segmental necrotizing glomerulonephritis. Changes are primarily ischemic, with fibrinoid necrosis and minimal proliferation. Immunofluorescence microscopy is usually negative. In the healing phase, thickening of the vessel wall may resemble that induced by chronic

hypertension; however, in hypertension the internal elastic lamina is preserved.

Patients present with systemic symptoms including fever, weight loss, arthralgias, and loss of appetite. Males are more commonly affected than females with a peak incidence in the sixth decade. There is a lack of eosinophilia or significant pulmonary involvement, which differentiates PAN from Churg–Strauss syndrome. Asymmetric polyneuropathy (mononeuritis multiplex—due to involvement of the vasa vasorum) strongly suggests the diagnosis of PAN. The only other disease causing mononeuritis multiplex is diabetes mellitus. Testicular pain is another common feature. Renal involvement is characterized by azotemia and hypertension. In general progressive renal failure is a late manifestation. Urine sediment is variable, and may be relatively benign if only larger vessels are involved, a setting in which there may be glomerular ischemia without significant necrosis. Dysmorphic red blood cells, red blood cell casts, and mild proteinuria are typically seen when there is focal proliferative glomerulonephritis. Nephrotic range proteinuria is unusual. Serum complement concentration is usually normal. Hepatitis B infection has been associated with the development of PAN.

The diagnosis is most commonly made by demonstrating typical vascular lesions on angiography of the celiac and renal arteries. Microaneurysms and irregular segmental constrictions are seen in larger vessels, with tapering and occlusion of smaller intrarenal arteries. Renal biopsy may be required if the angiogram is negative, and if no other easily biopsied affected tissue such as muscle or peripheral nerve can be identified.

The prognosis of untreated PAN is poor with survival rates of only 33% at 1 year, and 10% at 5 years. This improved dramatically with the advent of corticosteroids (50% 5-year survival). Mortality remains high secondary to renal failure, congestive heart failure, stroke, and mesenteric infarction. Long-term remissions are induced with cyclophosphamide in doses similar to those used for Wegener's granulomatosis. Patients with RPGN should also be given pulse corticosteroids.

As with Wegener's granulomatosis, improvement in renal function can be seen even in patients with far-advanced disease. Maintenance therapy should be continued for 1–2 years after remission.

CHURG–STRAUSS SYNDROME

Churg-Strauss syndrome is characterized by extravascular granulomas, eosinophilic infiltration of arteries and venules, and kidney involvement. Clinically the disease progresses through three stages. An allergic diathesis is usually the first clinical manifestation, beginning between age 20 and 30. Asthmatic symptoms are frequent in this stage. This is followed by peripheral eosinophilia. The final stage is systemic vasculitis. The time course required to progress from one stage to another is variable. The shorter the interval, the worse the prognosis. As systemic vasculitis develops, lung involvement becomes more prominent with noncavitating pulmonary infiltrates on chest radiograph. Often allergic and asthmatic symptoms improve as vasculitis develops. Coronary vasculitis is common, and the heart is often the most severely affected organ (resulting in 50% of deaths). Renal involvement is generally mild, with renal failure developing in less than 10% of patients. Despite the paucity of renal findings hypertension is relatively common (75%). The characteristic LM finding on renal biopsy is a focal segmental necrotizing glomerulonephritis. The interstitium is also involved with either a focal or diffuse interstitial nephritis with granuloma formation and eosinophilic infiltration. Patients with Churg-Strauss syndrome often respond to corticosteroids alone and generally are treated for 1 year; relapses are uncommon.

Type 3–Immune Complex Diseases

A variety of immune complex diseases can result in RPGN including postinfectious glomerulonephritis, lupus nephritis, IgA nephropathy, Henoch-Schönlein purpura, membranoproliferative glomerulonephritis, and membranous glomerulonephritis. Many of these disorders are covered in other sections of this chapter.

HYPERSENSITIVITY VASCULITIS

Hypersensitivity vasculitis primarily involves postcapillary venules. Skin lesions (palpable purpura) are the most predominant abnormality observed. Lesions vary in size from a few millimeters to centimeters and in severe cases ulceration may occur. Biopsy of affected skin reveals an intense neutrophilic infiltrate surrounding dermal blood vessels that is associated with hemorrhage and edema (leukocytoclastic vasculitis). Hypersensitivity vasculitis is often confined to skin but other organ systems including kidney may be involved. Vascular involvement in kidney occurs in the distal interlobular arteries and glomerular arterioles. In contrast to pauci-immune forms of glomerulonephritis such as Wegener's granulomatosis, IF shows diffuse granular deposition of immunoglobulin and complement. When the kidney is affected this is manifested as either Henoch-Schönlein purpura (HSP), essential mixed cryoglobulinemia (EMC), or serum sickness.

HENOCH-SCHÖNLEIN PURPURA

HSP is characterized by IgA-containing immune deposits at sites of involvement. Presenting symptoms include the characteristic tetrad of abdominal pain, arthritis or arthralgias, purpuric skin lesions, and kidney disease. Its annual incidence is 20 per 100,000 children. Skin lesions are most commonly seen on the extensor surfaces of the arms, legs, and buttocks. They are ultimately seen in all patients but on occasion are absent at initial presentation. Lesions can begin as urticaria and evolve into purpura. The most common joints involved are the ankles and knees. Gastrointestinal manifestations include vomiting, abdominal pain, and bleeding. Renal involvement is common and generally evident within days to months after the onset of initial symptoms. The urinalysis reveals microscopic hematuria, red cell casts, and mild proteinuria. On presentation the serum creatinine concentration is often normal or slightly elevated. Patients with more severe disease have nephrotic range proteinuria, hypertension, and elevated serum BUN and creatinine concentrations.

Immunofluorescence staining of purpuric skin lesions and occasionally normal skin is positive for IgA in endothelial cells of superficial blood vessels. Immune complexes may be absent from the vessel wall in older lesions. Therefore, the absence of immune complexes does not rule out Henoch-Schönlein purpura. Morphologic changes in the kidney are identical to those seen in IgA nephropathy. The most common lesion is a mild proliferative glomerulonephritis. In severe cases crescent formation and fibrinoid necrosis are observed. IgA and complement containing immune deposits are present on IF.

The diagnosis should be considered in a patient with skin lesions of hypersensitivity vasculitis, particularly in the presence of arthralgias and abdominal pain. Skin biopsy with immunoflourescence is often diagnostic. IgA deposition is found in dermal vessels in up to 75% of cases, however, early lesions must be biopsied. The absence of IgA in dermal vessels does not rule out HSP. Serum complement concentration is usually normal. Renal biopsy is only performed in patients with progressive increases in serum BUN and creatinine concentrations.

Henoch-Schönlein purpura is generally a benign self-limited disorder that resolves spontaneously. Adults tend to have more severe disease than children. Recurrences of purpuric skin lesions or glomerulonephritis can occur and recurrent disease does not imply a worse prognosis. The degree of renal involvement is the most important long-term prognostic factor. Prognosis is excellent in those with asymptomatic hematuria and proteinuria or focal glomerulonephritis. Poor prognostic signs include nephrotic range proteinuria and >50% crescents on renal biopsy. This group of patients is less likely to completely recover kidney function. In one study, patients with greater than 50% crescents had a 37% incidence of progressing to ESRD. Progressive kidney disease is uncommon in patients who present initially with mild disease. Skin lesions and kidney disease do not respond to corticosteroids alone. Therapy is often attempted with pulse steroids, cyclophosphamide, and plasmapheresis in patients with severe or progressive disease and crescentic glomerulonephritis. Its efficacy remains unproven due to the lack of randomized trials and the high spontaneous remission rate even in those with severe disease.

ESSENTIAL MIXED CRYOGLOBULINEMIA (TYPE II)

Cryoglobulins are antibodies that precipitate in cold and redissolve on warming. The biochemical characteristics responsible for this are not well understood. There are three different types of cryoglobulins. Type I cryoglobulins are monoclonal and are usually the result of multiple myeloma or Waldenstrom's macroglobulinemia. Type II cryoglobulins (essential mixed cryoglobulinemia) contain a polyclonal IgG and a monoclonal IgM rheumatoid factor directed against the immunoglobulin. Most cases are the result of infection with hepatitis C. Cryoglobulins are abnormally glycosylated and this may play a role in their cryoprecipitation. Type III cryoglobulins are composed of a polyclonal IgG and a polyclonal IgM rheumatoid factor. This may be the result of hepatitis C infection but can also be seen with SLE and lymphoproliferative malignancies.

Hepatitis C virus can bind to B lymphocytes and lower their activation threshold resulting in the production of autoantibodies. Cryoglobulins are also present in other forms of chronic liver disease including infection with hepatitis B and patients with other forms of cirrhosis. Liver disease may contribute to the development or persistence of cryoglobulinemia due to the fact that the liver is the primary clearance site of cryoglobulins.

Patients often present with systemic symptoms including fatigue and lethargy, as well as arthralgias.

Palpable purpura can also be the presenting complaint and commonly involves the lower extremities. Hepatosplenomegaly, lymphadenopathy, peripheral neuropathy, and Raynaud's phenomenon may be present. Serum complement concentrations are generally low. Renal involvement is present in approximately half of patients and ranges from asymptomatic hematuria and proteinuria to acute oliguric renal failure. Azotemia is present at onset of disease in a minority of patients. Hepatic enzymes are often elevated and may reflect underlying hepatitis B or C infection.

EMC should be considered in any patient with palpable purpura, especially if hypocomplementemia is present. The diagnosis is established by the presence of an IgM-IgG cryoglobulin with a monoclonal component by immunofixation electrophoresis. To test for the presence of cryoglobulins 20 mL of blood must be drawn in the fasting state and collected in a tube without anticoagulants. The tube is then placed in warm water for transportation to the lab. After serum is separated via centrifugation the sample is placed at 4°C and observed for cryoprecipitation.

The principal pathologic findings are found in skin and kidney. Skin biopsy reveals a leukocytoclastic vasculitis without IgA deposition. In the kidney LM resembles MPGN type I with lobular accentuation, diffuse mesangial and endothelial cell proliferation, and basement membrane thickening. On EM mesangial and subendothelial deposits are seen. The subendothelial deposits often have a characteristic "fingerprint" appearance. There are numerous intraluminal thrombi composed of precipitated cryoglobulin distinguishing EMC from MPGN type I. Immunofluorescence microscopy reveals the deposition of IgM and C3 in the glomerular basement membrane.

In most patients renal involvement is slowly progressive, with renal failure developing over months to years. Neither the cryoglobulin or complement concentration predicts those that will develop ESRD. Hypocomplementemia in the presence of renal failure, hypertension, and elevated serum BUN and creatinine concentrations are poor prognostic signs. The efficacy of treatment remains a question. Patients with fulminant disease (acute renal failure, progressive neuropathy, or distal necrosis requiring amputation) were often treated with plasmapheresis, prednisone, and cyclophosphamide before it became apparent that the majority of cases were related to hepatitis C infection. This regimen was successful in inducing remission in some patients. Reinfused plasma must be warmed or acute renal failure will be induced. Plasmapheresis is generally done three times per week for several weeks. Immunosuppressive therapy carries the risk of worsening viral replication and may further increase the risk of inducing non-Hodgkin's lymphoma. More recently combinations of interferon α and ribavirin were employed. Although this regimen is effective for the treatment of skin and joint involvement, there is little evidence that it is beneficial for the treatment of the renal lesion. In general ribavirin should not be used in patients with a GFR below 50 mL/minute. There is a high rate of recurrence of EMC in the renal allograft.

KEY POINTS
Rapidly Progressive Glomerulonephritis

1. Rapidly progressive glomerulonephritis is characterized by a rapid decline in renal function and crescent formation on renal biopsy. It is important to recognize since irreversible renal damage can occur over a span of weeks.

2. Rapidly progressive glomerulonephritis is subdivided into three types based on immunofluorescence microscopy: (1) anti-GBM antibody disease; (2) pauci-immune glomerulonephritis; and (3) immune complex disease.

3. Goodpasture syndrome is characterized by circulating antibodies to the GBM, glomerulonephritis and pulmonary hemorrhage.

Immunofluorescence microscopy reveals a linear deposition of IgG.

4. Pauci-immune glomerulonephritis is characterized by no or very little immunoglobulin deposition on immunofluorescence. This group of diseases is associated with ANCA and includes Wegener's granulomatosis, microscopic polyarteritis, classic polyarteritis nodosum, and Churg–Strauss syndrome.

5. Wegener's granulomatosis classically involves the kidney, as well as the upper and lower respiratory tract. Pathologic examination of lesions in the nasopharynx and lung reveals a necrotizing granulomatous vasculitis.

6. Classic polyarteritis nodosa is diagnosed by demonstrating typical vascular lesions on angiography of the celiac and renal arteries. Microaneurysms and irregular segmental constrictions are seen in larger vessels, with tapering and occlusion of smaller intrarenal arteries.

7. Churg-Strauss syndrome is characterized by extravascular granulomas, eosinophilic infiltration of arteries and venules, and kidney involvement. Clinically the disease progresses through three stages: an allergic diathesis; peripheral eosinophilia; and systemic vasculitis.

8. Henoch-Schönlein purpura presents with the characteristic tetrad of abdominal pain, arthritis or arthralgias, purpuric skin lesions, and kidney disease. Morphologic changes in kidney are identical to those seen in IgA nephropathy.

9. Essential mixed cryoglobulinemia should be considered in any patient with palpable purpura, especially if hypocomplementemia is present. The diagnosis is established by the presence of an IgM-IgG cryoglobulin with a monoclonal component by immunofixation electrophoresis.

Asymptomatic Abnormalities on Urinalysis

Abnormalities on urinalysis such as microscopic hematuria and proteinuria may also be the initial presentation of glomerular disease. Microscopic hematuria may result from bleeding anywhere in the urinary tract. The most common causes are nephrolithiasis, urinary tract infection, and malignancies. These disorders do not result in significant proteinuria. Hematuria in association with proteinuria is suggestive of a glomerular disease. Although any glomerular disease can initially present with an abnormal urinalysis, IgA nephropathy, Alport syndrome, and thin basement membrane disease are common glomerular lesions that often present initially with an abnormal urinalysis.

IgA Nephropathy

IgA nephropathy is the most common cause of glomerulonephritis worldwide. It is most common in Asians and Caucasians and relatively uncommon in African Americans. IgA nephropathy is unique among glomerular diseases in that it is defined not by its LM features but rather by the finding of immune deposits containing IgA in the mesangium and occasionally in the GBM on IF microscopy.

Approximately one-third to half of patients present prior to the age of 40 with intermittent macroscopic hematuria after respiratory infection. The majority of the remainder have asymptomatic abnormalities on urinalysis. Nephrotic syndrome and RPGN occur in a small percentage of patients. IgA nephropathy is associated with chronic liver disease, viral infections such as HIV and hepatitis B, rheumatoid arthritis, Reiter's syndrome, dermatitis herpetiformis, and gluten enteropathy.

Light microscopic findings vary from minimal changes to segmental or diffuse mesangial hypercellularity with an increase in mesangial matrix to segmental sclerosis. On IF microscopy the hallmark is the detection of IgA. Other immunoglobulins including IgG and IgM can also be seen, as well as C3. Focal thinning of the GBM is a common feature on electron microscopic examination. The only other glomerular disease associated with extensive glomerular deposition of IgA is lupus nephritis. In lupus nephritis, however, IgG deposition is often more prominent than IgA and C1q is detected due to activation of the classical complement pathway. In IgA nephropathy immune complexes activate the alternative pathway and do not bind C1.

Abnormal glycosylation of IgA1 plays a role in its deposition in the mesangium. IgA binds to mesangial cells and can induce proliferation and cytokine production. It also binds complement via the alternative pathway. Sublytic concentrations of C5b-9 are generated resulting in increased secretion of inflammatory cytokines, as well as the production of mesangial matrix.

End-stage renal disease develops in 20% of patients at 20 years. Predictors of a poor outcome include an elevated serum creatinine concentration, proteinuria >1 g/24 hours, hypertension, male sex, persistent microscopic hematuria, and young age at onset. On renal biopsy the presence of tubulointerstitial disease and crescents portends a poor prognosis. Treatment is generally reserved for patients with an elevated serum creatinine concentration, hypertension, and/or proteinuria greater than 1 g/24 hours. Angiotensin-converting enzyme inhibitors are more effective than other antihypertensive agents in slowing the progression of renal failure in patients with IgA nephropathy. Proteinuria can be further reduced with the addition of an ARB. Fish oil can be tried but studies are conflicting as to whether it is of benefit. Corticosteroids also reduce proteinuria and may improve outcomes in those with nephrotic syndrome and progressive disease despite ACE inhibitors or ARBs. Those patients with LM features typical of minimal change disease may be especially responsive to corticosteroids. Patients with RPGN are treated with intravenous pulse methylprednisolone, oral prednisone, and cyclophosphamide with or without plasmapheresis.

Alport Syndrome

Alport syndrome is an inherited disorder that results in the production of defective type IV collagen. Its incidence is approximately 1 in 50,000. Type IV collagen is a triple helix of alpha chains. Abnormalities in any one of the three chains results in an abnormal collagen molecule. Six alpha chains, COL4A1 through COL4A6, have been identified in humans. COL4A3, COL4A4, and COL4A5 are expressed in the glomerular basement membrane. Renal involvement (microscopic and gross hematuria, progressive rise in the serum BUN and creatinine concentrations, hypertension, proteinuria) is associated with sensorineural hearing loss and eye abnormalities (perimacular flecks and anterior lenticonus). The earliest change on renal biopsy is thinning of the GBM. As the disease progresses the GBM splits developing a laminated appearance.

In 85% of cases the mode of inheritance is X-linked dominant and is caused by mutations in COL4A5. Heterozygous females generally have mild disease. In 10–15% of cases inheritance is autosomal recessive and due to mutations in COL4A3 and COL4A4. Carriers generally have microscopic hematuria but rarely progress to renal failure or have hearing loss. In a few cases an autosomal dominant mode of inheritance is described.

Large deletions and frame shift mutations are associated with a more severe phenotype. Greater than 90% of these patients develop ESRD and deafness by age 30. The abnormality of alpha-5 chain synthesis leads to an abnormal GBM that is also deficient in the alpha-3 chain (Goodpasture's antigen). A deficiency of both alpha-3 and alpha-5 results in a higher incidence of ESRD and a higher risk of anti-GBM nephritis after renal transplant.

Thin Basement Membrane Disease

Thin basement membrane disease or benign familial hematuria is manifested by persistent microscopic hematuria, minimal proteinuria, and the absence of ear or eye involvement. Rarely do patients progress to renal failure. Inheritance is autosomal dominant. There is diffuse thinning of the lamina densa of the GBM (<200 nm). Some of these patients are heterozygous for mutations in COL4A3 and COL4A4 suggesting that thin basement membrane disease is the heterozygous state of autosomal recessive Alport syndrome.

KEY POINTS
Abnormal Urinalysis

1. IgA nephropathy is the most common cause of glomerulonephritis worldwide.
2. IgA nephropathy is unique among glomerular diseases in that it is defined not by its LM features but by the finding of immune deposits containing IgA on IF microscopy.
3. Abnormal glycosylation of IgA1 plays a role in its deposition in the mesangium. IgA binds to mesangial cells, induces proliferation and cytokine production, and binds complement via the alternative pathway.
4. Alport syndrome is an inherited disorder that results in the production of defective type IV collagen. The earliest change on renal biopsy is thinning of the GBM.
5. Thin basement membrane disease or benign familial hematuria is manifested by persistent microscopic hematuria, minimal proteinuria, and the absence of ear or eye involvement.

Additional Reading

Cameron, J.S. Lupus nephritis. *J Am Soc Nephrol* 10:413–424, 1999.

Cattran, D.C. Idiopathic membranous glomerulonephritis. *Kidney Int* 59:1983–1994, 2001.

Floege, J., Feehally, J. IgA nephropathy: recent developments. *J Am Soc Nephrol* 11:2395–2403, 2000.

Hricik, D.E., Chung-Park, M., Sedor, J.R. Glomerulonephritis. *N Engl J Med* 339:888–899, 1998.

Kamesh, L., Harper, L., Savage, C.O. ANCA-positive vasculitis. *J Am Soc Nephrol* 13:1953–1960, 2002.

Kluth, D.C., Rees, A.J. Anti-glomerular basement membrane disease. *J Am Soc Nephrol* 10:2446–2453, 1999.

Korbet, S.M. Treatment of primary focal segmental glomerulosclerosis. *Kidney Int* 62:2301–2310, 2002.

Lin, J., Markowitz, G.S., Valeri, A.M., Kambham, N., Sherman, W.H., Appel, G.B., D'Agati, V.D. Renal monoclonal immunoglobulin deposition disease: the disease spectrum. *J Am Soc Nephrol* 12:1482–1492, 2001.

Moake, J.L. Thrombotic microangiopathies. *N Engl J Med* 347:589–600, 2002.

Remuzzi, G., Schieppati, A., Ruggenenti, P. Clinical practice. Nephropathy in patients with type 2 diabetes. *N Engl J Med* 346:1145–1151, 2002.

Ritz, E., Orth, S.R. Nephropathy in patients with type 2 diabetes mellitus. *N Engl J Med* 341:1127–1133, 1999.

Rosenstock, J.L., Markowitz, G.S., Valeri, A.M., Sacchi, G., Appel, G.B., D'Agati, V.D. Fibrillary and immunotactoid glomerulonephritis: distinct entities with different clinical and pathologic features. *Kidney Int* 63:1450–1461, 2003.

Ross, M.J., Klotman, P.E. Recent progress in HIV-associated nephropathy. *J Am Soc Nephrol* 13:2997–3004, 2002.

Schwarz, A. New aspects of the treatment of nephrotic syndrome. *J Am Soc Nephrol* 12(Suppl. 17):S44–S47, 2001.

Vora, J.P., Ibrahim, H.A., Bakris, G.L. Responding to the challenge of diabetic nephropathy: the historic evolution of detection, prevention and management. *J Hum Hypertens* 14:667–685, 2000.

Mark A. Perazella

Tubulointerstitial Diseases

Recommended Time to Complete: 1 day

Guiding Questions

1. How does one diagnose tubulointerstitial disease?

2. The development of tubulointerstitial disease is characterized by what two circumstances?

3. Tubulointerstitial disease is characterized by what histopathologic findings?

4. What are the common clinical manifestations of tubulointerstitial disease?

5. Are there laboratory tests that suggest a diagnosis of tubulointerstitial disease?

6. What are the common categories of tubulointerstitial disease?

7. What is the basic model of the pathogenesis of tubulointerstitial disease?

Introduction

Structural abnormalities of the renal parenchyma that involve primarily the tubules and interstitium are called tubulointerstitial disease. In contrast to acute interstitial nephritis (AIN), diseases that cause tubulointerstitial disease, discussed in this section, are more often chronic processes (Table 18.1). Diseases of the tubulointerstitium are best thought of as either primary or secondary processes. Primary causes of tubulointerstitial nephritis typically occur due to systemic diseases or following exposure to environmental or therapeutic agents. In this circumstance, the glomeruli and vasculature are typically spared or have only minor structural changes until late in the course of disease. In general, approximately 10–20% of end-stage renal disease (ESRD) in the United States occurs from primary chronic tubulointerstitial disease. A secondary form of chronic tubulointerstitial disease may also result from progressive glomerular disease or vascular injury with associated renal parenchymal ischemia. A significant number of disease states cause this form of chronic tubulointerstitial injury, with diabetic nephropathy and hypertensive nephrosclerosis being most common. Tubulointerstitial disease with fibrosis and scarring significantly determine the progressive nature of these lesions and their ultimate outcome, the outcome being chronic kidney disease (CKD) and ESRD requiring renal replacement therapy.

Histopathology of Tubulointerstitial Disease

In chronic tubulointerstitial disease, a cellular infiltrate and variable amounts of fibrosis are noted within the architecture of the interstitium.

Table 18.1

Etiologies of Tubulointerstitial Disease

Immunologic causes
Systemic lupus erythematosis
Vasculitis
Amyloidosis
Cryoglobulinemia
Sjögren's syndrome
Therapeutic agents
Analgesics
NSAIDs
Chemotherapy (cisplatin, nitrosoureas)
Immunosuppressive agents (calcineurin inhibitors)
Lithium
Chinese herbs (aristolochic acid)
Occupational/environmental agents
Heavy metals (lead, cadmium, mercury)
Mycotoxins
Neoplastic/hematopoietic diseases
Lymphoma/leukemia
Multiple myeloma
Light chain deposition disease
Sickle cell disease
Hereditary diseases
Medullary cystic disease
Polycystic kidney disease
Karyomegalic interstitial nephritis
Vascular diseases
Renal atheroemboli
Radiation nephritis
Hypertensive nephrosclerosis
Infections
Bacterial pyelonephritis
Xanthogranulomatous pyelonephritis
Malacoplakia
Metabolic disorders
Hypercalcemia
Hypokalemia
Hyperoxaluria/oxalosis
Hyperuricemia
Cystinosis
Other conditions
Sarcoidosis
Obstructive uropathy
Balkan nephropathy
Tubulointerstitial nephritis uveitis (TINU)

Abbreviation: NSAIDs, nonsteroidal anti-inflammatory drugs.

The characteristic lesion is an inflammatory cellular infiltrate composed of lymphocytes, usually T cells and, to a lesser degree, plasma cells. Early in the course of disease, the acute cellular infiltrate is accompanied by interstitial edema, tubulitis with tubular basement membrane disruption, and dissolution of the normal tubulointerstitial architecture. Over time, the acute process transitions to a chronic tubulointerstitial lesion. The chronic histology is characterized by interstitial fibrosis with increased extracellular matrix, tubular ectasia and atrophy, and tubular dropout. The severity of this process typically advances over time until the entire tubulointerstitium is overtaken by fibrosis. In far advanced disease, glomerulosclerosis develops and blood vessels become involved by fibrosis and sclerosis. At this point in time, the patient often manifests clinically advanced CKD.

KEY POINTS
Histopathology of Tubulointerstitial Disease

1. Tubulointerstitial disease is classified as primary or secondary to another disease process.
2. In primary tubulointerstitial disease, the glomeruli and vasculature are normal early in the course of disease.
3. The characteristic lesion is a lymphocytic infiltrate.
4. Early in tubulointerstitial disease, interstitial edema accompanies the cellular infiltrate while tubular injury and interstitial fibrosis develop as the process progresses.

Clinical Presentation

More often than not, patients with tubulointerstitial disease have few clinical symptoms suggestive of CKD. In general, symptoms and signs reflect the extent of tubulointerstitial disease. For example, focal areas of injury are minimally symptomatic, whereas diffuse disease causes several tubular defects in electrolyte, acid-base, and mineral handling. Also, the area of the kidney involved by disease leads to disturbances characteristic of the loss of function of the injured tubular segment. Injury to the proximal tubule is associated with impaired absorption of sodium, glucose, phosphorus, amino acids, potassium, uric acid, and several low molecular weight proteins. In contrast, disease of the loop of Henle and distal convoluted tubule causes sodium and potassium wasting (salt wasting, hypokalemia, and hypotension). Involvement of the cortical and medullary collecting ducts may be associated with hyperkalemia and metabolic acidosis (hyperkalemic distal renal tubular acidosis) due to defects in potassium and ammonia (buffers acid) secretion by this segment. Another important determinate of the clinical manifestations of tubulointerstitial disease is the degree of compensation by the remaining normal (or less severely impaired) nephron segments. With mild-to-moderate disease, compensatory hypertrophy may eliminate or substantially reduce symptoms of renal disease.

Often times, chronic tubulointerstitial disease is discovered when blood testing reveals abnormal kidney function (increased blood urea nitrogen [BUN] and serum creatinine concentration) that is otherwise fairly asymptomatic. The presence of certain systemic diseases may also prompt investigation of kidney function and potential kidney disease. As is discussed later, several systemic diseases promote the development of chronic tubulointerstitial disease. The most common symptom associated with disease of the tubulointerstitium is polyuria. Two mechanisms account for this symptom including salt wasting and the inability to maximally concentrate the urine. Dizziness from low blood pressure (salt wasting), weakness from either severe hypokalemia or hyperkalemia, and bone pain/fractures from osteopenia induced by metabolic acidosis can also occur. Advanced chronic tubulointerstitial disease results in the development of usual manifestations of CKD approaching ESRD. These include anorexia, nausea, vomiting, lethargy, somnolence, fatigue, restless legs, and other uremic manifestations.

Laboratory Findings

As noted in the previous section, tubulointerstitial disease often manifests with various renal tubular and urinary disorders (Table 18.2). Examination of blood and urine chemistries often provide insight into the disease. Proximal renal tubular acidosis (RTA), as noted by a hypokalemic, nonanion gap metabolic acidosis, may occur in this setting. In this case, the urine is acid (pH ≤5.5) in steady state acidosis, but becomes alkaline (pH ≥7.0) when therapy to correct the metabolic acidosis with bicarbonate is attempted. A full-blown Fanconi's syndrome can develop with chronic tubulointerstitial disease involving the proximal

Table 18.2

Laboratory Manifestations of Tubulointerstitial Disease

Proximal tubular defects
Proximal renal tubular acidosis
Fanconi's syndrome
Distal tubular defects
Hypokalemic distal renal tubular acidosis
Hyperkalemic distal renal tubular acidosis
Concentrating defect
Salt wasting nephropathy
Sterile pyuria
White blood cells
White blood cell casts
Tubular proteinuria
Albuminuria (<1 g/day)
β_2-microglobulinuria
Retinol-binding protein excretion
Enzymuria
N-acetyl-β-glucosaminidase excretion
Alanine aminopeptidase excretion
Intestinal alkaline phosphatase excretion

tubule. This syndrome is characterized by the presence of a proximal RTA that also demonstrates phosphaturia, aminoaciduria, glycosuria, enzymuria, and uricosuria. Salt wasting (urinary sodium >20 meq/L) despite hypotension may indicate tubulointerstitial disease of the loop of Henle. Hypokalemia due to urinary potassium wasting may also occur with a lesion in this segment. An acidification defect in the distal nephron may cause a hypokalemic distal RTA that is characterized by hypokalemia, nonanion gap metabolic acidosis, and alkaline urine (first morning void pH >5.5). A hyperkalemic distal RTA (hyperkalemia with nonanion gap metabolic acidosis) may be seen with tubulointerstitial disease. Inability to concentrate the urine leads to a low urine osmolality and, if the patient is unable to gain free water access, may cause hypernatremia.

The urinalysis yields variable results in the setting of chronic tubulointerstitial disease. A couple of generalizations, however, can be made. Tubulointerstitial disease rarely has marked proteinuria, most often there is trace to 1+ protein on quantitative examination of the urine. A 24-hour urine collection or spot protein/creatinine ratio usually contains less than 1 g of total protein. Examination of the urine sediment under the microscope often reveals a preponderance of white blood cells (WBCs), occasionally with some WBC and granular casts. Red blood cells (RBCs) and RBC casts are extremely unusual. Urinary crystals may be present with certain disorders associated with chronic tubulointerstitial disease (calcium oxalate crystals with hyperoxaluria, uric acid crystals with uric acid nephropathy).

Examination of proteinuria (low molecular weight proteins) and enzymuria may provide insight into disease limited to the tubulointerstitium, however, they are not widely employed as clinical tools. High molecular weight proteins (>40,000–50,000 Da) in the urine are typically a marker of glomerular disease. Included in this group is albumin (69,000 Da), transferrin (77,000 Da), and IgG (146,000 Da). In contrast, small amounts of low molecular weight proteins are normally excreted in the urine. They are considered markers of "tubular" proteinuria (versus glomerular proteinuria). β_2-microglobulin (11,800 Da) and retinol-binding protein (21,400 Da) are the markers of tubular injury most commonly employed. Both substances are freely filtered; approximately 99.9% is reabsorbed in the proximal tubule where they are catabolized. When the reabsorptive capacity of proximal tubular cells is impaired, increased amounts of various low molecular weight proteins can be demonstrated in the urine. Thus, levels increase in urine when disease injures proximal tubular cells. Although both β_2-microglobulin and retinol-binding protein are used to evaluate tubulointerstitial disease, the assay employed for retinol-binding protein is more stable in an acid urine and is preferred.

Urinary enzymes also reflect tubular dysfunction and act as markers of tubulointerstitial disease. The basis for measuring high molecular weight enzymes in urine stems from the knowledge that the only source of enzymes is injured tubular cells. Despite this premise, however, the use of measuring enzymuria is hindered by a lack of correlation with specific disease states and the disconnect between severity of tubular injury and the magnitude of urine enzyme levels. Urinary enzyme activity is also affected by the presence of urinary enzyme inhibitors and activators, as well as urine pH and osmolality. A few enzymes accepted as useful urinary biomarkers are used in clinical studies to assess tubular damage. They include N-acetyl-β-glucosaminidase, alanine aminopeptidase, and intestinal alkaline phosphatase. Enzymuria remains a valuable research tool, but has not gained widespread use in the clinical arena.

Diagnosis of Tubulointerstitial Disease

The clinical diagnosis of chronic tubulointerstitial disease is considered when other possible causes of kidney disease are excluded, in particular intrinsic renal disease such as glomerular lesions, as well as obstructive uropathy. An in-depth history

of prescribed or over-the-counter medications ingested by the patient and any at risk occupational or environmental exposures suffered are key to assess causes of tubulointerstitial disease. Evidence of systemic disease associated with this form of kidney disease helps support the diagnosis. In addition to the history, the laboratory findings described above point to disease in the tubulointerstitium. In particular, evidence of tubular dysfunction is suggestive of chronic tubulointerstitial disease. These include a renal tubular acidosis, salt wasting, a urinary concentrating defect, and a urinalysis demonstrating pyuria with little or no protein. Ultrasonography of the kidney reveals normal-to-large size kidneys with acute interstitial nephritis, while small echogenic kidneys are present with chronic tubulointerstitial disease. The only exception to this caveat is certain infiltrative diseases where the Kidneys are often large and echogenic. Examples include sarcoidosis, lymphomas and leukemias, amyloidosis, and cystic kidney disease. The renal biopsy helps to establish the diagnosis. The classic lymphocytic infiltrate, the variable degrees of interstitial fibrosis, and tubular ectasia/atrophy characterize chronic tubulointerstitial nephritis. In the absence of a definable cause of chronic tubulointerstitial disease when the renal biopsy supports this diagnosis, an idiopathic form of disease or presumed substance exposure (drug or toxin) is often implicated as the underlying cause.

KEY POINTS
Clinical Presentation of Tubulointerstitial Disease

1. The clinical manifestations of chronic tubulointerstitial disease depend on the extent and severity of the process, the nephron segments most severely involved, and the compensatory response of the remaining normal nephron segments.
2. Renal tubular acidosis, salt wasting, and a urinary concentrating defect are some of the

3. The urinalysis in chronic tubulointerstitial disease often reveals pyuria with WBCs and occasional WBC casts in the urine sediment.

4. Measurement of β_2-microglobulin and retinol-binding protein in the urine are sometimes helpful to document "tubular" proteinuria and implicate a tubulointerstitial disease process.

5. Enzymuria reflects disruption of tubular cell integrity, but it has limited clinical use.

common manifestations of chronic tubulointerstitial disease.

Tubulointerstitial Diseases

Analgesics

Chronic tubulointerstitial nephritis, sometimes associated with papillary necrosis, has been considered a complication of high-dose, long-term analgesic ingestion. In particular, combination analgesics containing phenacetin are thought to induce chronic tubulointerstitial damage. It is less clear whether chronic ingestion of analgesics such as nonsteroidal anti-inflammatory drugs (NSAIDs) or aspirin alone will cause analgesic nephropathy. The diagnosis of this entity is suggested by a history of chronic headaches and other forms of chronic pain that promote long-term analgesic ingestion. Concomitant anemia may signal peptic ulcer disease from chronic aspirin or NSAID intake. Somatic complaints such as malaise and weakness are also present on history. Most patients have no symptoms referable to the urinary tract, although hematuria and flank pain may develop from a sloughed or obstructing papilla. The presence of CKD with minimal or no proteinuria signals tubulointerstitial disease. More prominent proteinuria, however, can occur with

advanced CKD, a reflection of hemodynamically-mediated glomerular injury and sclerosis. Intravenous pyelography is a highly sensitive radiographic test in the detection of papillary necrosis (Figure 18.1) (total or partial). Partial necrosis is characterized by a cavity extending out from the calyces. Findings in complete papillary necrosis include a ring shadow in the calyx and loss of the entire papillary surface (claw-like appearance). It is not sensitive, however, in the diagnosis of analgesic nephropathy because other diseases may cause papillary necrosis such as diabetes mellitus, obstructive uropathy, sickle cell disease, and renal tuberculosis. Given the limited sensitivity of intravenous pyelography in diagnosing analgesic nephropathy, as well as the associated

Figure 18.1

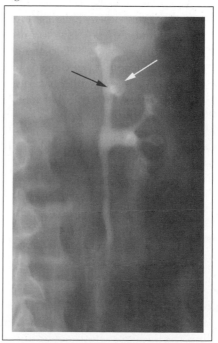

Papillary necrosis. Intravenous pyelogram of the kidneys reveals a cavity extending out from a renal calyx (shown by the white arrow) consistent with partial sloughing of the papilla. Calcification of several renal papillae is evident (one is shown by the black arrow).

nephrotoxicity of the large contrast load, other imaging modalities are employed. Renal ultrasound may show small-sized kidneys with increased echogenicity. This test is not sensitive enough to reveal subtle medullary calcifications or papillary defects from sloughed papillas. Computed tomography (CT) scan is a better imaging test for analgesic nephropathy. It can demonstrate calcifications in the medulla and papillary areas. Also, it may reveal lobulated or "bumpy" renal contours and decreased kidney size. All of these CT findings are suggestive of analgesic induced injury. Thus, this imaging modality is recommended to evaluate patients with a history and clinical findings consistent with analgesic nephropathy.

Treatment is supportive. The course of renal disease is determined by the severity of kidney dysfunction at the time of diagnosis as well as, whether the toxic medication is continued or not. Renal decline is expected if analgesic consumption continues, whereas stabilization or mild improvement in kidney function can occur with withdrawal of nephrotoxins. In addition to discontinuation of all culprit nephrotoxins, control of blood pressure in those with hypertension is important. In patients with advanced CKD, progression of renal failure often occurs despite analgesic discontinuation. In addition to implementation of renal replacement therapy, evaluation for uroepithelial malignancy and diffuse atherosclerotic disease should be undertaken.

Lead Nephropathy

Intoxication with lead is an illness that has plagued mankind since ancient times. Lead toxicity leads to disturbances in multiple organ systems, including the kidneys. Both acute and chronic kidney disease develop with lead intoxication. The focus of this discussion will be lead-associated chronic tubulointerstitial nephritis. Environmental lead exposure was described from ingestion of contaminated foodstuffs (lead in soil) or water (lead

pipes, lead pottery). Outbreaks of lead toxicity were reported in southern states in association with moonshine ingestion and remain a source of lead exposure to this day. Moonshine, which is homemade corn liquor, is fermented in stills that are often welded with lead solder and use automobile radiators (contaminated with leaded gasoline) as the condenser. Occupational exposure to lead occurs in workers who manufacture storage batteries, pottery, and pewter. Also, lead intoxication can develop in smelters, miners, and plumbers. In children, exposure to lead-based paint chips and dust can cause acute and possibly chronic lead intoxication.

Chronic lead intoxication presents with varying degrees of severity depending on the total amount of cumulative lead burden. Patients may have vague nonspecific symptoms including irritability, anorexia, insomnia, and myalgias. More severe lead exposure generally produces more pronounced neurologic, abdominal, rheumatologic, and renal-related symptoms. Hypertension, gout, and a tubulointerstitial nephropathy are the most common renal effects of lead. Tubulointerstitial nephropathy is often manifested by CKD associated with tubular dysfunction manifested as polyuria (due to salt wasting and a urinary concentrating defect), hyperkalemic distal renal tubular acidosis, absent or low-grade proteinuria, and sterile pyuria. Markers of lead nephropathy include increased urinary β_2-microglobulin, retinol-binding protein, and N-acetyl-β-glucosaminidase, and alanine aminopeptidase. Recent data suggest that even chronic low-level lead intoxication can lead to progressive CKD.

The renal lesion in chronic lead nephropathy consists of tubulointerstitial fibrosis mixed with a lymphocytic cellular infiltrate, tubular atrophy, and arteriolar thickening. Intranuclear inclusions in proximal tubular cells are not present, as they are found only in acute lead nephropathy. The degree of fibrosis varies with the severity and chronicity of lead exposure. Treatment requires discontinuation of lead ingestion, however, the reversibility is limited by lesions formed from previous exposure. Blood pressure control is important in hypertensive patients while the nephroprotective effect of an antagonist of the renin-angiotensin-aldosterone system (RAAS) is unknown in this disease. Lead chelation with ethylene diamine tetra acetate (EDTA) was shown to benefit patients with early CKD. In a study of subjects with chronic low-level lead exposure and kidney dysfunction, chelation therapy stabilized renal function as measured by changes in glomerular filtration rate (GFR).

Autosomal Dominant Polycystic Kidney Disease

The inherited cystic kidney disease, autosomal dominant polycystic kidney disease (ADPKD), is primarily a disease of the tubulointerstitium. It is a relatively common disorder, occurring in approximately 1 in every 400–2000 live births. The majority of patients with ADPKD have an abnormality on chromosome 16 (86%) that is linked to the alpha-globin gene locus (PKD1). The remaining families have a defect that involves a gene on chromosome 4 (PKD2), while some patients have an abnormality on an entirely different locus. Genes for both polycystic diseases were identified; PKD1 encodes the protein, polycystin-1 whereas the PKD2 gene product is polycystin-2. Polycystin-1 is localized in renal tubular epithelia, hepatic bile ductules, and pancreatic ducts and is found in plasma membranes. These sites of expression are also sites of cyst formation. Polycystin-1 is overexpressed in most renal cysts. Polycystin-2 is expressed in distal tubules, collecting duct, and thick ascending limb in normal fetal and adult kidneys and localizes to endoplasmic reticulum. Similarly, it is overexpressed in renal cysts.

Cyst formation is thought to result from a weakening of the tubular basement membrane or intratubular obstruction from hyperplastic cells. The primary defect, however, may be related to either abnormal cellular differentiation and maturation or altered function of renal cilia. Dilated tubules form early cysts that are filled by glomerular filtrate. Subsequently, cysts enlarge by secretion of fluid by cyst epithelium. Cyst growth is associated with both fluid secretion and hyperplasia of the cyst epithelium. Unidentified growth factors present in the cyst fluid likely contribute to cyst growth and disease progression in ADPKD patients.

Diagnosis of ADPKD requires documentation of cysts in kidney. Age determines the criteria. Patients younger than 30 years require at least two cysts (unilateral or bilateral), those 30–59 should have at least two cysts in each kidney, while patients greater than 60 years of age require four or more cysts in each kidney, pancreas, and spleen. Cysts may also be present in the liver. Clinical manifestations of ADPKD include hypertension, hematuria, proteinuria, nephrolithiasis, flank pain, and progressive kidney failure. Hypertension is associated with activation of the RAAS, as well as sodium retention when CKD is present. Hematuria is common (up to 50% of patients), and is due to renal infection, cyst rupture, and nephrolithiasis. Proteinuria is typically less than 1 g/day. Kidney stones occur in up to 20% of patients. They are composed of both calcium oxalate and uric acid. Acute flank pain is common, most often due to renal stones, cyst infection or pyelonephritis, or hemorrhage within cysts. Chronic flank pain is troublesome and probably caused by distension of the renal capsule by enlarged cysts (Figure 18.2). At times, cyst decompression or nephrectomy is required for intractable pain. Development of CKD and progression to ESRD occurs in up to 75% of patients by age 75 years. Factors associated with progression include younger age at diagnosis, male gender, African American race, presence of the PKD1 genotype, hypertension, gross hematuria, and rapid renal volume (cyst) growth. It is speculated that kidney disease progresses due to vascular sclerosis and tubulointerstitial fibrosis, rather than compression of normal renal tissue by enlarging cysts. This may be due, in part, to enhanced apoptosis of glomerular and tubular cells by cysts.

Treatment of ADPKD is directed at slowing progression to ESRD and reducing the morbidity of the other described clinical manifestations.

Figure 18.2

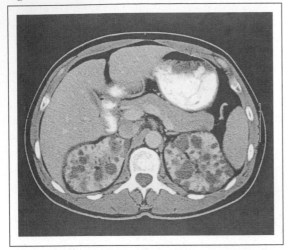

Autosomal dominant polycystic kidney disease. CT scan of the kidneys demonstrates bilateral renal cysts in a patient with ADPKD.

Blood pressure is controlled with drugs that modify the RAAS. Therapy directed at cyst growth is intuitive and supported by animal models, but no data are available in humans. Appropriate management of CKD (Chapter 16) and preparation for renal replacement therapy is required for these patients. Renal transplant is recommended; some patients require pretransplant nephrectomy to accommodate the allograft or remove a potential source of infection. Management of cyst and parenchymal infection requires antimicrobials that penetrate cysts well (quinolones, trimethoprim-sulfamethoxazole) and sometimes percutaneous cyst drainage. Stone therapy is more difficult than in patients with idiopathic nephrolithiasis. Percutaneous nephrostomy is complicated by the presence of large cysts. Extracorporeal shock wave lithotripsy is useful for stones less than 2 cm in diameter, but is associated with a higher frequency of residual stone fragments. Cyst decompression has been used to treat both acute and chronic flank pain and can ameliorate hypertension in some cases. There is no evidence, however, that this procedure slows progression of kidney disease.

Sarcoidosis

Chronic tubulointerstitial disease may complicate sarcoidosis. This systemic disease involves the tubulointerstitium of the kidneys through nephrocalcinosis from hypercalcemia/hypercalciuria, an effect related to excess 1,25-vitamin D_3 production by sarcoid granulomata. Diffuse infiltration with noncaseating granulomata and tubulointerstitial nephritis also occurs. The presence of disseminated disease, where lung involvement (hilar nodes, interstitial infiltration/fibrosis), uveoparotid disease, skin lesions, and liver lesions are present allow renal sarcoid to be easily identified. Limited sarcoidosis may require a renal biopsy to diagnose the cause of kidney disease. The clinical manifestations of renal (tubulointerstitial) sarcoid include absent or mild proteinuria, concentrating and/or acidifying defects and sterile pyuria. Hypercalcemia and hypercalciuria may also be present. A high serum angiotensin-converting enzyme concentration supports sarcoidosis in the proper clinical setting. Treatment of tubulointerstitial sarcoidosis includes a course of oral corticosteroids. Corticosteroids similarly correct vitamin D-associated hypercalcemia and hypercalciuria. Ketoconazole is employed to treat hypercalcemia in patients unable to tolerate steroid therapy.

Obstructive Uropathy

Obstruction of the urinary system leads to chronic tubulointerstitial injury and fibrosis. As will be discussed more fully in chapter 19 on obstructive uropathy, uncorrected chronic obstruction promotes irreversible tubulointerstitial disease and CKD. In unrelieved complete obstruction renal fibrosis evolves fairly rapidly (approximately 2 weeks), while partial urinary obstruction may occur insidiously over months. The pathogenesis underlying this process includes a combination of pressure-induced tubular injury and formation of various proinflammatory and profibrotic mediators. The end result of urinary obstruction is tubular atrophy, tubulointerstitial fibrosis, and loss of renal parenchymal mass.

Clinical signs of urinary obstruction include polyuria alternating with oliguria in partial obstruction and anuria with complete urinary obstruction. The presence of associated disease processes also provides clues. A history of kidney stones, prostate disease, and certain types of malignancies (cervical, uterine, prostate and lymphoma) suggest the possibility of obstructive uropathy. Any patient presenting with renal failure must have obstructive uropathy excluded. Suggestive laboratory tests include a hyperkalemic distal renal tubular acidosis and bland urine sediment. Renal ultrasound is the preferred test to assess for urinary obstruction. Dilatation of the pelvis and calyces (hydronephrosis) signal urinary obstruction (Figure 19.1). At times, however, CT scan may be required to improve accuracy and provide more information about etiology of the obstructing process. Treatment to relieve the obstructing process depends on the cause. It should be undertaken rapidly to reduce renal injury and preserve kidney function.

Sickle Cell Disease

Sickle cell nephropathy constitutes a number of different renal lesions that affect the glomerulus and tubulointerstitium. The relative hypertonicity and hypoxia of the renal medulla predispose patients to red blood cell sickling with microcirculatory occlusion and ischemic renal damage. Tubular deposition of heme filtered at the glomerulus contributes to tubulointerstitial injury and fibrosis. Clinical manifestations of sickle-related tubulointerstitial disease include hematuria, urinary concentrating defect, hyperkalemia, an incomplete distal renal tubular acidosis (associated with or without hyperkalemia), and papillary necrosis. Polyuria from the concentrating defect contributes to RBC sickling by increasing plasma tonicity (hypernatremia). At times, hematuria is profuse and prolonged. Often no obvious explanation for this type of hematuria is found, but sometimes it is due to papillary necrosis. Supportive therapy and sometimes bladder lavage to prevent obstructive

blood clot formation is undertaken. Obstruction of the urinary tract by necrosed papillary tissue can result and may cause acute renal failure if bilateral in the ureters or in the urethra.

Limiting the development of sickle-associated tubulointerstitial disease is not an easy task. During childhood, exchange transfusions reversed many of the tubular defects. Over time, however, many of the tubular disturbances become permanent and the patients will need to avoid dehydration from the urinary concentrating defect by drinking large volumes of fluid. This also reduces sickling in the renal medulla. Supportive care for hematuria is the usual treatment, although severe bleeding unrelated to papillary necrosis may require cautious antifibrinolytic therapy with epsilon-aminocaproic acid. Obstruction of the urinary collecting system with sloughed papilla or blood clots necessitates routine urologic therapies. These include retrograde cystography with stent placement and irrigation with saline.

Lithium

Lithium is employed widely to manage bipolar (manic-depressive) disorders. Tubular dysfunction clearly occurs with this drug. Nephrogenic diabetes insipidus and an incomplete form of distal renal tubular acidosis are associated with lithium therapy. Treatment with lithium also causes a chronic tubulointerstitial lesion in a small number of patients. It is somewhat controversial, however, whether lithium therapy truly causes chronic tubulointerstitial disease. It is likely that long-term lithium therapy is required to cause this renal lesion. Most cases are associated with mild CKD. Some studies suggest that 15–20% of patients develop a slowly progressive reduction in renal function, with the glomerular filtration rate reaching a plateau of approximately 40 mL/minute/1.73 m^2. The renal lesion is characterized histologically by tubular drop out with dilatation of tubular lumens, a mononuclear infiltrate in the interstitium, and varying degrees of interstitial fibrosis.

Treatment of CKD associated with lithium requires discontinuation of the drug. In most cases kidney function improves modestly or stabilizes. The course is often unpredictable, however, and some patients with advanced CKD progress to ESRD. Again, this may reflect secondary hemodynamic glomerular injury, resulting in glomerulosclerosis. Hypercalcemia, due to lithium-associated upward resetting of the calcium setpoint and suppression of parathyroid hormone secretion, may contribute to hemodynamic renal failure and polyuria in patients with underlying tubulointerstitial disease. Correction of hypercalcemia and any associated intravascular volume depletion reverses these renal disturbances.

Chinese Herb Nephropathy

An outbreak of renal failure was noted in Belgium, which was traced to the ingestion of a Chinese herb. Contamination of a Chinese herbal slimming (weight loss) regimen with aristolochic acid (or other unknown phytotoxins) promoted the development of a characteristic tubulointerstitial lesion. Chronic ingestion of these Chinese herbs is associated with CKD and ESRD. More commonly, the loss of kidney function followed a rapidly progressive course. Many patients required renal replacement therapy. The pathology of this renal lesion is characterized by a hypocellular tubulointerstitial fibrosis with marked tubular atrophy. Although aristolochic acid is the offending agent in most cases, other phytoxins may cause a similar lesion. These substances are mutagens and are associated with the development of transitional cell carcinomas. Patients exposed to this mutagen who develop genitourinary tract disease need to be evaluated for the possibility of cancer.

Treatment requires discontinuation of further aristolochic acid exposure and general supportive care appropriate for patients with CKD. Some patients stabilize kidney function while others have a progressive course to ESRD requiring renal replacement therapy or renal transplantation.

Renal Malacoplakia

Malacoplakia is an unusual chronic granulomatous disorder that can cause disease in the kidney. Although the actual pathogenesis is unknown, it is associated with renal parenchymal infection with gram-negative organisms. Due to abnormal macrophage function, impaired eradication of infection by organisms such as *Klebsiella oxytoca*, *Proteus mirabilis*, and *Escherichia coli* leads to chronic tubulointerstitial damage and granuloma formation. Malacoplakia occurs in patients with debilitating diseases marked by an underlying immunologic defect. It is associated with diabetes mellitus, alcoholism, tuberculosis, and treatment with immunosuppressive agents for organ transplantation. Diffuse infiltration or discrete intrarenal masses are seen on gross pathology. Histology reveals tubulointerstitial granulomas with clusters of PAS-positive histiocytes that contain Michaelis-Gutmann bodies (lamellated iron and calcium inclusions). These inclusions are believed to result from incomplete digestion of engulfed bacteria (bacterial debris) by abnormal macrophages. Residual intralysosomal debris acts as a nidus for mineralization and leads to the development of complex lysosomal bodies demonstrable by Prussian blue (iron) and von Kossa (calcium) stains. Treatment of genitourinary tract infection is key to preventing malacoplakia in susceptible hosts. At times, nephrectomy is indicated.

Hyperoxaluria/Oxalosis

Deposition of calcium oxalate crystals in the tubules and interstitium can lead to chronic tubulointerstitial nephritis and fibrosis. Hyperoxalosis can be divided into two clinical categories. One is the primary hyperoxalurias (types I and II) that are due to hereditary disorders inherited recessively. Both of these disorders are characterized by tubular calcium oxalate deposition, which often extends into the renal interstitium and is associated with fibrosis and scarring. Type I develops from a deficiency of α-ketoglutarate:glyoxalate carboligase (cytosolic enzyme), leading to the excessive accumulation of oxalate, glyoxalate, and glycolate. Clinical manifestations of type 1 disease are the direct result of end-organ deposition (kidney predominantly) of calcium oxalate crystals. At a young age, patients develop hematuria, nephrolithiasis, renal colic, pyelonephritis, and CKD. End-stage renal disease and death often ensue by age 20. Type II, which is much less common, results from a deficiency of leukocyte D-glyceric dehydrogenase. Formation of calcium oxalate stones is very common, however, CKD is unusual. Marked urinary excretion of oxalate occurs with both disorders associated with primary hyperoxaluria. As an example, urinary excretion often averages 240 mg/day compared with the normal total of 10–45 mg/day. Gross examination of these kidneys reveals dilated urinary systems, nephroliths, and infection while interstitial fibrosis and scarring are present histologically.

Acquired or secondary forms of hyperoxaluria are commonly due to excessive intake or absorption of oxalate or oxalate precursors. Poisoning with ethylene glycol, found most commonly in antifreeze, is a clinical example of a precursor that ultimately is metabolized to oxalate with tubulointerstitial calcium oxalate deposition. Similarly, anesthesia with methoxyflurane can result in calcium oxalate deposition in the kidney. Intravenous high-dose vitamin C (ascorbic acid), which is metabolized to oxalate, also induces renal deposition of calcium oxalate. Xylitol and E-ferol can cause tubulointerstitial disease from oxalate deposition. Short small bowel syndrome is a well known gastrointestinal cause of secondary hyperoxaluria. Clinical disorders include small bowel resection or bypass, Crohn's disease, celiac sprue, chronic pancreatitis, and Wilson's disease. Excessive absorption of oxalate occurs by the following mechanism. There is a high concentration of bile acids in the small intestine and colon. In the small intestine, bile acids saponify calcium, allowing unbound oxalate (which is usually complexed with calcium) to enter the large bowel. In the large bowel, bile acids increase the intestinal permeability to free oxalate

entering from the small bowel. Certainly, volume contraction from associated malabsorption and diarrhea contributes to renal calcium oxalate crystal formation and deposition.

Correction of the underlying cause of hyperoxaluria is the most obvious treatment. Liver and/or renal transplantation may be required for the primary forms of hyperoxaluria. Elimination of exogenous sources of oxalate such as excessive vitamin C, ethylene glycol, and methoxyflurane is intuitive. General management of all disorders of hyperoxaluria includes generous hydration to maintain high urine flow rate (and reduce calcium oxalate saturation) and reduced ingestion of foods high in oxalate. Oral calcium supplementation may reduce gastrointestinal absorption of oxalate by complexing with oxalate and reducing the amount of free oxalate available for absorption in the large bowel. Oral citrate (potassium or sodium) reduces crystal formation through blocking calcium-oxalate interaction in urine. Routine urologic procedures are required for large and/or obstructive calcium oxalate stones.

Medullary Sponge Kidney

An anatomic malformation in the terminal collecting ducts in the pericalyceal region of the renal pyramids leads to the kidney lesion characteristic of medullary sponge kidney. This relatively common renal disorder is associated with the formation of both small and large medullary cysts. The cortex is always spared. The cysts are most often bilateral and diffuse, but may sometimes only involve one kidney and a few calyces. Although medullary sponge kidney is not considered a genetic renal disease, some families exhibit an autosomal dominant inheritance.

Most patients are asymptomatic. Medullary sponge kidney is recognized when an intravenous pyelogram (IVP) demonstrates characteristic radiographic findings. The major clinical manifestations are isolated hematuria, urinary tract infection, and nephrolithiasis (flank pain, hematuria). Kidney stones in these patients are composed of calcium phosphate and calcium oxalate. Factors that increase stone formation include hypercalciuria, hyperuricosuria, hypocitraturia, and occasionally, hyperoxaluria. Excessive amounts of calcium in urine are likely due to impaired reabsorption of calcium by damaged collecting tubules. More importantly, urinary stasis and increased urine pH in cystic terminal collecting ducts contribute to calcium phosphate precipitation. An incomplete distal RTA, which is associated with an alkaline urine pH, may also increase calcium phosphate stone formation. Gross or microscopic hematuria develops from stones or urinary crystals. Episodes can be single or repetitive. Urinary tract infection occurs with increased frequency in medullary sponge kidney. Urinary stasis in collecting duct cysts and obstructing stones enhances infection risk. The diagnosis of this renal disorder is established by IVP. This imaging test demonstrates cystic dilatations of the terminal collecting ducts as a "brush" radiating outward from the calyces (Figure 18.3). Enlargement of the pyramids and intraductal concretions are also seen. When present, calcium stones appear as small clusters in the calyceal regions.

In general, medullary sponge kidney is a benign condition with an excellent long-term prognosis.

Treatment revolves around management of stones and urinary tract infections. Stones that obstruct the urinary system can cause renal failure and need to be appropriately managed by the urologist. Antibiotics that target the infecting organism and penetrate renal tissue (ciprofloxacin, trimethoprim-sulfamethoxazole, chloramphenicol) should be employed during urinary tract infection.

Tubulointerstitial Nephritis Uveitis Syndrome

An idiopathic form of chronic tubulointerstitial disease associated with uveitis (TINU) represents an autoimmune process. This syndrome is characterized by visual impairment (uveitis), fever, anemia, and tubulointerstitial renal disease (renal failure, minimal proteinuria, pyuria). The kidneys typically are normal or large and highly echogenic when examined by ultrasonography. Corticosteroid therapy often reverses the renal dysfunction, but the disease process frequently recurs. Due to the relapsing nature of TINU syndrome, chronic therapy with steroids or another immunosuppressive agent is required.

Figure 18.3

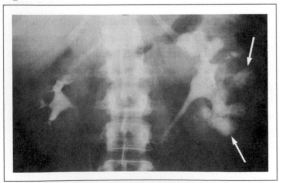

Medullary sponge kidney. Intravenous pyelogram (IVP) of the kidneys reveals a classic finding (cystic dilatations of the terminal collecting ducts shown as a *brush* [shown by the arrows] radiating outward from the calyces) of medullary sponge kidney.

KEY POINTS
Tubulointerstitial Diseases

1. Many diseases through various mechanisms can cause tubulointerstitial disease.
2. Tubulointerstitial disease can develop from medications, toxins, systemic diseases, immune-mediated processes, infection, malignancy, hereditary diseases, and metabolic disorders.
3. The most common causes of tubulointerstitial disease are those induced by therapeutic agents and vascular disease.
4. Treatment of the various causes of tubulointerstitial disease is directed by the underlying mechanism of injury.

Pathogenesis of Tubulointerstitial Disease

The tubulointerstitium comprises the majority of renal parenchyma. Approximately 80% of total kidney volume is composed of tubular epithelial cells and cells within the interstitial space. The vast majority of nonepithelial cells are associated with the rich vascular network found within the kidney. The rest of the cells consist of a small number of resident mononuclear cells and fibroblasts. Recognizing that the tubulointerstitium is such a large component of the kidney makes it easy to understand why inflammation within this compartment, leading to fibrosis, is a major factor in progressive loss of renal function.

The basic model that underlies the development of chronic tubulointerstitial disease, regardless of the inciting disease or event, is one that involves cellular infiltration, fibroblast differentiation and proliferation, increased extracellular matrix protein deposition, and atrophy of tubular cells. The pathogenesis of tubulointerstitial injury is similar whether the initiating process is a primary disease injuring the tubulointerstitium or is secondary to a primary glomerular or vascular disease process. Examples of such secondary causes include primarily glomerular diseases such as diabetic nephropathy and vascular diseases such as hypertension and calcineurin inhibitor toxicity. Activation of multiple proliferative pathways within the epithelial cells in an attempt to maintain integrity of this cell type occurs in response to tubular injury. An interplay between homeostatic proliferative and reparative forces and aberrant proinflammatory and overexuberant cell proliferation ensues. If the injurious factors overwhelm the normal cell processes, apoptotic pathways overrun the ability of tubular epithelial cells to survive. This results in tubular atrophy and interstitial fibrosis.

The initiating event that causes either primary or secondary injury to the tubulointerstitium promotes tubular atrophy and interstitial collagen deposition and fibrosis through various intrarenal and systemic factors. These include vasoactive substances such as angiotensin II (AII), endothelin, thromboxane A2, and vasopressin. These compounds induce reductions in renal blood flow after 24 hours of ureteral obstruction and likely contribute to ischemic injury. In addition to hemodynamic effects, AII has profibrotic effects mediated by binding to the angiotensin type 1 (AT_1) receptor. In fact, more than 50% of the fibrosis that develops in a mouse model of obstruction is dependent on expression of the angiotensinogen gene. This same process occurs in other forms of renal injury. Angiotensin II upregulates the expression of factors such as TGF-β, nuclear factor-κB, basic fibroblast growth factor, vascular cell adhesion molecule-1 (VCAM-1), TNF-α, and platelet-derived growth factor (PDGF). It is important, however, to recognize that increased expression of many of these chemoattractant compounds, adhesion molecules, and cytokines also occur independently of AII. Other types of renal disease and injury induce these processes through other mechanisms including pressure-associated injury (obstructive uropathy), hyperglycemia (diabetic nephropathy), infiltrative diseases (sarcoidosis), and induction of oxidative stress. Resident nonepithelial cells, such as the fibroblast, undergo proliferation/differentiation and produce interstitial fibrosis. Also, it is believed that renal epithelial cells undergo a process of dedifferentiation/redifferentiation into myofibroblastic cells expressing α-smooth muscle actin and collagen following exposure to the various factors noted above. Ultimately, the balance between homeostatic effects and harmful effects tips the balance in favor of the pathologic consequences, leading to collagen deposition, tubular atrophy, and interstitial fibrosis.

KEY POINTS
Pathogenesis of Tubulointerstitial Disease

1. The tubulointerstitium comprises approximately 80% of total renal mass.

2. The major cells of the tubulointerstitium are tubular and interstitial cells.

3. The basic model of tubulointerstitial disease consists of cellular infiltration, fibroblast differentiation and proliferation, increased extracellular matrix protein deposition, and atrophy of tubular cells.

4. Primary disease of the tubulointerstitium or secondary insults, such as glomerular or vascular disease, cause the same cascade of injury.

5. Vasoactive factors (angiotensin II, thromboxane, and endothelin), cytokines (TGF-β and TNF-α), adhesion molecules (VCAM-1), and chemoattractant compounds (monocyte chemoattractant peptide-1) contribute to tubulointerstitial inflammation and fibrosis.

Additional Reading

Dodd, S. The pathogenesis of tubulointerstitial disease and mechanisms of fibrosis. *Curr Top Pathol* 88: 117–143, 1995.

Eddy, A.A. Experimental insights into the tubulointerstitial disease accompanying primary glomerular lesions. *J Am Soc Nephrol* 5:1273–1287, 1994.

Jones, C.L., Eddy, A.A. Tubulointerstitial nephritis. *Pediatr Nephrol* 28:572–586, 1992.

Nath, K.A. Tubulointerstitial changes as a major determinant in the progression of renal damage. *Am J Kidney Dis* 20:1–17, 1992.

Sedor, J.R. Cytokines and growth factors in renal injury. *Semin Nephrol* 12:428–440, 1992.

Richard Formica

Chapter 19

Obstruction of the Genitourinary Tract

Recommended Time to Complete: 1 day

Guiding Questions

1. How does the bladder empty normally?
2. What are the common causes of urinary tract obstruction?
3. What is the pathophysiology of acute renal failure associated with urinary tract obstruction?
4. Which tests are most useful to diagnose urinary tract obstruction?
5. How much time does one have to relieve urinary tract obstruction before permanent renal damage ensues?

Introduction

Obstruction of the urinary tract is a common medical condition and an important cause of reversible renal failure. It affects all age groups. The cause of obstruction varies by age. Pediatric patients most commonly have anatomic abnormalities that lead

to obstruction such as stenoses of the ureter at the ureteropelvic or ureterovesicular junction, urethral valves, or strictures. Renal calculi are the most common cause of urinary tract obstruction in young adults, whereas in the elderly population renal calculi remain a prominent cause but benign prostatic hyperplasia (BPH) and neoplasm, as well as other pelvic carcinomas, are also important causes.

Urinary tract obstruction can be either unilateral or bilateral, partial or complete. An understanding of this is important because the presence of urine flow does not exclude obstruction. In the case of unilateral obstruction the unobstructed kidney continues to function normally. With partial obstruction urine flow can be decreased, normal, or even increased. The increased urine flow from a partially obstructed kidney results from tubular injury and loss of concentrating ability. Anuria most commonly results from profound shock or complete obstruction. Therefore, anuria in a patient who is hemodynamically stable should prompt an immediate search for obstruction.

With partial or unilateral obstruction the decline in glomerular filtration rate (GFR) may be mild. Therefore, an elderly patient or a patient with a history compatible with obstruction and unexplained chronic kidney disease should be evaluated for obstruction. Acute renal failure acquired in the hospital is rarely caused by obstruction; however, in some studies the incidence is as high as 10%, therefore evaluation of these patients should be done on a case-by-case basis.

Physiology of Micturition

Normal Bladder Function

The bladder is a smooth muscle reservoir lined by transitional epithelium. When fully contracted, it is only a potential space. In the absence of obstruction or bladder dysfunction there is no residual urine after voiding. The bladder fills at a rate of one mL/minute. This gradual filling allows the bladder to slowly expand and accommodate increasing volume by progressive relaxation. This allows intravesical pressure to remain between 0 and 10 cm H_2O during filling. When capacity is reached, approximately 400 mL, the

ability to accommodate additional volume is exceeded and the intravesical pressure rises rapidly to 30–40 cm H_2O. This results in stimulation of pressure receptors in the trigone that send impulses to the micturition center in the spinal cord at S2-S4. This results in detrusor contraction, bladder neck opening, and relaxation of the external sphincter.

Multiple spinal cord levels are involved in bladder function. Nuclei within the sacral spinal cord innervate the bladder and striated sphincter. The micturition center transmits signals to the brain as an urge to void that can be activated or suppressed through facilitator or inhibitor pathways in spinal cord. Parasympathetic fibers at the level of S2 and S3 stimulate contraction of the detrusor muscle and empty the bladder. Contraction is inhibited by alpha-adrenergic sympathetic fibers. The sphincter controlling continence is composed of voluntary muscles in the perineum innervated by the pudendal nerve (S2, S3) and an inner sleeve of smooth muscle extending from the bladder neck through the prostatic and membranous urethra innervated by alpha-adrenergic sympathetic nerve fibers. The micturition center coordinates contraction of the detrusor muscle (parasympathetic activation) and relaxation of sphincter muscles (pudendal nerve and sympathetic inhibition). During voiding, intravesicular pressure rises to 40–50 cm H_2O, and urine is expelled at a flow rate of 25 mL/second.

KEY POINTS
Physiology of Micturition

1. The bladder is a smooth muscle reservoir under both voluntary and involuntary control.
2. Normal micturition involves the coordinated action of many different levels of the central nervous system and disruption of any one can lead to bladder dysfunction and obstruction.

Signs and Symptoms

Symptoms

Signs and symptoms experienced by the patient with urinary tract obstruction depend on the rapidity and degree of obstruction. If obstruction occurs suddenly as in nephrolithiasis, distention of the ureter, kidney, and surrounding fascia causes intense pain. The pain is associated with other visceral symptoms such as nausea, vomiting, and diaphoresis. This is referred to as renal colic. If the onset of obstruction occurs slowly, as with prostate cancer, the patient may be asymptomatic. An important exception to this rule is the patient with partial obstruction. In this setting, a fixed amount of urine can bypass the obstruction without causing back pressure and hence distention of the renal pelvis and ureter. When urine flow increases, ureteral distension can occur proximal to the point of narrowing and result in symptoms similar to acute obstruction.

Renal colic is a sharp, pulsatile pain that waxes and wanes. The location of the pain, while not diagnostic of the site of obstruction, can provide clues to its location. Obstruction that occurs at the ureteropelvic junction or in the proximal ureter produces flank pain and tenderness. Obstruction in the distal ureter or at the ureterovesicular junction produces pain that radiates into the ipsilateral groin.

With chronic obstruction such as occurs with BPH, symptoms can be either obstructive or irritative. Obstructive symptoms include decreased force of urination, hesitancy, intermittency, and postvoid dribbling. Postvoid dribbling occurs due to a loss of pressure at the end of detrusor contraction. Irritative symptoms are the result of the effects of obstruction on the detrusor muscle. These include frequency, urgency, urge incontinence, and nocturia. Frequency results from a loss of bladder compliance and decreased bladder

capacity due to the retention of residual urine. Intravesicular pressure increases at low urine volumes and results in the sensation to void. Urgency is the result of hyperreactivity of the detrusor muscle. There is a sudden increase in the force of contraction that raises intravesicular pressure and an abrupt sensation of having to void ensues.

Signs

Only two entities, bilateral obstruction and profound shock, cause anuria. Therefore, anuria in a patient who is hemodynamically stable points almost exclusively to obstruction. The presence of normal to increased urine flow, however, does not rule out obstruction. In the case of unilateral complete obstruction urine flow remains normal. With partial obstruction, urine flow may increase because of loss of concentrating ability that results in a form of nephrogenic diabetes insipidus. Finally, in some patients with partial obstruction there can be alternation between oligoanuria and polyuria.

Chronic kidney disease can result from obstruction. Renal failure can either be acute with a rapidly rising serum creatinine concentration suggesting near complete loss of renal function or mild suggesting a partial loss of kidney function. The latter is particularly important in the outpatient setting, as this may be the only indication that obstruction is present.

Hypertension may be a presenting sign of urinary tract obstruction. Acute unilateral obstruction can activate the renin-angiotensin-aldosterone system (RAAS) and cause a sudden and acute rise in blood pressure in a similar fashion that renal artery stenosis causes hypertension. Bilateral obstruction does not activate the RAAS. The loss of ability to clear solutes, however, leads to volume overload and results in volume-mediated hypertension. It remains unclear why some patients with obstruction develop hypertension while others do not.

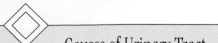

Causes of Urinary Tract Obstruction and Its Diagnosis

Causes

When considering the causes of urinary tract obstruction it is helpful to distinguish between complete and partial obstruction. Complete obstruction primarily occurs at the level of the bladder and is caused by prostatic enlargement or an atonic bladder. Complete obstruction results from retroperitoneal or pelvic tumors that arise near the bladder and involve both ureters. Complete obstruction may also develop from any cause in the patient with a solitary kidney. Neuropathic or atonic bladder, as in a diabetic or a patient with spinal cord injury, can result in complete obstruction. Proper bladder function requires complex coordination between multiple levels of the spinal cord and the detrusor muscle and sphincters. A defect in any of these results in loss of detrusor contraction, bladder overdistention, and finally loss of muscle function. As bladder volume increases, pressure is transferred to the collecting system and causes a decrease in glomerular filtration rate. The most common cause of complete urinary tract obstruction is BPH. Therefore, complete urinary tract obstruction is primarily a problem of men and not women. Benign prostatic hyperplasia is characterized by an increased number of epithelial and stromal cells in the periurethral area of the prostate. Epithelial gland formation is normally seen only in fetal development. This observed increase in cell numbers may be the result of epithelial and stromal proliferation or of impaired programmed cell death leading to cellular accumulation. Possible causes of this process are androgens, estrogens, stromal-epithelial interactions, growth factors, and other neurotransmitters. Hyperplasia of the prostate causes increased urethral resistance and results in compensatory changes in bladder

function. The elevated detrusor pressure required to maintain urinary flow in the presence of increased outflow resistance results in decreased bladder storage capacity. Therefore obstruction induces a change in bladder function that results in higher filling pressure and transmission of this pressure back to the renal parenchyma.

Partial obstruction of the urinary tract is caused most commonly by nephrolithiasis. Other causes are retroperitoneal fibrosis and ureteral tumors, as well as pelvic tumors that involve one ureter. Less commonly, blood clots that result from pathology within the kidney, shed papillae from papillary necrosis, and fungal infections resulting in fungus balls cause unilateral ureteral obstruction. In young male children, congenital urethral strictures and posterior urethral valves are rare forms of obstruction that must be considered. Adult males acquire urethral strictures from infections and trauma from indwelling catheters.

Diagnosis

It is important to rapidly diagnose urinary tract obstruction to avoid permanent kidney damage. The initial diagnostic maneuver is bladder catheterization. Even in the patient still producing urine this should be performed since an enlarged prostate may cause partial obstruction resulting in significant transmission of back pressure to the kidney. Urine flow continues because of the increased pressure generated by the overdistended bladder in order to overcome the increased resistance at the bladder neck. Bladder catheterization in this setting is diagnostic and curative. The initial rate of bladder drainage is discussed below.

Renal ultrasound is the test of choice to diagnose urinary tract obstruction because it can be obtained rapidly, is noninvasive, and does not require potentially nephrotoxic agents. Classic findings of obstruction are a dilated ureter and renal pelvis on the affected side (Figure 19.1). These findings may not be present in the setting

Figure 19.1

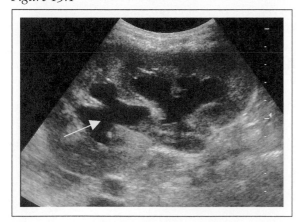

Renal ultrasound of obstruction. Shown by the arrow is the dilated renal pelvis surrounded by the kidney. This finding is referred to as hydronephrosis.

classic sonographic findings of obstruction (dilation of the collecting system) are not present and an elevated resistive index may be the only finding. The sensitivity and specificity of ultrasound for obstruction is 90%.

Computed tomography (CT) scanning is useful if renal calculi are suspected as the cause of obstruction (Figure 19.2). In this situation not only is the CT diagnostic but it also provides insight as to whether the stone will pass spontaneously because it can demonstrate the stone's size and position. Additionally, a CT scan provides

of acute obstruction before dilation occurs, for patients who are severely volume depleted and in settings where the kidney and collecting system are externally compressed as with retroperitoneal fibrosis or with scarring and fibrosis in a transplanted kidney. In this setting, a Doppler flow study of the kidney is useful because it allows calculation of a resistive index. An elevated resistive index suggests obstruction. The resistive index is calculated by subtracting the rate of diastolic blood flow from the systolic blood flow divided by the systolic blood flow. The resistive index rises as the rate of diastolic blood flow declines due to increased pressure and tissue edema. In extreme cases where diastolic blood flow is absent the resistive index is one. An elevated resistive index is a nonspecific finding and occurs in many types of acute renal failure such as acute tubular necrosis, renal vein thrombosis, hypotension, external compression of the kidney, and ureteral obstruction. The resistive index is most helpful in the diagnosis of obstruction in the setting of retroperitoneal fibrosis or malignancy. In this circumstance the

Figure 19.2

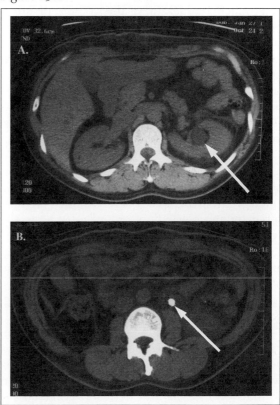

Computerized tomography scan of a kidney stone causing obstruction. Shown in panel A is the dilated renal pelvis (arrow) and in panel B the obstructing calculus in the ureter (arrow).

information about retroperitoneal processes such as lymphadenopathy, tumor, and hematoma.

Intravenous pyleography provides additional information in settings where papillary necrosis is suspected, with staghorn calculi, and for patients with multiple renal cysts. Additionally, it is used in association with the CT scan to further define the level of obstruction. Its use is limited, however, because a prolonged period of time is required to visualize the collecting system of the obstructed kidney and intravenous contrast is required.

Diagnosis of partial obstruction secondary to benign prostatic hyperplasia or abnormalities in micturition is accomplished with urodynamic studies. Uroflowmetry is simple to perform and provides useful information. Urine flow rate is determined by measuring the volume of urine expelled over time. Normal urine flow rate is 20–25 mL/second for a male and 20–30 mL/second for a female. Lower flow rates suggest an outlet obstruction, such as benign prostatic hyperplasia and higher flow rates indicate bladder spasticity or excessive use of abdominal muscles to overcome outlet resistance. This test is useful to assess the functional state of the lower urinary tract and to monitor therapy.

Cystometry uses gas or water to inflate the bladder while measuring intravesicular pressure. Often electromyographies of the external urethral sphincter and pelvic floor are included to assess synchrony of bladder and sphincter musculature. Cystometric studies provide information about many aspects of bladder function including total bladder capacity, the ability of the patient to perceive fullness, and the volume at which voiding occurs. Normal bladder capacity is 400–500 mL. The first sensation of fullness is usually felt at 150–250 mL but the sensation of definite fullness does not occur until 350–450 mL. Cystometric studies can also diagnose premature detrusor contraction. Premature detrusor contractions occurring prior to reaching true bladder capacity are the result of a hyperreflexic bladder or uninhibited behavior. Finally, the residual volume in the bladder can be detected. Under normal circumstances complete emptying of the bladder

should occur without higher than normal (up to >50 cm H_2O) voiding pressures.

Pathophysiology

Ultrastructural

On the ultrastructural level, acute renal failure in urinary tract obstruction is the result of increased pressure transmitted from the obstruction retrograde through the collecting system to the glomerulus. As tubular pressure rises the transcapillary pressure gradient decreases. This pressure gradient drives ultrafiltration and, therefore, as it declines so does glomerular filtration. The rise in intratubular pressure leads to reflex vasoconstriction of the intrarenal blood vessels and decreases glomerular blood flow. Thromboxane and angiotensin II (ATII) mediate the increase in intrarenal vasoconstriction. This response is physiologic since it shunts blood away from nonfunctioning nephrons. The initial component of renal injury is the result of increased tubular pressure followed by local ischemic injury.

Molecular

The second component of renal injury in urinary tract obstruction results from inflammatory cells recruited into the obstructed kidney. The obstructed kidney releases chemotactic agents. On a molecular level much is known about the role of cytokines in the molecular pathophysiology of urinary tract obstruction. In most cases of obstructive uropathy angiotensin II concentration rises. Angiotensin II (ATII) is important in the progression of many renal diseases including urinary tract obstruction. Angiotensin II is produced both systemically and locally. Tissue concentrations of ATII are 1000 times greater in the kidney than in plasma. There are two types of ATII receptors. The type 1 receptor (AT_1) mediates vasoconstriction and myocyte and fibroblast activation and proliferation. The type 2 receptor (AT_2) causes vasodilation and is antiproliferative. Therefore, inhibition of AT_1 receptor signaling is potentially beneficial while AT_2 receptor blockade is potentially detrimental.

It is important to fully understand the mechanism of action of angiotensin converting enzyme inhibitors (ACE-I). Initially ACE-I cause ATII concentrations to fall; however, after 3 months ATII levels return to pretreatment values. This "escape" from ACE-I results from local tissue production of ATII. Despite this, ACE I limit and cause regression of fibrosis. In addition to converting ATI to ATII, ACE degrades bradykinin. Blockade of ACE by ACE-I results in increased concentrations of bradykinin that has antifibrotic effects. Furthermore, the affinity of AT_1 and AT_2 receptors for ATII is similar, although perhaps there is a greater density of AT_1 receptors. The ATII receptor blockers (ARBs), such as losartan, selectively bind AT_1 receptors with 1000-fold greater affinity than AT_2 receptors. It is these differences between ACE-I and ARB that underlie the theoretical advantage of using them in combination. ACE-I increase

bradykinin concentration with its positive effects. Angiotensin receptor blockers inhibit the detrimental pathway induced via the AT_1 receptor but leave the AT_2 receptor unblocked. Therefore, ATII, which returns to normal concentration in the patient treated with ACE-I, only signals through the beneficial AT_2 receptor in the patient treated with combination therapy.

Increasing ATII concentration in urinary tract obstruction upregulates transforming growth factor-β_1 (TGF-β_1), tumor necrosis factor-α (TNF-α), platelet derived growth factor (PDGF), insulin-like growth factor (IGF-1), vascular cell adhesion molecule-1 (VCAM-1), nuclear factor-κB (NF-κB), monocyte chemoattractant peptide-1 (MCP-1), and intercellular adhesion molecule-1 (ICAM-1). These recruit inflammatory cells into the renal parenchyma that perpetuate the damage, repair, and fibrosis process leading to chronic scarring of the kidney.

Transforming growth factor-β_1 has multiple roles in the pathogenesis of renal disease. It promotes fibrogenesis in kidney by stimulating endothelin production, a potent stimulator of glomerulosclerosis and fibrogenesis, increases the activity of tissue inhibitors of metalloproteinases (TIMP), and directly decreases the activity of metalloproteinases, which in concert result in increased matrix deposition.

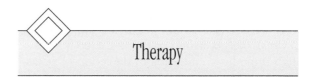

Therapy

The primary goal is rapid diagnosis. Once the level of obstruction is identified, therapy is targeted at the cause. In cases of bladder outlet obstruction insertion of a Foley catheter is initially curative. There is controversy regarding how quickly an overdistended bladder should be drained. Two potential consequences of rapid bladder drainage are gross hematuria that is caused by rapid reexpansion of veins in the bladder wall once pressure is relieved and the occurrence of reflex hypotension. Because of these concerns, it is advocated that after the first 500 mL of urine is removed the Foley catheter should be clamped and the remaining urine drained slowly over many hours. This approach is not supported by available data, however, since pressure in a distended bladder falls rapidly with small volume removal. Intravesicular pressure is reduced by 50% when 100 mL is removed and by 75% when 250 mL is removed.

With bilateral obstruction the concentrating gradient in renal medulla is lost. Renal failure causes a retention of osmoles and fluid. Once obstruction is relieved and renal function begins to recover there is often brisk diuresis. This is referred to as postobstructive diuresis. Initially urine output can be as high as 500–1000 mL/hour. The diuresis is a result of many factors. During the acute renal failure phase there is retention of excess fluids and osmoles. As filtration improves these osmotically active molecules are cleared and cause an osmotic diuresis. While obstructed, the kidney loses its medullary concentrating gradient, therefore, when filtration increases there is an inability to reclaim filtered free water. Finally there is direct tubular injury during obstruction that must recover. Replacement of urinary losses milliliter for milliliter only serves to perpetuate the diuresis. Normal replacement fluids are prescribed and the patient monitored for signs and symptoms of volume depletion. In this setting, daily weights are critical and an admitting weight to which daily weights can be compared is a must. High urine flow rate leads to depletion of potassium and magnesium and their concentrations should be monitored twice daily and replaced as required until urine output slows to 2–3 L/day. Angiotensin converting enzyme inhibitors and angiotensin II receptor blockers interrupt the pathogenic processes that cause renal injury on a molecular level. Given this there are theoretical reasons to employ combination therapy in the treatment of obstructive uropathy to prevent scarring and fibrosis. While data in humans do not exist, animal data show this approach is effective when started up to 3 days after the onset of obstruction.

With benign prostatic hyperplasia outlet obstruction results in hypertrophy of the detrusor muscle and the nonstriated sphincter at the bladder neck. This results in both obstructive and irritative symptoms. Since the inner sphincter is innervated by alpha-1 adrenergic sympathetic nerves, alpha-1 blockers may decrease outlet resistance. Alpha-1 receptors are abundant in the base of the bladder and in the prostate. The density of these receptors is increased in BPH. Terazosin, doxazosin, alfuzosin, and tamsulosin are long-acting alpha-1 blockers that can decrease bladder outflow resistance. The major side effect of these medications is orthostatic hypotension which is least with tamsulosin. Drugs that decrease the size of the prostate such as the 5-alpha-reductase inhibitor finasteride block the conversion of testosterone to dihydrotestosterone. The prostate shrinks due to atrophy of the glandular portion. Fibromuscular hyperplasia is unaffected but obstructive symptoms may improve because there is less prostate bulk to impinge on the urethra. Combined therapy with an alpha-1 blocker and a 5-alpha-reductase inhibitor was more effective than either alone in one trial. Invasive therapy should be considered for patients with severe symptoms. The most common surgical intervention is transurethral resection of the prostate (TURP). In the Veterans Cooperative Study TURP reduced symptom scores and decreased residual urine volume. Reduced and/or retrograde ejaculation is common after TURP. Alternative therapies for patients who are poor surgical candidates include transurethral incision of the prostate and prostatic stents.

KEY POINTS
Pathophysiology and Therapy

1. Rapid diagnosis is the most important aspect of therapy for obstructive uropathy.

2. After relieving obstruction the patient should be monitored for a postobstructive diuresis, because this may result in volume depletion and further renal injury.
3. Combination therapy with angiotensin converting enzyme inhibitors and angiotensin II receptor blockers has a theoretical role in the treatment of obstructive uropathy.

Expected Outcomes

Recovery from urinary tract obstruction is variable and dependent on the duration of obstruction. With total ureteral obstruction, complete recovery of glomerular filtration rate can occur if the obstruction is relieved within 1 week. Little or no recovery occurs if complete obstruction remains for greater than 12 weeks. Glomerular filtration rate may overestimate the degree of recovery. In animal models of obstruction up to 15% of nephrons from the obstructed kidney remain nonfunctional 60 days after the relief of obstruction despite the normalization of GFR. The normal GFR is likely due to hypertrophy of the uninvolved kidney. With partial obstruction the course is less predictable because obstruction may be present for a prolonged period prior to detection. Most functional recovery occurs within 7–10 days after relief of obstruction. In cases of severe renal

failure, dialysis may be necessary to support the patient until sufficient recovery occurs. In these patients, complete recovery is unlikely and they are often left with chronic kidney disease.

KEY POINTS
Expected Outcomes

1. Recovery from urinary tract obstruction is variable and dependent on the duration of obstruction.
2. If obstruction is relieved within 1 week complete recovery of renal function is expected; however, if the obstruction persists for more than 12 weeks no recovery occurs.
3. Most functional recovery occurs within 7–10 days after relief of obstruction.

Additional Reading

Gillenwater, J.Y. Clinical aspects of urinary tract obstruction. *Semin Nephrol* 2:46–54, 1982.

Klahr, S. Urinary tract obstruction. *Semin Nephrol* 21:133–145, 2001.

Tanagho, E.A., Lue, T.F. Neuropathic bladder disorders. In: Tanagho, E.A., McAninch, J. (eds.), *Smiths General Urology.* McGraw-Hill, New York, NY, 2004.

Wright, F.S. Effects of urinary tract obstruction on glomerular filtration rate and renal blood flow. *Semin Nephrol* 2:5–16, 1982.

Yarger, W.E., Buerkert, J. Effect of urinary tract obstruction on renal tubular function. *Semin Nephrol* 2:17–30, 1982.

Sergio F.F. Santos and
Aldo J. Peixoto

Essential Hypertension

Recommended Time to Complete: 2 days

Guiding Questions

1. How common is essential hypertension (HTN) and what factors predict its prevalence? How effective are current awareness, treatment, and control of hypertension in the United States?

2. What are the principal mechanisms of essential hypertension?

3. What can we learn from monogenic forms of hypertension to explain the origins of essential hypertension?

4. What is the general framework of the role of the kidneys and sodium retention in the pathogenesis of hypertension?

5. What is pressure natriuresis?

6. What are the goals of the clinical evaluation of the hypertensive patient?

7. What tests are indicated in the initial evaluation of the hypertensive patient?

8. How low should blood pressure (BP) be lowered by antihypertensive therapy?

9. What is the preferred class of drugs to be used in the treatment of the uncomplicated hypertensive patient?

10. How do comorbid conditions affect the choice of antihypertensive agents?

11. What is the difference between hypertensive urgencies and emergencies, and how is management different?

Introduction

HTN as defined by current standards afflicts more than 50 million Americans, and is thus—not surprisingly—the most common reason for a physician visit in this country. The magnitude of the problem has generated multiple public health efforts in the past 25 years leading to the present levels of awareness (70%) and treatment (59%). These levels are not optimal, however, especially because the rates of BP control are still quite low (34%), thus minimizing the potential protective effects that are obtained from effective therapy. These low rates are not only based on patient factors, but are also often related to lack of initiative on the part of the clinician. Therefore, it is imperative that we focus continued attention on education not only of the public, but also of medical professionals. The Joint National Committee on Prevention, Detection, Evaluation and Treatment of High Blood Pressure are the most prominent representatives of this educational effort, and its seventh report (The Seventh Report of the Joint National Committee on Prevention, Detection, Evaluation, and Treatment of High Blood Pressure [JNC 7]) was recently published. We urge everyone interested in hypertension to read the full report, which is referenced in the bibliography. In this chapter, we will review general aspects of HTN related to epidemiology, mechanisms, diagnostic evaluation, complications, and therapy.

Epidemiology

Current estimates of the worldwide prevalence of HTN are as high as one billion individuals (50 million in the United States). Its prevalence increases with age (Figure 20.1), and the BP rise is steeper in men

Figure 20.1

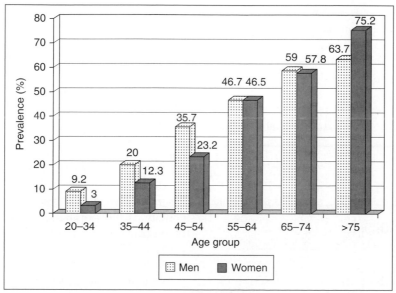

Age and sex-specific prevalence of hypertension in the United States. Hypertension was defined as BP >140/90 mmHg or the use of an antihypertensive agent. NHANES III. *Source:* Public use data file on www.cdc.gov web site.

than in premenopausal women. Women show a greater rise in BP following menopause, and the absolute prevalence of HTN is higher in women than men. HTN is a more pervasive problem in the Western world, and there is a relationship between average populational sodium intake and the prevalence of HTN. Other factors associated with a greater prevalence of HTN include ethnicity, lower socioeconomic status, lower dietary potassium intake, higher body mass index, and larger amounts of habitual alcohol use. The prevalence is greater in African Americans and non-Black Hispanics than in Caucasians. These two subgroups also have poorer control rates than Caucasians, which further amplify the cardiovascular burden of BP. Another important point is the fact that migration from a rural to an urban setting or from a nonindustrialized to an industrialized country increases the risk of HTN. These effects are primarily mediated by changes in dietary and psychosocial factors.

KEY POINTS
Epidemiology of Hypertension

1. The prevalence of HTN in the United States increases with age, female gender, and African American ethnicity.
2. Although awareness of HTN is now 70%, treatment and control rates are still very low (59 and 34%, respectively).
3. Limited physician intervention is an important cause of low treatment and control rates.

Pathophysiology

Essential HTN is the term used to describe elevated BP without a readily detectable cause. The term was coined at a time when high BP was thought to be required (essential) to surmount the established vascular disease in order to achieve target-organ perfusion. In the past, vascular disease was thought to precede HTN, and not be a result of it. Therefore, most experts discouraged physicians from treating high BP. It was not until the 1960s that it became clear that HTN was itself a major risk factor for vascular disease, and that its treatment resulted in improved outcomes. Only then was it determined that the need for higher BPs was not really "essential"—on the contrary!

The operative mechanisms in essential HTN are multiple, intersecting, and represent an attempt at a balance between vasopressor and vasodilator mechanisms. The formula, BP = cardiac output × vascular resistance, provides a valuable guide to the understanding of the pathophysiology of HTN. Changes in cardiac output usually result only in transient changes in BP, therefore, most of the chronic changes in BP control are dependent on the relationship between one of the determinants of cardiac output—blood volume (BV, the content)—and systemic vascular resistance (SVR, the container). For the sake of this discussion, BV will be referred to here as a surrogate for extracellular volume (ECV), even though an increase in ECV does not always result in increased BV, and vice versa. Because the vasculature has a great ability to accommodate blood volume due to its large capacitance bed (veins and venules), an inappropriate increase in vascular tone is necessary to result in HTN when BV is increased. Therefore, abnormalities in vascular resistance, either as a net increase or an insufficient decrease, are an essential part of HTN in almost all patients. An incomplete list of relevant mechanisms that impact on BP regulation and vascular function is shown in Figure 20.2. These systems are affected to different degrees in different individuals. Discrepancies are the result of the genetic heterogeneity of the population, and different degrees of exposure to environmental factors (sodium and potassium intake, alcohol use, and psychosocial stressors).

Genetic approaches to essential HTN have been difficult. It is estimated that heredity accounts for approximately 20–25% of one's BP and the determinants of this effect are polygenic

Figure 20.2

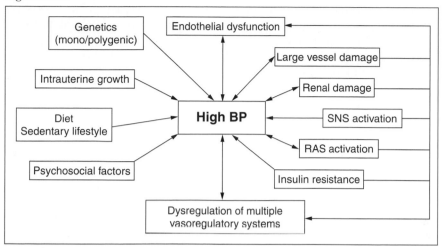

Relevant mechanisms involved in the genesis of hypertension. Abbreviations: RAS, renal artery stenosis; SNS, sympathetic nervous system.

and highly variable. Thus, the current understanding of the genetic mechanisms of HTN at large is poor, and restricted to the analysis of certain gene polymorphisms affecting the function of certain key mechanisms, especially the renin-angiotensin-aldosterone system (RAAS) (e.g., the angiotensinogen, angiotensin-converting enzyme [ACE], aldosterone synthase, and 11β-hydroxysteroid dehydrogenase genes) or salt sensitivity (e.g., the α-adducin gene). The relative importance of these polymorphisms is small.

Of greater relevance is the approach to monogenic disorders. Though rare, the understanding of the mechanisms related to HTN in these conditions leads to a better understanding of essential HTN in general. Examples of these disorders are listed in Table 20.1. The findings related to their different mechanisms indicate that single gene mutations altering renal sodium handling are able to produce sustained, severe HTN.

The aforementioned genetic studies lend support to a much older postulate related to the central role of the kidneys in the genesis of HTN. Multiple experimental and clinical models reveal that the development of HTN always depends on an abnormality in renal sodium handling. Even if the primary change is related to increased cardiac output or peripheral resistance, these

Table 20.1

Causes of Monogenic Hypertension and Their Respective Pathophysiologic Mechanisms, all with a Common Link to Increase Sodium Reabsorption

Liddle's syndrome (mutation in the epithelial sodium channel gene): decreased rate of removal of the epithelial sodium channel from the apical membrane

Syndrome of hypertension exacerbated by pregnancy (mutation in the mineralocorticoid receptor [MR] gene): increased MR activity with increased sensitivity to progesterone

Gordon's syndrome (mutation in WNK genes): increased Na-Cl cotransporter activity

Glucocorticoid-remediable aldosteronism (chimeric mutation in the aldosterone synthase gene leading to enhanced ACTH stimulation of aldosterone synthesis): increased aldosterone and some hybrid steroids (18-oxocortisol, 18-hydroxycortisol)

Apparent mineralocorticoid excess syndrome (mutation in the 11β-hydroxysteroid dehydrogenase type 2 gene): increased glucocorticoid availability for activation of the mineralocorticoid receptor

Abbreviation: ACTH, adrenocorticotrophic hormone; WNK, with no lysine (K).

abnormalities result only in transient increases in BP *unless* a change in the renal pressure-volume relationship occurs (see below), which will result in the need for a higher BP to guarantee sodium balance. Additionally, it is argued that HTN does not occur in the absence of kidneys, as long as salt and fluid overload do not occur. In a classic paper published in 1961, Merrill and coworkers demonstrated that the anephric state (surgically-induced) was associated with normotension in patients who restricted sodium and fluid intake, whereas the insertion of a transplanted kidney in the same subjects resulted in HTN. Furthermore, extensive data from hemodialysis patients dialyzed with long/slow dialysis techniques show that normotension can be achieved in more than 90% of patients as long as fastidious control of extracellular volume occurs. In addition, bilateral native nephrectomy results in improvement in BP

control in dialysis patients, as well as renal transplant recipients. These observations speak strongly in favor of the role of the kidney and ECV control in the genesis of HTN.

As mentioned above, abnormalities in renal sodium handling commonly result in elevated BP through interactions that were first championed by Guyton (the *Guyton Hypothesis*). In this now widely accepted hypothesis, the most relevant mechanism used by the body to regulate BP is to alter renal sodium handling, thereby controlling extracellular fluid volume and cardiac output. In the normal state, increased sodium intake causes an increase in extracellular fluid volume and blood pressure. Because of a steep relationship between volume and pressure (Figure 20.3, *normal*), small increases in BP produce natriuresis that restores sodium balance and returns BP to normal. This response becomes abnormal whenever there is

Figure 20.3

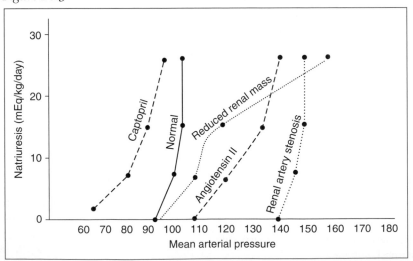

The renal pressure-volume control relationships. In normal individuals an increase in sodium intake leads to a rapid increase in BP, which in turn results in brisk natriuresis until sodium balance is restored and BP returns to normal. Increases in vasoconstrictor substances, or abnormalities in renal function or renovascular tone result in increased BP sensitivity to salt (right shift of the curve). In contrast, use of an ACE inhibitor can improve the pressure-volume relationship (left shift of the curve). (Modified from Guyton, A.C. *Hypertension* 19 (Suppl. 1):I2–I8, 1992, with permission from Lippincott, Williams & Wilkins.)

Figure 20.4

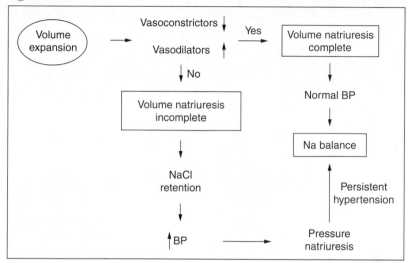

The concept of pressure natriuresis. If appropriate renal and vascular mechanisms exist, BP increases minimally and the excess volume is excreted completely, rapidly returning BP to normal (*volume natriuresis*). If adaptation is not normal, sodium retention occurs resulting in substantially increased BP, which then induces a pressure-natriuresis in order to achieve sodium balance (at the cost of chronic HTN).

impediment to sodium excretion. In such a case, the BP rise necessary to restore sodium balance is greater and the pressure-volume curve is reset to the right (Figure 20.3). The result is a state of increased sensitivity to dietary salt wherein the ability to excrete sodium becomes pressure-dependent. In this situation, sodium balance is achieved only at higher BP levels that are required to excrete the ingested sodium load, a process called pressure natriuresis (Figure 20.4). This chronic state of high BP generated by sodium retention is not related to increased BV, which is only minimally increased (if at all) in most hypertensive patients, but to sodium-related increases in SVR. The mechanisms underlying this vascular effect are not completely understood, but we know that sodium overload leads to increased sympathetic outflow and abnormalities in cation flux, especially calcium. Volume expansion decreases extracellular calcium and stimulates the production of parathyroid hormone (PTH), 1,25-dihydroxy vitamin D_3, and ouabain-like factors

that lead to an intracellular calcium shift, increased intracellular calcium, and thus elevated vascular resistance. Thus, abnormalities in pressure-volume relationships lie at the center of essential HTN, and also occur as an important part of the maintenance phase of most other causes of hypertension (such as hyperaldosteronism, renal artery stenosis, Cushing's syndrome, coarctation of the aorta, and even pheochromocytoma).

The current understanding of the interplay between renal sodium retention and HTN is illustrated in Figure 20.5. The inciting event is an increase in arteriolar tone in the renal vasculature (e.g., from increased activity of the RAAS or the sympathetic nervous system), subtle renal injury of any type, or the effects of inherited or environmental factors that lead to a sodium retentive phenotype. The sensitivity of an individual to salt/volume overload and the BP response observed with changes in sodium intake can be improved or corrected by modifying some of the factors that modulate salt sensitivity, especially the RAAS

Figure 20.5

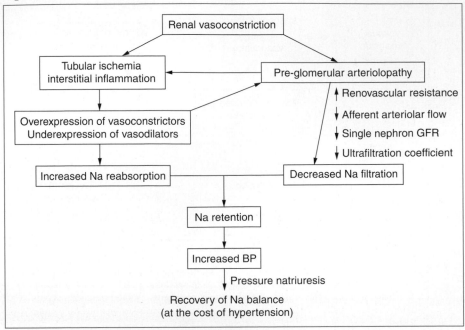

Hypertension as a result of insidious, subtle renal injury. (Modified from Johnson, R.J., Herrera-Acosta, J., Schreiner G.F., Rodriguez-Iturbe B. *N Engl J Med* 346:913–923, 2002, with permission from the Massachusetts Medical Society.)

(Figure 20.3). Obviously, in any individual who has increased sensitivity to salt (30–50% of the hypertensive population), sodium restriction can decrease BP effectively.

The sympathetic nervous system is important in BP control, and its activation may be an important early step in the process of increased renovascular resistance (increased arteriolar tone) that leads to sodium retention. Multiple strategies are available to block sympathetic overactivity in HTN, both at the central level, to limit central nervous system (CNS) sympathetic outflow, and at the effector level, with direct alpha- or beta-receptor antagonism.

The balance between vasopressor and vasodilator mechanisms is difficult to interpret in any individual patient. A summary of humoral systems that can be abnormally increased or decreased in HTN is shown in Table 20.2. Their relative role in the

Table 20.2

Humoral and Cellular Factors Related to Vascular Function in HTN

Catecholamines
Angiotensin II, aldosterone
Sex steroids
Prostaglandins
Endothelin-1
Bradykinin
Natriuretic peptides
Nitric oxide
Reactive oxygen species
Insulin and insulin resistance
Intracellular Na, Cl, K, Ca, Mg
Parathyroid hormone, vitamin D
Adrenomedullin
Calcitonin gene related peptide

pathogenesis of HTN varies substantially, and a detailed discussion is beyond the scope of this text. The vasculature is not only abnormal in its responses related to vascular tone, but also in its structure. Hypertensive subjects have diffuse capillary rarefaction, as well as a progressive decrease in the lumen of small arteries and arterioles. These structural changes limit organ perfusion (especially important in the kidney), and also impair vascular responses to vasodilatory substances.

An important pathophysiologic mechanism gaining recent attention is increased arterial stiffness, a problem that is particularly relevant to older individuals (and isolated systolic HTN [ISH]). Arterial stiffening is caused by loss of elastic fibers of large arteries, and is strongly associated with aging (especially after the sixth decade), smoking, diabetes mellitus, and kidney disease. As shown in Figure 20.6, this process leads to increased pulse wave velocity (PWV), which in turn results in faster reflection of the incident pulse wave. Faster reflection implies that the reflected wave returns to the heart before the end of systole, resulting in augmentation of central BP and increased systolic BP (SBP). This abnormality is relevant to left ventricular performance, as increased impedance to left ventricular (LV) ejection is an important factor in generating left

ventricular hypertrophy (LVH) and subendocardial myocardial ischemia, two common complications of HTN. Abnormalities in arterial structure also alter the shape of decay of the diastolic BP (DBP) curve resulting in a decrease in diastolic BP and wider pulse pressure.

KEY POINTS
Pathophysiology of Hypertension

1. HTN is the result of an imbalance between vasopressor and vasodilatory systems. A multitude of such systems are variably affected in any individual patient.
2. The kidneys have a prominent role in the genesis of HTN due to its effects on sodium handling. An abnormality in sodium excretion is a part of virtually all types of sustained HTN.
3. Arterial stiffness is an important cause of systolic HTN and widened pulse pressure in older patients.

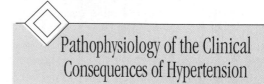

Pathophysiology of the Clinical Consequences of Hypertension

Figure 20.6

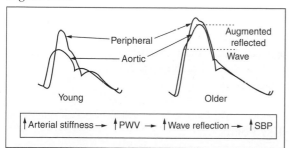

Effect of age and arterial stiffening on systolic blood pressure. Increased arterial stiffness results in faster pulse wave velocity (PWV) and wave reflection. Faster wave reflection augments the reflected pulse wave, thus increasing systolic BP (SBP). The relative magnitude of this effect is greater in the central blood vessels (aorta).

Hypertension is marked by diffuse vascular injury. If left untreated, elevated BP results in cardiovascular complications in as many as 50% of patients. Progressive damage affects several vascular territories, with a particular predilection for the cerebral vasculature, retinal vessels, coronary arteries, renal circulation, and arteries of the extremities. The heart is not only affected by way of coronary disease, but also due to pressure overload that leads to left ventricular hypertrophy.

Cerebrovascular disease is a frequent complication of HTN. At any given age, the risk of developing a stroke is increased by the presence of HTN, and the magnitude of this risk is directly related to the degree of BP rise. Vessels supplying the basal ganglia, brainstem, and cerebellum are exposed to higher BP levels, and there is a large drop of BP over a short distance in these short resistance vessels. Thus, these vessels sustain most of the damage in HTN, which develops as arterial hyalinosis and/or microaneurysms of the perforating branches. Occlusion of hyalinized vessels results in the small lacunar infarcts due to focal ischemia, and rupture of microaneurysms leads to the classic hypertensive hemorrhagic strokes of any of these sites, particularly the basal ganglia (more than half of all hypertensive cerebral hemorrhages are putaminal). In the neocortex, longer arteries with many branches act as a step-down transformer, protecting the cortex from more extensive HTN damage.

Damage to retinal vessels is extensive, and examination of these changes with an ophthalmoscope provides valuable information on the state of the microvasculature in HTN (see the Section *Diagnostic Evaluation*). Although hypertensive retinopathy is an infrequent cause of visual problems, there is an increased risk of central retinal vein occlusion in HTN, and high BP accelerates the progression of other eye diseases, especially diabetic retinopathy.

Cardiac involvement in HTN is extensive and complex. On the one hand, HTN leads to accelerated coronary atherosclerosis, a process mediated by shear stress, oxidative stress, and the coexistence of the metabolic syndrome (obesity, insulin resistance with or without diabetes mellitus, dyslipidemia, and HTN). This leads to clinical coronary disease and loss of myocardial mass due to ischemia and infarction. Additionally, the state of pressure overload results in concentric LV hypertrophy, which is the most common clinically relevant target-organ complication of HTN, and is associated with worse outcomes in HTN. LV hypertrophy and changes in the shape of the diastolic decay of the central BP curve (see above) lead to relative subendocardial ischemia, amplifying the effects induced by atherosclerotic changes. Long-term pressure overload and LV hypertrophy are maladaptive, and chamber dilatation and systolic dysfunction ultimately result, especially in patients with associated coronary disease and myocardial infarction. This course is responsible for the increased occurrence of congestive heart failure in HTN.

The kidneys are commonly affected by untreated HTN. Hypertensive nephrosclerosis is the result of progressive parenchymal ischemia due to narrowing and hyaline sclerosis of arterioles and small arteries. In addition, the larger interlobular arteries develop marked thickening of the media due to a reduplication of the elastic lamina (fibroelastic hyperplasia). This abnormality also results in areas of parenchymal ischemia and interstitial fibrosis. Nephrosclerosis causes a decline of glomerular filtration rate in as many as 5% of patients with HTN, and is most common in patients with long-standing uncontrolled BP, especially in African Americans.

Atherosclerosis of the peripheral vasculature is accelerated by HTN, though other factors seem more relevant, such as smoking, diabetes, hyperlipidemia, and hyperhomocystenemia. Nevertheless, HTN is a participant in the development of atherosclerotic plaques and its control is associated with small decreases in the incidence of peripheral arterial disease.

In patients who develop "malignant phase hypertension," a process in which BP is very high and there is evidence of target-organ dysfunction, diffuse endothelial damage leads to a microangiopathic picture (intravascular hemolysis, consumptive thrombocytopenia) and acute loss of renal function. Endothelial damage is caused by shear trauma, as well as toxicity induced by the RAAS (angiotensin II is a major pathogenetic factor). Histologically, there is extensive arteriolar damage and occlusion, a process named arteriolar fibrinoid necrosis.

KEY POINTS
Pathophysiology of the Clinical Consequences of Hypertension

> 1. Chronic hypertensive target-organ damage is mediated by direct injury to the vessel wall resulting in organ hypoperfusion or hemorrhage (retina and brain).

2. Left ventricular hypertrophy is the most common target-organ complication in HTN and it carries a worse prognosis.
3. Malignant hypertension presents with signs of diffuse endothelial injury and organ dysfunction.

Diagnostic Evaluation

The diagnostic evaluation of patients with high BP has five major goals:

1. Confirm the presence of HTN.
2. Stage the severity of the HTN.
3. Assess the extent of HTN-related organ damage.
4. Rule out causes of secondary HTN.
5. Identify factors that may impact therapy.

Confirming the Presence of Hypertension

The diagnosis of HTN is arbitrarily made when BP is >140/90 mmHg on repeated measurements. The expression "repeated measurements" should be emphasized; it is a mistake to label patients as having HTN based on an isolated reading. Therefore, clinicians caring for such patients must obtain repeated measurements of BP on different occasions. This can be done in the office or with the use of home BP measurements. When using office measurements, it is important that the individuals checking the BP observe the necessary techniques to obtain the readings, as these values will ultimately guide therapy. Patients should have at least 5 minutes of rest and no conversation should take place when obtaining the measurements. The arm should be at the level of the heart during the measurement, with the patient seated comfortably. No tobacco or caffeine intake should occur in the 30 minutes preceding the visit.

It is imperative that there is a good fit between arm circumference and cuff size. Small cuffs overestimate BP by as much as 20 mmHg. Korotkoff sounds 1 and 5 should be used to define systolic and diastolic BP in all patients, including pregnant women. The presence of an auscultatory gap must be ruled out, especially in older patients. This is easily done by obtaining the systolic BP by the palpation method before proceeding with the auscultatory technique. At least two readings should be obtained and averaged, and the label of HTN should only be applied after high BP readings are obtained on two or more occasions. Recent restrictions on the use of mercury sphygmomanometers have led to the widespread use of electronic oscillometric devices and aneroid manometers. In this respect, two cautionary notes apply: one should ascertain that the electronic device in use has been adequately validated according to Association for the Advancement of Medical Instrumentation (AAMI) standards (this information can be obtained from the manufacturer); and both aneroid and electronic devices should be calibrated at least every 6 months to guarantee continued accuracy.

Self-measurement of BP is a very useful technique to confirm the presence of HTN. These values provide information on the behavior of BP outside the physician's office and may represent the overall burden of BP better than office readings. Multiple monitors are available at reasonable prices ($50–$80), though only a handful have been adequately validated. The attention to technique should be the same as that in the office, thus the physician must spend some time explaining it to patients. Normalcy parameters for home readings are still a matter of debate, though most experts would agree that home readings should be no higher than 135/85 mmHg. Although there are no studies linking the use of home readings to improved cardiovascular outcomes, home monitoring is associated with greater involvement with one's own treatment and improved BP control. Therefore, we encourage most patients to purchase a home BP cuff, if they can afford it.

The burden of BP is best assessed by ambulatory BP monitoring (ABPM). In this technique, the patient wears an automated cuff that records BP

Table 20.3

Clinical Uses of Ambulatory Blood Pressure Monitoring

To rule out white-coat HTN in patients with high office BP and normal out-of-office BP, or in patients with HTN without target-organ damage
To evaluate patients with high-normal (*borderline*) HTN to better define BP averages to help make treatment decisions
To better define prognosis in patients with resistant HTN
To delineate the profile of BP in patients with labile HTN
To evaluate orthostatic symptoms in patients on antihypertensive therapy or in patients with autonomic neuropathy

Abbreviations: HTN, hypertension; BP, blood pressure.

every 10–30 minutes throughout a 24-hour period. ABPM provides readings outside the office and during sleep and wakefulness. This complete assessment affords a stronger ability to stratify risk, and indeed, many studies show ABPM to be a much better predictor of cardiovascular complications in HTN than office BP. The equipment is, however, expensive ($2000–$3000 per monitor), and is usually available only at referral practices. Despite the acknowledged value of ABPM in the evaluation of multiple situations in the hypertensive patient (Table 20.3), current reimbursement schedules approve its use only in the evaluation of white-coat hypertension (patients with office readings >140/90 mmHg and out-of-office readings consistently below this level with no evidence of target-organ damage). Accepted levels of normalcy for ABPM are <135/85 mmHg for the awake BP average.

Staging the Severity of Hypertension

After following the appropriate steps outlined above, we can stage the degree of HTN. JNC 7 has proposed a new classification that we will use for uniformity. In this new classification there are four categories:

1. Normal   <120/80 mmHg
2. Prehypertension   120–139/80–89 mmHg
3. Stage 1 hypertension   140–159/90–99 mmHg
4. Stage 2 hypertension   >160/100 mmHg

The most controversial category is prehypertension. It was created due to observations that cardiovascular risk increases as BP enters this range. There are, however, no definitive data showing that treatment alters the outcome of such patients, and this is a category that encompasses a large proportion of the adult population in the Western world. Despite this, it is reasonable that individuals who fall into this category engage in lifestyle practices that decrease their overall cardiovascular risk (see below). The classification of stages 1 and 2 HTN has a few specific ramifications, which we will review later in this chapter.

Assessing the Extent of Hypertensive Damage

The initial contact with a patient with suspected or confirmed HTN must provide a good assessment of target-organ damage that has already occurred. The history and physical examination focuses on unraveling signs and symptoms of coronary disease, congestive heart failure, cerebrovascular disease, peripheral vascular disease (including the aorta), and renal disease. The fundoscopic examination is a valuable tool as it provides a direct observation of small blood vessels. It is important to account for two separate components of retinal vessel damage: those related to arteriosclerosis; and those related to acute BP increases and altered vascular permeability. Chronic arteriosclerotic changes in retinal vessels are due to long-standing (months to years) pressure-induced damage and include progressive increases in arteriolar wall thickness (copper wiring and the advanced silver wiring appearances), arteriovenous crossings, which are due to perivascular fibrosis, and arteriolar microaneurysms.

Changes related to acute changes in BP are more dramatic and can occur over the course of hours to days. These changes include arteriolar spasm, retinal flame hemorrhages, exudates, and papilledema.

Judicious use of laboratory tests (urinalysis, serum creatinine concentration, and electrocardiogram) further adds to the assessment of organ damage in HTN. In patients with symptoms or abnormal tests, further evaluation is indicated with a focus on the involved organ system.

Ruling Out Secondary Hypertension

All patients with HTN should receive at least a basic evaluation in search of possible secondary causes of HTN, since these causes may lead to a specific, sometimes curative therapy (see Chapter 21). In the initial visit, the clinician should inquire about a family history of HTN or renal disease, history of established peripheral vascular or coronary artery disease to suggest renal artery stenosis, symptoms possibly related to primary aldosteronism (muscle weakness, cramps), pheochromocytoma (paroxysms of hypertension, headache, sweating, and palpitations), Cushing's syndrome (weight gain, new onset diabetes mellitus, changes in appearance with Cushingoid features), sleep apnea (snoring, witnessed apneas during sleep, daytime somnolence), and thyroid disease (hypo- or hyperthyroidism). A detailed evaluation of medications and over-the-counter preparations must also be performed in an attempt to identify any hypertensogenic substances (see Chapter 21). Finally, the basic laboratory evaluation advocated for patients with HTN can provide clues to secondary causes, such as the serum creatinine concentration (renal disease, renal artery stenosis), urinalysis (renal disease), serum potassium concentration (hypokalemia of primary aldosteronism and Cushing's syndrome), and hematocrit (polycythemia of sleep apnea). More specific searches for secondary causes are not warranted at the initial evaluation of the hypertensive subject. If any of the above steps are positive, specific screening tests are ordered targeting the disorders under suspicion.

Identifying Factors That May Alter Therapy

It is essential to approach hypertensive patients not only as it relates to their BP, but from a broad vascular risk perspective. Accordingly, the initial visit must include an assessment of other cardiovascular risk factors, such as diabetes mellitus, obesity, smoking, sedentary lifestyle, hyperlipidemia (a fasting lipid profile is recommended as part of the initial laboratory profile), and the presence of vascular disease in any territory. This stratification of risk is important in designing the aggressiveness of therapy. As discussed under "treatment," thresholds for initiation of pharmacologic therapy, BP targets, and drug choice vary substantially according to prevalent comorbid conditions in the individual patient.

Risk stratification is performed objectively using any of the many available risk prediction tables. The European hypertension guidelines make stronger statements on risk stratification than JNC 7, and we agree that overall risk assessment is important as an additive to risk estimation based on BP alone. Our personal preference is the Framingham risk calculator (calculates the 10-year risk of coronary heart disease based on age, sex, BP level, total cholesterol concentration, high density lipoprotein (HDL)-cholesterol concentration, diabetes mellitus, and smoking status) due to its easy calculation using free software for personal digital assistants (PDAs) or free online calculation at the NHLBI website (http://hin.nhlbi.nih.gov/atpiii/calculator.asp?usertype=prof).

KEY POINTS
Diagnostic Evaluation

1. HTN should be diagnosed only after high BP levels are reproduced several times.
2. Accurate technique for blood pressure measurement is essential to minimize errors in the assessment of hypertensive patients.
3. Home BP and ambulatory BP monitoring are valuable tools in the assessment of BP levels.

4. Evaluation of prevalent comorbidity and overall risk of future cardiovascular disease is an essential part of the initial evaluation of hypertensive patients.

5. The fundoscopic examination provides a direct examination of the structure of small arteries in HTN.

6. Possible secondary causes of HTN should be ruled out in the initial visit through the judicious use of the medical history, physical examination, and basic laboratory studies.

Treatment

The primary goal of hypertension treatment is to decrease cardiovascular and renal morbidity and mortality. If left untreated, HTN leads to one or multiple cardiovascular complications in as many as 50% of patients, and it is now undisputed that BP lowering leads to an improvement in patient outcomes in all domains of HTN-related injury. Estimates based on clinical trial data indicate that antihypertensive therapy results in an approximate 40% reduction in the risk of stroke, 20% reduction in coronary disease, and a 50% decrease in heart failure. The progression of chronic kidney disease to end-stage kidney disease is decreased by 50% with better BP control. Peripheral vascular disease is the least affected outcome. Lowering BP leads to minimal improvements in symptom scores and no change in objective measures of peripheral vascular disease. Table 20.4 summarizes treatment effects using the number-needed-to-treat (NNT) approach from the large National Health and Nutrition Examination Survey I Epidemiologic Follow-up Study (NHEFS). The benefits are obviously greater in patients with higher baseline BP and cardiovascular risk categories. What is also noticeable is that the NNT for patients with baseline BP in the JNC 6 high-normal range (130–139/85–89 mmHg) are well within the values of justifiable therapy, comparable to or lower than the numbers observed for other cardiovascular interventions, such as lipid-lowering therapy. Because these data were, however, observational (and not from a treatment trial), current guidelines do not yet recommend drug therapy in patients with BP levels lower than stage 1 HTN.

Table 20.4

Effects of a 12-mmHg Reduction of Systolic Blood Pressure on the Number Needed to Treat (NNT) to Prevent Clinical Outcomes in Hypertension According to Baseline BP Level and Overall Cardiovascular Risk

	RISK GROUP								
BP GROUP	**NNT FOR CV EVENTS**			**NNT FOR CV DEATHS**			**NNT FOR ALL DEATHS**		
	A	B	C	A	B	C	A	B	C
130–139/80–89 mmHg	25	13	10	486	36	21	81	19	14
140–159/90–99 mmHg	20	11	9	273	27	18	60	16	12
>160/>100 mmHg	10	7	8	34	12	11	23	9	9

Abbreviations: NNT, number needed to prevent one event; BP, blood pressure; CV, cardiovascular.
Note: Risk group A is the absence of cardiovascular risk factors. Group B is the presence of at least one cardiovascular risk factor other than diabetes mellitus (male gender, postmenopausal female, age >60, smoking, hyperlipidemia, or family history of coronary disease). Group C represents overt cardiovascular disease, target-organ damage, or diabetes mellitus. *Source:* Data compiled from the NHEFS Study.

The approach to HTN treatment is multifaceted, including risk factor modification, lifestyle changes, and drug therapy if needed. First, one must recognize HTN as a cardiovascular disorder whose morbidity is mediated not only by BP levels, but also by associated risk factors. Because the ultimate therapeutic goal is the prevention of cardiovascular disease, management of other risk factors is imperative regardless of their impact on BP levels per se. Accordingly, aggressive risk factor modification is an integral part of treatment of the hypertensive patient. Counseling and therapy should be provided regarding smoking cessation, weight loss, hyperlipidemia, and diabetes mellitus. Reduction of BP can be achieved with lifestyle changes and antihypertensive medications. We will discuss these approaches in detail in the sections that follow.

Lifestyle Modifications

Several lifestyle factors impact BP and are effective in preventing HTN in normotensive persons, as well as in lowering BP in those with HTN (Table 20.5). Weight reduction is an important step in those who are overweight (body mass index >25 kg/m^2) or obese (body mass index >30 kg/m^2) and should involve a combined effort including caloric restriction and increased physical activity. Unfortunately, significant weight loss is required to reduce BP enough to obviate the need for antihypertensive drugs, and such reductions are often not sustained over time. Pharmacologic adjuncts are of limited value in reducing weight as well as BP, but are worth trying in some patients who have difficulties losing weight despite proven adherence to diet and exercise. Orlistat is usually well tolerated, but sibutramine, the other approved agent for chronic (weight maintenance) use, needs close observation as it is a sympathomimetic agent that can result in BP elevation. Finally, surgically induced weight loss (bariatric surgery) results in improved BP in a substantial number of morbidly obese patients, but there are questions regarding the long-term durability of the BP effect despite relative weight stability. At this time, bariatric procedures cannot yet be recommended in the management of HTN accompanied by obesity, except in the group of morbidly obese patients (BMI of at least 35 kg/m^2).

The dietary approach to lowering BP should address not only calories (weight reduction), but also other strategies that may improve BP, such as low sodium and high potassium and calcium contents, and a low fat (especially saturated fat) to maximize cardiovascular risk reduction. The Dietary Approaches to Stop Hypertension (DASH) diet is the preferred plan, as it produces BP lowering results (8–14 mmHg) that are better than those historically observed with sodium restriction alone (2–8 mmHg). The DASH plan is the combination of low sodium, low saturated fats, and large amounts of fruits and vegetables (details of the plan are found at http://www.nhlbi.nih.gov/health/public/heart/hbp/dash/). It is our practice to recommend the DASH diet to all patients with HTN, with the exception of those with hyperkalemia (especially in chronic kidney disease), in whom potassium intake must be curtailed.

Increased physical activity is modestly effective in decreasing BP. It is also an important adjunct

Table 20.5

Lifestyle Modifications and Their Effects on Blood Pressure in Patients with Hypertension

MODIFICATION	APPROXIMATE SYSTOLIC BP REDUCTION (RANGE)
Weight reduction	5–20 mmHg/10 kg weight loss
Adopt DASH eating plan	8–14 mmHg
Dietary sodium reduction	2–8 mmHg
Physical activity	4–9 mmHg
Moderation of alcohol consumption	2–4 mmHg

Abbreviation: BP, blood pressure; DASH, Dietary Approaches to Stop Hypertension.
Source: From Joint National Committee 7. National Heart, Lung, and Blood Institute, National High Blood Pressure Education Program.

to weight loss, and is associated with decreased cardiovascular disease, depression, and osteoporosis. Thus, engagement in frequent aerobic activity for at least 30 minutes on most days of the week is advisable for all patients who are capable of doing so. Anaerobic (isometric) exercise is not associated with significant BP reductions or cardiovascular protection, and should not be used as a primary intervention in HTN.

Heavy alcohol use is associated with increased BP. The thresholds for this association vary according to population, gender, and type of alcohol, thus making precise recommendations difficult. If one uses a conservative approach however, hypertensive individuals should limit alcohol consumption to no more than two drinks (20–30 g ethanol) per day for men and 1–1.5 drinks (10–20 g ethanol) per day for women.

KEY POINTS
Lifestyle Modifications

1. The general approach to treatment of HTN is multifaceted, targeting not only BP values per se, but also other variables that modify cardiovascular risk.
2. Lifestyle modifications should be advised to all patients.
3. The most effective lifestyle interventions are weight loss (in overweight subjects), use of the DASH diet, and increased physical activity.

Antihypertensive Drug Therapy

Multiple large prospective, randomized clinical trials show that drug treatment of HTN improves outcomes, most prominently a decrease in the major cardiovascular complications of HTN. Individuals with higher baseline BP derive greater benefit from therapy than those with lower baseline BP. As an example, patients with malignant HTN have a four-fold decrease in mortality after

just 1 year of therapy, a remarkable demonstration of the value of BP control in severe HTN. In subjects with lesser degrees of HTN, results of therapy vary, but overall, there is about a 50% reduction in the incidence of CHF, 40% decrease in stroke, and 20% decrease in coronary artery disease and mortality. These observations justify the use of pharmacologic therapy as needed to bring BP to values under 140/90 mmHg.

HOW LOW SHOULD BP BE LOWERED?

Several observations link low achieved BPs to worse coronary prognosis and overall mortality. These led to the concept of a "J effect" in the treatment of HTN, and the "J point" would be around diastolic BPs less than 75 mmHg. In the only study to prospectively address this question (the hypertension optimal treatment [HOT] study), 18,790 subjects were randomly assigned to a target DBP of 90, 85, or 80 mmHg. No significant differences were noted in cardiovascular morbidity and mortality as the BP was lowered below 139/83 mmHg, except in diabetic patients, who benefited from a BP lower than 130/80 mmHg. No J effect reaching statistical significance was observed, but closer scrutiny of the data reveals an increase in most measured events for patients with diastolic BP <70 mmHg. This risk pattern was not noted for systolic BP. Therefore, current recommendations are to lower BP to <140/90 mmHg in most patients and to <130/80 mmHg in patients with diabetes mellitus. A separate recommendation to lower BP to <130/80 mmHg in patients with chronic kidney disease is reasonable but supported by less strong data (see Chapter 21).

DRUG CHOICE IN UNCOMPLICATED HYPERTENSION

The treatment of patients with uncomplicated HTN is based on multiple trials that compare individual antihypertensive drugs with placebo or among each other. Thiazide diuretics, beta-blockers, angiotensin-converting enzyme (ACE) inhibitors, calcium channel blockers, and angiotensin receptor blockers (ARB) are all effective in improving out-comes, and are considered appropriate initial choices. Not all members of each class of drugs were tested in large clinical trials, and many experts argue that interchangeable use of any one member of a class is not an acceptable practice. Despite this controversy, current guidelines rec-ommend the use of classes of drugs rather than individual agents.

The drugs with the best documented track record are thiazide diuretics. Because of their reproducible efficacy in reducing BP and improv-ing outcomes in all subgroups of patients, well known safety profile, and low cost, they are rec-ommended as first choice in most patients with HTN without a comorbid condition that would invoke the use of another specific drug class. The other classes are equivalent in preventing out-comes and reducing BP, but uniformly at a higher cost. Table 20.6 presents a list of all available drug classes, relevant indications for their use, class-specific side effects, and representative agents from each group.

In most trials, a substantial number of patients (up to two-thirds) require more than one drug to achieve BP targets, which reminds us of the importance of effective drug combination in the treatment of HTN. In most cases, the combination should involve a thiazide diuretic and another agent, as there is a synergistic effect between diuretics and most other antihypertensive drugs, with the possible exception of calcium channel blockers. In the process of drug escalation, it is important to note that most drugs have a progres-sive flattening of the dose-response curve within the recommended dose range. In addition, as the dose is increased, the occurrence of side effects is often increased. Thus, it is our preference to add a second drug before reaching the maximal recom-mended dose of the first. This combination hastens the achievement of BP targets and decreases the likelihood of side effects. Only after the combina-tion is in place do we push the drugs to the maxi-mal recommended doses. Figure 20.7 presents a useful tool to build effective drug combinations up

to the use of a third drug. The "Birmingham Hypertension Square" does not take into account, however, the need to use specific drugs due to "compelling indications." Thus, as an example, the combination of an ACE inhibitor and a beta-blocker would be a very reasonable initial combi-nation in a patient with diabetes mellitus and coronary artery disease even though it may not provide the most in terms of additive BP-lowering effect. Patients who do not achieve BP control with three intelligently combined drugs at maxi-mal doses, one of them being a diuretic, are con-sidered to have resistant HTN and should be referred to a hypertension specialist for a more detailed evaluation.

DRUG CHOICE IN ISOLATED SYSTOLIC HYPERTENSION IN THE ELDERLY

ISH in the elderly was extensively evaluated in clinical trials, and it is clear that a reduction in systolic BP effectively decreases cardiovascular events, particularly heart failure and stroke. Treatment of ISH was not shown to decrease mortality in individual trials, but a metaanalysis of available trials showed a small but significant reduction in both total and cardiovascular deaths. The targets for treatment are difficult to establish, and there is no evidence that lowering systolic BP to below 140 mmHg is beneficial, even though this is the target suggested by JNC 7. Thus, it is reasonable to try to reach a systolic BP as close to 140 mmHg as possible, but further low-ering should only be done when taking comor-bidity (see below) and symptoms (especially orthostasis) into account. The issue of orthostatic hypotension is a particular concern, as it is a common complication of drug therapy in older patients. All patients should be checked for orthostasis with seated and standing BP regard-less of symptoms, and titration should be stopped in the presence of significant positional BP changes.

Drugs proven effective in ISH include thiazide diuretics and dihydropyridine calcium channel

Table 20.6

Antihypertensive Drug Classes

CLASS	SPECIFIC INDICATIONS	RELEVANT SIDE EFFECTS	REPRESENTATIVE AGENTS
Diuretics			
Thiazides	Most patients with ISH, poststroke, osteoporosis, hypercalciuria (calcium stones)	Hypokalemia, impotence	Chlorthalidone, hydrochlorothiazide, indapamide, metolazone
Loop	CKD	Hypokalemia	Bumetanide, furosemide, torsemide
Potassium-sparing	Hypokalemia, CHF (spironolactone and eplerenone only)	Hyperkalemia, decreased libido, gynecomastia (spironolactone only)	Aldosterone antagonists: eplerenone, spironolactone Na channel blockers: amiloride, triamterene (should not be used as single agents)
ACE inhibitors	CHF, post-MI, DM, CKD, high cardiovascular risk, poststroke	Common: cough Rare: hyperkalemia, acute renal failure, angioedema	Captopril, benazepril, enalapril, fosinopril, lisinopril, moexipril, perindopril, quinapril, ramipril, trandolapril
Angiotensin II receptor blockers	CHF, LVH, DM, CKD, ISH, headaches	Best side-effect profile. Hyperkalemia, rare angioedema	Candesartan, eprosartan, irbesartan, losartan, olmesartan, telmisartan, valsartan
Calcium channel blockers			
Dihydropyridines	ISH, CAD (angina), Raynaud's phenomenon	Flushing, headache, edema, constipation	Amlodipine, felodipine, nifedipine, nisoldipine
Nondihydropyridines	Tachyarrhythmias, proteinuria, migraines (verapamil)	Constipation, bradycardia	Diltiazem, verapamil
Beta-blockers	Post-MI, CAD (angina), tachyarrhythmias	Bradycardia, sedation, depression, impotence, impaired perception of hypoglycemia	Cardioselective: atenolol, metoprolol, betaxolol

(continued)

Table 20.6

Antihypertensive Drug Classes (continued)

CLASS	SPECIFIC INDICATIONS	RELEVANT SIDE EFFECTS	REPRESENTATIVE AGENTS
	Hyperthyroidism, migraines, essential tremor (propranolol)		Nonselective: propranolol, nadolol Combined alpha/beta-blocker: labetalol, carvedilol
Alpha-blockers	BPH Should not be used as single agent (not first-line therapy)	Orthostasis (*first-dose reaction*), palpitations, nasal congestion	Terazosin, doxazosin
Central anti-adrenergics agents	Fourth-line combination therapy, autonomic diarrhea (clonidine) Intolerance to oral therapy: clonidine is the only agent available in patch form Should not be used as single agent (not first-line therapy)	Sedation, dry mouth, withdrawal syndrome and depression	Clonidine, methyldopa
Direct vasodilators	Fourth-line combination therapy Should not be used as single agent (not first-line therapy)	Edema, tachycardia (should be used in combination with a diuretic and a negative chronotropic agent)	Hydralazine, minoxidil

Abbreviations: ISH, isolated systolic hypertension; CHF, congestive heart failure; LVH, left ventricular hypertrophy; DM, diabetes mellitus; CKD, chronic kidney disease; MI, myocardial infarction; BPH, benign prostatic hyperplasia; CAD, coronary artery disease.

blockers. In one study of ISH accompanied by left ventricular hypertrophy, therapy with an angiotensin receptor blocker was very effective as well. Other agents, such as beta-blockers and ACE inhibitors have been effective in older patients with HTN, but not specifically in ISH. Thus, their use is reserved for compelling indications due to comorbidity (see below) or as second or third agents in combination therapy.

Drug Choice in Patients with Comorbid Conditions

Hypertension is often accompanied by other conditions that modify cardiovascular risk. In many of these conditions, specific agents were studied and shown to perform better than others. Remarkable examples include the value

Figure 20.7

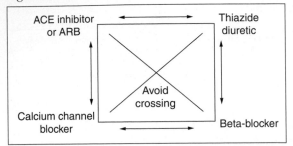

Effective antihypertensive drug combinations. The "Birmingham Hypertension Square" is a useful teaching tool to remind the clinician of how to best combine drugs. Sequential additions are based on combinations that result in maximal additive effects. Additions should be "lateral," not crossing the center. Thus, the most effective combinations include (1) diuretics with ACE inhibitors, angiotensin receptor blockers (ARB) or beta-blockers and (2) ACE inhibitors or ARB or beta-blockers with calcium channel blockers. (Adapted from Felmeden, D.C., Lip, G.Y. *Curr Hypertens Rep* 3:203–208, 2001, with permission from Rapid Science).

of ACE inhibitors in heart failure, coronary disease, diabetes mellitus, and proteinuric kidney diseases; angiotensin receptor blockers and ACE inhibitors in diabetic nephropathy; angiotensin receptor blockers in left ventricular hypertrophy; and beta-blockers after myocardial infarction. The second column in Table 20.6 presents a summary of these comorbidities and drugs that deserve specific consideration in each case. In these cases, the first choice of antihypertensive agent should be driven by the indication, rather than by general clinical trial results as described previously for the "uncomplicated" patient.

Several other comments apply to drug choice. In some patients, the comorbid condition is not one that alters cardiovascular risk, but may be important enough as to affect choice, either by avoiding or preferring specific agents. For example, patients with reactive airways disease (asthma) should not receive nonselective beta-blockers, though cardioselective beta-blockers are safe in stable patients with chronic obstructive

pulmonary disease. Patients with diabetes mellitus should have their glucose control monitored more closely when placed on a diuretic. Additionally, because the identification of hypoglycemic symptoms is dependent on adrenergic hyperactivity (tachycardia, diaphoresis, tremors), use of a beta-blocker may mask hypoglycemia, and patients and their families should be advised about this potential risk. Gout can be exacerbated by any type of diuretic. Finally, diuretics and beta-blockers may have mild adverse effects on the lipid profile, which should be monitored. Some agents may improve other diseases, such as the favorable effects of alpha-blockers on prostate hyperplasia; the prophylactic effects of nonselective beta-blockers and verapamil on migraines; the prevention of headaches by angiotensin receptor blockers; decrease in vasospasm in Raynaud's disease by calcium channel blockers; improvement of autonomic diarrhea by clonidine; or the prevention of calcium-containing stones and improvement in bone mineral density by thiazide diuretics.

KEY POINTS
Drug Therapy

1. Drug therapy is required in a large majority of patients with HTN.
2. Target BP values are <140/90 mmHg for most patients, and <130/80 for patients with diabetes mellitus.
3. Thiazide diuretics are the preferred initial agent in most patients with uncomplicated HTN due to demonstrated efficacy, safety, and low cost. ACE inhibitors, calcium channel blockers, beta-blockers, and angiotensin receptor blockers are reasonable alternatives.
4. Thiazide diuretics or dihydropyridine calcium channel blockers are the preferred agents in elderly patients with isolated systolic HTN.
5. Comorbid conditions strongly affect drug choice. When present, conditions such as

diabetes mellitus, coronary disease, heart failure, left ventricular hypertrophy, kidney disease, or stroke dictate preferred drug choices.

6. Only 40% of patients achieve BP targets on a single agent. Thus, effective combination therapy is an essential part of antihypertensive drug treatment.

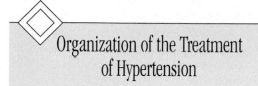

Organization of the Treatment of Hypertension

Putting It All Together

Hypertension is a condition that usually demands lifetime therapy. To counter this need, it is most often asymptomatic, thus the clinician needs to work hard with the patient in providing a good understanding of why treatment is needed. It is essential to spend time, explain the clinical consequences of long-standing HTN, and use techniques that are appropriate to the level of education of the patient. The importance of lifestyle changes needs to be emphasized to all patients. Ideally, patients should meet with a dietician to learn about the practical aspects of implementing the DASH diet. Drug therapy should focus not only on the drug choice directives described above, but also on cost, which is such an important limitation to therapy in uninsured or partly insured patients; using generic drugs may help achieving this goal. In order to improve adherence to treatment, the use of long-acting drugs with single daily dosing is the best alternative. In addition, patients should be warned of common side effects of therapy so that timely communication can occur in order to minimize patient discomfort and risk. Lastly, choosing drugs with favorable side-effect profiles is essential in

improving adherence: HTN is not symptomatic, treatment should not be symptomatic either!

After therapy is commenced, patients should be seen every 4–8 weeks until the target BP is achieved. There is clear evidence that "clinician inactivity" is a common factor in precluding the achievement of target BP values, and we should strive to be proactive in making adjustments in therapy whenever BP is not at target. These changes should consist of either an increase in dose of one agent or the addition of another agent. Once at target, it is reasonable to see patients twice a year to review persistence of control, adherence, and tolerance to therapy and to screen for the development of complications.

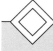

Hypertensive Urgencies and Emergencies

Whereas most patients with HTN have only mild-to-moderate elevations in BP, and few succumb to the dreaded cardiovascular complications of uncontrolled BP, a small number of patients have acute elevations of BP that demand immediate intervention. These acute events include hypertensive urgencies and emergencies. Hypertensive urgencies are those clinical situations in which the BP is severely high (arbitrarily defined as >180/120 mmHg) in the absence of end-organ dysfunction. If end-organ dysfunction is present, the term hypertensive emergency is applied, and emergency therapy is required to limit end-organ damage. Examples of acute end-organ dysfunction include hypertensive encephalopathy, intracerebral hemorrhage, acute myocardial infarction, unstable coronary syndrome, acute heart failure, aortic dissection, and eclampsia. Severe HTN in the immediate postoperative period of major cardiac or aortic surgery, or perioperative HTN in patients with an untreated pheochromocytoma should also be faced as hypertensive emergencies.

In hypertensive urgencies, patients often present without symptoms or with nonspecific symptoms such as headaches, epistaxis, dyspnea, atypical chest pain, palpitations, or anxiety. It is important to assure that BP reduction is not brisk, especially in older patients, who may develop an acute ischemic event due to excessive BP reduction. It is our preference to use long-acting drugs to treat acute elevations of BP that are asymptomatic. If the patient is undergoing chronic therapy, we usually resume their previous agent giving them a dose under our observation. We allow the patients to go home after their BP is safely under 180/110 mmHg, and we see the patient in follow-up in 2–7 days. For the previously untreated patients, our practice is to treat them with a short-acting drug (see below) while starting them on a long-acting agent. Patients who are symptomatic deserve the use of faster-acting agents to alleviate symptoms. Many agents were studied with similar results and recommendations are mostly based on opinion and personal preference. Our preference is to use clonidine (0.1 mg PO every 30 minutes up to three doses) or labetalol (200 mg PO every 30 minutes up to 600 mg). Short-acting nifedipine, once the most commonly used agent, should be avoided due to its unpredictable, often large reductions in BP that are associated with acute ischemic strokes and coronary events. These patients are best managed in an emergency room or urgent care setting. If improved, they can be discharged on a long-acting drug with early follow-up as described above. Although JNC 7 calls for combination therapy in patients with stage 2 HTN, we prefer to use only one agent at a time for patients with hypertensive urgencies, as "overaggressive" therapy may lead to excessive, symptomatic BP reduction.

The management of hypertensive emergencies demands placing the patient in an ICU setting and treatment should consist of an intravenous agent. Intraarterial continuous BP monitoring may be indicated in patients with difficult-to measure-BP or in those in whom very tight BP titration is needed, such as patients with aortic dissection, hypertensive encephalopathy, cerebral hemorrhage, or in the postoperative period of cardiovascular procedures. The choice of agent is based on the clinical condition and personal preference. Table 20.7 summarizes drug choices, dose ranges, and key clinical concerns for the most commonly used drugs. Sodium nitroprusside has a long-standing safety record and is our initial choice in most situations, with the exception of patients with increased intracerebral pressure (preferred agent is labetalol), eclampsia (delivery, hydralazine, magnesium sulfate), or acute coronary syndromes (nitroglycerin, beta-blockers). In aortic dissection, it is paramount to decrease the heart rate as well as BP, thus the combination of a beta-blocker (metoprolol or esmolol) with nitroprusside is the standard approach.

In tailoring the treatment of hypertensive emergencies, we must understand the importance of autoregulation of blood flow to target organs, especially the brain. The presence of long-standing HTN leads to functional adjustments to blood flow that protect the organ from hypertensive damage. If BP is decreased excessively, organ hypoperfusion may occur despite "normal" systemic BP. Therefore, the goal of therapy in most circumstances is to lower mean arterial pressure by no more than about 25% in the first hour of intervention. This is usually well tolerated, and BP can then be further reduced to levels of 160–180/100–110 mmHg in the ensuing 4–6 hours. Normal levels can be safely reached in 24–48 hours. Similar to hypertensive urgencies, long-acting agents are initiated immediately to shorten the need for intravenous therapy and to provide a bridge to chronic therapy. There are two important exceptions to this general rule: in patients with aortic dissection, the lowest BP tolerated should be aggressively sought in order to limit shear stress and further dissection. Conversely, patients with acute stroke call for more conservative treatment, since acute decreases in mean arterial pressure by more than 15% have been associated with worsening cerebral ischemia, and normalization of BP should be delayed until several days after the acute event.

Table 20.7

Drugs Commonly Used in the Treatment of Hypertensive Emergencies

	DOSE RANGE	INDICATIONS	CAUTIONS	COMMENTS
Continuous infusions				
Sodium nitroprusside	0.25–10 µg/kg/minute IV drip	Most emergencies	Impaired renal function (thiocyanate and cyanide intoxication), high intracranial pressure	Rapid onset and extinction (1–2 minutes) of action
Labetalol	20–80 mg IV boluses every 10 minutes or 0.5–2 mg/minute IV drip	Most emergencies Excellent choice in increased intracranial pressure	Heart failure, bradycardia/heart block	Rapid onset but prolonged duration of action (3–6 hours)
Esmolol	250–500 µg/kg bolus followed by 50–100 µg/kg/minute IV drip	Aortic dissection (with nitroprusside), perioperative HTN	Heart failure, bradycardia/heart block	Rapid onset and extinction (10 minutes) of action
Fenoldopam	0.1–0.3 µg/kg/minute IV drip	Most emergencies	Glaucoma	Rapid onset, but extinction may take up to 30 minutes Expensive
Nitroglycerin	5–100 µg/minute IV drip	Acute coronary syndromes, heart failure	Right ventricular infarction (severe hypotension)	Rapid onset and extinction Tolerance with prolonged use
Bolus dosing				
Hydralazine	10–20 mg IV every 15–20 minutes, then every 3–4 hours	Eclampsia	May worsen coronary ischemia (*steal*)	Duration of action <4 hours
Enalaprilat	1.25–5 mg IV every 6 hours	Acute heart failure	Acute renal failure, acute myocardial infarction	Duration of action 6–12 hours
Metoprolol	5–10 mg IV every 15–30 minutes, then every 4–6 hours	Acute coronary syndromes, perioperative HTN	Heart failure, bradycardia/heart block	Duration of action 4–6 hours

Abbreviations: IV, intravenous; HTN, hypertension.

KEY POINTS

Hypertensive Urgencies and Emergencies

1. Hypertensive urgencies are situations in which BP is severely elevated (>180/120 mmHg) without evidence of end-organ dysfunction. Treatment should be started immediately with oral drugs and early outpatient follow-up.
2. Hypertensive emergencies are accompanied by end-organ dysfunction and demand immediate BP lowering with intravenous therapy in the intensive care unit.
3. Nitroprusside is safe and effective in most hypertensive emergencies.

Additional Reading

ALLHAT Collaborative Research Group. Major outcomes in high-risk hypertensive patients randomized to angiotensin-converting enzyme inhibitor or calcium channel blocker vs. diuretic. The Antihypertensive and Lipid-Lowering Treatment to Prevent Heart Attack Trial (ALLHAT). *JAMA* 288:2981–2997, 2002.

August, P. Initial treatment of hypertension. *N Engl J Med* 348:610–617, 2003.

Elliott, W.J. Management of hypertensive emergencies. *Curr Hypertens Rep* 5:486–492, 2003.

Guidelines Committee. 2003 European Society of Hypertension-European Society of Cardiology guidelines for the management of arterial hypertension. *J Hypertens* 21:1011–1053, 2003.

Hajjar, I., Kotchen, T.A. Trends in prevalence, awareness, treatment, and control of hypertension in the United States, 1988–2000. *JAMA* 290:199–206, 2003.

Hansson, L., Zanchetti, A., Carruthers, S.G., Dahlof, B., Elmfeldt, D., Julius, S., Menard, J., Rahn, K.H., Wedel, H., Westerling, S. Effects of intensive blood pressure lowering and low-dose aspirin in patients with hypertension: principal results of the Hypertension Optimal Treatment (HOT) randomized trial. *Lancet* 351:1755–1762, 1998.

Hill, M.N., Sutton B.S. Barriers to hypertension care and control. *Curr Hypertens Rep* 2:445–450, 2000.

JNC 7 guidelines (Complete version). Chobanian, A.V., Bakris, G.B., Black, H.R., Cushman, W.C., Green, L.A., Izzo, J.L. Jr., Jones, D.W., Materson, B.J., Oparil, S., Wright, J.T. Jr., Roccella, E.J. Seventh report of the Joint National Committee on Prevention, Detection, Evaluation, and Treatment of High Blood Pressure. *Hypertension* 42:1206–1252, 2003a.

JNC 7 guidelines (Summary version). Chobanian, A.V., Bakris, G.B., Black, H.R., Cushman, W.C., Green, L.A., Izzo, J.L. Jr., Jones, D.W., Materson, B.J., Oparil, S., Wright, J.T. Jr., Roccella, E.J. The Seventh Report of the Joint National Committee on Prevention, Detection, Evaluation, and Treatment of High Blood Pressure: the JNC 7 report. *JAMA* 289:2560–2572, 2003b.

Oparil, S., Zaman, A., Calhoun D.A. Pathogenesis of hypertension. *Ann Intern Med* 139:761–776, 2003.

World Heath Organization/International Society of Hypertension Writing Group. WHO/ISH statement on management of hypertension. *J Hypertens* 21:1983–1992, 2003.

Sergio F.F. Santos and
Aldo J. Peixoto

Chapter

21

Secondary Causes of Hypertension

Recommended Time to Complete: 1 day

Guiding Questions

1. What is the prevalence of secondary hypertension?
2. What are the most common causes of secondary hypertension?
3. When should secondary causes of hypertension be investigated?
4. Which drugs/chemicals can cause hypertension and/or impair the effect of antihypertensive agents?
5. What are the clinical findings in a hypertensive patient with obstructive sleep apnea (OSA)?
6. When should renovascular disease be suspected?
7. How should renovascular disease be investigated?
8. Who benefits from interventions in renovascular disease?
9. What are the screening tests used to investigate primary aldosteronism?
10. What are the metabolic tests used for the diagnosis of pheochromocytoma?
11. What are the characteristics of hypertension in thyroid and parathyroid diseases?
12. What is the differential diagnosis of hypertension in pregnancy?

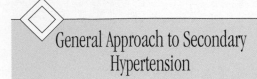

General Approach to Secondary Hypertension

Secondary hypertension (HTN) is defined as HTN that has a known etiology and is potentially reversible by specific treatment. The prevalence of secondary HTN is approximately 5–10% of all hypertensive patients, but several factors resulted in a recent increase in these estimates. More aggressive screening and better laboratory methods led to a higher rate of identification of certain conditions, especially primary aldosteronism; advances in the knowledge of mechanisms involved in the pathogenesis of HTN uncovered new causes of secondary HTN; and changes in the characteristics of the hypertensive population increased the prevalence of secondary HTN if the above definition of "potentially reversible" HTN is followed. For example, obesity is now "epidemic," is associated with HTN, and its successful treatment improves or normalizes blood pressure (BP). Likewise, essential HTN is a common cause of chronic kidney disease (CKD), and thus both essential and secondary HTN may coexist in the same patient as CKD progresses. The same is true for the aging population where the prevalence of HTN and macrovascular atherosclerotic disease increase concomitantly; making it more likely that renal artery stenosis (RAS) complicates the evolution of essential HTN. Lastly, secondary causes of HTN are frequently responsible for cases of resistant HTN. It is estimated that up to one-third of patients referred to specialty clinics for the evaluation of resistant HTN have secondary HTN; consequently, a very detailed screening for secondary HTN is imperative in the assessment of these patients. Other clinical circumstances (Table 21.1) also point to the need of more aggressive evaluation for secondary causes of HTN.

The initial evaluation of any hypertensive patient must include enough elements to provide an adequate screen for secondary causes. After all, it is in that initial encounter that the clinician has the

Table 21.1

Factors Associated with Secondary Hypertension

Hypertension resistant to appropriate therapy
Worsening of previously controlled hypertension
Onset of hypertension in patients younger than 20 or older than 50
"Malignant" or accelerated hypertension
No family history of hypertension

unique opportunity of identifying a potentially curable process. The history should include specific inquiry for symptoms of diseases that may cause HTN (Table 21.2), as well as for the use of substances that elevate blood pressure. The physical examination should include a search for differences in blood pressure and pulses between the upper and lower extremities; an evaluation of peripheral vascular disease (auscultation for carotid, abdominal, and femoral bruits, and palpation of the abdomen for aortic aneurysms); palpation of the thyroid gland; and examination of the abdomen for enlarged polycystic kidneys or masses. Laboratory tests must include an evaluation of renal function (serum creatinine concentration and urinalysis), serum glucose concentration, hemoglobin concentration, serum potassium and calcium concentrations. These simple and inexpensive procedures will be enough to raise the suspicion of secondary causes of HTN in most patients. In the paragraphs that follow we will present a more detailed discussion of the most relevant causes of secondary HTN.

KEY POINTS

General Approach to Secondary Hypertension

1. Secondary causes of HTN have been identified more frequently.
2. Primary and secondary HTN may coexist in the same patient.

Table 21.2

Clinical and Laboratory Clues for Relevant Secondary Causes of Hypertension

	SYMPTOMS AND SIGNS	BASIC LABORATORY TESTS
Obstructive sleep apnea	Snoring, obesity, large neck circumference, daytime fatigue	Respiratory acidosis
Renal parenchymal disease	Edema, pallor, hematuria	Elevated serum creatinine concentration, hematuria, proteinuria, anemia
Renovascular disease	Diffuse atherosclerotic disease, abdominal bruits, unexplained heart failure	Elevated serum creatinine concentration, hypokalemia
Pregnancy	Pregnancy-related	Proteinuria in preeclampsia
Primary aldosteronism	Muscle weakness, cramps	Hypokalemia, hypernatremia, metabolic alkalosis
Pheochromocytoma	Headache, palpitations, diaphoresis	Nonspecific
Cushing's syndrome	Truncal obesity, moon facies, purple skin striae	Hyperglycemia, hypokalemia
Thyroid disease	Hyperkinetic or hypokinetic state, enlarged thyroid, thyroid nodules	Nonspecific screening tests, abnormal TFTs.
Primary hyperparathyroidism	Constipation, kidney stones	Hypercalcemia with high PTH concentration
Coarctation of the aorta	Hypertension in the arms and low BP in the legs	Nonspecific
Drug-induced or drug-related	Nonspecific	Nonspecific

Abbreviations: TFTs, thyroid function tests; PTH, parathyroid hormone.

> 3. Clinical and laboratory findings in a basic screening in newly diagnosed HTN may suggest secondary causes.

include prescription and over-the-counter medications, as well as abused substances. It is important to remind clinicians to actively inquire about these chemicals when obtaining the history from a hypertensive patient.

Drugs and Chemicals

Many chemical substances used for a variety of reasons may cause HTN or lessen the effect of antihypertensive agents (Table 21.3). These

Oral Contraceptives

Oral contraceptive drugs commonly raise BP. These effects, however, are mild. No more than 10–15% of patients using oral contraceptives fulfill the diagnosis of HTN. The pathophysiology of BP elevation with oral contraceptive use is unknown. The incidence of HTN has decreased with the

Table 21.3

Commonly Used Substances That May Cause Hypertension and/or Mitigate the Effects of Antihypertensive Drugs

Oral contraceptives

Nonsteroidal anti-inflammatory drugs (NSAIDs, selective, and nonselective)

Sympathomimetic/sympathoactivating agents

    Pseudoephedrine, phenylpropanolamine

    Sibutramine

    Yohimbine

    Cocaine, amphetamines (prescription or illegal)

Selective serotonin reuptake inhibitors (SSRIs)

Monoamine oxidase inhibitors (MAOIs)

Cyclosporin and tacrolimus

Erythropoietin

Corticosteroids

Licorice

Ethanol

use of modern low-estrogen formulations in combination with new synthetic progestogens. It is recommended that every woman taking oral contraceptives have their blood pressure measured regularly. Most cases of HTN related to oral contraceptives are cured with drug withdrawal, though it may take several months until BP normalizes. Therefore, if HTN is diagnosed in patients who use oral contraceptives, the pill is discontinued and another type of contraception recommended.

Nonsteroidal Anti-Inflammatory Drugs (NSAIDs)

NSAIDs are the most commonly prescribed class of drugs in the United States. Because their use is common in the elderly, the population at greatest risk for HTN, it is important to review the effects of these drugs on BP. Decreased prostaglandin synthesis results in decreased renal blood flow and sodium retention, thereby contributing to HTN. Available data demonstrate that NSAIDs cause modest increases in BP, but this effect is primarily noticeable in patients with underlying HTN. Of greater relevance is the fact that NSAIDs antagonize the effects of most antihypertensive drugs, with the exception of calcium channel blockers. Most NSAIDs have similar effects on BP, particularly nonselective agents. Selective cyclooxygenase-2 (COX-2) inhibitors are also associated with BP elevation. Rofecoxib appears to have a more prominent, dose-dependent effect than other similar agents, such as celecoxib. This may be related to differences in drug half-life. Rofecoxib, however, is no longer available as it was withdrawn from the market due to increased cardiovascular events.

Substances Enhancing Sympathetic Activity

Remedies to relieve cold symptoms (oral or nasal sprays) often contain sympathomimetic amines such as pseudoephedrine and phenylpropanolamine. All such agents are associated with BP elevation. Other medications containing sympathomimetic activity include amphetamines used in the treatment of attention-deficit hyperactivity disorder or depression (dextroamphetamine, methylphenidate), and sibutramine, which is used for the treatment of obesity. Ephedra was a common component of nutritional supplements and over-the-counter weight loss preparations until its ban from the United States market in late 2003. The BP effects of its new "substitutes," such as green tea extract, bitter orange, and guarana are not yet known.

Other drugs may enhance sympathetic nervous system tone and increase BP without direct sympathomimetic activity. These include selective serotonin reuptake inhibitors (SSRIs), the most commonly prescribed antidepressant agents, and monoamine oxidase inhibitors (MAOIs). An important over-the-counter substance is yohimbine, which has resurged in the market of supplements for improved male sexual performance.

Finally, cocaine and ecstasy (methylenedioxymethylamphetamine–MDMA) are two illicit drugs that activate the sympathetic nervous system and may precipitate hypertensive crises.

Licorice

Licorice is a bush native to Southern Europe and Asia, the roots of which are sweeter than sugar and are used in candies and tobacco flavoring. In this country, the most common source of licorice extract is nutritional "energy" supplements. Glycyrrhizic acid is the active ingredient of licorice extract; it inhibits type II 11β-hydroxysteroid dehydrogenase, the enzyme that converts cortisol to cortisone, thus increasing the concentration of cortisol available to activate the mineralocorticoid receptor. It causes a form of pseudohyperaldosteronism with HTN, sodium retention, and potassium wasting, similar to the syndrome of apparent mineralocorticoid excess (AME) discussed later in this chapter. HTN generally reverses with stopping its ingestion.

Cyclosporin and Tacrolimus

Cyclosporin and tacrolimus are calcineurin inhibitor immunosuppressive agents commonly used in transplantation and in the treatment of certain immune-mediated diseases. In kidney transplantation the prevalence of HTN increased from 50 to 80% after the introduction of cyclo-sporin. Calcineurin inhibitors induce functional and morphologic changes in kidneys that are directly related to the pathogenesis of HTN. They produce renal vasoconstriction and decrease glomerular filtration rate (GFR) that impairs sodium excretion, and long-term use may cause interstitial fibrosis. Nephrotoxicity, however, is not the only mechanism for calcineurin inhibitor-related HTN. Activation of the sympathetic ner-vous system, impaired nitric oxide production, and increased endothelin release are other relevant factors. Although some publications suggest that calcium channel blockers are superior in the treatment of calcineurin inhibitor HTN, any antihypertensive agent can be used. Importantly, previous concerns about concomitant ACE inhibitor use are unfounded, and these drugs can be safely used to treat patients with HTN on a calcineurin inhibitor.

Erythropoietin

Recombinant human erythropoietin (EPO) is used for treatment of anemia in CKD, human immunodeficiency virus (HIV), postchemotherapy, and in certain hematologic disorders. Most patients have a mild BP increase when they initiate EPO therapy, and frank HTN can become manifest or made worse in about 30%. The BP rise is attributed to increased blood viscosity and direct EPO effects on vascular resistance, where it causes increased cytosolic calcium, increased endothelin-1 concentration, and resistance to nitric oxide. Because BP elevations are usually mild and benefits of EPO outweigh this side effect in most patients, routine measures to control BP should take place while continuing EPO therapy.

Corticosteroids

Corticosteroids used either for anti-inflammatory or immunosuppressive purposes may cause HTN. The proposed mechanism is the same as described for Cushing's syndrome (see below), and usually occurs with high-dose therapy or long-term use.

KEY POINTS
Drugs and Chemicals

1. A large number of substances may cause HTN. These include prescription and non-prescription drugs.
2. The mechanism of HTN depends on the substance used.

Obstructive Sleep Apnea

A good example of "new" causes of secondary HTN is OSA. OSA is a frequent sleep disorder (20% of adults have at least mild OSA), characterized by partial or complete closure of the upper airway during sleep. Blood pressure increases not only during apneic episodes, but OSA is also independently linked to daytime HTN. The odds of daytime HTN increase with the number of apneic episodes and the magnitude of nocturnal O_2 desaturation.

Pathogenesis

Hypoxemia, CO_2 retention, acute changes in intrathoracic pressure, and arousal from sleep trigger neural and circulatory responses such as sympathetic activation and increased levels of endothelin-1. Other known risk factors for cardiovascular disease, such as oxidative stress, chronic inflammation, and hypercoagulability also coexist in OSA, thus amplifying the cardiovascular risk of these patients.

Diagnosis

Patients with OSA are habitual snorers, have increased neck circumference, are uniformly overweight, and have daytime somnolence. In a hypertensive patient, knowledge of the neck circumference (>17 in.) and two features of the medical history (presence of habitual snoring or witnessed nocturnal choking or gasping) can predict polysomonographic abnormalities and select patients for further investigation. Polysomnography is the best procedure to evaluate OSA, as it provides not only the diagnosis but also information on the severity of the problem. The number of obstructive events (apneas or hypopneas) per hour is commonly used to quantify OSA: mild = 5–15 events/hour; moderate = 15–30 events/hour; severe = >30 events/hour. Patients with more than 15 events/hour are more commonly hypertensive and are more refractory to antihypertensive drug therapy.

Treatment

Weight reduction is essential in obese patients. Avoiding the supine position during sleep also reduces OSA episodes (a tennis ball sewn to the back of pajamas is a useful tool). Nasal continuous positive airway pressure (CPAP) is the best available treatment for OSA. CPAP forces air down the nose and throat under positive pressure, thus keeping the upper airways open, eliminating apneas. Effective CPAP treatment significantly reduces BP. In one study, nasal CPAP with effective positive pressure (9–12 cm H_2O) decreased BP by 10/10 mmHg, compared to a negligible decrease (1/1 mmHg) in the group receiving subtherapeutic CPAP (3–4 cm H_2O). The main problem with CPAP is patient compliance, which prevents long-term use in a substantial subgroup of patients.

KEY POINTS
Obstructive Sleep Apnea

1. Obstructive sleep apnea (OSA) is a frequent sleep disorder that causes HTN and is associated with other cardiovascular risk factors.
2. Overweight, large neck circumference, snoring or witnessed nocturnal choking or gasping, and daytime somnolence are strong indicators of OSA.
3. Nasal continuous positive airway pressure abolishes OSA and improves blood pressure.

Renal Parenchymal Disease

Renal parenchymal disease is the most frequent cause of secondary HTN (5% of all HTN cases). Most patients (80%) with progressive kidney diseases develop HTN, and the prevalence of HTN increases with worsening renal function. Unilateral parenchymal renal disease (cysts, tumors, reflux, hydronephrosis) may infrequently cause HTN.

Pathogenesis

The primary mechanism of HTN in bilateral kidney disease is impaired fluid and sodium balance, leading to increased plasma volume. A compensatory increase in BP occurs to augment sodium and water excretion (see Chapter 20). Furthermore, complex mechanisms involving activation of the sympathetic nervous system, increased intracellular calcium, inappropriate stimulation of the renin-angiotensin-aldosterone system (RAAS), altered balance of endothelium-derived vasoconstrictor and vasodilating factors (especially endothelin-1 and nitric oxide, respectively), and increased arterial stiffness are also operative in these patients. In unilateral renal disease, activation of the RAAS is the cause of HTN in renin-secreting tumors. The RAAS is also involved in HTN associated with unilateral reflux nephropathy and unilateral hydronephrosis.

Diagnosis

Edema, hematuria, and/or foamy urine may be present. Physical examination may disclose abdominal masses representing polycystic kidneys, hydronephrosis, or renal tumors. More importantly, the diagnosis of parenchymal kidney disease is made by laboratory evaluation with elevated serum concentrations of blood urea nitrogen (BUN) and creatinine and/or abnormalities in the urinalysis (hematuria, proteinuria). Because serum BUN and creatinine concentrations may underestimate the degree of renal dysfunction, formulas that estimate glomerular filtration rate are used to assess renal function more accurately (Chapter 16). In adults, the Modification of Diet in Renal Disease (MDRD) equations or the Cockcroft-Gault equation are most often used. They may be complemented by a 24-hour urine collection and the determination of the endogenous creatinine clearance. A more detailed diagnostic evaluation of kidney disease is found in Chapter 16.

Treatment

HTN is the most important factor in the progression of most parenchymal kidney diseases. A decrease in BP is associated with a fall in the rate of loss of glomerular function. Furthermore, BP control to <125/75 mmHg leads to substantial protection of renal function in patients with proteinuria. BP targets for patients with nonproteinuric kidney diseases are not well established. Recommendations for BP <130/80 mmHg were made by a National Kidney Foundation Task Force, and this is a reasonable target.

Drugs that act on the RAAS, angiotensin-converting enzyme inhibitors (ACE-Is) and angiotensin II receptor blockers (ARBs), are more effective than other agents in renal protection and proteinuria reduction at the same level of BP control. Therefore, patients with chronic kidney disease should receive an ACE-I or an ARB as the first pharmacologic option for the treatment of HTN. Close follow-up of renal function and serum potassium concentration must take place after initiation of any of these drugs. We routinely obtain serum chemistries 1 week after initiation and after each dose titration. It is well established that declines in GFR in the 25–30% range can be tolerated, as long as it stabilizes on repeat testing within 30 days. Hyperkalemia in the 5.5 meq/L range is safe and acceptable. It can be achieved with dietary intervention and diuretics.

In order to reach BP targets of 125–130/75–80 mmHg, a combination of two to three drugs is often needed. In this decision-making process, the increased cardiovascular risk represented by kidney disease and the frequent cardiovascular comorbidity afflicting these patients must be considered. Therefore, a diuretic may be indicated due to its cardiovascular protective effects or as part of the management of volume overload or heart failure. β-blockers are needed for coronary disease or heart failure. Calcium channel blockers may be helpful in coronary disease, and nondihydropyridine calcium channel blockers (verapamil and diltiazem) have antiproteinuric properties that are additive to ACE-Is or ARBs. Combining an ACE-I and ARB may further decrease proteinuria, and may decrease the progression of kidney disease in nondiabetic patients. In the absence of any compelling reason to choose one class over another, the first agent to be added to an ACE-I or ARB is a diuretic, which is often essential to achieve BP targets in patients with kidney disease. The choice of diuretic type is dependent on GFR: thiazide diuretics can be effectively used with GFR >30–50 mL/minute; when below this range, a loop diuretic is usually required, though our anecdotal experience with metolazone is positive. Third-line drugs are usually a calcium channel blocker or a β-blocker.

In the unusual cases of unilateral disease with HTN, nephrectomy is indicated for HTN associated with unilateral renal tumors. In other unilateral parenchymal diseases, nephrectomy must be evaluated carefully especially in kidneys with residual function. Surgical results are variable and often poor. Most patients can be managed successfully with drug therapy.

KEY POINTS

Renal Parenchymal Disease

1. Strict blood pressure control is recommended for patients with chronic kidney disease.

2. Angiotensin-converting enzyme inhibitors and angiotensin receptor blockers are preferred for the treatment of HTN in chronic renal disease.
3. The increased cardiovascular risk of chronic kidney disease must be taken into account when antihypertensive treatment is chosen.

Renovascular Disease

The prevalence of renovascular disease in the hypertensive population is approximately 1–5%. Increases in the aging population, however, may lead to an increment in the numbers of renovascular HTN due to atherosclerosis in the future. The main types of renovascular HTN are atherosclerosis (90%) and fibromuscular dysplasia (FMD) (10%).

Pathogenesis

Two classical animal models demonstrate the role of the RAAS in the pathogenesis of HTN after partial interruption of renal blood flow. In the Goldblatt I model (one kidney, one clip) there is unilateral arterial stenosis and nephrectomy of the contralateral kidney. In the Goldblatt II model (two kidneys, one clip), unilateral arterial stenosis is created, while the other kidney remains intact. Both models demonstrate that the RAAS is activated after constriction of the renal artery resulting in increased BP. In the Goldblatt I model blood volume expands and there is a "reset" of the RAAS (angiotensin II concentrations often return to normal), making chronic HTN primarily dependent on volume. In the Goldblatt II model the nonstenotic kidney promotes salt excretion (pressure natriuresis) and the RAAS remains activated in the underperfused kidney. Thus, chronic HTN is directly related to angiotensin II concentration. In both models natriuresis induced by diuretics reactivates the RAAS even if blood pressure is stable at high levels. Goldblatt I is the animal model for human bilateral renal artery stenosis (or unilateral stenosis in a patient with a single kidney). Goldblatt II is the animal model for human unilateral renal artery stenosis.

The cause of FMD is unknown; smoking is a prominent risk factor. Fibromuscular dysplasia has several different subtypes and may affect the arterial intima, media, or adventitia. It occurs predominantly in patients under age 30 and 75% are females. Atherosclerotic renovascular disease increases with age, and affects predominantly males, patients with diabetes mellitus and/or preexisting HTN, individuals who have other vascular disease, and smokers.

Diagnosis

Some clinical features may suggest that renovascular disease is the cause of HTN. Some of these features are those clues to the presence of secondary causes of HTN (Table 21.1). Others are unexplained azotemia, hypokalemia (due to secondary aldosteronism in unilateral stenosis), worsening of renal function with use of ACE-Is or ARBs (in bilateral disease, unilateral stenosis in a single kidney, or unilateral stenosis accompanied by underlying parenchymal disease), unilateral small kidney, abdominal and/or flank bruits, generalized atherosclerosis, and unexplained pulmonary edema.

Once renovascular disease is suspected, several techniques are used to confirm the diagnosis. Renal arteriography is the gold standard for the diagnosis of renovascular disease, but is invasive and has associated risks most importantly contrast nephrotoxicity and atheroembolic disease. Therefore, noninvasive techniques are the most commonly used options in the screening of RAS. Of the available techniques, three can be used as effective screening tools: computed tomography angiography (CTA); magnetic resonance angiography (MRA); and duplex ultrasonography.

Magnetic resonance angiography (especially when the images are enhanced by gadolinium) and CTA have the highest accuracy (specificity and sensitivity uniformly >90%) and are the most widely used noninvasive methods to detect renovascular disease. MRA is readily available in the United States, has excellent sensitivity and specificity, and easy interpretation. Computed tomography angiography provides excellent resolution and good detail of accessory vessels. It has high sensitivity and specificity but is less available than MRA and uses a large volume (~150 mL) of iodinated contrast, making it an undesirable option in patients with underlying kidney disease. Duplex ultrasonography shows the contour of the renal arteries through its two-dimensional images and grades the blood flow velocity at different segments of each renal artery via Doppler sampling. The presence of RAS is detected by an increase in flow velocity at the stenotic segments. It is easily available, and has good sensitivity and specificity. It is, however, strongly dependent on operator experience, is limited in obese patients, and is not suitable for accessory vessels. Because of these limitations, this test has not fared as well as MRA and CTA in comparative studies. In our opinion, this modality should be used only in institutions where the radiology service is committed to spending the time and effort required for the acquisition of optimal images. Figure 21.1 displays representative images of diagnostic modalities to diagnose RAS.

Other techniques used as screening methods for RAS include ACE inhibitor-stimulated peripheral plasma renin activity and ACE inhibitor-stimulated nuclear scintigraphy. Presently, none of these techniques has a role in the diagnosis of RAS in view of their limited sensitivity and specificity, especially in patients with underlying renal dysfunction.

One of the most difficult parts of the evaluation of RAS is to establish whether the identified anatomic lesion is physiologically significant. At present, no clinical or laboratory test is precise enough to predict whether correction of the RAS will result in improvement of BP (i.e., confirm that renovascular disease translates into renovascular

Figure 21.1

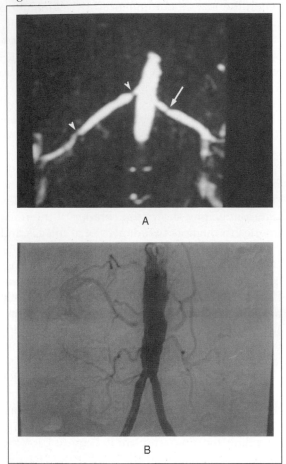

A

B

Imaging techniques in renal artery stenosis. Panel A shows an MR angiography revealing proximal left-sided RAS (arrow) and proximal as well as mid right-sided RAS (arrowheads). Panel B shows tight right-sided RAS on aortography; the left renal artery is occluded. Abbreviations: MR, magnetic resonance; RAS, renal artery stenosis.

HTN in the individual patient). Though inadequate as screening tests, ACE inhibitor-scintigrams (using Technetium diethylenetriaminepentaacetic acid (DTPA) or technetium 99 mertiatide MAG-3 as the radionuclide) may be useful as functional tests in patients with HTN, RAS, and preserved renal function. These tests must be done when the patient is off an ACE inhibitor or angiotensin receptor blocker for at least 2 weeks. Patients who show lateralization

in radionuclide uptake following administration of an ACE inhibitor (usually captopril) tend to have more favorable BP responses to revascularization, whereas those who do not lateralize on the scintigrams usually do not respond. It must be stressed that the literature on the use of these functional tests is not consistent, and personal preference (opinion) still guides most of this decision-making process.

Any patient who has a positive noninvasive test and an indication for intervention (see below) should undergo a renal arteriogram. The arteriogram will provide precise anatomical information, as well as some functional data, especially the systolic pressure gradient across the stenosis, which is considered functionally significant when >20 mmHg.

Treatment

The only effective treatment for RAS is revascularization to restore normal blood flow to the kidney, either operatively or percutaneously. Not all patients, however, should be revascularized. In patients with HTN and RAS, revascularization is indicated in patients who have not achieved BP control on three or more drugs and those with progressive loss of renal function during follow-up. Patients with bilateral disease benefit more from intervention than those with unilateral RAS. One other group found to benefit from intervention is patients with RAS and recurrent pulmonary edema that cannot be explained by cardiac causes.

Percutaneous transluminal renal angioplasty (PTRA) with or without stenting is currently the most commonly used technique for revascularization. In patients with FMD, PTRA alone usually suffices, and is curative in up to 60% of patients. Atherosclerotic disease, which preferentially involves the more proximal segments of the renal artery, uniformly requires the deployment of a stent for optimal results. There are no long-term studies comparing PTRA alone with PTRA plus stenting, but the short-term technical results and restenosis rates are substantially better with stenting than with PTRA alone. Technical results do not guarantee clinical

Figure 21.2

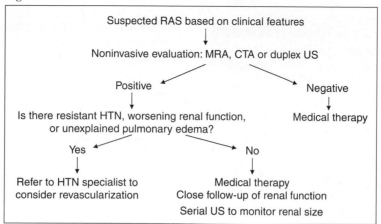

Algorithm for the evaluation of suspected renal artery stenosis. Abbreviations: RAS, renal artery stenosis; MRA, magnetic resonance angiography; CTA, computed tomography angiography; US, ultrasound; HTN, hypertension. Abbreviations: MR, magnetic resonance; RAS, renal artery stenosis.

response, and cures are extremely rare. Nevertheless, most patients do have a decrease in BP levels and/or a decrease in number of antihypertensive drugs. Older studies comparing surgical correction with PTRA indicate that surgery is better in the treatment of bilateral RAS, as it affords greater long-term patency. Current practice, however, reserves surgical revascularization for those cases where PTRA is not feasible or unsuccessful due to the complexity of the lesion. This trend was generated primarily by the improved long-term patency results with the use of stents.

Medical therapy with antihypertensive drug combinations may achieve BP control in many cases of atherosclerotic renovascular HTN, but RAS may progress on the diseased side or develop in the contralateral kidney despite BP control and the use of other strategies to prevent the progression of atherosclerosis. Patients who are managed medically should have their renal function monitored regularly. We also obtain renal ultrasounds (US) every 6–12 months to follow changes in renal length as evidence of renal ischemic atrophy, as these changes may occur before a rise in serum creatinine concentration (or decline in estimated GFR). Patients who

lose more than 1 cm over the course of 12 months are referred for revascularization. Figure 21.2 summarizes our approach to the management of RAS.

KEY POINTS
Renovascular Disease

1. The prevalence of atherosclerotic renovascular disease has increased and must be considered in patients with resistant HTN and generalized vascular disease.

2. Magnetic resonance angiography and computed tomography angiography are noninvasive methods with the best sensitivity and specificity for the diagnosis of renovascular HTN.

3. Percutaneous transluminal angioplasty with stenting is the most commonly used treatment for renovascular HTN.

4. Medical therapy may achieve blood pressure control in renovascular HTN, but atherosclerotic lesions may progress and renal function worsen.

5. Interventional therapy must always be con-
    sidered in patients with refractory HTN,
    worsening renal function, unexplained con-
    gestive heart failure, and in those with bilat-
    eral renovascular disease.

Primary Aldosteronism

In 1955, Conn published the case of a patient with
HTN and hypokalemia cured after the surgical
removal of an adrenal adenoma. Since then, laboratory and imaging screening tests have greatly
enhanced the identification of cases, and some
studies reported an incidence of primary aldosteronism in as many as 14% of all cases of HTN.
While such a number is likely to be an overestimate, it is clear that primary aldosteronism is
much more common than previously recognized.
Furthermore, the appreciation of the toxic effects
of excess aldosterone to heart and kidneys suggests that the overproduction of aldosterone is
clinically important. Interest in this disease caused
by autonomous hypersecretion of aldosterone has
increased significantly over the past several years.

Pathogenesis

Primary aldosteronism is caused by aldosterone-
producing adenomas (APA), bilateral idiopathic
adrenal hyperplasia, aldosterone-producing adrenal carcinoma, and familial aldosteronism. Excessive
aldosterone synthesis causes increased renal sodium
reabsorption and potassium excretion. Sodium
reabsorption causes plasma volume expansion,
which is the primary initiating mechanism of HTN in
this disease. Chronically, the hemodynamic profile
of patients with primary aldosteronism varies, and
elevated systemic vascular resistance in the absence
of volume expansion is common.

Diagnosis

Hypokalemia in a hypertensive patient is the most
common clinical clue to the presence of primary
aldosteronism. Normal serum potassium concentration, however, is present in more than 30% of
patients with primary aldosteronism, especially
in those with adrenal hyperplasia or familial
hyperaldosteronism. In patients with resistant
HTN, serum potassium concentration lower than
3.8 meq/L is very suggestive of primary aldosteronism, and we often encounter patients with concentrations >4 meq/L. Renal potassium wasting is
the cause of the hypokalemia. Once excessive
renal potassium loss (>30 meq/ 24 hours) is demonstrated, the plasma aldosterone concentration
(ng/dL) to plasma renin activity (ng/mL/hour) ratio
(ARR) is performed as the guiding screening test
(Figure 21.3). This test is performed in random
conditions while the patient is on most antihypertensive agents (with the exception of spironolactone), and is best obtained in a morning blood
draw. Values over 20 are suggestive of primary
aldosteronism, and values over 50 are highly
indicative of this diagnosis. The most common
cause of a false-positive ratio is chronic kidney
disease; other causes include potassium loading
and the use of β-blockers. Diuretics, ACE inhibitors,
and angiotensin receptor blockers may cause
false-negative results. If the clinical suspicion is
high and the patient is taking one such drug, the
more prudent strategy is to remove it for at least
2 weeks and repeat the test.

Because it is the variation in plasma renin activity that accounts for most of the variance in the
ARR, other tests are necessary to confirm excessive nonsuppressible aldosterone secretion. The
most commonly used confirmatory tests involve
the measurement of aldosterone production
under salt-loading conditions. Our preference is
the oral salt-loading test, wherein 24-hour urinary
aldosterone excretion is measured after 3 days of
oral sodium loading (at least 200 mmol sodium/
day), and an excretion greater than 12 µg/24 hours
is considered evidence of primary aldosteronism.
Another technique is to measure plasma aldosterone

Figure 21.3

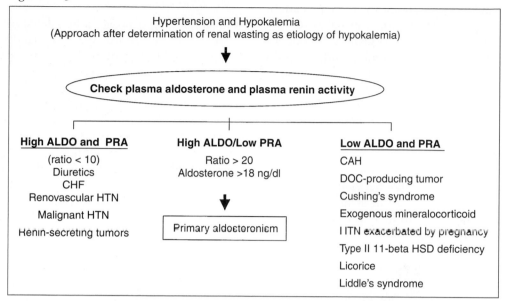

Evaluation of the patient with hypertension and hypokalemia. Abbreviations: ALDO, aldosterone; PRA, plasma renin activity; CAH, congenital adrenal hyperplasia; DOC, deoxycorticosterone; HSD, hydroxysteroid dehydrogenase.

before and after saline infusion (2 L over 4 hours). A positive test is the failure to lower plasma aldosterone levels to less than 10 ng/dL. Several other techniques are available to confirm the presence of autonomous aldosterone production (*fluodrocortisone* suppression test, captopril, or furosemide-stimulated plasma renin and aldosterone), but we find the two former tests the easiest and safest to perform in clinical practice.

Once the diagnosis of autonomous production of aldosterone is made, the next step is subtype differentiation. Imaging of the adrenal glands with thin-cut adrenal computed tomography is the principal means of distinguishing between the two main causes of primary aldosteronism, APA, and idiopathic bilateral adrenal hyperplasia (IAH). Adenomas were traditionally responsible for 70% of cases, but more recent data reveal a change in prevalence related to the more frequent diagnosis of milder cases, among which IAH is the most common cause. Therefore, current trends show IAH being at least as common

as APA. Aldosterone-producing adenoma is almost always unilateral and presents as a nodule generally smaller than 3 cm (Figure 21.4). Adrenal CT scans or magnetic resonance imaging (MRIs)

Figure 21.4

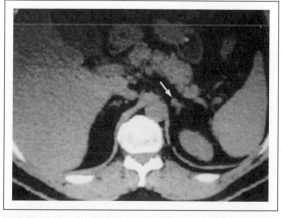

Radiologic appearance of an adrenal adenoma (arrow).

are able to detect lesions as small as 0.6 cm, and virtually all lesions larger than 1 cm can be detected by these techniques. Focal or diffuse hyperplasia of the ipsilateral gland is a common finding, while the contralateral gland is usually atrophic. In IAH imaging may be normal or show bilateral hyperplasia. Unfortunately, imaging may provide an incorrect diagnosis, especially because of the common occurrence of nonfunctional adrenal adenomas (*incidentalomas*), which may be present in as many as 4% of the general adult population. This has led many experts to argue for the necessity of plasma aldosterone measurement in samples obtained from adrenal veins (adrenal venous sampling [AVS]) to confirm the unilateral nature of the aldosterone hypersecretion (lateralization). This is the current gold standard for the differential diagnosis of APA and IAH. Because AVS is technically difficult and is fraught with possible complications, other "physiologic" methods are used in its place to help confirm the subtype. These include iodocholesterol adrenal scans (which we consider of little value), and biochemical tests including plasma 18-hydroxycorticosterone concentration (high in APA, normal in IAH), and the behavior of plasma aldosterone in response to 2 hours in the upright position (normal increase in IAH, paradoxical decrease in APA). Figure 21.5 summarizes the sequential approach to the diagnosis of primary aldosteronism.

Treatment

Unilateral laparoscopic adrenalectomy is the treatment of choice for APA. It cures the hypertension in 30–60% of cases. Cures are more common in younger patients with shorter duration of HTN and less severe HTN prior to intervention. Hypokalemia uniformly resolves after adrenalectomy.

Mineralocorticoid receptor blockers are the treatment of choice for IAH. Spironolactone has been used for many years and has an excellent track record in the control of HTN and hypokalemia in patients with IAH. Due to antagonism of androgen and progesterone receptors, however, spironolactone is often poorly tolerated, especially in men, in whom it may cause breast pain, gynecomastia, and decreased libido. Eplererone is a new mineralocorticoid receptor antagonist with minimal affinity for androgen and progesterone receptors, and no sexual or antiandrogenic side effects. Therefore, eplererone is a promising option for the treatment of mineralocorticoid-dependent HTN.

KEY POINTS
Primary Aldosteronism

1. Hypertension and hypokalemia due to renal potassium wasting suggests primary aldosteronism.
2. The sequential approach to primary aldosteronism consists of screening (plasma aldosterone to renin ratio), confirmation of autonomous production (salt-loading tests), and subtype differentiation (adrenal imaging and physiologic testing).
3. Plasma aldosterone concentration to plasma renin activity ratio greater than 20 is the best screen for primary aldosteronism.
4. Laparoscopic adrenalectomy is the treatment for aldosterone-producing adenomas.
5. Mineralocorticoid receptor blockers are the treatment for idiopathic adrenal hyperplasia.

Figure 21.5

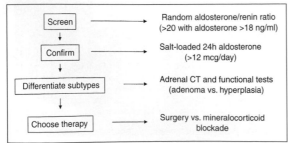

Summary of the clinical approach to primary aldosteronism.

Pheochromocytoma

Pheochromocytomas are catecholamine-producing tumors that develop from chromaffin cells of the adrenal medulla or sympathetic ganglia (extra-adrenal pheochromocytoma). Pheochromocytoma is a rare cause of secondary HTN, with an estimated incidence of 1 in 20,000 hypertensive patients each year. Because they are potentially fatal, however, they should be considered in all hypertensive patients. Approximately 10% of all pheochromocytomas are associated with familial syndromes, which include multiple endocrine neoplasia type 2 (MEN2a: pheochromocytoma, medullary thyroid carcinoma, and parathyroid adenoma; MEN2b: pheochromocytoma, medullary thyroid carcinoma, and mucocutaneous neuromas), von Hippel-Lindau's syndrome (retinal and/or cerebellar hemangioblastoma, renal cell carcinoma), and von Recklinghausen's disease (neurofibromatosis). Histologically, most pheochromocytomas are benign, though malignancy can occur in 10% of cases, more frequently among extraadrenal pheochromocytomas.

Pathogenesis

Most adrenal pheochromocytomas secrete epinephrine, whereas extraadrenal pheochromocytomas secrete predominantly norepinephrine. Most clinical manifestations of pheochromocytomas are caused by activation of adrenergic receptors by circulating catecholamines. In addition, there is an elevation of baseline sympathetic tone in this disease, which may explain the poor correlation between catecholamine concentrations and HTN in pheochromocytoma. Neuropeptide Y concentrations are increased in plasma and tumors of patients with pheochromocytoma. This transmitter has direct and indirect (potentiates norepinephrine) vasoconstricting effect on small arterioles. Lastly, it is important to remember that chronic elevation in sympathetic activity may lead to renal microvascular injury and sodium retention, which is part of the mechanisms of HTN in pheochromocytoma.

Diagnosis

A myriad of symptoms and signs related to catecholamine release may be present in patients with pheochromocytoma. The most common symptoms are episodes of intense headache, palpitations, and diaphoresis. This triad in a hypertensive patient has a sensitivity of 91% and a specificity of 94% for the diagnosis of pheochromocytoma. The major differential diagnosis is with anxiety and panic attacks and the use of exogenous sympathomimetic drugs. "Classic" cases have paroxysmal HTN with interspersed periods of normotension. Sustained HTN with or without superimposed paroxysms, however, is the most common presentation (about two-thirds of all cases). Paroxysms are triggered by a number of stimuli including exercise, smoking, urination, defecation, palpation of the abdomen, induction of anesthesia, or the use of drugs that affect catecholamine metabolism (worsening HTN after initiation of a β-blocker is a classic presentation). Rarely, patients with a predominantly epinephrine-secreting pheochromocytoma may present with paroxysmal hypotension rather than hypertension. This does not occur with norepinephrine-secreting tumors.

Biochemical tests are used to demonstrate catecholamine production by the tumor. The determination of plasma-free metanephrine concentrations, plasma catecholamine concentrations, urine fractionated and total metanephrines, urine catecholamines, and urine vanillylmandelic acid have been used, usually in combination. Plasma-free metanephrines and normetanephrines have excellent sensitivity and specificity with the convenience of a single blood draw and no specific requirements to stop medications. In fact, the only relevant interactions are with acetaminophen, which should not be used for 24 hours prior to testing, tricyclic antidepressants and phenoxybenzamine. Urine tests perform just as well but are more time demanding and affected by drug use (most commonly tricyclic antidepressants, β-blockers, and clonidine). Urine collections are particularly useful in patients with paroxysmal symptoms. It is useful to give these patients a collection bottle to take home with instruction to start a collection immediately following a paroxysm. This approach maximizes the likelihood of identifying excessive catecholamine production. Provocative (glucagon or histamine) or suppression (clonidine) tests may be used in patients with borderline levels. The clonidine suppression test is most commonly used, as provocative tests expose the patient to an unwarranted risk of severe hypertension and tachycardia.

Once the biochemical diagnosis is made, the next step is localization of the tumor. Both CT and MRI have high sensitivity, but they have low specificity due to the common presence of adrenal tumors. Most pheochromocytomas (about 95%) are found within the abdomen, but the possibility of multiple sites justifies the use of extensive scanning. An MRI from the neck to the pelvis (to include the bladder) is the initial imaging of choice; a CT scan is an alternative. Extraadrenal tumors are predominant in patients younger than 20 years old. Bilateral adrenal tumors occur more frequently in patients with familial tumors. A scintigraphy using ^{121}I- or ^{131}I-labeled metaiodobenzylguanidine (MIBG) should be obtained in patients with abnormal hormonal tests but a negative MRI. It will show increased uptake at the site of the tumor (or tumors if multicentric).

Treatment

The treatment of choice is surgical resection. In a hypertensive crisis the nonselective α-adrenergic blocker phentolamine should be used intravenously for BP control. All patients should receive medical therapy with oral phenoxybenzamine before surgery to avoid a hypertensive

emergency at the time of manipulation of the tumor.

Patients who cannot be treated by surgery receive chronic medical therapy. Long-term therapy with the nonspecific α-adrenergic blocker phenoxybenzamine or with the α_1-receptor blockers prazosin, terazosin, or doxazosin is the cornerstone of treatment. Tachycardia is a common side effect of phenoxybenzamine that demands the association of a β-blocker. β-blockers should be started only after α-blockade is established. Blood pressure and symptoms may be controlled by calcium channel antagonists.

KEY POINTS

Pheochromocytoma

1. Pheochromocytoma is characterized by episodes of HTN along with intense headache, palpitations, and diaphoresis.
2. Most cases have sustained hypertension with or without superimposed paroxysms.
3. Measurements of plasma and/or urinary catecholamines and/or their metabolites are used to confirm the diagnosis of pheochromocytoma.
4. Although most pheochromocytomas are intrabdominal, extended scanning is recommended to rule out extrabdominal sites.

Cushing's Syndrome

Cushing's syndrome is the result of excessive production of cortisol. The overproduction of adrenocorticotropic hormone (ACTH) by a pituitary adenoma is the most common form of the disease and is called Cushing's disease. Tumors of diverse origins and locations may secrete ectopic ACTH and cause Cushing's syndrome, most commonly lung carcinomas. ACTH-independent excessive cortisol secretion may be caused by adrenal adenomas and carcinomas. HTN is present in approximately 80% of patients with Cushing's syndrome. Because several other clinical features of the syndrome are more prominent, however, HTN rarely is the reason for investigation of the disease.

Pathophysiology

HTN in Cushing's syndrome is the result of sodium and fluid retention due to the mineralocorticoid action of cortisol. When present in high concentrations, cortisol saturates the enzyme type II 11β-hydroxysteroid dehydrogenase that converts cortisol to the inactive cortisone. As this enzyme system is saturated, more cortisol becomes available for activation of the mineralocorticoid receptor, which results in sodium avidity and volume expansion.

Diagnosis

Patients with Cushing's syndrome may display truncal obesity, the typical moon facies, facial plethora, purple skin striae, hirsutism, muscle weakness and fatigue, and wide mood swings. Glucose intolerance, amenorrhea, impotence, and decreased libido may also be present. Patients with Cushing's syndrome caused by ectopic ACTH secretion may have severe hypokalemia.

The laboratory diagnosis is first made by measurement of 24-hour urine free cortisol. This test has a high sensitivity, but false-positive results may occur in stress, obesity, alcohol abuse, and psychiatric disorders, especially depression. The overnight suppression test with a single dose of dexamethasone (1 mg) is a useful screening test to augment the specificity of urinary cortisol determination. Low-dose and high-dose dexamethasone tests are confirmatory tests that may also help to distinguish adrenal from pituitary cases. CT scan or MRI of the pituitary and adrenal glands add to the hormonal diagnosis to localize the causative tumor.

Treatment

The treatment of choice is surgical removal of the tumor. For Cushing's disease, transsphenoidal adenomectomy is the most common procedure, but in some cases total hypophysectomy may be necessary. Unilateral or bilateral adrenalectomy is performed for adrenal tumors. Chemotherapy may be necessary for malignant tumors. Drug therapy may be used before surgery, in failure of surgical treatment, and as a palliative treatment for incurable malignant tumors. Drug approaches may target different aspects of the disease, such as decreasing ACTH secretion (serotonin antagonists, dopamine agonists, gamma aminobutyric acid agonists, and somatostatin analogues), suppressing adrenocortical steroid synthesis (aminoglutethimide, etomidate, ketoconazole, metyrapone, mitotane, and trilostane), or antagonizing glucocorticoids on a receptor level (mifepristone).

KEY POINTS
Cushing's Syndrome

1. Increased production of ACTH by a pituitary adenoma is the most common cause of Cushing's syndrome.
2. Truncal obesity, moon facies and facial plethora, hirsutism, and purple skin striae are physical signs that suggest Cushing's syndrome.
3. Determination of 24-hour urine free cortisol is the diagnostic test of choice.

Thyroid and Parathyroid Disorders

Thyroid hormone has effects on the cardiovascular system and blood pressure regulation. HTN may be observed both in hypothyroidism and hyper-thyroidism, but the characteristics of the blood pressure profile differ with the metabolic disorder. The prevalence of HTN in hypothyroidism is high (~40%). Hypertension is predominantly diastolic and is associated with increased systemic vascular resistance and decreased arterial compliance. The decreased cardiac output of hypothyroidism may result in a narrowed pulse pressure. HTN in hyper-thyroidism is primarily systolic and is related to an increased cardiac output. Vascular resistance is decreased in hyperthyroidism, which results in a wide pulse pressure. Specific treatments for each thyroid disturbance are sufficient to normalize blood pressure in most patients.

HTN is commonly present in primary hyper-parathyroidism (prevalence as high as 70%). Increased cytosolic calcium resulting in increased vascular resistance and cardiac output would be rational pathogenetic mechanisms for the elevated BP. No correlation between calcium or parathy-roid hormone concentrations and blood pressure, however, are found in these patients. Removal of the adenoma-related gland cures or improves BP in most hypertensive hyperparathyroid patients.

KEY POINTS
Thyroid and Parathyroid Disorders

1. Hypertension is predominantly diastolic in hypothyroidism, whereas systolic HTN pre-dominates in hyperthyroidism.
2. Hypertension is frequent in hyperparathy-roidism, and is unrelated to serum calcium and parathyroid hormone concentrations.

Coarctation of the Aorta

Coarctation of the aorta is a constriction of the descending thoracic aorta, most commonly distal to the left subclavian artery. It is a relatively common congenital malformation (~7% of all congenital heart disease), but an unusual cause of HTN in the adult. The classic findings are HTN in the arms, diminished femoral pulses, and low arterial blood pressure in the lower extremities.

HTN in the upper extremities is a consequence of the mechanical obstruction to blood flow. Furthermore, renal ischemia may cause activation of the RAAS. Headache, chest pain, and pain in the legs with exercise are symptoms of coarcta-tion of the aorta, but many patients may be asymptomatic, particularly when the constriction is small. A systolic murmur may be heard on chest examination.

The chest radiography can show the "3 sign" appearance of the left superior mediastinal border representing the pre- and poststenotic dilation of the aorta separated by the indentation represented by the constriction itself. Notching of the ribs of the posterior lower aspect of the third to eighth ribs due to erosion by the large collateral arteries can be observed as well. Magnetic resonance imaging can define the loca-tion and severity of coarctation, which decreases the need for angiography for diagnostic purposes. Echocardiography is an alternative method to make the diagnosis and assess disease severity, though not as precise as magnetic resonance. Surgery is the preferred treatment, although there is growing experience with balloon angio-plasty with or without stenting as a viable alter-native, especially in individuals with high surgical risk.

KEY POINTS
Coarctation of the Aorta

1. Hypertension in the upper extremities along with low blood pressure in the lower extremities are the characteristic findings in coarctation of the aorta.
2. Magnetic resonance imaging or echocardio-graphy can be used to confirm the diagnosis.

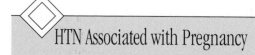

HTN Associated with Pregnancy

Hypertensive disease of pregnancy is one of the most important causes of maternal and perinatal mortality. Hypertension in pregnancy is also associated with prematurity and intrauterine growth retardation. The incidence of HTN in the first pregnancy is estimated to be 10%. Patients who are hypertensive before pregnancy or develop HTN before the 20th week of gestation are more likely to have HTN due to causes other than a hypertensive disorder of pregnancy.

Preeclampsia and Eclampsia

Preeclampsia is a syndrome where HTN is diagnosed for the first time after the 20th week of gestation along with proteinuria of at least 0.3 g/24 hours. It occurs in about 5% of pregnancies and affects predominantly nulliparas. Eclampsia is the syndrome of hypertension and seizures, usually occurring as a progression of preeclampsia, though 20% of eclamptic women do not have proteinuria. Decreased placental perfusion is the key mechanism of preeclampsia. It is caused by impaired endovascular trophoblastic migration and invasion. Recent data show that soluble fms-like tyrosine kinase 1 (sFlt-1), a circulating antiangiogenic protein, is increased in the placenta and serum of women with preeclampsia. This protein acts by adhering to the receptor-binding domains of placental growth factor and vascular endothelial growth factor, preventing their interaction with endothelial receptors on the cell surface and thereby inducing endothelial dysfunction. Differently from normal pregnant women, preeclamptic women are hyperresponsive to vasoactive agents such as angiotensin II and norepinephrine, and there are abnormalities in vasoactive substances such as nitric oxide, relaxin, and endothelin-1. Hypertension in preeclampsia is marked by increased peripheral resistance. The characteristic renal lesion in preeclampsia is glomerular endotheliosis. The glomeruli are enlarged with hypertrophy and swelling of the glomerular endothelial cells. Intravascular coagulation may be present in severe preeclampsia. HELLP syndrome (*h*emolysis, *e*levated *l*iver enzymes, *l*ow *p*latelet count) is a serious complication of preeclampsia.

The diagnosis of preeclampia is clinical. HTN in late gestation is defined as blood pressure levels of ≥140/90 mmHg. Proteinuria of 300 mg or more may be detected in a 24-hour urine collection. The protein-creatinine ratio in a random urine sample may estimate proteinuria and substitute for the 24-hour urine collection. Most cases resolve within 6–12 weeks following delivery.

Chronic and Transient HTN of Pregnancy

Hypertension diagnosed before the 20th week of pregnancy is usually a preexisting condition and not a specific complication of pregnancy. Preexisting HTN predisposes to preeclampsia. If HTN is diagnosed for the first time after the 20th week of pregnancy, without proteinuria, and the blood pressure normalizes postpartum, the diagnosis is transient HTN of pregnancy. The pathogenesis of this disorder is not well understood, and these patients have higher rates of HTN later in life.

Overview of HTN Treatment in Pregnancy

Treatment of HTN in pregnancy requires a tight balance between protection of the mother from elevated BP and preserved perfusion of the fetoplacental unit. In addition, concerns about fetotoxicity of different drugs dictate the use of time-honored therapies and avoidance of certain agents. Methyldopa is the drug of choice for chronic control of BP due to its long track record of safety in pregnancy. Alternatives include β-blockers (especially atenolol), combined α-β-blockers (especially labetalol), calcium channel blockers (especially nifedipine), and hydralazine. Diuretics are relatively contraindicated because they may induce volume depletion and electrolyte imbalance, but should be used whenever volume overload is present. Angiotensin-converting enzyme inhibitors are associated with a specific fetopathy and fetal death due to second and third trimester exposure and their use is contraindicated in pregnancy. Similar concerns apply to angiotensin II receptor blockers. It is important to remember that pregnant women with recent exposure to HTN are more susceptible to target-organ damage at lower BP levels. It is well established that BP levels as low as 170/110 mmHg can be associated with intracerebral hemorrhage in pregnancy, and BPs above this threshold are considered an emergency in the setting of pregnancy. In such situations, intravenous hydralazine is the drug of choice, though intravenous labetalol is a useful alternative. Fetal delivery is the specific treatment for pregnancy-induced HTN. Magnesium sulfate is indicated to control seizure activity in eclampsia.

KEY POINTS

HTN Associated with Pregnancy

1. Hypertension in preeclampsia is diagnosed after the 20th week of gestation.
2. Hypertension before pregnancy predisposes to preeclampsia.
3. Treatment of HTN in pregnancy requires a tight balance between protection of the mother from elevated BP values and preserved perfusion of the fetoplacental unit.
4. Methyldopa is the time-honored drug of choice in the management of HTN in pregnancy.

Inherited Renal Tubular Disorders

These are rare causes of HTN characterized by increased renal sodium reabsorption as a result of single gene mutations. They are useful to illustrate the role of the kidney in the pathogenesis of HTN (see Chapter 20). Though not actual secondary causes of HTN, they are discussed in this chapter due to the unique nature of their clinical presentations.

Glucocorticoid Remediable Aldosteronism (GRA)

Glucocorticoid remediable aldosteronism is an inherited autosomal-dominant disorder that imitates adrenal hyperplasia. Onset of HTN is in childhood with normal or elevated aldosterone concentration along with suppressed plasma renin activity. Marked HTN complicated by cerebral hemorrhage are hallmarks of this condition, whereas hypokalemia is not a prominent finding. Glucocorticoid remediable aldosteronism is caused by a gene duplication arising by unequal crossing over between two genes that lie next to one another on human chromosome 8. The genes encode aldosterone synthase and 11β-hydroxylase. The resulting hybrid gene encodes the ectopic expression of aldosterone synthase in the zona fasciculata. Its activity is thus regulated by ACTH rather than angiotensin II; therefore, administration of a glucocorticoid suppresses ACTH production and results in decreased aldosterone secretion. This is used as a diagnostic and therapeutic test. There is also increased excretion of 18-oxocortisol and 18-hydroxycortisol in the urine. Specific genetic diagnosis is made by the identification of the chimeric gene. Suppression of ACTH with exogenous glucocorticoid can be used as treatment, although most patients respond well to mineralocorticoid receptor antagonists or amiloride, and these drugs are the cornerstone of the chronic management of HTN in these patients.

Apparent Mineralocorticoid Excess (AME)

AME is a rare autosomal recessive disease. Affected individuals show impaired conversion of cortisol to the inactive cortisone due to absence of the enzyme 11β-hydroxysteroid dehydrogenase type II due to mutations of its gene on chromosome 16. In vitro, cortisol activates the mineralocorticoid receptor with potency similar to that of aldosterone. Therefore, normal subjects are protected from the mineralocorticoid effects of cortisol by the action of type II 11β-hydroxysteroid dehydrogenase. In its absence, there is a marked increase in the availability of cortisol in target epithelia (especially kidney) resulting in an "apparent" mineralocorticoid excess. Similar results are produced by licorice (glycyrrhizic acid), which inhibits the enzyme, and Cushing's syndrome, which results in overwhelming the enzyme system. The clinical features are the onset of HTN early in life, hypokalemia, metabolic alkalosis, low plasma renin activity, and suppressed aldosterone. Mineralocorticoid receptor blockers are the best treatment for patients with preserved renal function. Renal transplantation cures the disease.

Liddle's Syndrome

Liddle's syndrome is an autosomal-dominant disorder. There is a mutation in one of the genes in chromosome 16 coding for the β or γ subunits of the epithelial sodium channel. These mutations lead to a reduction in the clearance of sodium channels from the cell surface. The result is sodium retention, early-onset HTN, hypokalemia, metabolic alkalosis, suppressed plasma renin activity, and low plasma aldosterone concentration. It responds well to amiloride.

HTN Exacerbated in Pregnancy

This is an autosomal-dominant form of early-onset HTN that is exacerbated during pregnancy. It is caused by a mutation of the mineralocorticoid receptor, and compounds that normally bind but do not activate the mineralocorticoid receptor are potent agonists of the mutant receptor, particularly

progesterone. As progesterone concentration increases more than 100-fold in pregnancy, patients with this mutation develop accelerated HTN during pregnancy. No specific treatment is available. Spironolactone, however, has an activating effect on the mutant receptor, and may paradoxically result in worsening hypertension in these patients and should be avoided.

Gordon's Syndrome (Pseudohypoaldosteronism Type 2)

This is an autosomal-dominant syndrome caused by mutations in genes coding for the serine-threonine kinases WNK1 and WNK4, which result in enhanced sodium and chloride reabsorption via increased activity of the thiazide-sensitive Na-Cl cotransporter. Potassium secretion is reduced due to decreased activity of the ROMK potassium channel. The syndrome is characterized by HTN, suppression of the RAAS, and hyperkalemia. The phenotype is completely corrected by the administration of thiazide diuretics.

Congenital Adrenal Hyperplasia (CAH)

CAH can be caused by mutations in the genes coding for the 17α-hydroxylase or the 11β-hydroxylase enzymes, whose expression is deficient. Both are autosomal recessive disorders that present early in life in females with virilization and hypertension. Affected males have signs of hyperandrogenism such as acne, infantilism, and phallus enlargement. Hypokalemia is a rare finding. The underlying pathogenesis of the HTN involves feedback activation of ACTH leading to increased deoxycorticosterone (DOC), which in turn stimulates the mineralocorticoid receptor and produces HTN. Because of this DOC effect, CAH patients have suppressed renin and aldosterone levels. Treatment consists of glucocorticoid use to shut down ACTH production and normalize androgen and DOC production.

Patients with residual HTN respond well to mineralocorticoid receptor antagonists.

KEY POINTS
Inherited Renal Tubular Disorders

> 1. Mutations of a single gene that provoke increased sodium reabsorption are causes of HTN.

Additional Reading

Bravo, E.L., Tagle, R. Pheochromocytoma: state-of-the-art and future prospects. *Endocr Rev* 24:539–553, 2003.

Chemaitilly, W., Wilson, R.C., New M.I. Hypertension and adrenal disorders. *Curr Hypertens Rep* 5:498–504, 2003.

Danzi, S., Klein, I. Thyroid hormone and blood pressure regulation. *Curr Hypertens Rep* 5:513–520, 2003.

JNC 7 guidelines. (Complete version). Chobanian, A.V., Bakris, G.B., Black, H.R., et al. Seventh report of the Joint National Committee on Prevention, Detection, Evaluation, and Treatment of High Blood Pressure. *Hypertension* 42:1206–1252, 2003.

JNC 7 guidelines. (Summary version). Chobanian, A.V., Bakris, G.B., Black, H.R., et al. The Seventh Report of the Joint National Committee on Prevention, Detection, Evaluation, and Treatment of High Blood Pressure: the JNC 7 report. *JAMA* 289:2560–2572, 2003.

Lenders, J.W., Pacak, K, Walther, M.M., et al. Biochemical diagnosis of pheochromocytoma: which test is best? *JAMA* 287:1427–1434, 2002.

Lifton, R.P., Gharavi, A.G., Geller, D.S. Molecular mechanisms of human HTN. *Cell* 104:545–556, 2001.

Mansoor, G.A. Herbs and alternative therapies in the hypertension clinic. *Am J Hypertens* 14:971–975, 2001.

Myers, J.E., Baker, P.N. Hypertensive diseases and eclampsia. *Curr Opin Obstet Gynecol* 14:119–125, 2002.

Safian, R.D., Textor, S.C. Renal-artery stenosis. *N Engl J Med* 344:431–442, 2001.

Shamsuzzaman, A.S., Gersh, B.J., Somers, V.K. Obstructive sleep apnea: implications for cardiac and vascular disease. *JAMA* 290:1906–1914, 2003.

Young, W.F. Jr. Minireview: primary aldosteronism-changing concepts in diagnosis and treatment. *Endocrinology* 144:2208–2213, 2003.

Richard Formica

Urinary Tract Infection

Recommended Time to Complete: 1 day

Guiding Questions

1. How has the epidemiology of urinary tract infections (UTIs) changed?

2. What are the differences between asymptomatic bacteriuria, cystitis, and pyelonephritis?

3. What distinguishes an uncomplicated UTI from a complicated UTI and how do treatments vary?

4. Are particular patient populations at increased risk for UTI and are adverse outcomes a concern?

5. What is the pathogenesis of UTI?

6. What impact does bacterial antibiotic resistance have on UTI?

7. What are two important types of complicated renal infections?

Introduction

UTIs are one of the most common bacterial infections in the United States. The clinical presentation ranges from completely asymptomatic to septic shock. All ages are affected and certain subgroups of the population are particularly vulnerable.

A national survey in the mid-1990s estimated that UTIs resulted in seven million office visits, one million emergency department visits, and 100,000 hospital admissions per year. It is an illness that primarily affects women. One in three women by age 24 are treated with antibiotics for a UTI, and 50% of women have UTI symptoms at some point in their life. The incidence of UTI throughout life is shown in Figure 22.1. Early in life (circle 1) females are at higher risk than males due largely

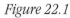
Figure 22.1

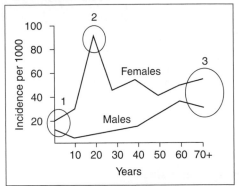

Incidence of UTI in the general population throughout life. Circles 1, 2, and 3 highlight three periods of urinary tract infection in life.

the bladder trigone occurs with cystitis. Pain on defecation results from compression of the inflamed prostate. Finally, patients may report symptoms of systemic infection such as fever, rigors, malaise, nausea, vomiting, general muscle and joint ache, and lassitude. These symptoms suggest a blood-borne bacterial infection. Nausea and vomiting are also the result of increased vagal activity because vagal nerve fibers innervate the renal capsule, as well as the stomach. Stretching of the capsule is sensed as gastric distention and triggers nausea and vomiting.

Site of Infection

The urinary tract is composed of the kidney and ureters, bladder, prostate and epididymis in men, and urethra. Infection in any of these results in the above symptoms and causes the patient to seek medical attention. It is important to accurately diagnose the site of infection, as the type and duration of therapy differs.

The most common form of UTI in both men and women is cystitis. There is a distinction between asymptomatic bacteriuria and a symptomatic infection of the bladder or cystitis. The patient with asymptomatic bacteriuria has a sufficient number of bacteria to be consistent with infection, greater that 10^5 colony forming units (CFU)/mL of a pathogenic bacteria, but no symptoms. Asymptomatic bacteriuria requires therapy only in specific patient populations. Cystitis refers to a symptomatic bladder infection that in addition to having a significant number of urinary bacteria is associated with dysuria, lower abdominal cramping, urinary frequency, and urgency. Cystitis is not associated with fever. If fever is present an invasive tissue infection exists. This implies infection of the renal parenchyma and is referred to as pyelonephritis.

When discussing cystitis or any infection of urinary tract components, it is useful to think in terms of uncomplicated versus complicated infection. Criteria that define a complicated UTI are shown in Table 22.1. An uncomplicated

to ureteral reflux. During the reproductive years women are at much higher risk than men (circle 2). With advancing age (circle 3) the gap narrows as the incidence of UTI in men increases due to benign prostatic hyperplasia. The term UTI in this chapter refers generically to an infection in any of the components of the urinary tract—kidney, bladder, prostate, and urethra. Each is discussed individually. Additionally, UTI is referred to as uncomplicated or complicated depending on the presence of risk factors that predispose the patient to an adverse outcome.

Symptoms and Signs

UTI refers to bacterial infection of the urinary tract. Patients, however, present with symptoms referable to the site and nature of infection. They complain of urinary frequency and urgency resulting from spontaneous bladder contractions due to irritation of the trigone. Dysuria is caused by inflammation of the urethra that causes pain or a burning sensation when further irritated by urine. Flank pain results from stretching and irritation of the renal capsule that causes pain in the area of the costovertebral angle. Irritation of

do not mention vaginal symptoms spontaneously and, therefore, should be questioned specifically. As with urethritis, a negative urine for leukocytes and a negative culture should raise suspicion of this diagnosis.

KEY POINTS
Urinary Tract Infection

1. Infections in different locations within the urinary tract present with similar symptoms.
2. Fever in a patient with UTI means tissue invasive infection.
3. The duration of therapy and the pathogens responsible for UTI are different in uncomplicated and complicated UTI.
4. Infection of the urinary tract with *Staphylococcus aureus* requires evaluation for a hematogenous source of infection.

Risk Factors for and Pathogenesis of UTI

Patient-Specific Factors

In order for a UTI to occur bacteria must first gain access to the urogenital system. This happens through introduction into the urethra during sexual intercourse or insertion of urinary catheters or other objects. The exception to this rule is infection with *Staphylococcus aureus* that results from hematogenous spread. Infection of the urinary tract with *Staphylococcus aureus* should prompt a search for an endovascular infection. Women are at greater risk for UTI because the vaginal introitus can become colonized with fecal bacteria. Use of spermacides and diaphragms increase the risk of UTI by altering the vaginal

flora and allowing overgrowth of pathogenic bacteria. Sexual intercourse mechanically introduces bacteria into the bladder. Men are at low risk for UTI compared to women because the periurethral environment is drier and not colonized by bacteria, their urethra is longer, and prostatic fluid contains antibacterial substances.

Once in the bladder, inadequate emptying of the bladder, as occurs with prostatism or patients with neurogenic bladder allows bacteria to multiply. This is illustrated in Figure 22.3. With small residual volumes (1 mL), over time, bacteria are cleared from the bladder. As the residual volume increases (8 mL), this is no longer the case. Anatomic abnormalities or nephrolithiasis provide sites for bacterial adherence and prevent expulsion. Why one individual is susceptible to UTI while another is not is dependent on genetic, biologic, and behavioral factors shown in Table 22.2. Women with recurrent UTIs have three times more *Escherichia coli* adhering to vaginal, buccal, and voided uroepithelial cells. Additionally, uropathogenic *Escherichia coli* can colonize the colon. Previous antibiotic use can alter protective vaginal and perineal flora and allow overgrowth of pathogenic organisms.

Figure 22.3

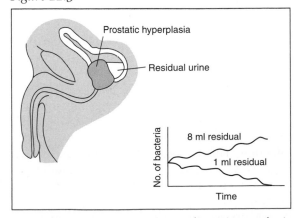

Urinary retention and UTI. Urinary obstruction results in incomplete emptying of the bladder. The presence of residual urine prevents clearance of organisms from the bladder and allows bacteria to multiply.

Table 22.2

Inherited or Acquired Host Susceptibility Factors for UTI

GENETIC	BIOLOGIC	BEHAVIORAL	OTHER
Blood group antigen	Congenital abnormalities	Sexual intercourse	Decreased mental status
Nonsecretor status	Urinary obstruction	Use of diaphragm	
Increased adhesion receptors	Calculi	Use of spermicides	
	Diabetes mellitus	Antimicrobial use	
	Anatomic abnormalities		
	Residual urine		
	Atrophic vaginitis		
	Urinary incontinence		
	Prior history of UTI		
	Maternal history of UTI		
	Childhood history of UTI		
	Catheters/stents/ foreign bodies		
	Condom catheters		
	Immunologic abnormalities (HIV)		
	Renal transplant		

Abbreviations: UTI, urinary tract infection; HIV, human immunodeficiency virus. Modified from Ronald, A. *Am J Med* 113:14S–19S, 2002 with permission.

Pathogen-Specific Factors

Bacteria contain virulence factors that contribute to pathogenicity. The primary virulence factor is the ability of bacteria to adhere to cell surfaces. It is important to note that microbial virulence is not related to antimicrobial resistance. The most adherent bacteria, unless acquired in the hospital setting, are sensitive to antibiotics. Bacteria that do not have an adhesion system do not cause infection. This is because enteric bacteria have negatively charged cell surfaces and are, therefore, repelled by the negatively charged cell membrane. The primary adhesion system used by bacteria is adhesins, which are lectin molecules located on their fimbriae. Adhesins bind oligosaccharides on epithelial cell surfaces and mediate internalization of bacteria into epithelial cells, where they replicate avoiding the host immune system. Other virulence factors include flagella that are necessary for motility and the production of an enzyme, hemolysin, that forms pores in the cell membrane. These pores allow bacteria to gain access to the cytosol of the renal epithelial cell where they multiply in an environment shielded from local defense mechanisms. Finally, the presence of aerobactin, which is necessary for iron acquisition, is an additional virulence factor. Iron is responsible for many processes in bacteria including upregulation of genes that enhance virulence and the formation of superoxides that degrade cell walls.

A virulence factor unique to *Proteus mirabilis* is urease. This enzyme converts urea into ammonia and carbon dioxide. The ammonia buffers hydrogen ions in the urine increasing pH. The alkaline pH results in the precipitation of phosphate, carbonate, and magnesium forming struvite stones. These stones allow *Proteus mirabilis* to colonize the genitourinary tract and cause obstruction and urinary stasis further promoting bacterial multiplication.

KEY POINTS
Risk Factors for and Pathogenesis of UTI

1. Patient-specific risk factors for UTI can be modified to decrease the incidence of infection.
2. Pathogen-specific virulence factors are not the cause of antibiotic resistance.

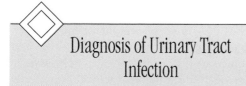

Diagnosis of Urinary Tract Infection

The diagnosis of UTI is based on the history and a few simple laboratory tests. In men the symptoms of dysuria (pain or difficulty on urinating), frequency (frequent voiding of small amounts of urine), and hematuria (presence of blood in the urine) is relatively diagnostic of UTI. Other diagnoses to consider are prostratitis and urethritis. A diagnosis of acute prostatitis is made when signs and symptoms of UTI are present and there is prostate tenderness on rectal examination.

The physical examination in the evaluation of a patient with UTI is of limited value. As stated above, tenderness on prostate examination aids in differentiating prostatitis from cystitis. Additionally, palpation of the lower abdomen can reproduce symptoms in cystitis helping to confirm the clinical suspicion of cystitis as opposed to urethritis. Finally, eliciting tenderness over the costovertebral angle suggests that if pyelonephritis is present inflammation in the kidney is severe enough to result in significant capsular swelling.

Laboratory Examination

Laboratory examination is usually limited to the urinalysis. In an uncomplicated UTI the presence of pyuria and bacteriuria makes the diagnosis. A urine culture and sensitivity is obtained for any patient with a fever or a patient meeting criteria for complicated UTI. Urine culture is the gold standard for diagnosing UTI. In a patient with symptoms suggesting UTI a quantitative urine culture of $\geq 10^2$ CFU/mL is highly sensitive (95%) and specific (85%). In an asymptomatic patient a quantitative culture of $\geq 10^5$ CFU/mL is considered diagnostic of UTI. The diagnosis of UTI is made when the proper signs and symptoms are present and there are leukocytes in the urine and a bacterial colony count of $\geq 10^5$ CFU/mL. It should be stressed that in the setting of a history of symptomatic UTI, if the colony count is $\leq 10^5$ CFU/mL the patient should still be treated. Other processes such as prostatitis or urethritis should be considered and are discussed below. The importance of the colony count is primarily in the setting of asymptomatic bacteriuria in a patient other than the pregnant woman. In the asymptomatic patient a risk-benefit decision must be made taking into account the potential for developing true infection versus exposure to unnecessary antibiotic therapy.

In a woman, the same symptoms are again suggestive of a UTI but the diagnoses of urethritis and vaginitis are more difficult to distinguish. A history of vaginal discharge strongly suggests a vaginal disorder, while its absence greatly increases the probability of UTI. The presence of hematuria on urinalysis directs the diagnosis toward UTI. In the nonpregnant woman, leukocyturia and bacteria cultured from the urine at $\geq 10^5$ CFU/mL confirms the diagnosis. In pregnancy, asymptomatic bacteriuria of $\leq 10^5$ CFU/mL is considered to represent an infection.

The diagnosis of chronic prostatitis is more difficult because symptoms are similar to cystitis. Complicating the diagnosis is the fact that bacteria within the bladder may be different than the bacteria causing infection within the prostate. In addition, bacteria in the bladder often outgrow prostatic bacteria. Therefore, it is necessary to perform a split urine collection. After cleaning the periurethral area, the patient voids an initial amount that is discarded and collects what would be considered a midstream collection. At this point, however, the patient is instructed to stop voiding prior to emptying the bladder and a prostatic massage is performed. Prostatic secretions are collected for culture and leukocyte count and the patient finishes voiding into a separate container. For a test to be positive, the midstream collection must have $\leq 10^3$ CFU/mL and the postmassage collection must have greater than 12 leukocytes per high power field. Bacterial cultures from prostatic secretions and postmassage urine guide antibiotic therapy.

The diagnosis of urethritis is made by a high index of suspicion and a sample from the urethra. *Chlamydia trachomatis* is diagnosed using a ligase chain reaction test performed on urine or urethral discharge. *Neisseria gonorrhoeae* is diagnosed through culture. A urethral swab is performed. The sample is taken several millimeters up the urethra and, therefore, a calcium alginate tip swab is used. The specimen is immediately plated onto room temperature culture medium such as Thayer-Martin agar.

KEY POINTS
Diagnosis of Urinary Tract Infection

1. For an uncomplicated patient, a history consistent with UTI and pyuria on urinalysis establishes the diagnosis.
2. For a complicated patient, a culture and sensitivity must be performed.

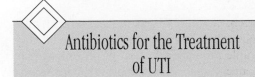

Antibiotics for the Treatment of UTI

The treatment of uncomplicated UTIs was straight forward until recently. This is because the causative agents, *Escherichia coli* and *Staphylococcus saprophyticus*, were largely sensitive to trimethoprim-sulfamethoxazole (TMP-SMX). Additionally, antibiotic concentrations in urine greatly exceed those in plasma. This made the concern about in vitro resistance at traditional serum minimal inhibitory concentrations (MICs) less relevant because a clinical cure could still be achieved. Therefore, empiric therapy with TMP-SMX 160/800 mg twice a day for 3 days resulted in both clinical and biologic cure and was the mainstay of therapy. At present resistance to β-lactam antibiotics, principally ampicillin and cephalothin, is too high, up to 40%, to recommend them for empiric therapy. Recently TMP-SMX resistance is increasing and approaches 20% in some regions of the country. This resulted in a shift in initial therapy.

Resistance to floroquinolones is very low, in the range of 1–2%. Ciprofloxacin is commonly used in a 3-day course for uncomplicated cystitis and a 7–14-day course for complicated cystitis or pyelonephritis. Gatifloxacin, a newer floroquinolone, has an advantage in that it has broader gram-positive organism coverage, can be administered once a day, has a urinary excretion rate of 70%, and it does not affect cytochrome P450-mediated metabolism. Gatifloxacin should be used with caution in diabetic patients as hypo- and hyperglycemic events were reported.

Resistance to nitrofurantoin remains low. It is used as a suppressive agent to prevent recurrent UTI at dose of 50–100 mg/day. It is especially useful in pregnancy because it has not been reported to be teratogenic. It can also be used as treatment for uncomplicated cystitis. Nitrofurantoin, however, does not achieve high enough serum concentrations to be employed for the treatment of acute pyelonephritis. Furthermore, it cannot be used in patients with chronic kidney disease.

Recurrent UTIs, which occur commonly in otherwise young healthy women, can be a source of considerable morbidity. As many as 27% develop a recurrence within 6 months of initial infection. These develop despite normal anatomy and physiology of the urinary system. Typical predisposing factors, such as urinary obstruction, bladder stones, and pregnancy need not be present. Most often, recurrent episodes represent reinfection (new infection after a cure) rather than relapse of a previously treated UTI. Factors associated with recurrent UTI include uropathogenic coliforms (p-fimbriated strains of *Escherichia coli*) that adhere to uroepithelial cells, frequent sexual intercourse and diaphragm-spermicide use, a short urethra, and the postmenopausal state. Once major anatomic problems are excluded, prevention is achieved through behavioral changes (reduced spermicide use, postcoital voiding), liberal fluid intake, and cranberry juice ingestion. Women who experience two or more symptomatic UTIs within 6 months or three or more over 12 months should receive antibiotic prophylaxis. Postcoital antibiotic prophylaxis or continuous prophylaxis (6 months duration) are effective but run the risk of antibiotic resistance developing over time.

The treatment of acute prostatitis, as distinct from chronic prostatitis, is based on the same principles as treating pyelonephritis. In most cases the patient is hospitalized because of systemic illness and broad-spectrum antibiotics are initiated until the causative agent is identified. The same precautions regarding antimicrobial resistance patterns apply as above. The inflamed prostate is freely permeable to antibiotics and in contrast to chronic prostatitis a variety of antimicrobial agents are used. The duration of therapy is 4–6 weeks in order to ensure that there are no bacterial foci remaining within the prostate.

Chronic prostatitis presents a therapeutic challenge because there is a barrier between the prostatic stroma and the microcirculation. This barrier is analogous to the blood-brain barrier formed by the meninges and makes passive diffusion the only route by which antibiotics can penetrate prostatic tissue. Therefore, only non-protein-bound, lipophilic drugs achieve therapeutic levels within the prostate. The two types of antibiotics that are effective in treating chronic prostatitis are the quinolones and trimethoprim-sulfamethoxazole. These antibiotics achieve predictable levels within the prostate and have excellent bioavailability, up to 80%, when administered orally. This is particularly advantageous because the duration of therapy must be 6–12 weeks to achieve durable results.

Treatment for urethritis is initiated empirically when the diagnosis is suspected prior to final culture results. Ceftriaxone (250 mg given intramuscularly as a one-time dose) will treat *Neisseria gonorrhoeae*. Doxycycline (100 mg orally twice a day for 7 days or azithromycin 1 gm given as a single oral dose) is equally effective at treating *Chlamydia trachomatis*. Both agents are also effective against *Ureaplasma urealyticum*.

KEY POINTS

Antibiotics for the Treatment of UTI

1. Antimicrobial-resistant bacteria are more common, therefore, broad-spectrum empiric coverage with a quinolone is appropriate.
2. In order to avoid inducing further antibiotic resistance, once culture and sensitivity results are available, antibiotic therapy is changed to the narrowest possible spectrum.

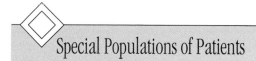

◇ Special Populations of Patients

Pregnant Women

Urinary tract infection in pregnancy, although occurring at only slightly increased frequency compared to similar age nonpregnant women, has a high morbidity. Bacteriuria complicates 6–7% of all pregnancies with multiparous women at highest risk. In pregnant women, UTI increases fetal morbidity and mortality. In a large study, bacteriuria and pyuria within 2 weeks of delivery resulted in a significant increase in perinatal mortality. Asymptomatic bacteriuria in pregnant women is associated with preterm deliveries and low birth weight and, therefore, must be treated.

Bacteria isolated from pregnant women with UTI and the virulence factors they possess are the same as those for the general population. This suggests that the mechanism by which bacteria gain access to the urinary tract is the same for pregnant women as for nonpregnant women. The hormonal milieu in pregnancy, however, results in smooth muscle relaxation and ureteral dilation that allows bacteria to reflux into the kidney. Therefore, if untreated up to 40% of patients with asymptomatic bacteria develop pyelonephritis. Because of this, cost-benefit analyses demonstrate that it is beneficial to screen pregnant women for asymptomatic bacteriuria.

For asymptomatic bacteriuria a 3-day course of antibiotics is effective. In pregnancy, penicillins and their derivatives are safe. Additionally, sulfonamides are safe with the exception of the last days of pregnancy and nitrofurantoin can also be used. Trimethoprim should be avoided. Floroquinolones and tetracycline are contraindicated.

KEY POINTS
Pregnant Women

> 1. Bacteriuria and UTI have negative consequences on the outcome of pregnancy.
> 2. All pregnant women must be treated.

The Spinal Cord Injury Patient

The spinal cord injury (SCI) patient averages 2.5 episodes of UTI and between 10 and 20 episodes of bacteriuria ($>10^5$ CFU/mL) per year. In this circumstance UTI refers to a true infection. There are many reasons for the increased risk and it is dependent on the level of the spinal cord injury and its effects on the normal micturition pattern. Spinal cord injury patients have impaired or absent micturition and often have chronic indwelling bladder catheters. For patients without catheter drainage, the increase in intravesicular pressure required to void causes reflux of contaminated urine into the renal collecting system and allows bacteria to seed the parenchyma. For patients with SCI vesicourethral dysfunction may present as high intravesicular pressure, increased residual volume, or both. The increased vesicular pressure is a result of dyssynergy between bladder contraction and the striated sphincter at the bladder neck. The usual response is for sphincter muscles to progressively fire as the bladder fills. This is the guarding reflex that prevents incontinence. Once urination begins the sphincter completely relaxes. In the SCI patient, as the bladder contracts, due to distention, the sphincter repetitively contracts forming an obstruction to the free flow of urine. The pressure generated by contraction of the bladder is transmitted backward into the kidney. Stasis is the result of not being able to empty the bladder due to loss of bladder contraction.

The risk of UTI is greatest with indwelling Foley catheters, being many times higher than intermittent catheterization and condom catheters. The risk is equivalent with condom catheters and intermittent catheterization. This reflects the trade-off between mechanically introducing bacteria from the perineal area into the bladder during each catheter insertion and providing a closed space in which bacteria can proliferate, as is the case with condom catheters.

Bacteria causing infection in SCI patients vary depending on the series, however, when compared to non-SCI patients the incidence of *Escherichia coli* and *Klebsiella* species is less common and *Pseudomonas*, *Proteus*, and *Serratia* is more common. Microbial resistance to antibiotics is frequent in these patients due to multiple antibiotic exposures and, therefore, culture of the urine is necessary. Relapse of infection or recolonization occurs most commonly with *Escherichia coli* and *Klebsiella pneumoniae* because these are two common bowel organisms that contaminate the perineal area. If the patient is felt to have a true relapse of infection as opposed to colonization, a source should be sought. Relapse is defined as reinfection with the same organism within two weeks after a course of antibiotic treatment. Common sources are stasis of urine, urinary calculus, and abscess of the urinary tract.

The treatment of SCI patients with asymptomatic bacteriuria is controversial because on the one hand chronic antibiotic exposure leads to antimicrobial resistance and on the other hand SCI patients are debilitated and may have less reserve to tolerate systemic infection. The decision to treat an SCI patient must be individualized. The most important factor is the patient's prior clinical course with similar episodes of asymptomatic bacteriuria.

KEY POINTS
The Spinal Cord Injury Patient

1. Spinal cord injury patients are at high risk for UTI because of chronic indwelling catheters and loss of coordinated micturition.
2. Antimicrobial-resistant organisms are common pathogens because SCI patients have multiple antibiotic exposures.

The Diabetic Patient

Few prospective studies address whether diabetic patients are at increased risk of UTI. Studies in diabetic women suggest that the rates of asymptomatic bacteriuria are higher than their nondiabetic counterparts. In one study, the difference was large with a prevalence of asymptomatic bacteriuria in diabetic women being 26% and 6% in nondiabetic women. This finding suggests a serious health risk because other research showed that asymptomatic bacteriuria in diabetic women is a risk for pyelonephritis and decline in renal function. In healthy, nonpregnant women without structural abnormalities of the urinary tract, diabetes mellitus, or immunosuppression such serious complications are rare.

Diabetes mellitus is also a risk factor for more serious complications of UTI, as well as infections with unusual pathogens. These serious complications include emphysematous cystitis and pyelonephritis, abscess formation, renal papillary necrosis, and xanthogranulomatous pyelonephritis (XGP). In diabetics, infections with gram-negative rods other than *Escherichia coli* are more common and the rate of fungal infection is also greatly increased.

There are several reasons postulated as to why patients with diabetes mellitus have a greater incidence of asymptomatic bacteriuria and UTI. The nature of these studies makes the hypotheses difficult to prove. Microvascular disease damages bladder function and, therefore, impairs bladder emptying. This results in outflow obstruction, urinary incontinence, and increased residual volume—all these allow colonization and bacterial overgrowth in urine. Diabetics may have decreased antimicrobial activity of urine and an increased adherence of bacteria to uroepithelium. Hyperglycemia impairs the function of lymphocytes and decreases cytokine production of monocytes. Whatever the etiology of the increased susceptibility to infection, the presence of diabetes mellitus makes a UTI complicated and it must be treated accordingly.

Urinary tract infections in diabetics are more likely to be caused by antibiotic resistant organisms. There is also a higher rate of complications and a higher rate of infection by unusual organisms. In a prospective surveillance study of hospitalized patients with funguria, diabetes was found to be present in 39% of the cases. Therefore, treatment of a diabetic with UTI should involve initial therapy with a broad-spectrum antibiotic such as a quinolone. Patients need to be monitored carefully and if there is no improvement in 3 days alternative pathogens should be sought and imaging studies such as ultrasonography performed to exclude abscess formation. Treatment is employed for a minimum of 7 days, longer as indicated by the progress of an individual patient. Pre- and posttreatment cultures are performed to ensure eradication of the infecting organism.

Diabetic Patient

> 1. Diabetic patients are at high risk for developing complications of UTI.
> 2. Antimicrobial-resistant pathogens are more common in diabetic patients.
> 3. Diabetics are at greater risk for atypical pathogens such as fungi.

The Transplant Patient

In the renal allograft recipient UTI and specifically pyelonephritis can cause acute renal failure. This is due to several factors including the following: the patient has only one kidney; calcineurin inhibitors decrease afferent arterial blood flow; and interstitial inflammation caused by infection diminishes renal blood flow. Furthermore, in the first 3 months posttransplant, the incidence of urinary tract infection is greater than 30%, and there is a relatively high rate of bacteremia and overt pyelonephritis of the allograft. The reason for this increased risk of infection is the high level of immunosuppression in the first 3 months after transplantation. In addition to decreased immune function in both sexes, there is increased vaginal overgrowth of bacteria and fungi in women. After transplantation a period of time is required for the bladder to stretch back to its normal size and regain adequate contractile function. During this period increased residual volume and incontinence predisposes to bacterial overgrowth. Finally, the transplanted ureter does not have a competent ureterovesicle valve and, therefore, reflux of urine into the renal collecting system is common.

Rates of UTI in renal transplant recipients are reduced by the prophylactic use of trimethoprim-sulfamethoxazole and by instructing the patient to void every 2 hours in the initial posttransplant period. Infections in renal transplant patients are treated as complicated UTI. Initial antibiotic selection is broad spectrum with the quinolones being

first choice. A patient with UTI without fever is treated for cystitis but receives 7–10 days of antibiotic. A patient with a fever is treated as pyelonephritis and receives 4 weeks of therapy. Posttreatment urine cultures are required to ensure eradication of the infection and surveillance cultures are recommended if the patient has more than one episode of UTI.

Transplant Patient

> 1. The incidence of UTI during the first three posttransplant months is 30%.
> 2. Pyelonephritis in a renal transplant patient can cause acute renal failure.
> 3. Treatment for cystitis is extended to 7–10 days and treatment for pyelonephritis is extended to 4 weeks.

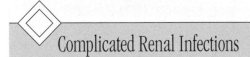

Complicated Renal Infections

Emphysematous Pyelonephritis

This form of pyelonephritis, which occurs most often in patients with diabetes mellitus, is a gas-producing, necrotizing infection involving the renal parenchyma and perirenal tissue. The mechanism of gas formation and pathogenesis of emphysematous pyelonephritis is unclear and is not entirely explained by simple gas production by the involved organisms. The clinical presentation is similar to other forms of severe, acute pyelonephritis. Fevers, chills, flank or abdominal pain, nausea, and vomiting are common. Patients manifest hyperglycemia, leukocytosis, elevated serum blood urea nitrogen (BUN) and creatinine concentrations, and pyuria. *Escherichia coli* is the most common organism followed by *Klebsiella pneumoniae*; bacteremia frequently accompanies this form of pyelonephritis. Diagnosis is made when plain radiograph of the abdomen reveals air in the renal parenchyma or surrounding tissue. Computed tomography (CT) scan is performed in this circumstance to define the extent of infection and evaluate the urinary tract for other lesions.

Treatment of emphysematous pyelonephritis often requires nephrectomy (or open drainage) and intravenous antibiotics. Recently, CT scan was employed to place gas-forming UTIs into four prognostic categories. They include the following classes:

1. Gas present only in the collecting system.
2. Gas within the renal parenchyma without extension to the extrarenal space.
3a. Extension of gas into the perinephric space.
3b. Extension of gas into the pararenal space.
4. Bilateral or solitary kidney with emphysematous pyelonephritis.

Therapy is based on class of the lesion. Antibiotics plus percutaneous catheter placement are sufficient for patients with Class 1 or 2 disease. Antibiotics plus percutaneous catheter placement is the initial treatment of choice for patients with Class 3 disease without organ dysfunction. Antibiotics plus immediate nephrectomy is needed for patients with Class 3 disease with organ dysfunction (renal failure, disseminated intravascular coagulation, shock). Percutaneous drainage is needed for patients with Class 4 disease. Nephrectomy is employed to treat drainage failures. The overall mortality rate approaches 20%.

KEY POINTS
Emphysematous Pyelonephritis

1. Emphysematous pyelonephritis occurs most commonly in patients with diabetes mellitus.
2. Gas-forming organisms such as *Escherichia coli* and *Klebsiella pneumoniae* are associated with this form of pyelonephritis.

3. Treatment is based on class of lesion. Antibiotics and either percutaneous drainage or nephrectomy are available therapeutic options.

Xanthogranulomatous Pyelonephritis

Xanthogranulomatous pyelonephritis is a relatively unusual form of chronic pyelonephritis characterized by formation of mass-like lesions in the kidney. Destruction and necrosis of the kidney necessitates nephrectomy. Approximately two-thirds of cases are complicated by obstruction of the urinary system with infected nephroliths. Renal cell carcinoma is often a concern on initial evaluation of the enlarged kidney. It is often unilateral, but can be bilateral. Xanthogranulomatous pyelonephritis frequently develops in middle-aged women with a history of recurrent urinary tract infections. Flank pain, fever, malaise, anorexia, and weight loss are often present at the time of evaluation. A thorough physical examination may reveal a unilateral renal mass. Anemia, liver function abnormalities, and an increased erythrocyte sedimentation rate (ESR) are nonspecific findings. Urinalysis demonstrates pyuria, bacteriuria, and white blood cell casts. Gram-negative organisms (*Escherichia coli, Klebsiella, Providencia, and Proteus mirabilis,*) are the most common culprits.

Imaging is key to the diagnosis of XGP. Computed tomography scan is the preferred diagnostic tool in the evaluation of XGP. Renal cell carcinoma is excluded by CT scan based on the finding of several rounded, low-density areas within the renal parenchyma that are surrounded by an enhanced rim of contrast medium (dilated calyces lined with necrotic xanthomatous tissue extending into the renal parenchyma). Kidney stones are present in the dilated calyces. Extension of this process into the perirenal area is visualized. Xanthogranulomatous tissue can also invade adjacent gastrointestinal tract and create fistulas into the colon or duodenum.

Grossly, XGP appears as an enlarged kidney with multiple mass-like lesions. The kidney is destroyed by inflammation as witnessed by necrotic renal tissue surrounded by layers of orange-colored material. Staghorn calculi and other nephroliths are often seen within the calyces and renal masses. Perirenal extension into and adherence to surrounding structures develops from the inflamed kidney. Microscopic examination of the renal tissue reveals necrosis, leukocytes, lymphocytes, plasma cells, and macrophages. Vascularized granulation tissue, hemorrhage, and lipid-laden macrophages (xanthoma cells), which give the yellow appearance are also present.

Surgery combined with antibiotics is the only therapy for XGP. Complete nephrectomy, where kidney and involved surrounding tissue are removed and all fistulas closed, is the mainstay of treatment. Localized disease without extension into surrounding tissue or bilateral XGP can sometimes be successfully treated with partial nephrectomy and antimicrobial agents.

KEY POINTS
Xanthogranulomatous Pyelonephritis

1. Xanthogranulomatous pyelonephritis can masquerade as a renal malignancy.
2. Gram-negative organisms underlie infection in XGP.
3. Computed tomography scan best demonstrates the extent of disease, excludes malignancy, and identifies the presence of renal stones.
4. The histopathology of XGP is characterized by necrotic tissue, cellular infiltration, and lipid-laden macrophages (xanthoma cells).
5. Antibiotics and nephrectomy (complete or partial) are required to treat XGP.

Additional Reading

Bent, S., Saint, S. The optimal use of diagnostic testing in women with acute uncomplicated cystitis. *Am J Med* 113:20S–28S, 2002.

Dairiki-Shortliffe, L.M., McCue, J.D. Urinary tract infection at the age extremes: pediatrics and geriatrics. *Am J Med* 113:55S–66S, 2002.

Foxman, B. Epidemiology of urinary tract infections: incidence, morbidity and economic costs. *Am J Med* 113:5S–13S, 2002.

Gupta, K. Addressing antibiotic resistance. *Am J Med* 113:29S–34S, 2002.

Hurlbut, T.A., Litttenberg B. The diagnostic accuracy of rapid dipstick tests to predict urinary tract infection. *Am J Clin Pathol* 96:582–588, 1991.

Nicolle, L.E. A practical guide to the management of complicated urinary tract infection. *Drugs* 53:583–592, 1997.

Nicolle, L.E. Urinary tract infection: traditional pharmacologic therapies. *Am J Med* 113:35S–44S, 2002.

Ronald, A. The etiology of urinary tract infection: traditional and emerging pathogens. *Am J Med* 113:14S–19S, 2002.

Schaeffer, A. The expanding role of fluoroquinolones. *Am J Med* 113:45S–54S, 2002.

Siroky, M.B. Pathogenesis of bacteriuria and infection in the spinal cord injured patient. *Am J Med* 113:67S–79S, 2002.

Stamm, W.E. Scientific and clinical challenges in the management of urinary tract infections. *Am J Med* 113:1S–4S, 2002.

Stapleton, A. Urinary tract infections in patients with diabetes. *Am J Med* 113:80S–84S, 2002.

Stapleton, A., Nudelman, E., Clausen, H., Hakomori, S., Stam, W.E. Binding of uropathogenic *E. coli* R45 to glycolipids extracted from vaginal epithelial cells is dependent on histo-blood group secretor status. *J Clin Invest* 90:965–972, 1992.

Index

Page numbers followed by italic *f* or *t* denote figures or tables, respectively.

X-FILES CONFIDENTIAL

The Unauthorized X-Philes Compendium

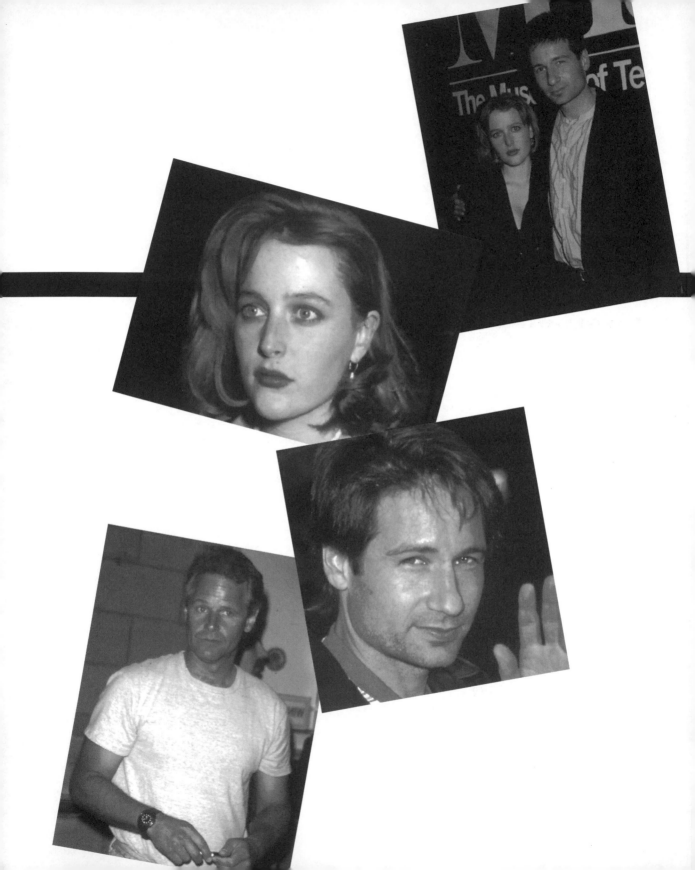

TED EDWARDS

X-FILES CONFIDENTIAL

The Unauthorized X-Philes Compendium

LITTLE, BROWN AND COMPANY

Boston New York Toronto London

A *Little, Brown* Book

Published simultaneously in the USA and Great Britain in 1996 by
Little, Brown and Company

Copyright © 1996 by Ted Edwards

The moral right of the author has been asserted.

This book has not been approved, licensed, or sponsored by any
entity involved in creating or producing *The X-Files*.

Photographs copyright © 1996 by Albert Ortega

Designed by Barbara Werden and Caroline Hagen

A CIP catalogue record for this book is available from the British
Library.

ISBN 0 316 88181 3

Printed and bound in Great Britain by
Hartnolls Ltd, Bodmin, Cornwall

Little, Brown and Company (UK)
Brettenham House
Lancaster Place
London WC2E 7EN

To Chris Carter and the crew of The X-Files,
*for bringing equal doses of quality
and terror to the tube*

The X-Files

Contents

The X-Files

Foreword
BY JEFF RICE

I'd had it in mind, back when I was a copyboy for the *Las Vegas Sun,* even before I became a reporter for that paper, to write a modern-day vampire novel that would do away with most of the clichés associated with such stories, eliminating the conventions such as people living in dread of the night; the fog that usually appears as "atmosphere"; the instant acceptance by a populace that there *is* a vampire stalking them, and the corresponding response of massed action in knowing just where to look for the vampire and what to do when the vampire is found — a story without the customary isolated settings, torchlit prowlings, and eerie castles.

By the time I was a reporter, I'd also had it in mind to write a novel about Las Vegas, but not about gambling or gamblers per se; one in which the city wasn't just the background setting but an integral part of the tale, a character in itself.

In addition to being a reporter in Las Vegas, I'd also had jobs in advertising and public relations there, and even some private investigative work from time to time.

By the time I started to write the novel, I'd also been a columnist and editorialist for a magazine in Las Vegas, done a few stints as a wire editor, field reporter, and fill-in newscaster for a radio station, and was doing more of the same in Los Angeles. While holding down a job as the copy director for an advertising agency, I also did some work as a reporter and critic for a small newspaper and some part-time investigative work as well.

Somewhere along the line, as I struggled to decide which of the novels to write, it occurred to me that I could combine both into a genre or subgenre of fiction that I didn't think had been tried: a thriller combining the vampire story with a police and political cover-up, all based on what I knew would be the logical bureaucratic response to the situation I could create: a threat not only to life but also to the all-important tourist trade of a city that existed on the strength of it.

In writing *The Kolchak Papers* (which chronicles an adventure in the life of reporter Carl Kolchak), and later rewriting it into *The Night Stalker,* I felt I'd succeeded fairly well at not only entertaining the reader but also showing some things about Las Vegas that didn't make it into the publicity generated by the hotels and casinos and into the feature stories greased by the Chamber of Commerce. Others must have felt that way, too, because it was very quickly picked up as a property to be adapted into a script for a 1971 TV movie, which became the highest-rated TV movie aired to that date and the fourth-highest-rated movie ever broadcast. Certain elements of my approach to the novel, such as the idea of keeping the news of the vampire from the public because it was bad for business, would crop up in later films like *Jaws,* and many of the elements of both the book and movie were so widely imitated

"Many of the elements of *The Kolchak Papers* and *The Night Stalker* were so widely imitated . . . that they became and have remained a kind of formulaic approach."

following the success of the movie that they became and have remained a kind of formulaic approach to such thrillers.

The Night Stalker, its book and TV movie sequel *The Night Strangler,* and the subsequent weekly series came out at a time when the American public was beginning to shake off the relative innocence of the 1950s (and I mean "relative") and the hopes of the brief Camelot era of the 1960s, and settle into the slowly dawning realization that the war in Vietnam and other matters the government said were in the national interest were not quite what they appeared to be. The release of what came to be known as the Pentagon Papers only served to fuel this growing awareness that our government, like any other government, had a double set of books, one for the insiders and one for the people, and their bottom lines didn't jibe.

Reporters were enjoying a period of increased appreciation that would peak for a few years with the near-canonization of Woodward and Bernstein, who nailed the story of the Watergate break-in and what Richard Nixon had really been up to in his near paranoid bid to gain re-election when, in his blindered insecurity, he ordered or allowed things to be done that were totally unnecessary in regard to a campaign he could not possibly have lost.

Kolchak, dealing with "monsters" every week, dealing with various forms of official denials and cover-ups, gave people a chance to root for someone who was, essentially, one of them, an ordinary guy who just kept on digging to get at the facts, to get at the truth, and to lay it out for his readers. Covert government activities — which have been going on since the dawn of governments — and their exposure had made people feel increasingly powerless and cynical, and Kolchak came along at just the right time to give them someone to identify with.

People often talk about the *X-Files* protagonists, Mulder and Scully, picking up the baton of Kolchak, in battling to get at the facts about the matter at hand — whether it be extraterrestrial contact and government involvement or other side issues. And with decades now of periodic revelations of other government cover-ups (most notably Iran-Contra), once again the ordinary citizen can focus on something fictitious yet see all the intense behind-the-scenes workings of agencies and departments and bureaucrats who work to serve their own ends. It's not only entertaining, of course, but it serves as a kind of safety valve for people's emotions, confirming their worst fears about malfeasance and misfeasance in matters more esoteric than skimming a little money from budgets or taking payoffs from lobbyists.

I don't think anyone has done more to foster the idea of picking up where Kolchak left off, at least in a general thematic way, than *X-Files* creator Chris Carter, who has repeatedly credited Kolchak, in his various incarnations from the novels to the TV series, as his inspiration. And his acknowledgments of me and my work are very gratifying.

who wish, at the least, that they'd just go away, and who will act, at the most and worst, to discredit or even destroy them. All three protagonists are after the truth.

But Kolchak operates *outside* the system, seeking to dig out facts and expose them to the American public. He rather oddly combines the skepticism and even cynicism of a reporter with the curious open-mindedness of a child who can accept what most adults refute, pro forma; that there are "more things in heaven and earth," as Shakespeare put it, "than are dreamt of in [our] philosophy." He is driven by a reporter's zeal to get the *story*, whatever it is, and lay it out for the public.

Mulder and Scully operate *within* the

"Kolchak gave people a chance to root for someone who was, essentially, one of them, an ordinary guy who just kept digging to get at the facts."

It has become something of a popular pastime for hard-core genre fans to compare and contrast the series *Kolchak: The Night Stalker* with *The X-Files,* and, to a degree, these efforts are valid. Certainly, they are fun. Kolchak and Mulder and Scully all have to deal with eerie situations and constantly find themselves up against officials at various levels

system, seemingly as an afterthought of some department head, trying to tie up loose ends — or dig them out and tie them up — and trying to make their part of the system work *for* the people, rather than against them. But, if one may push their analogous relationship to Kolchak a bit, they bifurcate many of the conflicting aspects of his character. Mulder is the open-minded one, the one who accepts the "infinite possibilities," as Gene Roddenberry characterized them; is fascinated with them, and approaches them eagerly, as a child would. Scully is the skeptic — not a cynic like Kolchak, but very, *very* solidly grounded in the world of hard facts, or science, and in what is known rather than suspected or dreamt-of. They work very well together (and with relatively little and generally productive friction), with Mulder inspiring Scully to take that "one step beyond," while Scully acts as a kind of grounding wire, a check and balance to Mulder's enthusiastic pursuits.

All of them — Kolchak, Mulder, and Scully — are constantly frustrated by official interference in just about every conceivable form, but none of them really ever quit trying to do what they see as their jobs: to get at the truth, whatever it may be.

If *The X-Files* has succeeded in terms of ratings and longevity, where Kolchak did not (at least in its single 1974–75 season as a series), it must be due in part to superior writing, in part to a willingness by Fox to stick by it, and in part due to a much more diverse and fragmented TV marketplace. There were only three networks when *Kolchak: The Night Stalker* was on the air, and very little original dramatic programming being syndicated for "local" TV stations. Today, thanks to the advent of cable broadcasting, there are so many TV venues that it is possible with much

lower ratings — relative to all the shows extant—for a series to survive and even to thrive and become not only a cult classic but a genuine phenomenon. Thus it is with *The X-Files,* and if *Kolchak* is due any credit at all, it may be because it first tapped in to a segment of the viewing audience that was, perhaps, undervalued in its day.

For the most part, *The X-Files'* writing quality has stayed very high, and though some purists (and I am not really quite in that category) may have become slightly disenchanted by the second season, and some of the stories in the third season have appeared to stray a bit from the main plotline of the show, *The X-Files* maintains its overall quality very well. The writers appear to work hard at not becoming too formulaic or predictable within the show's own necessary formula and style, but the bulk of the credit for its continued quality and ongoing success must go to Chris Carter, who is its creator and has kept up a grueling hands-on control since its inception.

Since its inception, I have greatly enjoyed *The X-Files* and consider myself a very definite fan. I try to never miss an episode, because I feel somehow cheated of one of the better things in life when I do, and await the next episode with eager anticipation. (Okay. I need my regular *X-Files* "fix.")

From what I've heard, *The X-Files* has continued to gather to it new viewers, and most viewers of *The X-Files* have (possibly because they have been inspired by the show) sampled, and become regular watchers of, the Sci-Fi Channel's offerings, which, I'm told, have included reruns of episodes of *Kolchak: The Night Stalker*. This brings my series to the attention of a new generation of viewers, which is always gratifying, and gives some of those in my own generation a chance for a second look at it. In regard to other venues, I've heard that *The X-Files* has done well in comic book form for Topps and as novels for HarperCollins.

I think it's become clear, certainly from Chris, that my Kolchak work, to some degree, inspired him to create *The X-Files* and, for my own part, I'm very pleased that he did and very pleased with the ongoing result.

If I may be allowed to express an overall opinion as to the success of *The X-Files*, I'd put it this way: Chris Carter has become, in his own right, the Robert Ludlum of series television. And, thanks to him, the genre of paranoia and conspiracy is alive and well. More power to him.

October 1996

The X-Files

Acknowledgments

This book has its origin in the vast research done by a variety of people who have come together to present an all-encompassing view of *The X-Files.* For their invaluable assistance, I would like to thank Joseph Rugg, Thomas Sanders, Edward Gross, Dexter Frank, Bill Planer, and John Raymond. Special thanks to Albert Ortega for use of his photographic materials. Thanks also to my agent, Laurie Fox, and my editor, Geoff Kloske.

I would also like to offer a very special thanks to Douglas Perry for his vast editorial skills.

The X-Files

An Introduction

Write what you know — that's been the mantra of creative-writing instructors for at least half an eon, and if it's a truism of all good writing, then *X-Files* creator Chris Carter has had a terribly traumatic life. "Good doesn't necessarily win," says Carter, who worked in sitcoms before devising the concept for his Fox network hit. "In fact, it wins a surprisingly paltry amount of the time — and we often try to live in denial of that."

Not anymore. *The X-Files* revels in the power of our darkest impulses; it gets down in the mud and rolls around with them. And we can't stop watching: Carter's stories of evil and violence, using black magic, demons, and aliens to represent very real fears, have turned *The X-Files* from an episodic curio into a cultural phenomenon. Of course, Carter and his writers probably have little firsthand knowledge of toxic monsters from Chernobyl, circus freaks with their siblings growing out of their chests, or rampaging manitous. But they understand that what's important in fantastic stories is the emotional validity of the characters who are facing those horrors. Then it becomes what writer Joe Haldeman calls "invented truth." And so Carter uses FBI agents Fox Mulder and Dana Scully to ground his show in reality: we see through their eyes, and experience their fear, their confusion, their desperation. Typically, *The X-Files* is described as science fiction, but a more accurate description might be "social-science fiction." It is, after all, fueled by the realities — and internal anxieties — of its time: the era of diminished expectations.

It is that grounding in the psychology of the 1990s that differentiates *The X-Files* from its closet relative, the noir film, which has had a resurgence recently but which, in most cases, is little more than the sum of its double crosses and knifing shadows. *The X-Files*, on the other hand, doesn't merely show us the symptoms of societal disintegration — corruption, hypocrisy, violence, fear — it attacks the cause. It concerns itself with the dark side of technology, competition, politics, ambition, and selfishness; it warns against the risks of abandoning an interior life or one's community. To be sure, it reinforces the notion that our attempts to combat evil are usually an exercise in futility. But Mulder and Scully also give us hope — however Sisyphean — that the effort alone is significant.

PART ONE

The X-Files

Given the skepticism — even condescension — their findings receive within the FBI hierarchy, special agents Fox Mulder and Dana Scully would be justified in feeling that they were blazing new ground with every alien encounter, vampire battle, and monster sighting. But *The X-Files'* investigators actually are relative latecomers to the paranormal beat, appearing on the scene twenty years after a boozing, burned-out journalist named Carl Kolchak first saw the netherworld where others just saw bizarre crimes in *The Night Stalker* — a direct progenitor of the later series.

The X-Files, winner of the 1994 Golden Globe Award for best television drama, is a phenomenon so large that it has generated spin-off products, on-line services, and serious talk of a feature film version within the next few years. "It was just one of those ideas that seemed to work on a number of levels," says series creator Chris Carter, recalling his initial concept. "Also, it just seemed like a TV series to me. Lots of stories to tell without having to be self-referencing, without having to rely on going into the lives of the characters. But, basically, I just wanted to do something as scary as I remember *The Night Stalker* being when I was in my teens."

The Night Stalker is the 1971 TV movie that introduced the character Kolchak (Darren McGavin), a newspaper reporter whose investigation of a series of murders in Las Vegas leads him to a vampire. Due to the popularity of both the film and the character, created by author Jeff Rice, Kolchak returned the following year for another TV movie, *The Night Strangler,* and then again in 1974 for a short-lived weekly series. In the series, Kolchak relocated to Chicago, where he took on werewolves, mummies, zombies, Indian demons, sewer-roaming creatures, and, of course, aliens.

As inspiration for the character, Rice cites old-time journalists such as Ben Hecht and Charles MacArthur, who wrote the play *The Front Page* and who, Rice points out, had been hard-nosed reporters themselves in the 1920s, when newspapers were practically the only source of information. But Rice didn't draw solely from the legends of the profession. "Part of the inspiration came from my chief mentor at the *Las Vegas Sun,* Alan Jarlson," the former journalist recalls. "He was probably one of the last of the generation of those reporters trained in a time when TV had not yet become the be-all, end-all of 'news,' which creates news as often as it reports it. [Kolchak was based in part on] what I saw of him and how he worked—how he reacted not only to news as it developed and he reported and edited it, but also how he handled the sneakier aspects of censorship when he encountered it. And, certainly, part of the inspiration was the projecting I did in my own mind of what I'd be like when I reached the age I am now, if I chose to remain a reporter."

As Rice points out, his effort, originally titled *The Kolchak Papers,* was the first and

"Mulder and Scully are equal parts of my nature," muses Carter.

only one to blend the newsroom and horror-fiction genres. "That wasn't my main consideration when I started the actual drafting," he says. "All I wanted to do was create a 'good read' of the type that I thought I would find entertaining; something for people to use to kill time in airports, on planes, or in hotels when stuck overnight in a strange town. Of course, I also felt I could use the book as a vehicle to say a few serious things about my town — to use it as an intrinsic part of the story rather than as a mere background setting — and to make a few pithy comments about the misuse of power, the latter being an underlying theme in the novel."

An interesting parallel between *The X-Files* and *Kolchak: The Night Stalker* is the employment of opposing emotional and intellectual perspectives about the bizarre things occurring in the story. In short, both shows counterbalance the believer and the skeptic to ground the story in a realistic milieu. On *The Night Stalker,* skeptics surrounded Kolchak

on all sides — except when the monsters had him cornered. On *The X-Files,* the conflict is more personal and less accusatory. Mulder is the believer and Scully is the skeptic.

"Mulder and Scully are equal parts of my nature, I guess," Chris Carter muses. "I'm a natural skeptic, so I have much of the Scully character in me, yet I'm willing to take leaps of faith, to go out on a limb. I love writing both those characters, because their voices are very clear in my head." He does admit, however, that as the series has progressed, Scully's skepticism has been somewhat eroded. "But she is a scientist first and foremost," he says. "What she sees, what is unexplainable, what seems fantastic to her, she believes, truly, can be ultimately explained scientifically. She is a scientist and will always be one, so she maintains a scientific distance from things, whereas Mulder leaps in and wants to believe."

In *The Night Stalker,* Kolchak is the sole believer against a world of skeptics, and it's his battle to get the truth out despite the odds that makes viewers root for him. But while audiences always cheer those who endure ridicule and worse in their fight against conventional wisdom — be it Galileo or the 1969 Mets — that isn't the only source of the show's enduring popularity.

"Maybe its appeal remains because it was

then, and remains now, a very different kind of show," Rice says. "Maybe people see, in the monsters and the way public knowledge and discussion are stopped, symbols for all those things various government entities wish the people not to know about. Maybe people — fans — admire Kolchak because he just keeps on trying to do what he sees as work that has value: trying to keep the public informed about what is going on."

Indeed, it sounds like Rice could be talking about *The X-Files*. But as much as he's a fan of *The Night Stalker*, Carter identified some fundamental misjudgments in the '70s series that he wanted to avoid when creating his own show.

"I saw what the limitations were," he says. "I think having a 'monster of the week' reduced the longevity of the storytelling capabilities. I thought there was a wide world of weird science, paranormal phenomena, and other kinds of stories to tell that were best explored by people who had a reason to explore them, and who actually could effect some outcome. Rather than being limited, as Kolchak was, to just writing about something and trying to convince people what the truth is, it seemed to me it was stronger using FBI agents. There

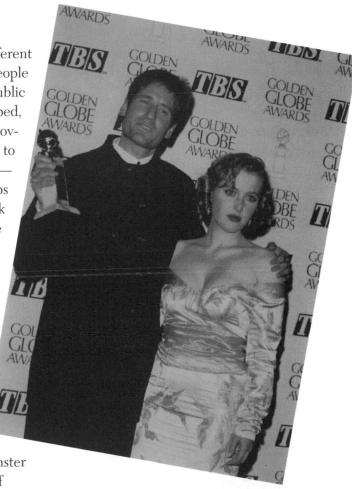

David Duchovny and Gillian Anderson at the 1994 Golden Globe Awards, where *The X-Files* won for best television drama.

must be somebody out there who responds to all the weird things we read about or hear about, even though the FBI says it doesn't have a so-called X-Files division. But one has to wonder."

In an attempt to expand the narrative format of *The X-Files*, Carter occasionally throws in episodes that have no supernatural threat whatsoever. In season two's "Irresistible," for example, the antagonist is a mortuary worker who likes to cuddle with the clientele, the rigor mortis the better. Looking for new thrills, he begins seeking breathing victims to kill, one intended cadaver being Scully.

"I think it's one of our scarier shows, and I think I was able to explore the character of Scully in a way I wouldn't have been able to with a supernatural theme," Carter says. "Sometimes even more scary than the things we can imagine are the things that are unimaginable, which is that the man standing next to you could be this kind of guy. Sometimes the face of evil can become frighteningly real and distorted through a prism of your own unconscious fears. That's what we were playing with. I thought it worked in its own way. You'll see more stuff like that. I think *The X-Files* works the best when it's closest to being real, and that allows us to go and cast our lines out farther into the supernatural at other times. I think, if anything, we have to keep the show fresh and keep reinventing it, or else it's going to become stale and fall into a 'ghost of the week' format."

Jeff Rice concurs with many of Carter's criticisms of the old *Night Stalker* series, particularly the monster-of-the-week tack.

"What I proposed to ABC lo these many years ago," he says, "was that Kolchak deal with more realistic issues of misfeasance and malfeasance in high office; I wanted to deal with people in power covering things up, things they didn't want made public, things they were dealing with badly or couldn't deal with at all because they didn't understand them. Now, Kolchak was only a reporter. It gave him a certain freedom of thought and mind-set, though it limited his access to everything. Carter has put his protagonists into a position that gives them some access to information and allows them to operate in ways Kolchak never could. And they do manage to have some effect on the outcome of situations, despite interference from those far more powerful, in ways Kolchak never could. Part of the appeal is that they care enough to try, and they do — over and over — and take their lumps for their efforts. My impression is that people like to think somebody gives a damn about the truth and is willing to risk all to get at it."

Mulder and Scully's Kolchak-like search for truth at almost any cost — along with the show's paranormal creepiness and gritty narrative realism — has given *The X-Files* the kind of broad-based popularity Kolchak never quite achieved.

"I feel we've been doing good work all along," Carter says. "Now, with the success, everybody is going to look at us closely. But I don't want the standard to change. I don't want people to expect *T2* [*Terminator 2*] or something like that. We're going to be doing the same good shows we've always done; we're not going to pump them up. I don't feel any reason to try and outperform myself. At the same time, what happens when the spotlight goes on you is that you are considered mainstream. I still think of this as being cultish in its feel, subversive. It worries me that all of a sudden the perception will change. I can guarantee you that the show won't."

One thing that has changed is the silence coming from Kolchak's typewriter, which has begun clacking to life again in a new novel and a forthcoming comic book line from Topps. Additionally, producer–director Dan Curtis (known to older genre fans for the '60s gothic soap opera *Dark Shadows*) is talking about resurrecting the character for either the big screen or TV. The common thread linking all these efforts is that Kolchak will be transplanted from the '70s to the '90s unaged, and he will continue to deal — in his own cynical way — with our fast-changing society.

"His reaction to the present-day situation won't be markedly different from what it was to the 1970s," Rice predicts. "He'll still be cynical (his best armor against the slings and arrows of outrageous fortune), sarcastic (his manifestation of that cynicism), and he'll still

be idealistic enough to keep plugging away at doing what he feels is his job, his calling: protecting the public's right to know what the hell is going on around them, whether or not they even want to know.

"Despite all the tremendous societal changes that occur within each decade," he

> **"When I was sitting in my office in my surf trunks, barefoot . . . writing the pilot for *The X-Files*, I never imagined that they would be making *X-Files* underwear."**

elaborates, "there are still constants: greed, the lust for power, prejudice, and so on. The late H. L. Mencken, a man of incredibly sharp eye and tongue and pen (and not without some damned ugly prejudices of his own), skewered all forms of pretense in his heyday, the 1920s and 1930s. Kolchak will have to be our Mencken for the nineties."

As *The X-Files* continues to see its audience swell, Carter occasionally pauses — awed by what his creation has become. "When I was sitting in my office in my surf trunks, barefoot, playing ball with the dog every twenty minutes, writing the pilot for *The X-Files*, I never imagined that they would be making *X-Files* underwear," he says with a laugh, "and that ten thousand people a week would be logging on to the Internet to talk about the show. You can't imagine that kind of growth or success. It's unreal.

"But the show itself and the stories have grown in ways that have been surprising," Carter says. "You set out to do something, and it's like Lewis and Clark in that you don't know what you're going to encounter. The surprise is in the discovery of where the show has gone and how the people I've hired have brought amazing things to it. Oftentimes, things can never be as good as you imagined them, [but] oftentimes on this show, things are better."

The X-Files

The Walt Disney Company bills itself as the happiest place on Earth, where the sun is always shining and smiles are handed out like Chiclets. Not the kind of place you'd expect Fox Mulder to cut his teeth. Or, for that matter, Mulder's alter ego.

"If you look at my résumé," says X-Files creator Chris Carter, "you won't find any clear connection between my previous work and The X-Files."

Until he became the Fox network's master of creepiness, Carter was a veritable poster boy for Mom, apple pie, and Chevrolet. Born and raised in the blue-collar Southern California town of Bellflower, Carter had what he terms a "fairly normal" childhood made up of Little League baseball and surfing. After graduating from Cal State Long Beach with a degree in journalism, he weighed the pros and cons of his two greatest ambitions — being a beach bum and being a writer — and decided to split the difference.

"I went to work for Surfing magazine, which is a big deal — an international magazine," Carter says. "It was really to postpone my growing up, and those were the best years of my life. I ended up working for them for thirteen years and was listed as senior editor when I was twenty-eight. So I went around

the world, surfing, and I got to write. I wrote constantly. I learned how to run a business. It was a wonderful, adventurous time. I did many other things, too. I was a potter during those times."

A what?

"Yes," he says with a laugh, "I did all those California cliché things. I actually made hundreds of thousands of pieces of pottery. I sat and made dinnerware. I threw most of it away because I got tired of looking at it, but I hope to do that again someday. It was wonderful, repetitious. There's a certain Zen thing that goes on when you make something with your hands, over and over."

Carter attributes his "settling down" to his wife, Dori Pierson, whom he met in 1983. It was Pierson who encouraged him to find something to be passionate about besides surfing, and suggested screenwriting. His first efforts were strong enough to attract the attention of then–Disney executive Jeffrey Katzenberg, who signed him to a multipicture deal. As a result, he wrote the TV movies B.R.A.T. Patrol and Meet the Munceys.

"When I went to Disney," Carter explains, "I actually became known as a comedy writer. So that was what people thought of me as: a person who had a certain handle on the voice of contemporary youth and the comedic voice. That's what people kept wanting me to write. I like that type of writing very much, and I think I can do it. But The X-Files really is more where my heart is: in scary, dramatic, thriller writing."

But it would take several years before he had the opportunity to prove it. While at Disney, Carter met with then–NBC president Brandon Tartikoff, who brought him to the network. There he wrote and produced a number of pilots, including *Cameo by Night,* a detective show starring *Sisters'* Sela Ward, and a sitcom called *A Brand New Life,* which was supposed to have been a modern take on *The Brady Bunch.* Carter followed that by producing the musical comedy series *Rags to*

"Sometimes the *Night Stalker* influence is overstated," explains Carter.

Riches, which starred veteran actor Joseph Bologna. "Basically, I took the job on *Rags to Riches* to learn how to produce television," he admits. "It was a terrific opportunity to do that. And I got to learn physical production."

Carter wrote and produced a Disney Channel pilot called *The Nanny* before drawing the attention of Stephen J. Cannell Productions president Peter Roth, who read and enjoyed Carter's script for *Cool Culture,* based on the writer's experiences working for *Surfing* magazine. Although the script was never purchased, Roth planned on utilizing Carter for the CBS series *Palace Guard.* But

when the executive shifted over to Fox as head of TV production in 1993, he hired Carter, along with several other producers, to develop programming. At that point, Carter began to nurture his idea for a series that would tap in to his childhood memories of *The Night Stalker* and *The Twilight Zone.*

"Sometimes the *Night Stalker* influence is overstated," Carter explains. "Somebody asked me in what way it inspired me and I said, 'I think I remember two scenes from the old show. One where Darren McGavin is confronted by a vampire and is able to drive a stake into his heart, and the other is in an alleyway.' I just remember being scared out of my wits by that show as a kid, and I realized that there just wasn't anything scary now on television. The inspiration is general rather than specific."

He also points out a distinction between *The X-Files* and Rod Serling's *Twilight Zone* that he feels is too often overlooked. "Rod Serling was telling fables, almost allegorically. You see a lot of that in *The X-Files,* too, but each of the episodes of *The Twilight Zone* had a bigger message, a bigger purpose, and that was to illuminate something about the human comedy. We don't set out to do that; we don't set out to be instructive — there's no message behind each *X-Files* episode. Although there is something you can take from it, we're not teaching."

Beyond the influence of *The Night Stalker* and *The Twilight Zone, The X-Files* began to take solid form in Carter's mind thanks to an old friend who was familiar with the work of Dr. John Mack of Harvard. "Mack, who has become famous in UFO circles, surveyed a big cross-section of American citizens and found that three percent of Americans believe they've actually been abducted by UFOs," Carter says. "That means if there are one hundred people in a room, three of them have actually been abducted, or believe they have. And this psychologist friend of mine, whose specialization is schizophrenia, told me that — and this is a sane, credible, believable person —he's looked into people's eyes and he's seen, whether it be multiple personalities or the schizophrenic himself, what he feels is not human. So he believes in the alien abduction syndrome, or in alien abduction. I thought that was a great leaping-off point for the series."

But this was going to be somewhat different from the typical alien premise. Carter decided to ground the show in reality by offering a counterpoint to the mysterious paranor-

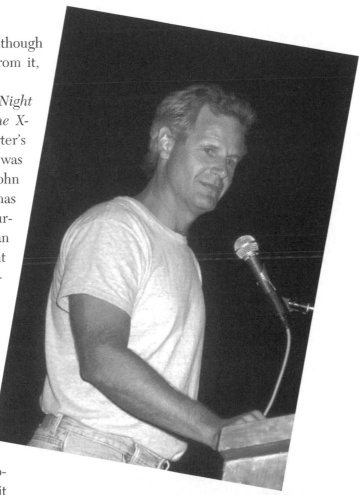

The surfer dude is actually Chris Carter, creator and executive producer of television's most frightening series, *The X-Files*.

mal happenings: that is, Scully's scientific skepticism. Mulder, who believes his sister was abducted by extraterrestrials, is obsessed with proving the existence of ETs. But Scully, originally assigned to partner with Mulder to

The X-Hoax

Like many a television series, *The X-Files* went through some changes between conception and hitting the airwaves. When the show was first presented to the press, series creator Chris Carter announced an idea that in fact never came to pass

"One character is a skeptic and one is a believer," he said. "The skeptic is going to be right as much as the believer is. They'll uncover hoaxes. There will be, indeed, more traditional FBI cases that involve what seem to be paranormal phenomena and we'll have evidence and MOs that seem otherworldly, if you will. But they won't always be alien abduction. Or it may turn out to be someone, as I say, perpetrating a hoax. I'd say about half the time these are going to play out as either hoaxes or traditional cases that appear to have paranormal aspects to them. Oftentimes you'll end up with a crook in handcuffs."

In the series's first three seasons, there was only one episode ("Jose Chung's *From Outer Space*") that could possibly be interpreted as a hoax.

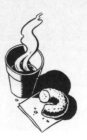

debunk his theories, finds more prosaic explanations for the cases they encounter.

❀ ❀ ❀

As originally conceived, the show wasn't so much *The Night Stalker* as, uh, *The Avengers*.

"I loved that show," Carter says of the classic '60s series starring Patrick Macnee and Diana Rigg. "I loved that relationship between Steed and Emma Peel, the intensity of the stories. It's the way I sort of instinctively write, so that has also fed in to my ultimate concept of the show. The character of Mulder came first, because he was the key to the series in that he was the person who wanted to believe. You need that before you can move ahead. Then Scully as his opposite. It's the nature of any interesting relationship. When someone forces you to justify what you believe in, you take that person more seriously and, in turn, that person really turns you into a better, clearer thinker, which is what Scully does for Mulder. I always felt that the show was from Scully's point of view. We would cut to her reaction to what Mulder was saying. She was the one who would pull Mulder back and say, 'Look what you're doing; look what you're saying.'"

And from the very beginning Carter has been adamant about one thing: Mulder and Scully — despite a tantalizing bedroom pictorial in *Rolling Stone* — will *not* be sweating up the sheets together. "I think a little sexual tension goes a long way," he says, "and I think the thing that makes this show unconventional in that way is that we're not going to have the characters jump into the sack for sweeps. The fact that their relationship is a cerebral one, first and foremost, actually is more interesting for me to write. I also think it'll carry us a long way, and it makes the show an interesting one because it is a suspense–mystery genre show. It's allowed us to play the stories rather than these characters' love lives. So it will never be *Moonlighting*. But with men and women, there is, whether by society's projection or by our natural biological projections on these things, a sexual tension between the two. I've always said that the best kind of sexual tension for me is when you put a smart man and a smart woman in a room. You've got immediate sexual tension, no matter if it's romantic."

❊ ❊ ❊

Creating credibility was the chief mandate from the start. "To make the show convincing, you do have to make it believable. I felt that the characters and the investigative process had to be really believable, so I set out to do just that. Credible, believable characters and credible, believable situations dealing with

incredible and unexplainable phenomena. I did as much research as I could through the FBI, and they were rather reluctant then. It was a limited resource. But I did research on all the things that I was writing about —

Carter decided to ground the show in reality by offering a counterpoint to the mysterious paranormal happenings: that is, Scully's scientific skepticism.

aliens, UFOs, and the FBI — just by reading about it."

Producer–director Daniel Sackheim, who took home the 1994 Best Directing Emmy for his work on *NYPD Blue* and who also produced the *X-Files* pilot, worked closely with Carter throughout the development of the series. "Chris wanted to do something that was scary and that felt real, and that's what attracted me to the project," Sackheim says. "In the initial stages, we had talked about two projects as stylistic sources, one of which was *The Thin Blue Line,* a documentary about a cop-killing in Texas back in 1976. The result of the documentary was that the case was reopened and the man convicted of the crime was found innocent by virtue of the material and evidence presented in the documentary, and the man who had identified him as the killer turned out to have actually committed the crime. It was an unusual film because it was the first of its kind to ever be presented in an intensely stylized fashion, with much emphasis being on the evidence produced: the letters being typed on a report or a piece of evidence being dropped on the street.

"To be fair," Sackheim continues, "Chris came up with the concept of the show, he wrote it, he really deserves all the credit for it, but I guess he was looking for someone to help him execute it — and that's where sources like *The Thin Blue Line* came in. We had also talked about the realism of something like *Prime Suspect,* which was the miniseries on PBS with Helen Mirren. There was much discussion of sort of mining the style for the show, but the reality is that *The X-Files* has sort of found its own style in that it doesn't have a confined style to it. Everybody who comes on the show attempts to make a little scary movie. I think it's a testament to the uniqueness of the show, unlike something like *NYPD Blue,* which is more rigid in its format. The *X-Files* style is distinctive and yet it is also fluid."

Sackheim admits he doubted the show could prosper for long, considering the inherent limitations of the character arcs of Scully as a doubting Thomas and Mulder as the believer, because every week Scully is exposed to situations that in all likelihood would make her a believer.

"Yet they manage to offer the appropriate point of view," he adds. "I think Chris is really smart in that he had a well-thought-out plan. He had a game plan going into the pilot and he knew where he would be halfway through year one, at the end of year one, halfway through year two, the end of year two, and the beginning of year three. He had a plan in his mind as to how it would develop and how the characters would develop. There was sort of an internal bible worked out. He said it to me when we were doing the pilot: 'The reason most series fail is that nobody has a long view of where the show is going to go,' and he felt that he did."

Carter himself believes humbly that the show's success has as much to do with viewers' fascination with UFOs as it does with the creativity of the show itself.

"The idea that there are visitors to the planet, that they are not only visiting now but have been visiting since prehistory, and how it affects us is a very interesting idea," he muses. "I suppose just looking up into the night sky at all those millions of stars up there, you wonder if it's possible. I have a pet theory that everyone wants to have that experience where they're driving through the desert at night, and they see something and can't explain what it is. I think it's all about religion. Not necessarily Christian religion, but it's about beliefs — and meaning and truth and why are we here and why are they here and who's lying to us. It's religion with a lowercase 'r.'

Encountering a UFO would be like witnessing a miracle."

The true miracle was that the show got on the air at all. The Fox executives were, to say the least, nervous about a show that explored the paranormal and UFOs, a premise that had a spotty track record on TV. They also wondered whether such a show — which Carter was selling to them as inspired (however minimally) by real-life events — could compete with such network stalwarts as *Unsolved Mysteries* and *Cops*. As Carter noted in the pages of the show's official companion, "Everyone thought this has got to be as real as possible. No one could understand why someone would want to watch a show if it weren't true."

The pilot script was delivered around Christmas 1992, and Carter was given the go-ahead for production. Robert Mandel, who had helmed the cult favorite *F/X* among other films, was hired to direct, with Sackheim serving as producer. The premiere episode had Mulder and Scully investigating a series of supposed abductions which, despite her best efforts, Scully cannot completely explain away scientifically.

Fox was willing to give this upstart Carter a chance to justify the kudos Roth was heaping on him, but it really had little faith in the *X-Files* concept. The network was convinced that another quasi-fantastic series, the Sam Raimi–produced *Adventures of Brisco County, Jr.*, would be their fall hit, and that *The X-Files* would last maybe half a season. But when the 1993–94 season began, it quickly became obvious that there was little audience interest in *Brisco*, while the core demographics, if not the initial ratings, for *The X-Files* were exceptionally promising. Vindication was Carter's, and he shares it enthusiastically with the crew that brings the show to life each week.

"People feel very invested in the show and they're proud to work on it," Carter enthuses. "My feeling is that most things fail in this business, and the powers that be always proceed as if what you're going to do is going to fail; they're always hedging. So we went boldly forward and showed them we knew what we were doing, what kind of stories we were telling, that we could tell them well. I think that boldness translated into a winning team. I'm sounding like a coach now, but in many ways it is like putting together a good team of people. And this is the best team you could hope for."

The X-Files

CHAPTER THREE
Two of a Kind: David
Duchovny and Gillian
Anderson

"It's weird," muses David Duchovny, who plays FBI agent Fox Mulder. "To me, *The X-Files* is like a wave and I'm on top of it looking down. And right now it's a *biiiiig* wave, so sometimes it's scary. I feel I've got ten more years of playing the guy. When I'm forty-five, I'll start thinking about what else I want to do."

Duchovny sometimes wishes he wasn't involved at all.

The ambitious Duchovny, who's starring in the feature *Playing God,* wasn't always so enthusiastic about an extended run as the obsessive G-man who warily sports the nickname "Spooky." "When you're trying to envision the career that you want to have — especially before your [career] has really taken a turn into reality and you're just living in possibility — you have everybody's career," he says. "You do all the parts. So there's a certain disappointment when your life becomes just one part."

That disappointment has been alleviated recently not only by the opportunity to pursue

other roles during *The X-Files'* summer break but also by a whopping $100,000 paycheck for each episode and greater creative involvement in the show. "Being offered the chance to submit storylines and to direct — it reminds me of playing with my dog," Duchovny says. "I'll give him a choice between a tennis ball and a Frisbee: whatever it takes to keep him involved."

And yet, Duchovny sometimes wishes he wasn't involved at all. Though the Ivy League–educated actor understood at the beginning of his career that fame was the price of success in the performing arts, he still wasn't prepared when his star went supernova.

"Privacy is something I have come to respect," he says. "And ultimately, you also come to realize that you're being appreciated for something that doesn't have that much to do with you. So it's not satisfying. It's perfume. Nothing goes inside. [The fame] doesn't give you anything deep or meaningful. You get Knicks tickets — that's about it. Being on TV and having so many people see you makes you self-conscious enough as it is. So there are two things I don't want to do in my spare time: One is talk about *The X-Files* and the other is to think about how people are perceiving me."

Gillian Anderson, who plays Mulder's partner Dana Scully, echoes her co-star.

"I think that with any success, there is a bittersweet quality to it," she offers. "In order

16

to produce the quality of show that we're producing, everybody who's involved has to do an incredible amount of work. Especially with all the attention we've received, the Golden Globe award, and the snowball effect that's going on. It [creates] a lot of pressure to keep doing more and to keep doing better. At the same time, we're working and we're on a quality show, and it can be incredibly enjoyable sometimes. It depends on the day, and the hour, and the mood. I wouldn't wish it on anybody, but it's also the most wonderful thing to have the opportunity."

Viewing the *X-Files* phenomenon from the inside, Anderson has developed her own ideas about the show's success.

"The series deals with many aspects of the paranormal, and one of the aspects is the spiritual one," she says. "That's very appealing to people. I'm less sure about what intrigues people about the horror side of it, because that never appealed to me. But on a spiritual level, some of the episodes deal with the possibility of coming back to life or some sort of spiritual awakening. And that offers hope, some way out of the fear and the pain of everyday life on this planet."

Duchovny concurs, adding: "I think *The X-Files* is very nineties, because everything is left in doubt. There's no closure, no answers. Most of the credit goes to Chris Carter. . . . Obviously, it's tapping in to something the nation wants. I think it has to do with religious

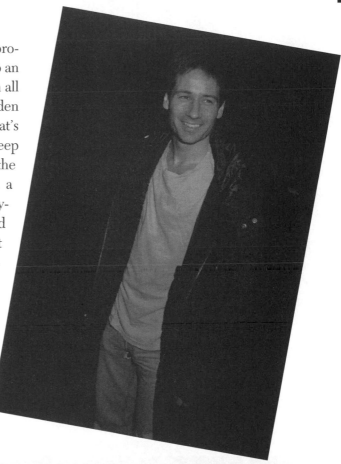

David Duchovny in an uncharacteristically giddy mood, which fans of the X-*Files* aren't used to seeing.

stirrings — a sort of New Age yearning for an alternate reality and the search for some kind of extrasensory god. Couple that with a cynical, jaded, dispossessed feeling of having been lied to by the government, and you've got a pretty powerful combination for a TV show.

and excellent production values offered by Carter's behind-the-scenes pros, *The X-Files* probably wouldn't be the monumental success it is today if the lead roles had gone to, say, Patrick Duffy and Heather Locklear.

"At first, I cast the roles separately," says Carter. "We cast David and then we cast Gillian. So they did have a chance to go into a room together and act together. And I saw the chemistry immediately, which is unusual. I said, 'These are our two people.' Honestly, I think you just get lucky with the chemistry. And I'm lucky to work with them, too, because they're both smart and good people. Both personally and professionally, we lucked out in getting the chemistry we did."

❊ ❊ ❊

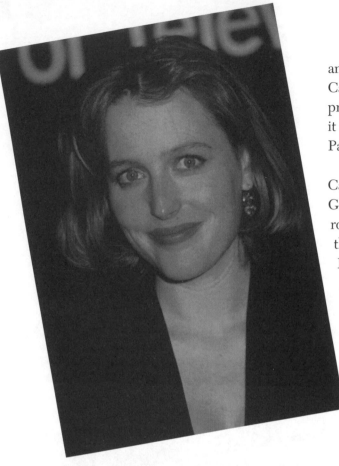

Gillian Anderson, probably not used to the attention, smiles nervously for the paparazzi.

Either that, or the Fox network has an *amazing* marketing department."

Fox's amazing marketing execs were no doubt aided in their task by Carter's casting of Duchovny and Anderson, who immediately clicked as a team. Screen chemistry is a nebulous, hard-to-predict quality, and the two leads of a weekly series must have it for the show to work. Even with the top-notch writing

Born and raised in Manhattan, Duchovny attended a boys' prep school in the city, where he excelled both in the classroom and on the playing field. After finishing up his secondary education with honors, he enrolled at Princeton University, where he played on the baseball and basketball teams. Next came Yale University, where he earned a master's degree in English literature while serving as a teaching assistant. But his march toward a life of rigorous academic study and tenured ease came abruptly to a halt in the mid-1980s, when an actor friend convinced him to try out for a Löwenbrau beer commercial. He landed the part and found his passion. In his case, the acting bug turned out to be a leech — he soon abandoned his PhD program and moved back to New York City, where he scored a few Off Broadway roles and bit parts in such films as *Working Girl, New Year's Day,* and *Beethoven.* Then came his breakthrough: playing a transvestite FBI agent in the David Lynch series *Twin Peaks.* For Duchovny, it was a significant experience beyond the career repercussions. People on the crew, he says dolefully, actually laughed at him. "The interesting thing is it hurt my feelings," he admits. "I have been lucky — or unlucky — enough to be an accepted human being. I'm white, I'm male, I'm straight. But now I know the constraints women feel when they dress, and what it's like to be ridiculed for being gay by unfeeling men. And on top of all that, my vanity kicked in. I felt so unattractive."

With *Twin Peaks* providing something meaty to put on his curriculum vitae, his career really started to move. He starred in Zalman King's sexy anthology series *The Red Shoe Diaries* on Showtime, and landed roles in the feature films *The Rapture, Julia Has Two Lovers,* and *Chaplin.* Then Chris Carter came into his life, though Duchovny didn't think he'd get much of a chance to become acquainted. "I thought I could go to Vancouver for a month and get paid, and then

go on and do my next movie. After all, a show about extraterrestrials — no matter how well made — how many can you do? I didn't see the show opening up to be about *anything* that's unexplained, which is limitless."

Carter, for his part, had greater faith in Duchovny than the actor had in Carter's show. "David read for the part and was perfect," the

"*The X-Files* is very nineties, because everything is left in doubt. There's no closure, no answers."

X-Files creator says. "We were obligated to give the network a choice of at least two actors, but we knew David was it from the start. He was just very, very right for the role."

Daniel Sackheim, who produced the pilot and directed three episodes, reflects: "I remember the first time we screened the pilot. Everybody thought David was a movie star. I think he offered a certain sense of vulnerability. He was handsome, but he was sort of like the boy next door. He was the brother that you wanted to comfort. That was the quality David brought that we were excited about."

✻ ✻ ✻

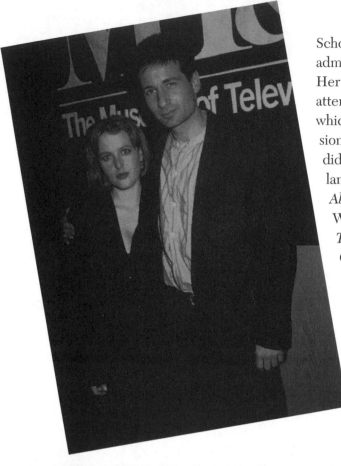

David Duchovny and Gillian Anderson attend an X-Files event at the Museum of Television and Radio.

School in Chicago and impressed the school's admissions committee with her raw talent. Her stage work at the university attracted the attention of the William Morris talent agency, which took her on as a client with the provision that she relocate to New York City. She did so, and while working as a waitress she landed the lead in the Off Broadway show *Absent Friends,* which won her a Theater World award. Roles in a production of *The Philanthropist* in New Haven, Connecticut, and in the feature film *The Turning* quickly followed. Then, in 1993, the then-twenty-five-year-old read the pilot script for *The X-Files* and auditioned the next day.

"It's very interesting," Anderson says, "because I remember exactly where I was when I read the script. I was enthralled by it. It was very different from anything I'd read, and certainly the character of Dana Scully was incredibly appealing to me. I had a very distinct feeling that the show would be a part of my life when I read it, even though in the process of going to the auditions, which took about a week and a half, there was certainly nervousness, fear, and questioning of my ability to land the role. I nonetheless still had a very strong feeling that it was going to be a part of my life."

She wasn't the only one. "When she came into the room, I just knew that she was Scully," says Carter. "She had an intensity

The road to fame for Gillian Anderson was more direct. An indifferent student in high school and given to punk-rock dress and attitudes, the rebellious, spiky-haired teen found the theater to be a sanctuary of sorts. After graduating from public school in Grand Rapids, Michigan, she auditioned for DePaul University's prestigious Goodman Theater about her, the kind of intensity that translates well across the screen."

The network's execs, however, still had some trouble with the interpretation. After viewing Anderson's filmed audition, Fox's honchos were nonplussed. She wasn't the bouncy, former-model type that typically fit into the second lead, they told Carter. Of course, they were right.

"Gillian is an attractive woman," says Daniel Sackheim, "but she is not what one would call a sex queen. She's not the classic sex symbol type — tall, blonde, big-breasted — you know, the kind of woman networks love to put in those kinds of roles. What appealed to me was Chris's desire to cast the role real, as opposed to casting it in the traditional way networks cast, which is to skew it to a certain level of sex appeal. Chris didn't want to do that, and that's one of the things that drew me into the project."

"When she came into the room, I just knew that she was Scully."

In the end, the network relented, and Carter got his Scully.

"I sort of staked my pilot and my career at the time on Gillian." Carter smiles. "I feel vindicated every day now."

PART TWO

The X-Files

The only thing we have to fear, said Franklin Roosevelt, is fear itself.

Our thirty-second president must not have gone to the movies very often. If he had, he would have known that there were horrors far darker than self-doubt and pessimism. There were vampires and giant gorillas and zombies and swamp creatures. And they all wanted to kill you in the most gruesome fashion imaginable.

From the medium's beginnings at the turn of the century, filmmakers have exploited our fascination with fear, using horrific creatures to represent everyday terrors. In 1910, when film was still just a hobby for geek tinkerers, Thomas Edison created a silent short of Mary Shelley's *Frankenstein*. And the manipulation of our fears has steadily gained in variety and sophistication since. In the 1930s and '40s, audiences were introduced to a multitude of monsters, most notably Bela Lugosi's Dracula, who flitted through a long series of successful films — even an Abbott

> **Most television fare is just eye candy, whereas *The X-Files* is "an intellectual exercise."**

and Costello comedy. In the '50s, the studios put Dracula on hold to make way for alien invaders, a threat more applicable to the Cold War era.

In the traditional horror film of the Red Scare years, the supernatural threat ultimately becomes known to the community at large, which rallies together — and around the flag — to put a stop to it. But as the Soviet menace receded (psychologically, if not tangibly), we became more concerned about the momentum of our own society, a technological behemoth that we feared alienated, or simply disposed of, individuals. Its antennae tuned to this shift, the horror genre became more internalized, examining the dark side of the soul and the consequences of moral decay. The result, at its best, was films like *Rosemary's Baby*, *The Omen*, and *The Exorcist*. And it's here, beginning with *The Invaders* and *The Night Stalker* in the late '60s and early '70s, that television began to outpace its big-screen parent.

Considerable influences on films and TV shows of this bent were the Vietnam War and the Watergate scandal. Trafficking in the public's loss of confidence in its representatives, films like *Three Days of the Condor* obliterat-

Shooting in Vancouver

Throughout its production history, *The X-Files* has appeared to be taking place in various locations throughout the world, but in fact all of it has been shot in Vancouver.

"The drawback is that I'm sitting in Los Angeles right now while they're shooting up there and I can't walk over to the stage to make changes and tweaks," Chris Carter explains. "The quality control suffers, so you hope you get what I have right now, which is Bob Goodwin, who has similar sensibilities to me. He does a great job up there. But there's a communication problem, first of all, by the very nature of the distance between us. There is a problem with weather — you get a lot of rain up there. If you want to shoot a day-for-day scene outside, chances are you're going to be doing it in the rain, and chances are you've got between the hours of nine and three to do it. The sun never gets too high in the sky. The opposite is true in the summer. You don't get much darkness. It gets dark like eleven at night and gets light at about four in the morning. Those are the hours you have to work if you want to get night scenes. Those are some of the drawbacks.

"On the positive side," he adds, "there are financial benefits. Obviously the exchange rate is something that works to our benefit, saving us twenty percent on the dollar. You can't argue the economics of going to Canada with a show like this, a two-lead show. More importantly, Vancouver turned out to be a very multipurpose city. It can double as almost anywhere in the U.S. There are only a few limitations. You can't do big desert scenes. So as far as the location, it's ideal and is a pretty negotiable city. Plus, there aren't any traffic jams to deal with."

ed the line between horror and realism. As public cynicism only grew in the following years, *The X-Files* almost seems inevitable.

Which is not to say it was easy to get the show on the air. Chris Carter brought a fresh, even radical, approach to supernatural horror, and TV executives embrace change with about as much enthusiasm as Russian pensioners do. But for the creative talent, it was a dream come true.

"Working on *The X-Files* was a relief," says writer Glen Morgan. "Jim Wong [Morgan's longtime writing collaborator] and I worked at Cannell Productions for so long on shows such as *21 Jump Street* and *The Commish*, and we were looking to move on. But then we sat down and watched the pilot for *The X-Files* and said, 'Wow.'"

Adds Wong, "In some ways, Glen and I have always liked suspense and the darker side of life. When we watched the pilot we said, 'You know, there are so many ideas that come to mind when you think about *The X-Files* versus anything else out there.' That's what appealed to us."

Once he had Morgan and Wong in the fold, Carter recruited Howard Gordon and Alex Gansa, best known to genre fans for their work on *Beauty and the Beast*. "I loved *Star Trek*, but I was not a hardcore SF fan," Gordon admits. "Except for films like *The Exorcist*, I wasn't a horror film fan. I didn't dislike it, but it certainly wasn't something that I'd ever given much thought to. Alex and

I found ourselves baffled and, frankly, a little bit out of our depth at first. We were more inclined towards straight-ahead dramas. We struggled mightily with our first script for the show. I didn't think the show was a perfect fit, but I was glad for the opportunity. I've often described it as feeling like I'm a miler being asked to do sprints. It's not really my event, but I've developed certain muscles that have enabled me to survive and thrive."

Filling out the core staff for the series's launch were co–executive producer Robert Goodwin, who was given the assignment of overseeing the physical production of every episode; director of photography John Bartley; special-effects pro Mat Beck; composer Mark Snow; co-producer Paul Rabwin; production designer Graeme Murray, a veteran of TV's *Wiseguy* and the feature films *Never Cry Wolf* and John Carpenter's remake of *The Thing;* and makeup artist Toby Lindala. Together, they crafted a new style of television storytelling.

"There are a lot of people involved in the production of the episodes," Carter says. "It's music, it's lighting, it's photography, it's production design and scripts, and, of course, the actors. My relationship with each of those people is very tight, and we work very closely

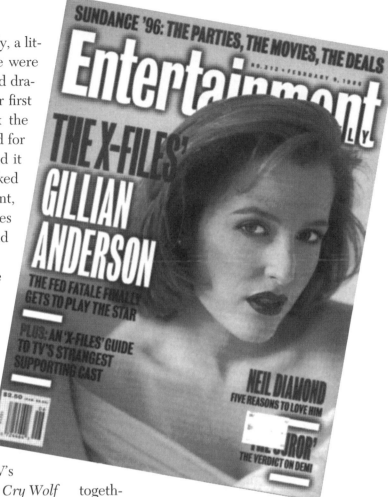

together. This is a rare case, I think, where when you give them the scripts, they come up with ideas to make them better. Everyone's stock rises with success, and so what usually happens is people want to take their stock and trade it up, and everybody wants to do something different or better, or maybe even a feature. Everybody thinks that features are the big thing. But I think we're doing feature-quality work on the TV show, week in and week out, and that's the reason that these people have stayed: it's an opportunity to consistently do good work.

"One-hour episodic drama is the hardest show in town," he continues. "Beyond that, when you have shows that succeed in the format — *Hill Street Blues, L.A. Law, Picket Fences* — they're usually ensembles, so you've got a lot of people to carry the workload. They're done as interiors on standing sets inside buildings. We are really doing a little movie each week. We are out usually about five or six of the eight days we're shooting; we can't go back to standing sets. This all takes a lot of intensive production attention. We have two characters who have to carry most of the workload. And we're all laboring to make it real for the audience."

That commitment to realism within a supernatural premise is what attracted director David Nutter to the series. "The key to the drama is making everything as real as possible," says Nutter, who directed the pilot episode of Carter's new series, *Millennium.* "To do this, you really have to get the characters' emotions and the environment of the story just right. You also have to get into the hearts and minds of people — not only those who are putting the show together, but the people who are at home, watching. I looked at the show as a strong, realistic drama. If the audience believed it and could relate to it, you could then turn it on its head and do the things that make the show what it is. That's

the key: to get the audience to go along for the ride. It's like locking them in to a seat of the roller coaster. Once you've done that, you've got them."

Michael Lange, who directed a pair of episodes during the first season, offers the opinion that most television fare is just eye candy, whereas *The X-Files* is "an intellectual exercise."

"I remember when I first started watching the show, which was before I even got an assignment to direct one, my first impression was that these were true stories taken from the deep files of the FBI," he says. "And I'm a fairly sophisticated viewer. And with the subjects it deals with, you can, for the most part, accept that maybe this *could happen.* One of my favorite Hitchcockisms is his saying that he didn't believe films had to be believable, merely plausible. That's the same thing with *The X-Files.*"

And the two people most responsible for making it plausible aren't the writers or directors, but David Duchovny and Gillian Anderson. The give-and-take between their characters provides the series with its analytical and moral code. Duchovny's Fox Mulder is the primary champion of the FBI's X-Files; he's obsessed with paranormal investigations. Anderson's Scully, a doctor and forensics expert, is assigned to the X-Files to temper Mulder's enthusiasms. It is the emotional reality of their characters that lets the audience accept the bizarre happenings. No other

Attracting Opposites

On *The X-Files*, Fox Mulder (David Duchovny) believes in UFOs and the paranormal, while his FBI partner, Dana Scully (Gillian Anderson), is a skeptic. But the actors who play Mulder and Scully see things differently from the way their characters do.

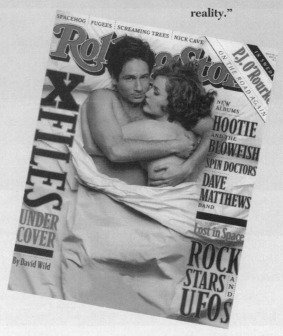

"Personally," Duchovny says, "I'm the kind of person who needs to be shown something before I can believe it, and I haven't had any personal experiences with UFOs. But, on the other hand, it's hard for me to believe that we're the only sentient life in this universe. I think there's got to be something else out there. I just don't know why they always seem to choose people in North Dakota. So I'm waiting.

"I guess I believe in the abstract, but not in the specific," he continues. "You know, if you ask me if I believe that the things we do on the show are possible, I say yes. But if you ask me if I believe that they actually have happened, I say no. *The X-Files* aims at a point where physics and metaphysics meet; where science and poetry come together. We take the real world and put imagined things in it. We're not science fiction and we're not cops and robbers. We have one foot in each."

Unlike Duchovny, Anderson is something of a believer. "I think the more I get comfortable with this character, the more she's becoming like me in some of her mannerisms," the actress says of Dana Scully. "But I am not that much of a skeptic. I do believe in UFOs, I do believe in certain paranormal phenomena like ESP and psychokinesis. In that respect, I think I'm different from Scully. I think I have a tendency to get as single-minded and obsessed with my work as Scully does, but in a different way. She's a medical doctor and an FBI agent, and I'm an actress. But the paranormal is something that I've always been fascinated with, and I think on a certain level, I've always just known or assumed it to be a reality."

One of the most hotly debated questions on the Internet these days is whether or not Fox Mulder and Dana Scully should — to quote Maddie and David in *Moonlighting* — "get horizontal." Despite the cover of *Rolling Stone*, which seems to say the opposite, Chris Carter emphasizes that it will never happen. "That's David and Gillian in bed, *not* Mulder and Scully," says Carter, regarding the *RS* cover.

series traffics so subversively in the unexpected, but Mulder and Scully make it all seem like just another day at the office.

Considering that the *X-Files* budget is significantly lower than that for such genre fare as *Lois & Clark* and the now defunct *seaQuest*, Robert Goodwin is amazed that the show is able to achieve all that it does. "I feel, with some pride, that what we're delivering is the best-quality television you can get. We don't skimp; we just find a way to do what we want within our budget. The first year, I almost had a nervous collapse every time I got a new script: 'Okay,' I would say to myself, 'here's a good one: This guy can relocate all the bones in his body and slither through tiny air vents and suck people's livers out of their bodies. Great. How do we do that?' Every episode there's something that's really amazingly challenging to create. From great fires to worms wriggling under the skin of people."

After an episode is shot, co-producer Paul Rabwin steps in and supervises all aspects of postproduction. "Many things that I do have to be done during the preproduction stage when, for example, there are television screens that have to be photographed. The film that is being projected on the TV screen has got to be processed so that it can be rephotographed by a camera. In one episode we have our guys watching film supposedly from the 1950s showing DDT being sprayed over kids in a swimming pool. I have to find and obtain the material, have it transferred in

In Praise of The Night Stalker

Not to belabor the point, but at this juncture it's pretty obvious that Chris Carter was inspired by night-stalking reporter Carl Kolchak to create *The X-Files*. The love affair doesn't stop at the top, however.

Although *The X-Files* is quite different from *The Night Stalker*, there are undeniable similarities between the experiences of agents Mulder and Scully and those of the journalist Kolchak.

"I recently saw *The Night Stalker* for the first time since the early seventies," says Glen Morgan, who has co-written many *X-Files* episodes, "and I was surprised how much we are similar to it. In the TV movie, they find a girl in a river of sand. Everyone else is stumped, and Kolchak is saying, 'There are no footprints. And all her blood is gone.' He's raising all these weird questions. That's what Mulder would do. I guess that type of show was long overdue. There was a hole in TV that needed to be filled."

Adds Morgan's writing partner James Wong, "I just remember watching *The Night Stalker* as a kid and being so scared. So it's great to be doing *The X-Files* as an adult, and to really be conscious of what we're doing: trying to scare a new generation."

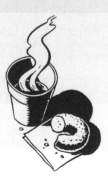

such a way that it can be rephotographed, and have it sent back up there in time for them to shoot the scene. So there are certain areas that are considered postproduction which actually happen prior to the filming taking place."

The bulk of Rabwin's work involves editing, music, sound effects, and special optical effects. Terming himself a "general overseer" of these areas, he notes that specific experts work in each of those departments.

"We have three editors who work in rotation," he explains. ""One would get all of the film on one episode and will spend three or four weeks working on it, then he finishes that and starts working on another. The three of them rotate. The editor works in conjunction with the director and the producers of the series, all of whom have a say in what will make the show better. Sometimes a show will be several minutes longer than network requirements, and we have to edit material out. On a rare occasion we have a show that actually comes in a little on the short side and we have to come up with creative ways to lengthen it.

"Generally, the main focus during the editing process is to get the show to work well, to make it interesting, to make it flow, to make it entertaining, and to drop a bombshell at the magic moment at the end of the act so that people will come back after the commercials."

One particularly difficult aspect of each episode of *The X-Files* is the use of special optical effects, supplied by Mat Beck during postproduction. "Those require a certain amount of time, and very often we need to have the film edited before we can start making the effects," Rabwin notes, "because with special effects very often you're paying for the amount of time spent in a particular kind of edit bay, where each frame has to be artistically rendered. You want to be as specific as possible as to where the special effects have to be. You can't just say, 'Let's just treat the entire scene and we'll just cut it.' You have to say, 'There are exactly three and a half seconds of this particular scene that needs to have this special effect.' If you made it four seconds, it could cost you another thousand dollars for that extra half second. So you need to have the show edited fairly substantially before you can begin many of the special effects.

"On a television schedule," he elaborates, "they're shooting eight working days, which is ten calendar days, but we're on the air every seven days. Eventually the law of averages catches up with you. As you get deeper into the season, you get closer and closer to the airdates from the time you finish shooting. The show is on the air Fridays. We've had some very madcap schedules where we have finished shooting a show on a Thursday, we look at all of our film on Friday, work all weekend, and then on Monday we finalize the show. We give it to the sound effects people on Tuesday and we deliver it a week later. That's the kind of a schedule we've had on occasion.

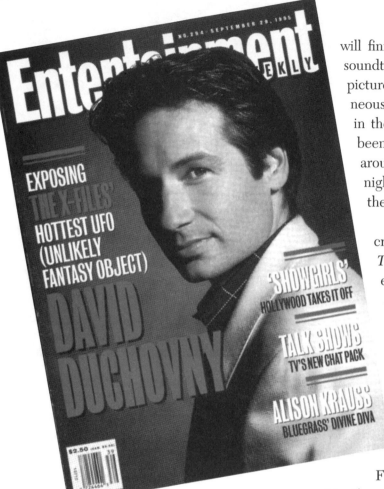

will finish on Wednesday night, take that soundtrack and put it onto the completed picture that has been worked on simultaneously with color correction and putting in the opticals and special effects we've been talking about. It all comes together around three in the morning Thursday night–Friday morning. We deliver it to the network and they air it that night."

Despite this kind of seemingly crushing schedule, in its first season *The X-Files* managed to offer a variety of supernatural or paranormal stories, ranging from liver-eating serial killers ("Squeeze" and "Tooms"), technology run amok ("Ghost in the Machine"), possession ("Ice," "Space," "Lazarus," "Born Again"), genetic experimentation ("Eve"), ghosts ("Shadows," "Beyond the Sea"), deadly insects ("Darkness Falls"), and faith healers ("Miracle Man").

"The composer will generally spend a week creating the score, the sound effects supervisor and his staff will spend a week collecting all of the sound effects and putting them into a package that will, in essence, have them all in sync with each other. Generally on the Tuesday and Wednesday of the week the show is airing, we will mix together all of the music and sound effects. It's a two-day process. We generally

But there is one theme above all others that everyone on the crew can count on regularly: space aliens and government conspiracies, the show's bread-and-butter subject.

Aliens arrived in the pilot episode, which brought Mulder and Scully together and launched them on their first case: the mysterious disappearance of several teenagers in Oregon. Upon investigation, evidence of possible extraterrestrial involvement is discovered. But such a traditional treatment of ET visitation was not indicative of the course of the series. Whereas the pilot dealt with standard UFO premises, the next episode, "Deep Throat," took a further step into the fantastic. Mulder sneaks onto a U.S. Air Force base, where he discovers that the military is conducting experiments with alien technology it has stumbled upon, hoping to develop an advanced aircraft.

In the character-driven "Conduit," Mulder and Scully investigate the disappearance of a young girl, which taps in to Mulder's memories of the abduction of his sister. "Fallen Angel" turns up the heat on the aliens-among-us premise. In this episode, an alien creature survives the crash of its ship and flees authorities, using its ability to become invisible to human eyes. Mulder and Scully, naturally, want to find it before the military does.

"E.B.E." begins with Mulder and Scully hearing that an alien craft has been downed, and that an extraterrestrial body has been found by the government. This time — thanks to Deep Throat's manipulations — Mulder *just* misses alien contact, probably by a moment or two. It all culminates with "The Erlenmeyer Flask," and its tale of experimentation with alien DNA, an alien embryo, the death of Deep Throat, and the closing of the

X-Files, all of which was designed to lead in to the show's second season. Together, these episodes bring Mulder and Scully, as well as the audience, ever closer to actual contact with extraterrestrials.

"I think it was a very conscious thing with

"It's easy to scare people," says Carter simply, "but it's hard to scare them in a way that has some resonance; that really makes them double-lock their doors at night."

us," Chris Carter says. "We realize you can't keep playing with the audience; you have to bring them closer. Actually, my feeling is that even by the end of season one we *had* had contact of a sort. We came closer than I had anticipated coming in the first twenty-four episodes."

Also accomplished during that first season was the establishing of some of the series's parameters on what would and would not work within the format.

"We're charting uncharted waters; we're figuring it out and telling the best stories that we can with our wonderful characters," Carter says. "I don't want it to be each week that we

The Death of Deep Throat

Guiding Fox Mulder through the treacherous waters of government intrigue during the debut season of *The X-Files* was Deep Throat, the shadowy inside informant who was dramatically knocked off in the first-year finale, "The Erlenmeyer Flask."

"The mystery of a character who has unlimited sources of information, but also has enemies, makes for interesting acting work," says Jerry Hardin, who played the enigmatic informant. "Since he wasn't clearly defined by the writers, I had a chance to pursue the role freely. That's interesting to do, because he could be a bad guy just as easily as a good guy. In TV, you're often dealing only with characters who are black or white, and the actor must make a big effort to somehow get a few specks of the other colors."

Deep Throat, who appeared in seven episodes of the first season, acquired a surprisingly strong cult following during his run. The character's death at the end of the season caught a lot of viewers off guard.

"When you kill a character like Deep Throat, it's almost like killing off Janet Leigh in *Psycho*," says co–executive producer and "Erlenmeyer Flask" director Robert Goodwin. "It affects people."

Although he enjoyed Hardin and his portrayal, series creator Chris Carter says, "The character had provided information in a very systematic and predictable way, and I was interested in exploring new ways of Mulder getting his information."

But Hardin blames himself for aiding his character's demise. "I was pushing to make the character a regular," he notes. "I think they felt they needed to accede to my desires or get rid of me. So they decided to get rid of me."

go for the expected. We'll take detours. I think we've got so many strong episodes that we can take chances. It's what I always try to do, and I think it's what makes a series fresh — you bear off in different directions and check them out."

His favorite catchphrase for the series is that every story has to take place within the realm of extreme possibility. "I just think it's a much more interesting show if it's believable. I think it's much more frightening. You know, if you look at Michael Crichton's *Terminal Man* or *Jurassic Park* or *The Andromeda Strain*, the most frightening part is that you actually believe that it *could* happen. The tricky part each week is taking these stories and rooting them in reality; making it believable that they could really be happening, therefore heightening the scare.

"It's easy to scare people," says Carter simply, "but it's hard to scare them in a way that has some resonance; that really makes them double-lock their doors at night."

The X-Files

SEASON ONE
Episode Guide

Episode 1.1
"The X-Files" (pilot)

Original airdate: September 10, 1993
Written by Chris Carter
Directed by Robert Mandel
Guest starring: Doug Abrams (Patrolman),
Zachary Ansley (Billy Miles), Alexandra Berlin
(Orderly), J. B. Bivens (Truck Driver), Ken
Camroux (Third Man), Charles Cioffi (Section
Chief Scott Blevins), William B. Davis
(Cigarette-Smoking Man), Cliff DeYoung (Dr.
Jay Nemman), Lesley Ewen (Receptionist),
Katya Gardener (Peggy O'Dell), Jim Jansen
(Dr. Heitz Werber), Sarah Koskoff (Theresa),
Stephen E. Miller (Truitt), Ric Reid
(Astronomer), Leon Russom (Det. Miles),
Malcolm Stewart (Dr. Glass)

FBI agent Dana Scully is assigned to be the partner of Fox Mulder, the agency's leading expert on the so-called X-Files: cases involving the unexplainable, from reported UFO abductions to the paranormal. Essentially given the task of debunking Mulder's discoveries by applying a scientific approach, Scully nevertheless finds it impossible to completely skewer her new partner's efforts through scientific reasoning.

Their first assignment brings them to
Oregon, where the death of a teenage girl and the disappearance of several other teens indicate that they have been abducted by aliens. At episode's end, the one piece of evidence obtained — a tiny metallic cylinder that had been inserted in a victim's nose — is given to the enigmatic Cigarette-Smoking Man, who places it in a storage house within the Pentagon.

❊   ❊   ❊

A justifiably proud Chris Carter states, "I think the pilot worked great, and I'm helped to that opinion by the response I've gotten to it. Also, when we tested it with test audiences,

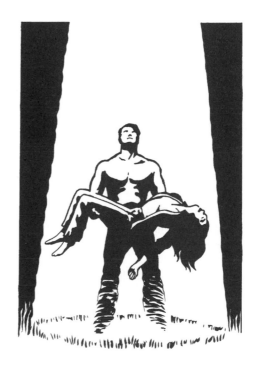

it was the kind of response that you only dream about. In fact, I remember when I first screened the pilot for Rupert Murdoch and the Fox executives, I'd finished the pilot at five in the morning and they saw it at eight in the morning. That's how close we were to deadline. But after the screening, there was spontaneous applause from the audience. These are people who usually watch to see how the boss responds, but it was an overwhelmingly positive response to the show. I think it succeeds on many levels.

"I was helped on the pilot by a very collaborative group consisting of director Bob Mandel and Daniel Sackheim, the producer. Dan also directed 'Deep Throat,' 'Conduit,' and 'The Host.' The two of them were instrumental in giving the pilot the quality and standard for what has become the series."

"What impressed me," notes former scriptwriter and co–executive producer Glen Morgan, who went on to co-create *Space: Above and Beyond* with James Wong, "was the merging of *Silence of the Lambs* and *Close Encounters of the Third Kind*. It got Jim and me aboard, and I liked the open ending. It was scary, and there's nothing scary on TV."

Howard Gordon, who along with partner Alex Gansa had produced the fantasy series *Beauty and the Beast*, was also impressed with the pilot and irresistibly drawn to the series itself. "The pilot set the tone of the show really successfully," he says. "It established Mulder and Scully's characters, as well as the aspect of Mulder's sister supposedly being abducted. There was also a good solid murder investigation. Pilots are a strange breed, because you have to tell a story while simultaneously introducing the characters the audience is going to love, and you have to do it all in forty-eight minutes. Although I think the series has improved on it, the pilot was a tremendous synthesis of all the parts."

Rating/Audience Share: 7.9/15

Episode 1.2
"Deep Throat"

Original airdate: September 17, 1993
Written by Chris Carter
Directed by Daniel Sackheim
Guest starring: Charles Cioffi (Section Chief Scott Blevins), John Cuthbert (Commanding Officer), Michael Bryan French (Paul Mossinger), Brian Furlong (Lead Officer), Seth Green (Emil), Jerry Hardin (Deep Throat), Doc Harris (Mr. McLennen), Andrew Johnston (Col. Budahas), Lalainia Lindejerg (Zoe), Vince Metcalfe (Kissell), Sheila Moore (Verla McLennen), Monica Parker (Ladonna), Michael Puttonen (Motel Manager), Gabrielle Rose (Anita Budahas)

Mulder is contacted by the mysterious Deep Throat, a government source who is willing to provide tidbits of information to help the agent in his quest to discover the truth about UFOs and a far-reaching government conspiracy. As a result, Mulder and Scully travel to

Idaho to investigate the disappearance of a pilot from Ellis Air Force Base. What they (Mulder in particular) discover is that the military is performing mind experiments on pilots who have been flying new vehicles apparently created from alien technology.

❄ ❄ ❄

"The character of Deep Throat of course came from the infamous Watergate figure, who may or may not have existed," offers Chris Carter, who also cites Donald Sutherland's portrayal of "Mr. X" in Oliver Stone's *JFK* as inspiration. "I felt that we needed a connection: somebody who would come from this mysterious, shadowy government; somebody who works in some level of government that we have no idea exists, and he comes to Mulder and Scully and leads them carefully, selectively, without giving them too much and making them work for the answers, but helping them when they reach a dead end or helping them when they make a wrong turn."

Also pleasing to Carter was the fact that Daniel Sackheim returned to direct the episode. "It was a natural and worked well," Carter enthuses. "We were of one mind as to what the show is about, so I wrote this episode that he thought was great and he did a wonderful job directing it. The episode also further served to establish the landscape we were going to be working in with *The X-Files:* the introduction of Deep Throat, and the idea

that the government knows even more than we established in the pilot and that they will go to any length to protect that information."

While the notion of the government utilizing alien technology to improve its own aircraft seems highly original, Carter demurs. "Believe me," he says with a laugh, "when you start reading the material that's out there, anything you can imagine has either been imagined or experienced by some folks."

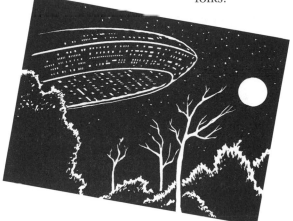

Howard Gordon views "Deep Throat" as part two of the pilot, with Carter attempting to reestablish the themes of a government UFO conspiracy. "The Army using alien technology is what made it most interesting," he opines. "The whole Roswell thing and Ellis Air Force Base are the pillars of UFO mythology, so it was an appropriate and smart first choice for Chris. And then the idea of the government doing mind control . . . People really responded to Mulder's putting his neck on the line, seeking the truth and then getting taken himself and having his brain subjected to the same thing these pilots were subjected to."

Co–executive producer Robert Goodwin, who supervises physical production of the series, found "Deep Throat" to be a particularly challenging episode.

"We had to put together a new crew, and

"We wanted to get right out of the box after 'Deep Throat' and do something that *wasn't* an alien story."

'Deep Throat' was a break-in period where everybody came to learn the kinds of demands of quality that we were making," he explains. "They'd worked on several shows prior to ours that hadn't been as challenging or demanding. There was a certain level of quality that they had to step up to, and in all honesty, virtually all of the departments did that. But it was a learning experience.

"My most vivid memory of the episode was a sequence in which Mulder is out on the tarmac at this Air Force base where this UFO hovers over him," Goodwin continues. "We had that, plus about three shots where this UFO hovers over him, and then a few more scenes where these two teenage kids show Mulder where the base is. We started shoot-

ing ten o'clock Friday morning and we finished shooting eight o'clock Saturday morning. It was amazingly difficult. We had one scene where these two kids lead Mulder to the edge of the base. Originally it was written that they would lead Mulder up to a certain point and say, 'We'll leave you here; we're not going any farther. Go through that part of the fence when it gets dark.' And we were supposed to dissolve to night. Well, as we were progressing we realized we weren't going to get it shot that afternoon and we had to turn it into a night scene. Then we had to turn it back into a day scene because we couldn't get it shot before the sun came out."

Rating/Audience Share: 7.3/14

**Episode 1.3
"Squeeze"**
Original airdate: September 24, 1993
Written by Glen Morgan and James Wong
Directed by Harry Longstreet
Guest starring: Henry Beckman (Det. Frank Briggs), James Bell (Johnson), Gary Hetherington (Kennedy), Doug Hutchison (Eugene Victor Tooms), Paul Joyce (Mr. Werner), Terence Kelly (George Usher), Donal Logue (Tom Colton), Kevin McNulty (Fuller), Rob Morton (Kramer), Colleen Winton (Lie Detector Technician)

Mulder and Scully travel to Maryland, where they go up against Eugene Tooms, a mutant who can squeeze his body through any space and who comes out of hibernation every thirty years to devour the livers of five victims. Tooms must be stopped before he vanishes again for another three decades.

❈ ❈ ❈

"Squeeze" was significant in the development of *The X-Files* in that it informed the audience that the show wasn't just going to be a UFO series. As Glen Morgan explains it, "I remember I read an article about Richard Ramirez, the Night Stalker of LA, in the middle eighties, and the rumors were that he was climbing in those little windows everyone has in their bathroom above their shower. Supposedly he would climb in through those windows and the dust and soap grime on the sill was undisturbed. He was a pretty big guy. I think we took it from there. That was when it was Jim and Chris and I sitting around saying, 'How about this, how about that?' Some things we thought would be too far out there."

"An okay episode," adds Jim Wong, "but I was very disappointed by its production. There were a lot of things that didn't work for us and we had to go back and reshoot. The production of it left such a nasty taste in my mouth that I've never really thought it was

that good, but we've gotten a lot of [positive] reaction to it. It *was* creepy, though, and in that way it worked really well. All I can see is what it should have been. It should have been more than it was, though it did do its job."

Morgan notes that the episode was truly saved in postproduction, and that editing made the show. "I think it's been so long since television has done horror, and it's been an area for low-budget features for so long, that people have forgotten how to do it well. We

"We found this Canadian contortionist named Pepper. We said, 'Here's the little opening, see what you can do.' All we added were some sound effects of bones snapping and cracking."

wanted certain things which weren't agreed with, and when we watched the episode it wasn't scary. It was a show that taught us all a lot."

The casting of Doug Hutchison as Tooms stands out in Morgan's mind. "When the actor came in to read," he recalls, "we said, 'No, no, he looks like he's twelve years old.' Then I said, 'Come to think of it, he looks forty.' Then the director said, 'Can I see you go from a neutral position to one of attacking me?' Doug just sat there and said, 'A neutral position?' a couple of times. And the director said, 'And then you're going to attack me.' 'I'm going to attack you?' Doug responded. All of us react-

ed, 'Oh, brother, here's a nut.' Then he was immediately into it and he really scared the shit out of us. He just started off as if he didn't understand what we were talking about. What he was really doing was showing us how he was building up to being a maniac. Naturally we said, 'He's the guy.'"

Chris Carter recalls that when the series was okayed by Fox, he had been on vacation with his wife in France and had to head back to California a week earlier than expected. "Which didn't go over well with my wife." He smiles. "So she stayed and traveled around the country while I came back and started to work with Glen and Jim. We wanted to get right out of the box after 'Deep Throat' and do something that *wasn't* an alien story. It was a story that expanded the realm of what an X-File could be. As far as the germ of the idea, I had eaten some foie gras in France and I thought, 'Wouldn't it be intriguing if some human was interested in eating the livers of other humans?' That was the kernel of the idea, and they turned it into a terrific, dramatic, and very scary episode."

From Robert Goodwin's point of view, the chief challenge of "Squeeze" was designing the scene in which Tooms climbs up onto the roof of a house, squeezes into a very small opening in the chimney (dislocating most of the bones his body), enters the house, and chows down on his victim's liver.

"Somehow," Goodwin says, "we found this contortionist named Pepper. So we brought Pepper to the set, thinking we could get at least part of the scene with him as a photo double. We said, 'Here's the little opening — see what you can do.' Well, Pepper squeezed right down inside the damn thing, right in front of us. He got his whole body inside of there. That's what you see. All we added were some sound effects of bones snapping and cracking. We didn't do any visual effects at all. It was amazing."

Despite the incredibly flexible Pepper, effects supervisor Mat Beck and his team did get some work. "Mat Beck did this wonderfully subtle computer effect of Tooms's fingers stretching as he climbs up the house," says co-producer Paul Rabwin, who supervises post-production. "The viewer actually had to wonder if those fingers really were stretching. I think that's a real key to our show. As opposed to saying with red lights and sirens that the fingers are stretching, you make the audience ask, 'Is that happening? Am I seeing that?' It's a very effective way of doing visual effects."

Referring to a later shot in which Tooms fluidly erupts from a heating vent, Beck explains that the show is careful not to take any effects shots over the top. "Hutchison came rocketing out of the vent we built six different ways from Sunday. It was pretty intense, even unstretched. We then shot a clean background plate of the apartment, added a bunch of blue-screen material around the grate, and shot him again coming out of the grate against the blue so we could stretch him [on the computer]. We squeezed him a bit when we put him back in the scene, but not a lot, because Chris Carter insists that less is more: just a hint of the unnatural is all that is required."

A hint was all that *was* needed, as most viewers felt that combination of terror and fascination Carter is always aiming for. Tooms became the show's most identifiable demonic figure — no small feat in a series devoted to such characters. Even the normally stoic Gillian Anderson was a bit unnerved. "It was just incredibly creepy to me." She laughs. "I think it was one of the first scripts I read where I was nervous afterward."

Rating/Audience Share: 7.2/13

Episode 1.4
"Conduit"
Original airdate: October 1, 1993
Written by Alex Gansa and Howard Gordon
Directed by Daniel Sackheim
Guest starring: Michael Cavanaugh (Sheriff), Charles Cioffi (Section Chief Scott Blevins), Taunya Dee (Ruby Morris), Don Gibb (Kip), Anthony Harrison (Fourth Man), Mauricio Mercado (Coroner), Akiko Morison (Leza Atsumi), Shelley Owens (Tessa), Joel Palmer (Kevin Morris), Glen Roald (M.E. Worker), Carrie Snodgress (Darlene Morris), Don Thompson (Holtzman)

In Sioux City, Iowa, Mulder's feelings for his abducted sister are reawakened when he learns of a teenage girl who has apparently been abducted as well. He and Scully check out the story of the girl's mother, Darlene Morris, who was an abductee herself but is reluctant to talk about it. At episode's end, Scully does her best to account for everything scientifically, but she is confronted with information that has no rational explanation.

☼ ☼ ☼

"Alex [Gansa] and I made an effort to play to our own strength, which is character," says Howard Gordon. "We thought this was an interesting place to reiterate Mulder's quest for his sister. We set out to tell a simple abduction story, which was played out behind the shadows. We wanted to create an air of tension. With everything that happened, we wanted to explain what it could be. At every point, everything can be explained. Was she taken or killed by her boyfriend, who she was seeing against her mother's wishes? Is it *Twin Peaks* or an alien abduction? That was the theme of the show.

"We also used UFO lore," he continues, "like the idea of repeat abductions and mother–daughter abductions. Apparently you're taken and sometimes several members of the family are taken as well. I think we're most proud of the ending: Mulder's quest is reestablished (and Daniel Sackheim directed it beautifully) with Mulder sitting alone in a church with only his faith. The story, again, was fueled by Mulder's belief and emotional connection with this case. Another girl taken from her family. And, in a way, the little boy who is the conduit, who is also perhaps touched by the aliens, is essentially Mulder. Those little touches the fans seem to respond to. It was difficult for us, but in the end satisfying. It came out of frustration on our parts, and creative uncertainty."

Most significant about "Conduit" for Glen Morgan was the fact that it drove home the notion of strength in diversity in terms of the writing staff.

"Alex and Howard worked on *Beauty and the Beast* and *Sisters*, and they have a better

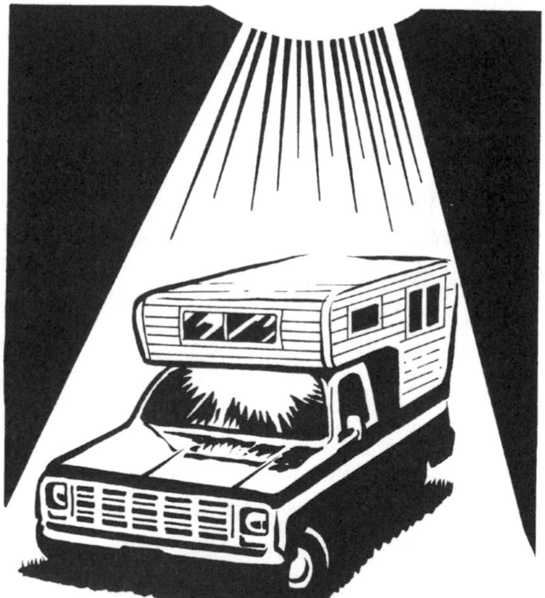

character-dramatic sense," he muses, "and I think 'Conduit' really helped define Mulder. Those guys are Princeton-educated, Ivy League, with a literature background. Jim and

I are more blue collar, from San Diego. I grew up on Hammer horror films and things like that. Everybody on staff was kind of teaching everybody else."

For Carter, one of the episode's highlights was its conclusion and "the realization by Scully that Mulder may not be a crackpot. The science that she so depends on points to an abduction. The girl's physiology and body chemistry at the end of the show says that she may have been in a state of weightlessness. It really helped to define something that was very important to the show, which was its point of view. It was, I think, a very defining episode in terms of how to tell these stories using these characters we had put in motion."

Rating/Audience Share: 6.3/11

Episode 1.5
"The Jersey Devil"

Original airdate: October 8, 1993
Written by Chris Carter
Directed by Joe Napolitano
Guest starring: Andrew Airlie (Rob), Bill Dow (Dad), Tamsin Kelsey (Ellen), Jayme Knox (Mom), Michael MacRae (Ranger Peter Boulle), Hrothgar Mathews (Jack), Gregory Sierra (Dr. Diamond), Claire Stansfield (Jersey Devil), Jill Teed (Glenna), Wayne Tippit (Det. Thompson)

A murder similar to one in 1947 leads Mulder and Scully to New Jersey, where Mulder

wants to investigate the legend of the "Jersey Devil," a supposed beast who has been stalking human prey for some time. They learn that the subject of their search is actually a primitive woman, a genetic mutation or throwback to humanity in its previous incarnation.

✿ ✿ ✿

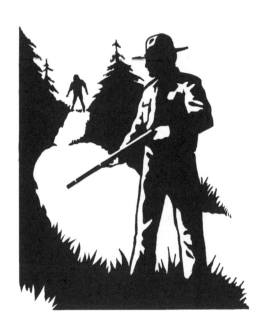

"I had read an essay by this guy E. O. Wilson, who writes about bugs — particularly ants — and he had written a story that posed the question of whether or not man is hellbent on his own extinction," Chris Carter recalls. "There's this idea that we, being carnivores, start to eat our own tails because we're so gluttonous. I mean that not in the eating sense but what we do to the land. I thought of the curious idea, 'What if evolution had provided us with an evolutionary mutation which is almost a throwback to the Neanderthal?' The idea that there's a de-evolutionary bent in nature that, in order to survive, we would actually go

One of the episode's highlights was its conclusion and "the realization by Scully that Mulder may not be a crackpot."

backwards. So I had the idea that we could do a sort of caveman in the woods of New Jersey. The little twist, of course, is that it's not a man, it's a woman. I think the episode was very well directed, and I think it was a little different approach for us. It was a little more poetic and didn't have the 'boo,' which is the big effect or the big scare.

"I also think it further established the relationship between Mulder and Scully," Carter continues, "and expanded the idea of what an X-File is and where it can take place."

James Wong didn't share Carter's enthusiasm for the episode. "Beautifully shot," he says, "it started off great, but I felt the story ran out of steam in the middle. It didn't go anywhere; there weren't enough complications to it."

"That was a difficult show because it was the death of a thousand cuts," Robert Goodwin recalls with a laugh. "To make that work, it required so much shooting, so much film at different angles. I do, however, remember a personal experience making that episode. We needed more footage of this wild woman stalking Mulder as he's walking through the forest at one particular point. I was sent off into the woods with a second unit and a six-foot-tall naked woman to do this filming. However, it was at this forest up here called the Greater Vancouver Regional District. It's not open to the public because it's a preserve. So I get to the gate and my two sons, who are at that time twelve and eight, are with me that day. I said, 'Come on, guys, we're going to shoot some film of the big, tall naked lady.' We get to the gate and the guard won't let the kids in because they're not covered for liability insurance. He said the kids were going to have to wait in the parking lot several miles from where we were shooting, and then he said, 'You don't want them in there, anyway, because we've had several mountain lion attacks over the last week and it was just spotted a half a mile down the road.' I said, 'You want me to leave my two kids standing in a parking lot, telling me that there are mountain lions half a mile down the road?' They wouldn't let them go, so I'm up there, and I should have been having the time of my life with this naked lady, and all I can think about is how my two little boys are stuck at the gate, about to be mauled by a mountain lion."

Adds Glen Morgan with a smile, "They had a naked woman running around the set, so people were pretty thrilled."

Rating/Audience Share: 6.6/12

Episode 1.6
"Shadows"
Original airdate: October 22, 1993
Written by Glen Morgan and James Wong
Directed by Michael Katleman
Guest starring: Anna Ferguson (Ms. Winn), Kelli Fox (Pathologist), Lorena Gale (Ellen Bledsoe), Deryl Hayes (Webster), Tom Heaton (Groundskeeper), Nora McLellan (Jane Morris), Tom Pickett (Cop), Barry Primus (Robert Dorland), Veena Sood (Ms. Saunders), Lisa Waltz (Lauren Kyte), Janie Woods-Morris (Ms. Lange)

A young woman named Lauren Kyte seems to be under the protection of a ghostly force. Mulder and Scully investigate and learn that Lauren's employer, Howard Graves, who was like a father to her, supposedly committed sui- *cide. In actuality, the man was murdered by his business partner and is reaching out from the beyond to make sure that justice is done.*

❆ ❆ ❆

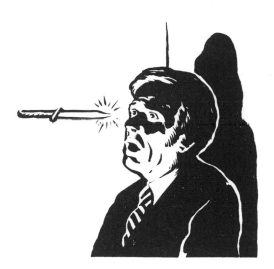

"It wasn't a great script," a candid James Wong admits, "although I thought the director did a good job with it. It was entertaining, but not my favorite episode. The network wanted a lot more relatable things. Originally we made this girl a lot more interesting, but because they wanted relatable things, we made her a secretary, and it wasn't really involving. An average episode."

Glen Morgan notes that a big influence on the episode was *The Entity*, though on the surface of things it looked like their take on *Carrie*. "That's what Chris wants, the idea: 'Can it be this thing and then become that?' I never realized that's what experts think poltergeists are. Usually poltergeists are around younger kids. They have a telekinetic ability

"A big influence on the episode was *The Entity,* though on the surface of things it looked like their take on *Carrie.*"

and don't know how to control it or don't realize it. That's another criterion in writing a script for this show: try and have a way for Scully to explain it. As a writer you're saying, 'If we go in this direction, it allows Scully to say this. If we go in that direction, it allows her to say that.'"

"A very popular show," says Carter. "Very well done, really great effects, and more of a meat-and-potatoes kind of story. An FBI sting and a good mystery that Mulder and Scully investigate. Overall, a really solid episode."

Michael Katleman, who went on to co-create the short-lived Fox series *VR.5*, directed the episode. "As a director," he explains, "you go into some things in episodic television where it's laid out very clearly. The great thing about *The X-Files* is that it *wasn't* laid out. There were a lot of ways to go from a directorial standpoint. You could shoot things in a lot of different ways because you were going into the psyche. You had a lot more freedom to

explore certain areas that haven't been explored yet. For instance, 'Shadows' was about a woman being haunted by her ex-boss. In the beginning it appears she's being haunted by him, but he's really protecting her. When you look at that situation, how do you show that? Which way do you show that someone is possessing someone or protecting them? It's really wide open as to the ways you can explore this psychological dilemma. In that sequence where the attackers come into her house, how do you tell that story? It's done from a psychological perspective, so there are many different ways to do it."

Rating/Audience Share: 5.9/11

Episode 1.7
"Ghost in the Machine"
Original airdate: October 29, 1993
Written by Alex Gansa and Howard Gordon
Directed by Jerrold Freedman
Guest starring: Gillian Barber (Nancy Spiller), Marc Baur (Man in Suit), Wayne Duvall (Jerry Lamana), Bill Finck (Sandwich Man), Jerry Hardin (Deep Throat), Rob Labelle (Brad Wilczek), Blu Mankuma (Claude Peterson), Theodore Thomas (Clyde)

46

Deep Throat informs Mulder that the Defense Department is extremely interested in computer genius Brad Wilczek, who has mastered computer intelligence. Proof of this comes in the form of the high-tech Eurisko building, whose Wilczek-developed computer command system has taken control of the building and is killing anyone who attempts to tamper with its programming.

❋　❋　❋

"My least favorite episode," offers Howard Gordon, who co-wrote the script with Alex Gansa. "I think Chris Carter and I argued what the worst episode of the first season was. Alex and I contend that it was 'Ghost in the Machine,' and Chris insists it was 'Space.' This is easily and clearly our worst. It's basically uninteresting. Some of the concepts may have been interesting, maybe the idea of artificial intelligence. But it's an old idea. There may have been a more interesting way of doing it."

Glen Morgan agrees. "I think parts of the episode worked. What maybe fell a little flat is that we were a little too afraid of doing HAL [from *2001*] and, in a sense, I think that's what the building needed: to have a scary personality. I think we could have given the building a little bit more of a mean-spirited personality to get it away from HAL. HAL, even when he was being dismantled, was very soft-spoken and was never angry.

There's a line between something being an influence and just taking an idea. I don't think we've taken. At least I hope we haven't."

"It had some neat stuff at the end," James

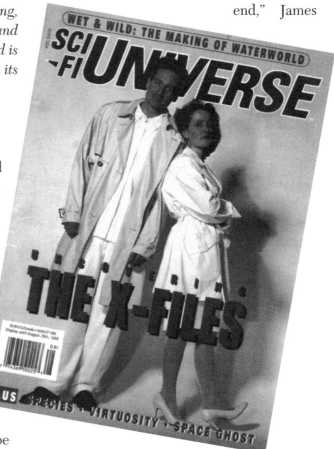

Wong adds, "although I think the ending was a little unsatisfying to me visually, as well as in terms of how Mulder comes to dismember the machine. It was either a little too easy or maybe we could have thought of something more fun to do with the machine. Actually the script was a lot more fun, but it ran into production problems in terms of the budget and we had to devise something that was a little more straightforward. They reprised some of the elevator stuff and it was just a lot more complicated. Overall a fun episode."

One major supporter of "Ghost in the Machine" is Chris Carter, who thought the script effectively addressed the question of just what made up an X-File. "It doesn't have to be paranormal," he notes. "In this case it's technology run amok. X-Files involve lots of different scientific and technological and natural anomalies, and this is just another case of that. I think the action scenes and the abduction of Scully were great. A very successful episode on many levels. Some people didn't think so, but I did. There are some computer buffs who question a few things we had done. Maybe they have some valid arguments, but I think as a dramatic piece it was strong and good."

One difficult aspect of the episode, according to Robert Goodwin, is the fact that the story is told primarily from the point of view of the computer that has taken over the building.

"It's almost like we were shooting two different shows," Goodwin says, "because in any given scene you're showing two or three monitors which show something different happening. So you're spending forever prefilming a scene, transferring it over to video, and playing it back over the monitor. It was a very complex show. Jerry Freedman directed that. If you didn't have a good strong director with

a lot of years of technique behind him, that could have easily been brought to its knees."

Rating/Audience Share: 5.9/11

Episode 1.8
"Ice"
Original airdate: November 5, 1993
Written by Glen Morgan and James Wong
Directed by David Nutter
Guest starring: Xander Berkeley (Dr. Hodge), Felicity Huffman (Dr. Da Silva), Steve Hytner (Dr. Denny Murphy), Ken Kirzinger (Richter), Jeff Kober (Bear), Sonny Surowiec (Campbell)

When communication is cut off with a research facility in Alaska — and the last words of anyone stationed there are, "We are not who we are" — Mulder and Scully, accompanied by a team of physicians and scientists, proceed to Alaska, where they discover a parasitic wormlike creature that takes control of the human mind and intensifies feelings of fear and paranoia, with deadly results.

✢ ✢ ✢

An early high-water mark for the team of Morgan and Wong, "Ice" inspires Carter to enthuse, "They took to the show like crazy, and they're one of the reasons we've done so well and are being so well received. They just outdid themselves on this show, as did director David Nutter, who really works so hard for us. They had worked with David before, and it was a nice partnership that came to *The X-Files*. I think they wrote a great script and he did a great job directing it, and we had a great supporting cast. I think that the cast, directing, and writing came together. 'Ice' was inspired by *The Thing*, as anyone who knows the genre will tell you, but I think it was even better as an X File. It pitted the characters of Mulder and Scully against each other in a way that was very interesting and a new look at their characters early on in the series. It's the stuff of great drama."

"To me," says Nutter, "the real great thing about 'Ice' is that we were able to convey a strong sense of paranoia. It was also a great ensemble piece. We're dealing with the most basic emotions of each character, ranging from their anger to their ignorance and fear. The episode also showed a real trust between Mulder and Scully. It established the emotional ties these two characters have with each other, which is very important. Scaring the hell out of the audience was definitely the key to the episode. The main thing is that it really had to scare the hell out of the actors on the show. Their fear

had to relate with [the audience's], and I think it did that."

Gillian Anderson can concur with that. "It was very intense. There was a lot of fear and paranoia going on. We had some great actors to work with, and the way the set was built was like a bunker almost. We felt like we were really in that place, as opposed to many of the sets, which are three-quarters walls. This was the Antarctic — for all we knew, that's where we were shooting. And it was cold. That particular studio was the old Spelling studio, and it doesn't have heat."

The script for "Ice" was inspired by an article in *Science News* about a group of scientists

" 'Ice' was inspired by an article in *Science News* about a group of scientists in Greenland [who] found these worms frozen that later came back to life."

in Greenland drilling into 250,000-year-old ice. "The Greenland Ice Project was taking core samples from deep within the ice to study," James Wong says. "We started with that. The amazing thing is that they apparently found these frozen worms that later came back to life. It was *after* we wrote the episode that we found it out, which was a little scary."

The entire Arctic complex was created by production designer Graeme Murray, who had worked on John Carpenter's remake of *The Thing.* "That kind of a one-set show works quite well for the series," Murray opines. "You

put a bunch of people into a claustrophobic space and set something loose in there. There's nowhere to go. They can't run. They have to stay and confront it, and that makes for a very tense and exciting episode."

Interestingly, "Ice" was originally conceived as a so-called bottle show, one that would take place in a single location, because it would be cheaper to produce.

"There was a budgetary concern at that point," Wong agrees. "Our shows were going over budget and we needed to do a show that was more contained. We were going to do this one later in the season, when there was the possibility of snow in Vancouver, so we could have some exteriors with snow. As it turned out, we were over budget and we liked this idea, so we had to do it all inside."

But did it save money? "It really didn't," Carter recalls with a chuckle. "We got such production value, and production value costs money. There's no tricks involved. Every dollar we spend shows up on the screen. That's why the show looks so good. We are actually a pretty low budget show, but we've brought a lot of folks together who have given us the most for our money."

Upon receiving the script, Robert Goodwin was immediately struck by its power and the question of how they were going to bring it to life.

"You've got these worms which are living inside of bodies and you can see one wriggling under the skin of a dog and then under a couple of people," he says with a sigh of mock exhaustion. "There's a scene where they pull one of the worms out of the guy's neck. It was a combination of rubber worms and, in some shots, those completely generated by computer. [Makeup artist] Toby Lindala really saved us. For the scene where you see the worms in the back of the neck, one process you can do is build an entire body from a mold made of the actor, so what you're shooting is a very detailed mannequin that looks very realistic. But Toby came in and said, 'Let me try something,' and he actually created a process in which he created false skin that went over the real neck of the person and he built a channel with this worm in it. Actually right there on the actor's neck you could see the worm. It was disgusting, but it was cool. It was one of those things where going in to it you didn't know how you were going to do it. What I was deathly afraid of was that we would do something that looked so cheesy that it would just take away from the story. But everyone delivered, and it's a classic episode."

Rating/Audience Share: 6.6/11

Episode 1.9
"Space"
Original airdate: November 12, 1993
Written by Chris Carter
Directed by William Graham
Guest starring: David Cameron (Young Scientist), Paul DesRoches (Paramedic), Alf Humphreys (Second Controller), Ed Lauter (Lt. Col. Marcus Aurelius Belt), Tyronne L'Hirondelle (Databank Scientist), Tom McBeath (Scientist), Terry David Mulligan (Mission Controller), Susanna Thompson (Michelle Generoo), French Tickner (Preacher), Norma Wick (Reporter)

When Mulder and Scully are secretly informed that a deliberate string of sabotage attempts on America's space shuttle program seems to be taking place, they come into contact with former astronaut and current head of the shuttle program Lieutenant Colonel Marcus Belt. This former hero, it turns out, may be possessed by an extraterrestrial spirit that does not want anyone to join it in outer space.

✿ ✿ ✿

"The conceit was taking a space shuttle up into space and saying that it was essentially hijacked by an alien," Chris Carter says. "It took a lot of research on my part, and I was under a tremendous amount of pressure to get that script done and do a lot of things that an executive producer has to do as well. I didn't know if it was going to work, and I'm still not very happy with some of the special effects in it. We were under a tremendous time crunch in postproduction. I was working until four in the morning two or three nights to make the effects right. I should mention that I was working with the guy who really means a lot to the show and added a lot to it in terms of special effects, Mat Beck, the special effects producer. He was responsible in the pilot for the wonderful vortex in the forest, which took more coordination than the invasion of Normandy. He has just continued to come through with great special effects. But we were both under time pressure here that didn't allow us to do what either of us would have liked to.

"The show comes down to scripts. They have to be really tight and well conceived in order to tell a good story so that you don't have to rely on the special effects. I think we've done that. 'Space' was the first time that I thought the effects didn't live up to my

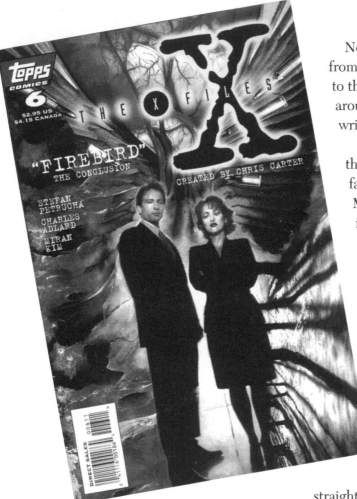

Noting that Carter likes to take his ideas from the newspaper, Glen Morgan points to the disappearance of the Mars Observer around the same time "Space" was being written.

"Chris wanted to use that as well as the other elements that maybe we're all familiar with, such as the face on Mars," Morgan says. "Even if you're not familiar with it, you kind of learn about it from the show. I thought it was a really great idea, that there must be a saboteur in NASA, because people must have wondered what the hell was going on. I think we maybe could have done a better job of conveying that the aliens were controlling this guy. Ed Lauter did a good job, though."

Referring to the lackluster special effects job on the episode, Morgan notes that in recent years Fox has produced straight series like *L.A. Law* and *Picket Fences*. "Suddenly they're doing an effects show and everyone thinks that you can have a regular postproduction schedule," he muses. "I think that was a nutty episode, with like four days for the effects. A lot of times you've got the show cut and you still don't know what the effects are — they run higher than you anticipated; sometimes they turn out crummy. In that case, we ran out of time and money and were stuck with some effects that didn't work. Hopefully we learned from that. I think

expectations, but I think the rest of the episode was very strong."

James Wong opines, "It was a great script and a pretty good episode. The problem came from the fact that some of the special effects were farmed out and they just didn't turn out well, so they looked cheesy and made the show less effective. I thought it was really neat the way they incorporated all the NASA footage in that episode. When I look at it, though, all I see are the problems."

on a show like this, when you really take chances, sometimes you're going to embarrass yourself and other times you hit a home run. You knew every week what *The Commish* was going to be, and it just wasn't as much fun."

For Robert Goodwin, the biggest challenge of the episode was re-creating NASA Mission Control in Houston, which involved video playback and machines with techno graphics. "Because everyone has seen so much of it on TV, you had to do something worthwhile or it would become a joke. In that show, I think the art department really came through. They vacuum-formed all these computers, stations, and everything else. I thought it was all very effective. A real tour de force for the art department."

About the set that became Mission Control, Graeme Murray explains: "It was an empty room in a public building here that is used, I believe, for theater presentations, that we converted. We got what photographs [of Mission Control] we could, and there's actually a fair amount of them. It's reasonably easy to re-create, like the Oval Office seems pretty easy to re-create. It was an interesting show, but a little confusing, because at the end you kind of say, 'Now what the hell was that about?'"

Rating/Audience Share: 6.5/11

Episode 1.10
"Fallen Angel"

Original airdate: November 19, 1993
Written by Alex Gansa and Howard Gordon
Directed by Larry Shaw
Guest starring: Marshall Bell (Commander Henderson), Scott Bellis (Max Fenig), Frederick Coffin (Chief Joseph McGrath), Jerry Hardin (Deep Throat), Jane MacDougall (Laura Dalton), William McDonald (Dr. Oppenheim), Tony Pantages (Lt. Fraser), Sheila Paterson (Gina Watkins), Freda Perry (Mrs. Wright), Michael Rogers (Lt. Griffin), Alvin Sanders (Deputy Wright), Bret Stait (Corp. Taylor), Kimberly Unger (Karen Koretz)

Mulder has twenty-four hours to prove that a spaceship has crashed — this despite a large military presence that is evacuating a small Wisconsin town, claiming that a toxic spill endangers the population. Things intensify when Mulder learns that Commander Henderson and his soldiers are in pursuit of the powerful alien pilot. Amid all of this, Mulder and Scully encounter Max Fenig, a man who claims that he has been abducted by aliens and that this situation mirrors that of Roswell, New Mexico, in 1947.

✤ ✤ ✤

"Right away we established that there was a cover story, that this town was being evacuated based on a supposed toxic spill," Howard Gordon explains. "This, of course, played right into the paranoid aspect of the show. And it was a pretty straight-ahead story, with Mulder operating covertly in a quarantine zone. It's an episode we're proud of. Alex and I like to dig our teeth into a character that interests us, where there's some emotional resonance. Scott Bellis was one of those discoveries we get sometimes in casting."

Notes Chris Carter with a wry smile, "Everyone keeps saying, 'This is my favorite episode.' Leaping forward, each one becomes people's favorite episode. I think we were helped by the great direction of Larry Shaw. And actor Marshall Bell, who played Henderson, was also great. I think it was very suspenseful right out of the box. You were headlong into the story and it never let up

"Something invisible is much more interesting. Certainly more than something that is very real and has a fur coat or a wagging tail."

until the end. We also got to expand Deep Throat's involvement, raising the question that he may not be what he appears to be. I think it really played into an expansion of his character — who he is and why he's doing

this, all of which was explored later. I think the episode had great effects, and it enlarged our alien repertoire."

Of Deep Throat, Gordon adds: "We took the character and pushed him forward a step. Is he ally or foe? We weren't sure at that point ourselves what he was, and we thought we'd couch it in the demise of the X-Files. So we had a frame within a frame that we worked in."

Robert Goodwin remembers writing a memo on the episode about the several sequences where the alien is on the loose and is invisible.

"You really can't see it," Goodwin says, "and then he goes through a laser beam that's up as protection around this Army base. As he goes through, the base buzzes and he becomes visible. Mat Beck, who does our visual effects, needed to create this thing as something actually there which he could take with his visual effects afterwards and completely change its appearance. But at least it gives him something to start with. Here's a memo I wrote on the show: 'Page 15. Shape that distinguishes itself. The effect we are after here is that as the alien moves towards the laser beams, we see its hazy aura approaching. As it crosses through the laser beams we'll see its central anthropological shape. It's a dinosaur-like shape with a large head, a humped back, wing-like webbed limbs as opposed to arms, and long skinny legs. It moves like a dinosaur. To

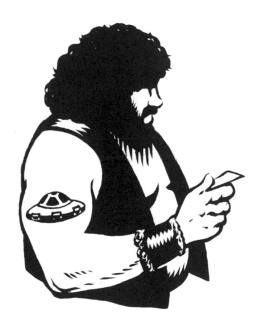

achieve this effect, Mat Beck needs an image of this creature on film that he can morph and distort in postproduction. He says the best color would be orange, so we need to hire a woman who can move well (probably a dancer) and create an orange-colored, hump-backed, big-headed, webbed-armed, pointy-butted outfit for her. And that's exactly what we did. If you could see the dailies of this woman in this orange outfit with a bicycle hat, her arms pinned back, humped over and stuffed full of pillows, you would be hysterical. It was the craziest thing you've ever seen. But the final effect was very good."

According to Carter, the invisibility of the extraterrestrial was quite deliberate. "I always think what you don't see is scarier than what you do see," he explains. "You need a good otherworldly effect; otherwise it's going to look like a monster of the week. As soon as you create a monster and give it shape, you can know it or you can catch it. Something invisible is much more interesting. Certainly more than something that is very real and has a fur coat or a wagging tail."

From a design standpoint, Graeme Murray recalls: "We did what was supposed to be a mountaintop surveillance center in Colorado that was seen in the opening of the show. It was a wall set with no walls to it that was really just kind of plunked into the middle of a black stage and we put up pieces of glass and made reflections of computer monitors and dials and gauges and that kind of thing and tried to build a set that didn't have any boundaries to it. In kind of the flipside to 'Ice,' which was one set, this was a whole bunch of different, interesting things. It's the only time we've done a UFO crash, although you weren't really sure if it was a UFO or an airplane crash."

Rating/Audience Share: 5.4/9

Episode 1.11
"Eve"

Original airdate: December 10, 1993
Written by Kenneth Biller and Chris Brancato
Directed by Fred Gerber
Guest starring: Garry Davey (Hunter), Tina Gilbertson (Donna Watkins), Jerry Hardin (Deep Throat), Harriet Harris (Dr. Sally Kendrick), Maria Herrera (Guard #2), Janet Hodgkinson (Waitress), David Kirby (Ted Watkins), Erika Krievins (Cindy Reardon), Sabrina Krievins (Teena Simmons), Robert Lewis (Officer), Joe Maffei (Guard #1), Tasha Simms (Ellen Reardon), Gordon Tipple (Detective), George Touliatos (Dr. Katz), Christine Upright-Letain (Ms. Wells)

A pair of men are murdered by their eight-year-old daughters in, respectively, Connecticut and California. What draws Mulder and Scully to the case is the fact that the two little girls are exact twins. Upon further investigation, they discover that both of their families had been involved in a 1950s genetic experiment known as the Litchfield Project, which resulted in the creation of boys and girls referred to as Adams and Eves, who have heightened strength and intelligence, and who are psychopathic in nature and look exactly alike.

✵ ✵ ✵

"A freelance episode, and Jim [Wong] and Glen [Morgan] came in at some point on and did an interesting rewrite on it," Chris Carter recalls. "We also had a first-time director in Fred Gerber, who brought some interesting stuff to it. I liked the episode, the casting in particular, with the twin girls. We had to cast in Vancouver and so you're limited in the twins you find up there, because the labor laws are different. It's just difficult to shoot with kids in any case. Also Harriet Harris was excellent."

Robert Goodwin agrees that the biggest challenge of the episode was the casting. "It's hard enough to find one good kid actor, but to find twins who can act is really tough," he says. "At one point I thought we should cast one actor and then do a photo double and split screen, but there was so much with the two of them together that it was impossible. It also would have been very expensive. We just got very lucky that we found these little girls who were terrific. 'Eve,' like most of the scripts, was so goddamned good that our job was not to screw it up. If we can do it without screwing it up and deliver what's on the page, we're going to have a good show. 'Eve' in particular was a very good show."

"I loved the teaser," Carter recalls with a smile, "where the little girl is hugging her teddy bear out in the street and two joggers come by and find that her daddy is sitting, slumped, in the swing set. It's kind of a horrific image and not something you see on your regular network TV show."

Rating/Audience Share: 6.8/12

Episode 1.12
"Fire"
Original airdate: December 17, 1993
Written by Chris Carter
Directed by Larry Shaw
Guest starring: Lynda Boyd (Bar Patron), Duncan Fraser (Beatty), Christopher Gray (Jimmie), Phil Hayes (Driver #1), Dan Lett (Sir Malcolm Marsden), Keegan Macintosh (Michael), Laurie Paton (Lady Marsden), Amanda Pays (Phoebe Green), Alan Robertson (Gray-Haired Man), Mark Sheppard (Cecil L'ively/Bob)

Mulder is visited by an old girlfriend, Phoebe Green, who is trying to protect a British lord after several members of Parliament have been burned to death. When Scully joins the investigation, they learn that the suspect is Cecil L'ively, the caretaker of the lord's Cape Cod retreat, who apparently has the ability to create flames from his mind.

❊   ❊   ❊

"This is an episode that people were mad at me from the beginning for because I wanted to do something with fire and it's very hard to work with," says Chris Carter with a laugh. "Fire is much hotter than you think it's going to be. Actually, it's amazingly frightening when you're around it and it's burning things down in your studio. Until you're actually confronted with those balls of flame, you can't imagine it. So that was an interesting thing. It's a very popular episode, and I'm just somewhat happy with the way it turned out. Having written it and imagined it in certain ways, I think it could have been a lot better. Although I thought it was generally well directed, the show felt very 'wide' to me — very loose and lacking some things."

"Boy," Robert Goodwin moans in mock weariness, "that was a hard one. Any kind of a fire stunt is a major undertaking, because it involves so many overlapping things. First of all, it is a stunt, so you have to have a stuntman who can work fire. A lot of them can't. We had two full body burns in that show and those were people inside those flames. If it's inside, which many of the film sequences were, because of natural concerns for safety and all the legal concerns by the fire department, you have to carefully design and build the sets in such a manner that they're fireproof and the fire can be controlled. It was a major feat, a real logistical and creative feat, because you wanted it to look good. Mark Sheppard is at the far end of the hall and Mulder is in the foreground. He waves with his arms and these flames come racing down the hallway and along the ceiling. It's just a spectacular moment, but it got to be so hot that the actor could not stand it any longer and had to duck

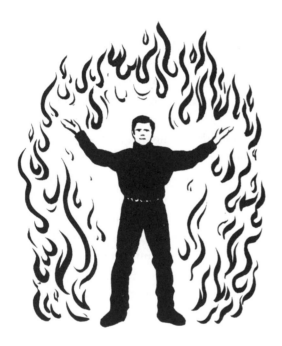

out of the show. I remember that there was a whole lot of trickery we had to pull off because he was supposed to be standing there when he wasn't. Director Larry Shaw, with very short time to prepare, was able to pull it off."

One aspect of the show that Carter did enjoy was the attempt to explore a little more of Mulder's background and personality. "I

thought it was interesting to show a little bit of Mulder's history by bringing an old girlfriend back," he notes. "I've always wanted to do a Scotland Yard detective who was a woman. I also thought it was an interesting chance to use Amanda Pays and to make a villainess of her."

James Wong doesn't feel that the relationship was conveyed effectively. "I thought there was so much more in the script in terms of emotions that Mulder and Amanda Pays's character were supposed to have. There's a lot more to their relationship in the script than there was on the screen. It didn't play at all, and that should have been the subtext of the whole show. We ended up cutting a lot of stuff that just didn't work."

"The weird thing about that script," adds Glen Morgan, "is that Chris had that concept and started writing it, and then LA started burning. I think that fueled him a bit. And I think Chris would acknowledge that Jim Wong is a very good editor. At one point the story was muddled and Jim, in editing, put things in a different way and it came out good. That was a situation where you didn't have the time to do an insert and fix it. People have written that they like it. I like that bit with the cigarette in the beginning where it lights itself. Little things like that are effective."

Rating/Audience Share: 6.8/12

Episode 1.13
"Beyond the Sea"
Original airdate: January 7, 1994
Written by Glen Morgan and James Wong
Directed by David Nutter
Guest starring: Katherynn Chisholm (Nurse),
Don Davis (Capt. William Scully), Brad Dourif
(Luther Lee Boggs), Fred Henderson (Agent
Thomas), Lawrence King (Lucas Jackson
Henry), Sheila Larken (Margaret Scully),
Randy Lee (Paramedic), Don MacKay
(Warden Joseph Cash), Len Rose (Emergency
Room Doctor), Lisa Vultaggio (Liz Hawley),
Chad Willett (Jim Summers)

Mulder and Scully, who is coping with the death of her father, take on a kidnapping case that leads them to a prisoner on death row named Luther Lee Boggs. Claiming to be psychic, Boggs tells the duo he'll help solve the case if they can get his sentence changed. In the midst of the investigation, Scully — the skeptic — sees visions of her dead father and, despite Mulder's claims she's being manipulated, she turns to Boggs as a possible channel to her father's spirit.

✵ ✵ ✵

"I'm uncomfortable talking about my own work, but I am proud of this episode," Glen Morgan admits. "Jim and I have written maybe thirty hours of television, and before working on this series there were maybe three *21 Jump Street*s which I can say I'm proud of. 'Beyond the Sea' is another show I'm proud of. We fought pretty hard for Brad Dourif, and Chris came through for us. [*One Flew Over the*] *Cuckoo's Nest* is a movie that means a lot, and to have Brad Dourif [a star of that movie] saying our lines just meant the world to me. If you had someone crummy in there, that's where the show would have fallen apart. The story provided us with a chance to deal with Scully and expand her role a bit and change the rules around. If people say it's derivative of *Silence of the Lambs*, that's just a brilliant idea Thomas Harris came up with. I hope it's not seen that way, and it's something I tried to avoid as much as possible. I just thought that Brad Dourif and Gillian's performances were great, and David Nutter did a great job directing."

For his part, Nutter is justifiably proud of the show. "To me," he says, "I think it's the most accomplished piece of directing of actors I have been able to do. I thought Brad Dourif was brilliant, and I thought I helped bring him to where he should have been, and we were able to capture what he could really do onscreen. I very much enjoyed working with Gillian on the show. I think she's a young actress with a lot of talent but not a lot of experience prior to this show. I think this episode really made a difference in how the audience looks at Scully. I think it brought a lot of dimension to her character, and for her as a person it definitely had a lot of impact. It also allowed us to explore the emotional side of things, which we don't talk that much about. To me it's right up there with 'Ice.' Certainly one of the most enjoyable shows I did."

Robert Goodwin recalls, "The whole thing was spellbinding. One of those episodes where a guy in my position just has to get the sets built, stick the actors in, let the director do his job and let the actors do theirs."

"My favorite episode of the first year," Chris Carter enthuses, "and one of my favorites overall, flipping the Mulder and Scully points of view. Actually, the network did not want to do that episode. They had turned it down because they thought it was too much like *Silence of the Lambs*. I was so sure this was a great episode that I remember running up to the executive building — literally running — into Dan McDermott's office and saying, 'These guys believe in this episode, I believe in this episode, we've got to do this episode.' They finally let us do it, although there was a question of whether or not we'd have Brad Dourif. I remember calling Peter Roth, the president of Twentieth Century Fox, at home on Thanksgiving and saying, 'This is the guy we need for this episode.' There was a money issue. He was the person who signed off on that. I pulled him away from the Thanksgiving table and he said, 'Just cast him,' and that was it. The tim-

ing to call him was perfect, though it was inadvertent."

Rating/Audience Share: 6.6/11

Episode 1.14
"Genderbender"
Original airdate: January 21, 1994
Written by Larry Barber and Paul Barber
Directed by Rob Bowman
Guest starring: Doug Abrahams (Agent #2), Paul Batten (Brother Wilton), Grai Carrington (Tall Man), Lesley Ewen (Agent #1), Michele Goodger (Sister Abigail), Brent Hinkley (Brother Andrew), Mitchell Kosterman (Det. Horton), Nicholas Lea (Michael), Aundrea MacDonald (Pretty Woman), Tony Morelli (Cop), Peter Stebbings (Male Marty), John R. Taylor (Husband), David Thomson (Brother Oakley), Kate Twa (Female Marty)

When five people die during sex — and there is evidence of an impossible amount of pheromones — Mulder and Scully proceed to a Massachusetts religious sect known as the Kindred. There, Scully nearly falls victim to one of the sect, but is rescued by Mulder. What they discover is that members of the Kindred have the ability to switch genders at will, with the implication at episode's end being that they are actually an alien race.

✿ ✿ ✿

"We had brought in a couple of writing producers, Paul and Larry Barber, who came up with the idea of gender-shifting characters in a sort of Amish setting," Chris Carter recalls. "I think the idea is pretty good, and there are some interesting visual moments. Rob Bowman really rose to the occasion and showed us what he is capable of, which is why he's on the show as a producer now. A terrific episode given real style and passion by Rob."

One bit of criticism Carter has received about the episode is its conclusion, with circular burn marks in a field that indicate a UFO may have been involved in the scenario. "I like that ending, though a lot of people complained," he says. "I think it's vague: Is it or isn't it? That ambiguity is a hallmark of some of our best episodes."

James Wong doesn't agree. "There were problems with the ending of the show," he says, "in that we pretty much wrapped it up relatively quickly and just threw in something [the burn marks]. Those things always seem like a little trick. It's like we tried to play a trick on the audience to make them say, 'Ooh, what the heck was that?' But when it's not integral to the story, it lessens the impact. You don't get a sense of a cathartic moment, because we kind of blew it."

"Initially," Glen Morgan adds, "we said we wanted an episode with more of a sexy edge, but it was difficult to find a story that shows sex as scary. As a result, it kind of veered off to, What if there are people like the Amish who are from another planet? I think people have said that we overstepped the bounds on that one. Maybe we went too far. At what point do we become unbelievable?"

Rob Bowman was the best of the early directors of *Star Trek: The Next Generation*, helming episodes in that show's first two seasons that were visually unlike those of anyone else working on the series. Feeling stifled, he left in the middle of year two and was creatively reborn when he joined *The X-Files*.

"At the time of 'Genderbender,' *The X-*

"We wanted an episode with more of a sexy edge, but it was difficult to find a show that shows sex as scary."

Files was a series that hadn't fully defined itself," Bowman explains. "The script I received was from outside writers who, in Chris's mind, hadn't fulfilled his wishes, whatever they were. The concept of the show was a low-tech episode where they didn't want to have any high-tech anything. They wanted

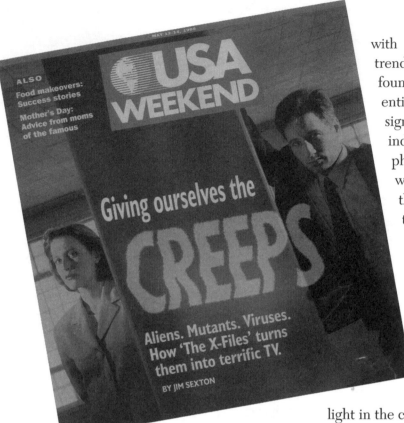

USA WEEKEND

Giving ourselves the

CREEPS

Aliens. Mutants. Viruses.
How 'The X-Files' turns
them into terrific TV.

BY JIM SEXTON

with its vanity and sex and what's trendy. That's what the Amish people found in the magazine the one guy is enticed by. Reproduction was a very significant part of their culture, as indicated by the cave and the very phallic, lubricated cave walls that were found. I suppose the trick that I had to pull off was to draw the greatest contrasts between the two worlds.

"The difficulties of shooting it were just that the cave was so small that we had guys crawling around there and there was no light. Lantern light is not enough to light up a face for film. Production-wise, it was very difficult to get enough light in the cave. I had to go back an extra day and fill out quite a bit of the stuff with Mulder and the cave because it took too long to get the stuff I needed. I'd say that seventy-five percent of the stuff with Mulder down in the caves was shot another day with a smaller unit."

For Robert Goodwin, "Genderbender" was an artistic triumph, primarily in terms of art direction. He also cites the female-to-male switch as being a technical challenge.

"One of these guys has gone haywire because he's tasted sex and he's off and his pheromones are so strong that they can kill anyone he has sex with. He/She doesn't care because they're overpowered by lust. To real-

mostly lantern light, and the only tech you would have would be the contrast between the city life and this very primitive farm life. There was a deliberate attempt to come up with swirling lights, multicolored things, people wearing shining clothes, lots of steel and shine and some Gigerisms with very sexual connotations, and you slam that against people carrying lanterns around in these monk-like outfits.

"It was a very bizarre story," Bowman elaborates, "especially for me, because it was my first episode. The story challenges were to examine the influence of a superficial society,

ly pay off the business about this person being able to change gender, we decided we'd have one shot where we would actually morph the female into the male. We wanted to be as believable as possible. We'd already cast the female, who had a very distinct look, and we searched around and found this wonderful young actor who looked very much like the girl. There was a very strong resemblance. In the scene, Mulder has trapped this person and she morphs into the male and comes out, knocks him down, and takes off. When we shot the two parts of the morph and put it together, the two actors really looked so much alike that it didn't look like a morph. It looked like this girl was just standing up. We were *too* good at casting, I think, and it zapped the energy out of the moment."

Graeme Murray notes that the design of this particular episode was a true hybrid. "We were working with an Amish kind of look, also a sleazy downtown look, and a kind of alien center where they brought people to be revived," he says. "It has a nice feel to it. That kind of Amish culture is sort of alien anyway, and combining real alien on top of that was interesting."

Rating/Audience Share: 7.2/12

Episode 1.15
"Lazarus"
Original airdate: February 4, 1994
Written by Alex Gansa and Howard Gordon
Directed by David Nutter
Guest starring: Christopher Allport (Agent Jack Willis), Alexander Boynton (Clean-Cut Man), Jay Brazeau (Professor Varnes), Lisa Bunting (Doctor #1), Brenda Crichlow (Reporter), Jackson Davies (Agent Bruskin), Russell Hamilton (Officer Daniels), Peter Kelamis (O'Dell), Callum Keith Rennie (Tommy), Mark Saunders (Doctor #2), Jason Schombing (Warren James Dupre), Cec Verrell (Lula Philips)

In a Maryland bank, Scully and FBI agent Jack Willis are drawn into a shoot-out with a robber named Warren Dupre. Both Willis and Dupre are wounded and brought to the emergency room. Willis dies, but suddenly "comes back" after Dupre jumps up and dies himself. Shortly thereafter, Willis begins acting differently, with Mulder concluding that Dupre's spirit has somehow taken over the agent's body.

❈   ❈   ❈

Chris Carter enthuses, "A very good and well-acted episode. I like it because it actually seemed so real to me. It played less as a paranormal science fiction show than as whether or not something could really happen. The entire cast was wonderful. Overall that was a terrific episode."

According to Howard Gordon, the story initially had Mulder possessed by the person he was hunting. Fox didn't really like the notion of their hero experiencing, firsthand, such a supernatural occurrence. "I think that was a wise decision," Gordon admits, "though at the time we were angry and up in arms."

Director David Nutter notes, "Pacing was the key for that show. It was the opposite of 'Beyond the Sea.' I thought a lot of movement had to happen. The camera was moving, the actors were moving, all of which was designed to move the script along. It wasn't one of the more involved scripts. Just a pretty basic, straightforward story."

Rating/Audience Share: 7.6/12

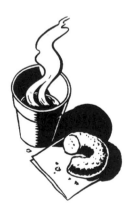

Episode 1.16
"Young at Heart"

Original airdate: February 11, 1994
Written by Scott Kaufer and Chris Carter
Directed by Michael Lange
Guest starring: Courtney Arciaga (Progeria Victim), Alan Boyce (Young John Barnett), William B. Davis (Cigarette-Smoking Man), Robin Douglas (Computer Specialist), Christine Estabrook (Agent Henderson), Merrilyn Gann (Prosecutor), Jerry Hardin (Deep Throat), Graham Jarvis (Dr. Austin, NIH), Robin Mossley (Dr. Joe Ridley), David Petersen (Old John Barnett), Gordon Tipple (Joe Crandall), Dick Anthony Williams (Reggie Purdue)

Mulder finds himself going up against a killer from his past, John Barnett, whom he had put behind bars several years earlier, prior to taking on the X-Files. Barnett supposedly died in prison, but all clues are indicating that he is back, stalking Mulder and his friends, primarily Scully. They ultimately discover that Barnett has actually been a participant in a genetic experiment that is reversing the aging process, supplying him with the perfect means of disguise.

❄ ❄ ❄

"I liked the script very much," recalls director Michael Lange, "and I think I stayed fairly close to the original draft. I liked it because it had a lot of good spookiness to it. To me, the intriguing part was the doctor's research into being able to reverse the aging process, which I wish we could have explored more.

"In my first meeting with Chris Carter on the tone of the show," he adds, "Chris said, 'Remember one thing: On *The X-Files*, the Devil is in the details.' I write it big on my script whenever I do the show, because it's the details that make it work, as opposed to broad strokes. As a director, you really have to pay attention to all those details, or else no one is happy."

One problem, according to Glen Morgan, was the fact that the episode aired right after "Lazarus," and there were certain similarities between the shows. "When I looked at my bulletin board at the time," he reflects, "I saw that there was a pattern of 'Shadows' through 'Space' where we were trying to scare people. Then starting with 'Beyond the Sea' I think we were trying to do more intellectual stories. Then we tried to go back to a little more visceral storytelling. I think we may have been a little off course on some of them. Chris had said, 'Where's the big boo? Where's the real scare scene?' And I don't know if they had those."

For Robert Goodwin, "Young at Heart" is one of the most emotional episodes of the first season. "When Mulder and Scully are finding out about this doctor, they're running this old scratchy black and white footage of him in the institute he ran back in the fifties and sixties, in which he was working with children who had progeria, the disease that aged them, so that by the time they're ten they're like seventy-year-olds. We needed that footage to run, and Paul Rabwin contacted the Progeria Society and we actually brought a darling little girl up from San Diego who had the disease. We shot this footage with her. Michael Lange directed. He has two little girls and I have a couple of kids, and it was a very, very touching moment for all of us. We felt it was good

> "Chris said, 'Remember one thing: on *The X-Files*, the Devil is in the details.'"

because it made the disease visible, so it helped create more public awareness of it. On an individual basis, when we contacted the parents we found out they were big fans of the show, as was the little girl. It was almost like a 'Make a Wish' kind of thing; it was wonderful."

Rating/Audience Share: 7.2/11

Episode 1.17

"E.B.E."

Original airdate: February 18, 1994

Written by Glen Morgan and James Wong

Directed by William Graham

Guest starring: Tom Braidwood (Frohike), Dean Haglund (Langly), Jerry Hardin (Deep Throat), Bruce Harwood (Byers), Peter LaCroix (Ranheim/Druse), Allan Lysell (Chief Rivers)

Claiming it's a means of protecting Mulder, Deep Throat sends Mulder and Scully on a wild UFO chase, diverting them from a military operation to contain an extraterrestrial retrieved from a UFO crash over Iraq. By the time Mulder figures out the truth, the E.B.E. (extraterrestrial biological entity) has been exterminated. Deep Throat reveals that he is one of three people who has participated in the extermination of extraterrestrials in the past, and his helping Mulder is an attempt to make amends for what he has done.

Note: This episode introduced the Lone Gunman, a conspiracy-obsessed organization that is well aware of Mulder's efforts.

❀ ❀ ❀

"When we tested 'Squeeze' with an audience," Glen Morgan recalls, "they said, 'Well, it was okay. I don't know if a person could stretch like that. But I like the UFO and conspiracy stuff,' so Jim and I had a chance to do one, and 'E.B.E.' was the result. A lot of that was from fan mail, what people wanted us to deal with. I think 'E.B.E.' was written for people who we felt were hardcore *X-Files* fans: people into UFOs and every conspiracy imaginable. The thing is, they screened 'E.B.E' and people were saying, 'I like the UFO episodes, but there was one where this guy kind of stretched . . .' C'mon, make up your mind. Anyway, the movie I kind of really looked at in order to catch the tone for 'E.B.E.' was *All the President's Men,* dealing with dark parking lots and that kind of paranoia."

James Wong isn't as pleased with the final product. "I really felt we didn't do a great job on the script," he says. "We wanted to do a show that's all about paranoia and a conspiracy theory, but at the end I felt like we didn't really gain a lot of new ground or learn a lot of new things. I think we played a lot of texture instead of substance."

"Another of our most popular first-season episodes," says Chris Carter. "Jim and Glen wanted to do an alien episode, and this is what they came up with. I thought it was well directed by Bill Graham. I thought there were some really memorable scenes in it, particularly Deep Throat and the shark tank, also the teaser with the Iraqi pilot. Some really wacky stuff: the UFO party, and the introduction of the Lone Gunman, and they've served us well since then. Glen and Jim had both gone incognito to things like UFO conventions and saw folks setting up their booths, selling rather paranoid literature. These guys represented a certain type that we had run across."

Says Graeme Murray, "A lot of the episode took place in a facility in Vancouver where they do high-voltage electrical research, which is where we created the containment facility where they hold the alien. That was a fascinating kind of place, where they create lightning and high-voltage electrical effects. A wonderful location for us. Then we built a couple of things. There was a forty-foot truck that transported the alien, and we built an interesting room in there, although you didn't see much of it actually in the show. It was like a traveling life support room for an alien."

Rating/Audience Share: 6.2/9

Episode 1.18
"Miracle Man"

Original airdate: March 18, 1994
Written by Howard Gordon and Chris Carter
Directed by Michael Lange
Guest starring: Scott Bairstow (Samuel), Lisa Ann Beley (Beatrice Salinger), Iris Quinn Bernard (Lillian Daniels), R. D. Call (Sheriff Daniels), Chilton Crane (Margaret Hohman), Alex Doduk (Young Samuel), George Gerdes (The Rev. Cal Hartley), Roger Haskett (Deputy Tyson), Campbell Lane (Margaret's Father), Dennis Lipscomb (Leonard Vance), Walter Marsh (Judge), Howard Storey (Fire Chief)

A faith healer named Samuel who, in 1983, brought a man back to life by praying over him, finds himself the subject of a Mulder and Scully investigation after he attempts to heal a woman who dies instead. Seeming miracles turn out to be quite man-made, and there is much skepticism over Samuel's "powers," even as he cryptically mentions Mulder's sister and the fact that she was taken away by strangers within bright lights. In the end, though, his true spiritual abilities are revealed.

✲ ✲ ✲

"Miracle Man" marked the first collaboration between Howard Gordon and Chris Carter, following Alex Gansa's departure from the series.

"Howard came to my house," Carter says, "and said, 'Help me out,' so we went to my living room and put up this bulletin board and in a matter of hours we came up with this story. Then Howard and I split up the scenes. It was a blast, because Howard and I had never written together before. We had a great time. And I think it set the tone and laid a foundation for what our relationship is. Besides that, we wanted to do something with the bright side of the paranormal, and of course we had to contrast it against the dark side, with this kid who had been able to heal people with his hands and believed he had lost his gift. It was really a story about human nature, jealousy, and the tragedy of this kid's death set against the idea of Mulder and Scully's faith and the appearance of Mulder's sister."

Of the scenario itself, Gordon adds: "We said, 'This is a show about belief, about possibilities.' We're all believers at some level. There's healing beyond what you get at your local MD. Given that, I think there's a power of faith, and so we set out right away to not do the obvious, which would be to make these people into buffoons. In a way, it was a kind of Jesus story. You don't have to look too hard to see the parallels. Samuel was a kid who was given a gift. Our premise was, What if a prophet or someone with special powers was set down on Earth? What would happen to him?"

"On an intellectual level," says director Michael Lange, "it really dealt with the subject of God — the power of God — and the power of man in kind of a neat way. There were a lot of things to think about, working on it as a director, and also for the viewer. If you want to go along with it, it can really take you to some neat places. I was trying to kind of create the image of the son of Jesus, basically. Some of the things I put in were actually pulled back by the network when they saw it. Networks, and I think human beings in general, always have a problem with compositing violence with religion. There was one scene where Samuel was beaten up by the guys in the jail cell and was killed, as we find out in the next scene. I had this one image that I shot, which was the silhouette of him against the wall with the bars, and he actually had

taken a crucifix pose, and that of course went bye-bye. Even the bold Fox network couldn't handle that one.

"All of the tent stuff with the faith healing was done in one day," he continues. "We had three hundred extras and managed to get it done in one day. I, myself, have a kind of skepticism about all these faith healers, but by the end of that day I could see how people would be drawn into it, because it's very compelling. There were some very inspirational things in there, and everyone became so infused with this fervor that you really could understand how it could all happen. It doesn't happen often on TV that you can explore an area of the human experience and feel it that much."

Glen Morgan is a little more critical of the episode. "I think it's kind of easy to pick on religion," he says, "especially one of the fundamentalist backgrounds. It's easy to portray them as Bible thumpers. To tell you the truth, there are a lot of people for whom it's their faith, and I would like to have had a little more respect towards that. Overall, my personal belief is that some of the phoniness needs to be exposed; however, it's just kind of easy to say this is all that it is. I think there is more to it. There are good people who have Christian faith in their background. They're not just on bad cable. It's a tough challenge because, really, on network TV they don't want you to deal with religion."

Robert Goodwin's difficulties with the episode were of quite a different nature. "The problem with 'Miracle Man' is always a problem when you shoot a show that's set in the South anywhere but in the South," he explains. "It's really easy to do a bad Southern accent. That, for me, was one of the bigger challenges, because a lot of the supporting actors come from Vancouver, but there are also people up here who come from the South. I hired a dialect coach to help even it all out so it didn't sound like they were coming from fifteen different parts of the South."

"Setting up the tent and getting that Southern atmosphere in Vancouver was kind of interesting," says Graeme Murray. "That episode was kind of difficult to put together logistically. There were a lot of different little places, and trying to get that Southern atmosphere was a little tough. It was a real location show. A lot of time in the shows like that is spent trying to put together a day of shooting where you have what are supposed to be four or five different locations and we don't really have the time to move during a day. You pretty much have to shoot a day in the location, so everything has to be found within walking distance of the major set of that day. 'Miracle Man' was particularly like that, and putting it all together was very tricky."

Rating/Audience Share: 7.5/13

Episode 1.19
"Shapes"
Original airdate: April 1, 1994
Written by Marilyn Osborn
Directed by David Nutter
Guest starring: Jimmy Herman (Ish), Michael Horse (Charley Tskany), Dwight McFee (David Gates), Paul McLean (Dr. Josephs), Ty Miller (Lyle Parker), Renae Morriseau (Gwen Goodensnake), Donnelly Rhodes (Jim Parker)

Reports of a strange beast that has attacked a man reach the desks of Mulder and Scully, who proceed to the Two Medicine Ranch in Browning, Montana. There they learn that rancher Jim Parker shot the beast that attacked his son, Lyle, and the creature turned out to be an Indian named Joseph Goodensnake. Eventually, Lyle — the victim of the beast's bite — finds himself transforming into an Indian manitou.

❀ ❀ ❀

"People would say to me, 'When are you going to do the vampire and werewolf thing?'" Glen Morgan recalls. "Well, here it is. Like a good rock band should be able to play standards by Chuck Berry, I feel we should be able to do the basics. I think there's room for the straight-out, scare-the-hell-out-of-people type of show."

"The network wanted a monster show,"

notes David Nutter, "and that's what they got. The main crux for me on that show was to create an atmosphere that would make it as different as possible from other episodes. Also, the manitou wasn't too much in your face. You only saw a little bit of the monster here and a little bit of it there, and it was all very well handled."

"The manitou is a combination of eleven or twelve different sounds of varying degrees, varying pitches, and varying speeds."

The visual execution of the manitou especially pleased Robert Goodwin. "That monster was put together in a combination of traditional and computer ways," he says. "We had a man in a suit with an articulated mask. Then we had a dog's-head mask that was also articulated for the teeth and the fangs, and those elements were brought together."

The final ingredient needed to bring the manitou to life came in postproduction, where Paul Rabwin supervised the sound effects. "We needed a combination of sounds in order to make it frightening," he recounts. "A sound that was part animal and part human. We had several groans and screams from different animals, ranging from a hawk's screech to a lion's roar. Then I had an actor who specializes in voices do a number of different screams and sounds. In the end, the manitou is a combination of eleven or twelve different sounds of varying degrees, varying pitches, and varying speeds. The sound was familiar in that we heard elements of the Wolf Man, but different in that it was definitely *The X-Files.*"

"I thought Jim and Glen, in rewriting Marilyn Osborn's script, did a terrific job of giving us a good sort of meat-and-potatoes werewolf story by calling it a manitou, which was our *X-Files* twist on it," says

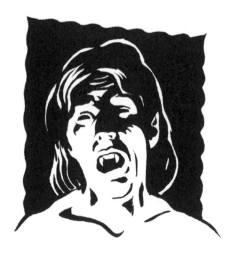

Chris Carter. "I thought it was very well directed by David Nutter. Glen's right in his feeling that this show should be able to deal with more traditional monsters. I defend that.

When you do twenty-five episodes a year, you are going to get some that are a little more down the pipe, and I think this one is an example of that."

Graeme Murray explains, "We were trying to re-create this big-sky Montana ranch country in Vancouver. We shot in a town that was created for a show called *Bordertown*. It was one of those shows where you just try and get it done on schedule and on budget."

Rating/Audience Share: 7.6/14

Episode 1.20
"Darkness Falls"
Original airdate: April 15, 1994
Written by Chris Carter
Directed by Joe Napolitano
Guest starring: Jason Beghe (Larry Moore), Barry Greene (Perkins), David Hay (Clean-Suited Man), Tom O'Rourke (Steve Humphreys), Ken Tremblett (Dyer), Titus Welliver (Doug Spinney)

Mulder and Scully are drawn to the Olympic National Forest in northwest Washington State, following up a report that loggers have been attacked and killed by a mysterious entity. Once there, they find themselves essentially trapped with several other people, the victims of phosphorous insects that have seemingly been unleashed from a recently felled tree, and that feast on human flesh.

❈ ❈ ❈

Chris Carter reflects, "This came right from my college biology class, where we studied the reading of tree rings. I thought, 'Let's go to the woods and cut open one of these big trees, which are really historical time capsules of everything that has gone on in the past couple of thousand years. What if there are these bugs that escape and hold everyone hostage?' It was supposed to be a bottle show, but in fact it turned out to be one of our hardest shows. The first day of that episode, I woke up and looked out the window and there was a blizzard and I thought they were never going to make it; that nothing would match from that day on. You see some scenes where the actors are just miserably soaked. *We* didn't make that rain."

Indeed, "Darkness Falls" is probably most noteworthy for the physical hardships it imposed on the cast and crew.

"It was the dead of winter," Robert Goodwin moans. "Out of eight days of shooting, six of them were in the forest. There were terrible rainstorms and mud, and it became a logistical nightmare. On a television series you don't usually tackle that kind of thing. That's usually reserved for big-budget features. In any case, at one point I just sent the company home because it was raining so hard. It was like trying to see through a waterfall. But it all came out in the end, and the episode was pretty scary."

"It was very tough on the crew," seconds

Glen Morgan. "No one wanted to go through that again. The next episode was 'Tooms,' and Bob Goodwin called me up and said, 'You know those keys on your typewriter that spell

"Rabwin cast 10,000 mites, which were very temperamental."

EXT for exterior? They're now broken.' So 'Tooms' had a lot of interiors."

Perhaps the producer with the most legitimate reason for complaining about the episode is Paul Rabwin, who had to cast 10,000 extras for the episode — without getting an increased budget. "I spent a lot of time trying to find the right stock footage of the thousands of insects we needed for the show," he says. "Ninety-five percent of the insects you see are computer generated, particularly the descending swarm and the specks in the corner of the room. But there were a couple of shots where we wanted to see thousands of bugs up close, and we couldn't find any stock footage that had the feel we were looking for."

Rabwin ultimately hooked up with a cameraman who specializes in microscopic photography, which in turn led to his "casting" 10,000 mites, which were extremely temperamental.

"They tend to shy away from the light," he points out. "And photographing them was difficult — they were so small you couldn't corral them. We finally figured out that they're slowed down by the cold, so we took this nitrogen solution and placed it on the bottom of the slide, and all these little buggers congregated around the nitrogen. Then we removed the nitrogen and quickly put it on the microscope, and we had about a thirty-second window of opportunity to photograph them before they started to disperse. It was an effects-heavy show, and there were a number of scenes that these insects were in, so it had to be staged properly."

Rating/Audience Share: 8.0/14

Episode 1.21
"Tooms"

Original airdate: April 22, 1994
Written by Glen Morgan and James Wong
Directed by David Nutter
Guest starring: Steve Adams (Myers), Henry Beckman (Det. Frank Briggs), Pat Bermel (Frank Ranford), Gillian Carfra (Christine Ranford), Andre Daniels (Arlan Green), Jan D'Arcy (Judge Kann), Glynis Davis (Nelson), William B. Davis (Cigarette-Smoking Man), Mikal Dughi (Dr. Karetzky), Doug Hutchison (Eugene Victor Tooms), Catherine Lough (Dr. Richmond), Mitch Pileggi (Assistant Director Walter S. Skinner), Frank C. Turner (Dr. Collins), Paul Ben Victor (Dr. Aaron Monte), Jerry Wasserman (Dr. Plith), Timothy Webber (Det. Talbot)

Eugene Tooms, who was arrested and placed in a sanitarium at the conclusion of "Squeeze," is released for good behavior, and attempts to go back to his old ways, doing his best to get Mulder out of the picture by making it seem that the FBI agent has been stalking and threatening him, resulting in the desired effect. However, when Tooms kills his doctor, chows down on the man's liver, and goes back into hibernation, Mulder and Scully discover his nest in an area beneath a building, where they have a final confrontation.

✵ ✵ ✵

"Here's the weird thing," muses Glen Morgan, "and I can't explain it. When we were finishing 'Shapes,' I said, 'This is really good; I like it.' When I saw it aired, I said, 'Kind of a letdown. I don't know why.' When we were doing 'Tooms,' I was disappointed, and then we were mixing in the sound and I thought, 'Man, I love this.' Doug Hutchison really stole the show. He had the character down.

"Jim and I had never done a follow-up to a show we had written. You have the challenge that you just assume that a lot of people hadn't seen the first one, so you have to quickly recap what this guy is about and that's why act one is at Tooms's trial. You could recap what the rules were with this monster. With this character, it's kind of like, 'What would you like to see him do?'

"The other thing was that the first show ['Squeeze'] had a director who was a problem, so this was a real chance to correct that part of it and do some of those things that were cut out of the first episode. I cannot tell you how unwatchable the first cut of 'Squeeze' was. When I watch it, I can't even follow the story. I just see where we solved problems, or hope that we solved problems."

Robert Goodwin says, laughing, "Nothing brilliant to say about the episode. We brought back Pepper, our contortionist from Seattle. My kids and their friends kept showing up at the set, because Tooms is their hero."

Chris Carter admits, "This was sort of the command performance of Tooms. We had had such a difficult time with 'Squeeze' — it took so much care in postproduction to make it what it was — that this was an opportunity to take the character and do a sequel using David Nutter, who that season was definitely our best director. To have him come in and give it his take. In a way, it was almost a vindication episode. I think it turned out very well, and Tooms remains a very popular character."

"The main thing for me on that show," says David Nutter, "was knowing how popular this character was, I felt it was important to give him his just deserts on the second show. The producers weren't so happy with how the first show turned out. The character caught on; they had worked very hard to make it work to the point they wanted. But for the second show, they really wanted to make it good. I'm lucky I was available to do that one. I think it's a real classic horror story; I think Tooms is a real classic character in the horror genre, and

I wanted to punch that up as much as possible. I think I'm really happy with the finale of that show."

Rating/Audience Share: 8.6/15

Episode 1.22
"Born Again"
Original airdate: April 29, 1994
Written by Alex Gansa and Howard Gordon
Directed by Jerrold Freedman
Guest starring: Leslie Carlson (Dr. Spitz), P. Lynn Johnson (Dr. Sheila Braun), Dwight Koss (Det. Barbala), Peter Lapres (Harry Linhart), Andre Libman (Michelle Bishop), Mimi Lieber (Anita Fiore), Brian Markinson (Tony Fiore), Richard Sali (Felder), Maggie Wheeler (Det. Sharon Lazard), Dey Young (Judy Bishop)

An eight-year-old girl with a penchant for disfiguring dolls is linked to a series of deaths, all of which are reminiscent of the work of a serial killer who is now dead. An investigation by Mulder and Scully seems to indicate that the serial killer has been reincarnated in the body of the little girl.

❊   ❊   ❊

Says Howard Gordon, "The idea of reincarnation hadn't been done yet, and there were parts of it that I think were interesting, but I don't think it was very well executed on any front. It was a pretty classic back-from-the-dead revenge tale, and not done particularly interestingly. And it had elements that were repetitive to one of my previous [*X-Files* episodes], 'Shadows.'"

"One of our least successful episodes," Chris Carter admits. "I thought the direction was a little sloppy, but it's one of those episodes that plays a little closer to reality and I like that about it. There's a nice twist in it about a man marrying the wife of another man he had killed. There were actually some nice effects. Just not one of my favorites."

Robert Goodwin's strongest memory of the episode was its teaser, in which a police officer went through a window. "We were shooting the exterior portion of the body exploding out this window. There were actually a pair of windows in this room. We took out the glass from one of them and put in what we call candy glass. And we used this cannon that blasted the debris out the candy-glass window. We had three or four cameras shooting the thing. They call 'Action,' the window blows out, and we realize that the force of the concussion from this cannon has also knocked a hole about three feet across and a foot high in the real window next to our phony window. Al Campbell, our key grip, sort of a Will Rogers kind of guy, says, 'I have a perfect solution for this. When the woman goes to the window, and looks down to see the dead guy, just pan over and next to him will be his dead dog.'"

Rating/Audience Share: 8.2/14

Episode 1.23
"Roland"
Original airdate: May 6, 1994
Written by Chris Ruppenthal
Directed by David Nutter
Guest starring: Garry Davey (Dr. Keats), Dave Hurtubise (Dr. Lawrence Barrington), Zeljko Ivanek (Roland Fuller), Sue Mathew (Lisa Dole), Micole Mercurio (Mrs. Stodie), Kerry Sandomirksy (Tracy), James Sloyan (Dr. Nollette), Matthew Walker (Dr. Surnow)

At a propulsion laboratory, a scientist is trapped in a wind tunnel and is killed through the actions of a severely handicapped janitor named Roland. Upon checking out the situation, Mulder and Scully learn that Roland's brother, Dr. Arthur Grable, recently died in an apparent accident and that the man's head is being kept in a jar of liquid nitrogen. When they learn that Grable's research is being pilfered by his fellow scientists, Mulder concludes that somehow Grable's brain is reaching from beyond the grave (or perhaps the liquid nitrogen) to control Roland's actions.

❈ ❈ ❈

"Probably the weakest script from start to finish that I got," David Nutter admits. "I was really fortunate to get a really fine actor named Zeljko Ivanek, who was wonderful. I thought he was just great. Basically when I knew I had him, I thought it was important to push that as much as possible, to help outweigh the frailties in the script. I felt like it was a real strong character piece. Some of the shows are going to be like that. You're not always going to get the best scripts in the world, but if you get a good actor involved with it and really push that aspect of it, it will definitely help to make it better."

Chris Carter concurs. "Just an amazing performance. This guy, Zeljko, should have won an award for this. I thought he was just fantastic. He was actually the first person to come in and read for this part, and then we had about ten people come in after him, but they just didn't get it. We cast this guy and he turned in a terrific performance which, for me, made the episode. Hats off to David Nutter and to the writing staff for falling in and making the episode really work."

Glen Morgan offers, "Overall, ultimately it probably wasn't completely effective, but I think the show should do some softer, so to speak, episodes; episodes that demonstrate the paranormal isn't always horrifying. It can offer different notions of hope, a life afterwards, consciousness, and things like that."

"You may not notice it in the episode, but there were a lot of scientific rooms and a wind tunnel to be created," says Graeme Murray.

"It was all kind of fun. It was interesting for us just learning some of these things; we spent a lot of time in some of the scientific research places around Vancouver and in the universities."

Rating/Audience Share: 7.9/14

Episode 1.24
"The Erlenmeyer Flask"
Original airdate: May 13, 1994
Written by Chris Carter
Directed by Robert Goodwin
Guest starring: William B. Davis (Cigarette-Smoking Man), Anne DeSalvo (Dr. Carpenter), Lindsey Ginter (Crew-Cut Man), Jaylene Hamilton (Reporter), Jerry Hardin (Deep Throat), Ken Kramer (Dr. Bérubé), Jim Leard (Capt. Lacerio), Phillip MacKenzie (Medic), Mike Mitchell (Cop), John Payne (Guard), Simon Webb (Dr. Secare)

Mulder and Scully investigate a government scientist, Dr. Bérubé, who has cloned extraterrestrial DNA recovered from an alien embryo and is injecting it into terminally ill humans. Those subjects return to complete health, but are stronger than they originally were. And the government's reasons for the alien DNA experiments go beyond the goal of advancing medical science. Guided by Deep Throat, both Mulder and Scully (seemingly no longer the skeptic she once was) are determined to reveal the truth before it's completely and ruthlessly covered up. Shockingly, the episode ends with Deep Throat's death, the disposal of the alien embryo, and the closing of the X-Files, with Mulder and Scully being reassigned.

❉   ❉   ❉

Says Chris Carter, "'Erlenmeyer Flask' brings back nothing but good memories. It just has terrific images in it; it really brought the series in its first year full circle. It was successful in doing what we wanted to do, which was to close down the X-Files. It shocked a lot of people. Glen told me he got a message on his machine when the show ended, a woman with a shaky voice saying, 'What have you done?' They couldn't believe we had killed off a very popular character and closed the X-Files. I think it led us into the second season in a very interesting way."

"That was another case where we had to fight the network," Glen Morgan notes. "They said, 'Closing the X-Files is completely unacceptable. We will not air it because people will believe the show's been canceled.' My response was, 'It's your job to let them know it hasn't, and this is the best way to end the season.'"

"That was a big show for us," says Graeme Murray, "creating all the tanks that the bodies were floating in. We tried to make this kind of life support facility that looked real but also had an eerie aspect to it as well. That was a big set show and pretty interesting; a show where the script really inspired everybody to do the best job they could do."

For Robert Goodwin, who directed this season finale, the episode held special meaning. "In terms of a challenge, and coming at the end of the season — after a real long, tough time — this was a very difficult show, demanding physically, mentally, and every other way. It's the hardest series I've ever worked on. At the end of a very long year, the cast and crew were so tired, yet they all took a deep breath and just said, 'Here we go, guys,' and they gave the finale a two-hundred-percent effort. There's not one department that fell down. Everything about that episode is absolutely first class. The acting, the art direction, the camera work. There's nothing in it that isn't the best you can get, and that's really a credit to a lot of very talented people."

A highlight of the production for Goodwin was a sequence in which Scully is sitting on a bridge, waiting for Deep Throat to show up. His car finally arrives and she crosses the bridge to reach him.

"She's now got the alien fetus she's taken from a top-secret facility," Goodwin explains, "and he says, 'Okay, give it to me, I'm going to make the exchange [for Mulder].' She says, 'No, I'm going to do it.' Scully's very distrustful of him. Mulder's disappeared, she's

stressed out. What happened was, the night we shot that scene, we had a little scene to shoot somewhere else and we had to move over to this bridge. The plan was to get there

> "'The Erlenmeyer Flask' shocked a lot of people. Glen told me he got a message on his machine when the show ended, saying, 'What have you done?'"

an hour before it got dark so we could block the scene, and I had one shot I wanted to do, which was way up high on this crane elevator. We got to the location to block the scene. One end of the bridge was handled by the Vancouver police, and they didn't show up. By the time they got there, I had lost an hour. My plan had originally been to shoot this high scene, get down on the bridge and shoot this dialogue scene, the little piece with the two of them at the car where she's not going to give him the embryo. Then we go and do all the physical stuff that was needed for the whole sequence.

"Because of the hour lost," Goodwin continues, "I realized that the one part of it I could shoot on a stage was the dialogue: essentially two close-ups of them talking. So I didn't do the dialogue. I did everything else first. What happened was, I finally got to the dialogue and it was five in the morning. All night long, all these actors have been running back and forth and getting shot and dropping dead and doing all the things they had to do. And Gillian was very tired. Now I wake her up — she's been sleeping in the back of the car — and I say, 'Okay, let's do the dialogue.' And she got angry, rightfully so. Actually, not really angry. She was tired. I said, 'Listen, we're about to lose the darkness. The sun is going to come up in about twenty minutes. Let's just shoot it. If it's no good, I promise you we won't use it.' She said okay. The same thing with Jerry. We shot the scene and the both of them were so tired and stressed that it came out so strongly on film and was great. It taught me a lesson. If I'm in a similar situation, I'm going to do the same exact thing. If you look at her performance, she's just wonderful. We never had to reshoot it."

The X-Files

"During our first year," says co-producer Paul Rabwin, "the industry said *The X-Files* was a cross between *The Twilight Zone* and *The Night Stalker.* By our second season, *TV Guide* said that a new show, *The Kindred,* was 'a feeble attempt to imitate *The X-Files.*' Now the industry is saying the other networks are trying to launch shows that will take the eighteen-to-forty-nine audience away from *us.* We were even spoofed in *Mad* magazine. I guess we've made it!"

Even the FBI opened its door, inviting Carter in from the cold.

They certainly have. But with all due respect to Alfred E. Neuman, *The X-Files'* arrival in the big time of network television probably had more to do with winning the 1994 Golden Globe award for best drama than it did with a *Mad* magazine parody. It marks one of the few instances where critical attention significantly altered public awareness.

Many television viewers who had only vaguely heard of the Fox network show decided that if it could win a prestigious industry award against such highly acclaimed competition as *Chicago Hope* and *NYPD Blue,* there must be something to it. "The Golden Globe made a lot of people take notice," explains Rabwin, who supervises postproduction of each episode of *The X-Files.* "When we won, you could hear a pin drop. It was like the longest shot in the world coming in, and everyone was dumbfounded. It's given us wonderful credibility."

The momentum quickly transformed the creepy cult show into a ratings juggernaut. Soon after the Golden Globe victory, Viewers for Quality Television nominated the series for best drama and David Duchovny and Gillian Anderson as best actor and actress. Public approval followed critical acclaim, and the series went up 42 percent in the ratings during its second season, the highest gain of any show. "We became contenders." Rabwin smiles. "Suddenly, we were in a very different position than we were during the first year."

Even the FBI, which had refused to help Chris Carter when he was researching the show for its launch, opened its door, inviting the *X-Files* inner circle in from the cold.

"It was funny," Carter says of his tour of FBI headquarters in Washington, D.C., shortly after the second season began, "because when I was first preparing the show, they were very reluctant to give me any information. They didn't know who I was or what I wanted or what I was doing, and they really wouldn't

Co-Executive Producer Robert Goodwin

"Essentially, I'm the commander of the invasion of Normandy, and at the same time I'm worrying about the forces in Italy."

Although this sounds like a bit of self-importance from an ego in overdrive, everything is put in perspective when one realizes that the speaker is Robert Goodwin, co–executive producer of *The X-Files*.

Goodwin, a veteran of such quality television fare as *Hooperman; Mancuso, FBI; Eddie Dodd;* and *Life Goes On*, is the guy who supervises all aspects of physical production of the Fox sensation, taking the various scripts and somehow seeing that they are brought to life on film.

"On a show like *Life Goes On*, the biggest problem we had was whether we were shooting the kitchen or the living room," says Goodwin. "We had two stages at Warner Brothers, the house on the back lot, and that's it. It was essentially the same cast every week. All of which means it was much easier to produce, as opposed to *The X-Files*, which is murderous. We have eight days of shooting, so we potentially have eight days to prepare each episode. I have casting to do, the locations, various and sundry meetings regarding special effects or stunts, then we use the last day to have a production meeting and go over the script page by page with all the heads of production to make sure everyone is prepared for what they have to do. Then we have a 'tone' meeting, which usually involves the writer, the director, myself, and Chris Carter. What we do in the tone meeting is go through the script and make sure that the director and writer are on the same page. Sometimes it's not completely clear what the writer had in mind, so this is an opportunity to take care of that. We discuss characterization, what the actors require, what we hope to get out of it. Then we have our final 'show and tells' with prop support and special effects, and then they're off shooting."

Part of the challenge for Goodwin is that there are two units usually shooting simultaneously, which means he is responsible for getting sets, wardrobe, props, actors, and directors to two different locations at the same time. "It's like doing the *New York Times* crossword puzzle every day," he says with a laugh. "For instance, on a day like today, [producer–director] Rob Bowman is finishing up an episode he's just done that involves a mysterious discovery at the bottom of the ocean, so we have a lot of underwater photography. We finished the principal photography last Wednesday; yesterday he was out on a boat in Vancouver harbor. Meanwhile, [producer–director] Kim Manners started principal photography on his episode yesterday, and he'll shoot for eight days. Then we have a bunch of other second-unit sequences being prepared for next week, all of which [producer] J. P. Finn has to keep in his head at once. And I have to oversee all of this to make sure that when the crew gets there, they have something to shoot."

Back in the 1970s, Goodwin was under contract at Paramount Pictures, where he supervised the production of a variety of television movies. Each movie, naturally, was an entirely different experience, which he credits for preparing him for the daily challenges of *The X-Files*.

"It's not difficult keeping the show new, because it always is new," he notes. "There are different genres of *X-Files* stories. There are funny ones, mythology stories, the monster/scary stories, and that sort of thing. The only thing repetitive about the show is some of its thematic material. But each week, you're always being faced with something new and different to work out. What makes it a little harder is that the natural tendency is that when you've done one thing, you want to try and top yourself. Because of that, the shows have gotten bigger. If you look at some of the first-year shows compared to what we're doing now, there's a *huge* difference in terms of the amount of work that has to be done. But I think we've got a lot more self-confidence than we used to have. Before, it seemed we were always teetering on the edge of a precipice and now, having done so many of them, the stress factor — for me, personally — is a lot less. For the most part, we handle whatever they give us.

"I've been fortunate to have a very long career, I think, because I know how to select material and I have always associated myself with shows that have tried harder," he adds. "Shows that have wanted to be more than just standard television."

One quality production Goodwin will probably *not* be involved with is the proposed *X-Files* feature film. The reason is simple: The film would have to be shot during the show's hiatus (likely between the fourth and fifth seasons), which means preproduction would have to begin during the television season, and there simply wouldn't be time for anyone involved in the show's production to work on the film.

"To be honest with you," Goodwin observes, "I find the pace of life on a feature film — prepping, production, and postproduction — a little too lethargic. I wouldn't have that much interest in it. Besides, on a very pragmatic level, this show takes almost eleven months a year to shoot. When I get those five or six weeks off, all I want to do is go lie down somewhere. The movie Fox just did based on *Power Rangers* didn't do very well, and that may support the line of thinking that if you can watch it on TV every week, why would you want to pay to see it at the movies? Of course, *The X-Files* does have a huge following and there would be tremendous interest.

"Whatever happens," he says with a grin, "I'll certainly go see it. Hey, I'm a big fan."

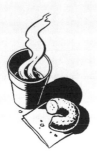

cooperate with me at all. So beyond a little protocol or procedure that they described to me, I didn't know this institution. I was sort of writing about it blindly, having only what I had read and the little they had told me. A year goes by, and all of a sudden the phone calls start coming from FBI agents who are secret fans, and we developed a few relationships with these people. Finally, at the end of the year, a couple of them became such big fans that they were able to coordinate an *X-Files* tour of the FBI for Gillian Anderson, David Duchovny, and me, and *TV Guide* was allowed to come in and document the whole thing.

"I made some notes," he adds, "but mostly it was just a chance to see up close what I had been writing about. I have developed contacts since then, so if I need to know something about ballistics or DNA testing or fingerprinting, I've been able to call and get good expert advice or information from these people. Still, officially they can't say they endorse the show or that they are in any way connected to the show."

Producer J. P. Finn, who works in collaboration with Robert Goodwin on the physical production of the series, acknowledges the critical kudos as a key to the show's becoming a mainstream hit, but he also says there was more to the ratings explosion than simply recognition of good work. "I think the success of the show has a lot to do with the quality, because we do great work. But I also think our timing was great. We arrived at the same time that prime-time episodic television is dominated by statistical concerns: age and wealth demographics and so forth. "That eliminates anything that's really a fringe or risky kind of idea," he says. "Being that *The X-Files* opened on Fox, which already likes to try different things, we were never intended to be anything except something dark, mysterious, intelligent, and fun. I don't think we ever expected to be as popular as *Melrose Place* or any of the shows like that. If that was the original goal, we wouldn't have the show we have."

Howard Gordon, who was promoted from supervising producer to co–executive producer in the third season, agrees with Bowman. "It's a fairly intelligent show," he observes. "People know they're going to be turned on to part of our world that they don't normally see. Whether it's government conspiracy or ghosts, they're going to see something that will take them to a place they don't usually see. There are so many shows on television, and so little that distinguishes one from the other. This is one of those shows that's different, and as long as you deliver on the product, people will come."

"A lot of it has to do with the stories we tell and how we tell them," Carter opines. "I think the writers on the show have hooked in to what really scares people. We try to stay away from horror conventions, and I think we've been very successful at that; I think we've been very successful at finding the universal, real scariness out there and plugging in to it."

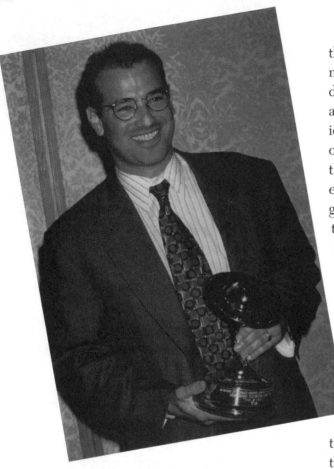

Howard Gordon.

the Internet took off. We were probably the first show to be adopted by the Internet, and that drove the underground word of mouth. Those good vibes permeated through the audience we first attracted, and Fox paid attention to it. It kept us going when the ratings weren't so great, and so we survived, and in the second year the general public became more aware of us."

Producer–director Rob Bowman observes

Despite ubiquitous press (*Entertainment Weekly* and *TV Guide* featured cover stories the same week *People* profiled Anderson on its cover) in the aftermath of the Golden Globe breakthrough, the show's creators didn't allow success to pull them away from the game plan.

"We don't listen to our own press," Carter proclaims. "We're still the same people, and we don't sit on our laurels. I think all of us realize we did real good shows as well as shows that could have been better. None of us likes to feel we've done anything less than our best, and there's a nice little competitive thing going on. We all want to one-up the other guy, in the most constructive way imaginable. We push each other, so all this attention doesn't necessarily bring any additional pressure. I pressure myself more than anyone or anything. I want to make sure we're happy with what we do. I just do what I feel is right and hopefully people will like it. You can't succumb to the pressure."

Co–executive producer Goodwin actually found himself more confident as the second season dawned, in spite of the sudden attention of the press and the public. Staying within the budget, he says, had never been a problem — the show's makers had proved themselves capable of consistently producing quality work for about $1 million per episode.

"I became immune to the pressure of accomplishing the impossible." Goodwin laughs. "After getting twenty-three impossible-to-produce scripts that first year, by the second year it didn't matter what they sent. So the stress level has changed. Second year we were so much more confident, because we had pulled so many amazing things off. Some

"*The X-Files* could be like an Ed Wood movie if you're not careful."

of the guest directors who come in start hyperventilating. They say, 'Oh my God, have you read this script?' and I would respond, 'Yes, you've got an easy one.'

"[The second-season episode] 'The Host' is a perfect example," he continues. "The script required a large humanoid flukeworm that's going to be moving through all these sewers and Russian freighters and so on. Sure, it was hard, but in the end we did it. There was none of the panic or disbelief that was there the first year. Now I say, 'Okay, if that's what you want, that's what we'll do.' But that doesn't mean we became complacent. If you don't do it right, it becomes laughable. It could be like an Ed Wood movie if you're not careful."

Hoping to avoid making *Plan 9 from Prime Time*, Carter instituted an unusual policy at the beginning of the second season, giving directors the additional authority and responsibility of producing. For half the season,

David Nutter was employed this way until he moved over to *Space: Above and Beyond.* He was followed by Rob Bowman and Kim Manners, both of whom have remained under contract with *The X-Files.*

"I think Chris Carter is starting a real smart trend here," says Manners. "I believe he feels that directors make good producers in a creative sense, which is really not normal network thinking. The truth is that a director has so much more knowledge of what it takes to bring it all together on a set, and he also has much more knowledge in the cutting room. Let's face it, from the time that script is written until the public sees it on the air, it's either been filmed on the set or redirected in the editing room."

Bowman notes that the difference between being a producer-director on a show as opposed to being a freelance director on assignment is a distinct and powerful one, both psychologically and practically. First of all, a producer–director has "made the roster" and is no longer a free agent, he says, thus removing the pressure of needing to sell his services to different series during the course of a season.

"As a result," Bowman says, "the only thing I've got to think about is *The X-Files.* My allegiance changed; this was now my show, and I was fully committed to it. So now I'm trying to keep my ears open for Chris Carter, Howard Gordon, and the other writers. How do we tell the stories better? Who are the directors I need to look at to hire on to the show? Who are the best storytellers? There are a lot of guys who can shoot nice film, but there aren't very many who can tell a story. I think the trick is to find directors who can think like writers. I need to talk to the newcomers, even though they may be twenty-five-year vets, and say, 'This is how we like to have it done on our show.' It's a highly creative show, and I don't want to stifle anybody's creativity, as long as they're paddling in the same direction we are, because we know how to get there."

"Gillian came back ten days after giving birth."

And if Robert Goodwin's stress level has dropped since the first season, it may be because he's spreading it around to more people. For the second season, the average episode of the series was still scheduled for just eight days of production, which Kim Manners terms "a joke," but by this time, cast and crew had figured out how to stretch production as much as possible. Second-unit photography, for example, typically has a separate deadline, which usually brings production up to about ten days. "Sure, it's second unit," Manners says of the crew that shoots backgrounds and various periphery scenes that usually don't include the principal actors, "but they've still got their own crew, and they're shooting with cast and sound." This core work

Designing The X-Files

Creating the impossible is the everyday objective of the cast and crew of *The X-Files*, which strives for, and often achieves, a feature-film-quality look with each new episode. While no single person is more important than another in bringing the show to life, one can't help looking to the series's production designer as playing an integral role in its success.

"I kind of ended up here semi-accidentally," says production designer Graeme Murray with a shrug. "I just feel like we're a bunch of little kids making forts in the woods. You get to build some weird stuff and you have the budget to kind of build the fort you want — plus, you're old enough to have girls in, too."

Upon graduating from art school, Murray, a Vancouver native, began his professional career as an illustrator with a serious interest in printing. "I enjoy fine typography and old-style engraving," he says. "I honestly thought I was going to do book illustrations and make my own books, but you start off one way and if the road goes a different way, you follow it."

The road first led him to a local television station in the days before computer graphics, when illustrators would create station slugs and promotional images. This ultimately led to his becoming art director of the Canadian series *Beachcombers*. From there he took on two projects he considers the most prestigious of his pre–*X-Files* career, the feature film *Never Cry Wolf* and the CBS crime series *Wiseguy*, starring Ken Wahl. Shot in Vancouver, *Wiseguy* brought Murray a tremendous amount of recognition that piqued the interest of other production companies shooting in Canada, and that eventually brought him to the attention of Chris Carter and co–executive producer Robert Goodwin.

"The art director they had for the first five or six shows wasn't getting along with Bob Goodwin," says Murray. "Once you don't get along with Bob, it's not Bob who's going to go. I met with him, and here we are."

But the road from "there" to "here" has been a challenging one as his imagination has been unleashed on a weekly basis. "Chris Carter's ambition has always been that these are little features," Murray says, "and we all try to approach it that way. For instance, I like layering things. I like to see things through glass or through doorways, and place other elements behind, so the set has a bit of depth and it's not just flat walls or anything real straight. As much as possible, we try to make it feel like there's a world beyond the little room you're actually in. The set also has to feel right for the story. We try to give each episode an individual look, so we use different colors or different moods to make each one stand by itself, which is unusual for most episodic stuff. I think that fits in with Chris's thinking. He's always felt that if he could get that kind of feature quality and as long as the show's popular, he can push. That's what he's been doing.

"But I'm not complaining," Murray concludes. "There's nothing else you can liken this show to, where you're in a completely different arena every time. It is never the same, and you get the opportunity to do things you've never had a chance to do before. Most series work, for example, kind of takes place in and around a police station where everything is street-related or police-related. This show just goes everywhere. It's the variety that keeps it interesting. I think there are a lot of shows you do so that you can pay the rent or buy groceries, but *The X-Files* is much more than that. It's a series you're proud to be a part of."

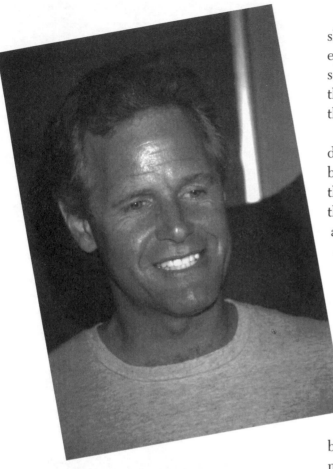

Chris Carter.

is mirrored by a separate shot-insert unit that can shoot up to five days a week. "The shows have just gotten enormous," Manners says. "When we had our second-season wrap party, Chris Carter commented, 'Man, there's a lot of people that work for me that I don't even know.' He thought he knew everybody, but there's the construction crew, the special-effects crew, the makeup crew. Frankly, these

shows are a huge undertaking. They are not episodic television shows in the traditional sense. These are small features or movies of the week that we're trying to turn out. That's the challenge we face."

It all works, says Manners, who began directing television almost two decades ago, because of the guidance and encouragement that come from the top. "Not only is it a vision that Chris shares, but also the opportunity to actually be a filmmaker. He encourages everybody — not just the directors — who works with him. 'Hey, you're a filmmaker, you have good ideas,' he tells us. 'Do your best work. Make this your best effort.' He inspires that from us."

Such testimonials would sound a tad disingenuous coming from an underling trying to snare a promotion, but that's pretty clearly not the origins of such kudos for Carter. From the top to the bottom of the creative ladder, the commitment to Carter and to *The X-Files* is complete.

"It's a seven-days-a-week job," says Rob Bowman. "I've totally sacrificed my personal life for the show. I was dating somebody for five years who had incredible patience, but still we couldn't hold on. You may ask if that kind of commitment is worth it. Well, to me, it is. It's an expensive personal contract, but I can't imagine anything else I'd rather be doing."

❋ ❋ ❋

All that dedication was to be tested in the second season, which saw the core premise of the series turned on its head by the events of the first season's finale as well as Gillian Anderson's real-life pregnancy. In "The Erlenmeyer Flask," the X-Files was closed down by the FBI bosses, and Mulder and Scully were separately reassigned, allowing Carter to write Anderson out of the show (via an apparent alien abduction in "Duane Barry" and "Ascension") during the latter stages of her pregnancy.

"In the beginning of the season," says Carter, "we did what producers are supposed to do, which is turn problems into assets. I thought it was really a testament to both David and Gillian's dedication to us. First of all, David had to carry a tremendous amount of work because Gillian's availability was limited. But Gillian was such a trouper in that she wanted more work and worked right up until she just couldn't anymore. Then she came back ten days after giving birth."

For Howard Gordon, Anderson's pregnancy brought back memories of his tenure on *Beauty and the Beast,* where star Linda Hamilton's similar announcement essentially sounded the death knell for that show.

"Obviously, there was an immediate feeling of déjà vu," Gordon says with a laugh.

"The difference — and it was a significant one — was that Gillian wanted to be on the show. We were clearly working with someone who would be game for doing whatever she could. We were able to block out not only the episodes that would have to exclude her, but

Scully's limited involvement [resulted in] increased exposure for some of the ancillary characters, which gave substance and depth to the *X-Files* universe.

ultimately it sort of was a blessing in disguise because it forced us to contrive something that has been grist for the mill and will continue to be, in terms of her abduction or disappearance. As it turned out, her pregnancy not only gave birth to [Anderson's daughter] Piper, but to a whole new avenue of possibilities on the show. I really love most of the first seven or eight episodes of the season, because they dealt so profoundly with the main characters: her disappearance, Mulder working with [Agent] Krycek, who was a Judas among them . . . it was all very exciting stuff."

Former co–executive producer Glen Morgan, who left *The X-Files* midseason with partner James Wong to create the Fox series *Space: Above and Beyond,* admits he was

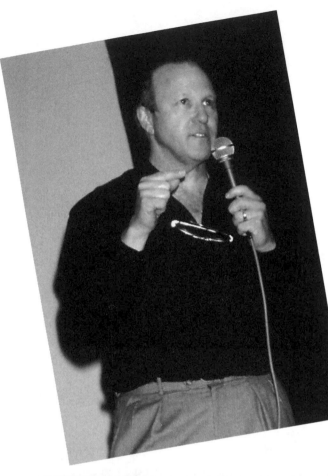

Paul Rabwin.

quite concerned about the temporary loss of Anderson.

"No matter how good David is, *The X-Files* is a two-person show; that's what makes it work," he says. "And suddenly we're turning it into a one-person show. We were really messing with the concept. The whole business of splitting them up is the kind of thing you would do at the beginning of year three. So we

crossed our fingers. We were just hoping that people would hang in there until she got back."

What Anderson's departure did allow for was a renewed enthusiasm for one of the show's staples: government conspiracies.

"What those episodes, and the show in general, made me realize was that *The X-Files* almost seems like the kind of show that would have gone over during the Reagan years," says Morgan. "Films like *JFK* and *Silence of the Lambs* — Scully, especially in the beginning, was very much like the Jodie Foster character — and older films like *Parallax View*, *The Conversation*, *Three Days of the Condor*, and *Klute* are all conspiracy-oriented, weird, paranoid movies that I think Chris tapped in to."

An additional result of Scully's limited involvement was the increased exposure offered to some of the ancillary characters, which gave substance and depth to the *X-Files* universe. Among the peripheral characters who stepped up in the second year were rogue agent Krycek (Nicholas Lea); his mysterious, enigmatic boss, the Cigarette-Smoking Man (William B. Davis); Mulder's superior, Assistant Director Walter S. Skinner (Mitch Pileggi); and Mr. X (Steven Williams), who replaced Deep Throat as Mulder's chief inside informant.

Strangely, the conspiracy arc that Carter so carefully charted during Anderson's pregnancy was shelved when she returned midseason. When Mulder and Scully were finally reunited in "Firewalker," the two agents largely left government intrigue behind and headed out into the hinterlands to pursue a wide variety of paranormal phenomena in a series of stand-alone episodes. Besides confronting Flukeman ("The Host"), they had close encounters with Vietnam veterans who hadn't slept in twenty-four years; sexy vampires; reincarnated serial killers; a boy-next-door necrophiliac; Satan worshipers who doubled as members of the PTA; deadly viruses and parasites; and a scientist whose experiment caused his shadow to suck unsuspecting passersby into a black hole.

But while the change of emphasis was jarring to many viewers, the show didn't completely abandon Mulder's search for the truth about UFOs and the government's efforts to suppress that information. The two-part "Colony" and "End Game" was probably as ambitious as *The X-Files* can get, with Mulder seemingly reunited with his long-missing sister, only to be forced to give her up to an alien bounty hunter. Samantha, he finally becomes convinced, isn't really his sister, but an alien clone. The season finale, "Anasazi," brought Mulder to a buried boxcar containing what appear to be alien corpses. Investigating further, he learns that they might be human beings who had been subjected to government experiments involving alien DNA.

Before he can uncover the truth, he is either killed in the boxcar or abducted by aliens, in either case paving the way for the third season and the frustrating problem of maintaining Scully's skepticism in the face of all she's encountered.

Once again citing his concern that success can breed complacency, Carter took a fairly unorthodox approach to forming the writing staff for the third year. Contributing writer Frank Spotnitz became story editor, and Carter added writers such as Darin Morgan (who brought a quirky sense of humor to the show with episodes like "Humbug"), *Northern Exposure*'s Jeff Vlaming, *Chicago Hope*'s Kim Newton, and John Shiban to the full-time staff. There was not one genre writer among them.

"I chose to go with unknown quantities," Carter says. "This isn't a sci-fi genre show, as far as I see it. It's a cross-genre show. It's some kind of a suspense thriller–espionage crossbreed. If I get [an established] science fiction writer, that could work to the show's disadvantage, because you can't approach *The X-Files* as straight science fiction.

"Ultimately," he concludes, "my goal then was the same that it's always been: to create twenty-two to twenty-four really scary shows. I just want to scare the hell out of the audience. That's all."

SEASON TWO
Episode Guide

Episode 2.1 (#25)
"Little Green Men"

Original airdate: September 16, 1994
Written by Glen Morgan and James Wong
Directed by David Nutter
Guest starring: Raymond J. Barry (Sen. Richard Matheson), William B. Davis (Cigarette-Smoking Man), Mike Gomez (Jorge Concepcion), Vanessa Morley (Samantha, age 8), Mitch Pileggi (Assistant Director Walter S. Skinner)

The X-Files remain closed, with Mulder and Scully given other assignments. At the same time, Mulder begins to lose faith in his own beliefs — that, essentially, the truth is out there — until he is contacted by Senator Richard Matheson and finds himself heading out to a supposedly abandoned SETI program site in Puerto Rico where a message has been received from the Voyager spacecraft. Scully arrives to help him, and together they must flee government agents who are out to capture them.

❅ ❅ ❅

"I thought it was a great first episode, coming off of 'The Erlenmeyer Flask,'" says Chris Carter, "and it established what was going to be the Scully–Mulder relationship for at least the first eight episodes. I thought the script by Glen and Jim and the direction of David Nutter were terrific, and that David and Gillian's performances were excellent. I'm very proud of that show as a season opener."

Glen Morgan explains that "Little Green Men" began life as a feature he and Jim Wong were attempting to write. "But we liked the idea so much," he explains, "that we decided to do it for Mulder. The other thing is that I was irked that the government had shut down the SETI project and I wanted to address that. Most important, I was on the set first season once when Duchovny was talking about the episode 'Beyond the Sea' [which focused on the Scully character] and he said, 'That was a pretty good episode. When are you going to write one like that for me?' Well, I liked him, he deserved it, and I thought that's what 'Little Green Men' was trying to be."

One interesting aspect of the show is that Mulder has waited years for contact, but when it's about to happen he freaks out.

"Although I don't think it came across as well as we wanted it to," Morgan says, "we were trying to work up the notion, 'Was that even there? Is this real?' At some point in editing I realized that it didn't play that way. Earlier in the show Mulder has said to Scully, 'I'm starting to doubt that my sister was abducted.' So you're trying to say, 'Is this in his head? Do we create these kinds of fear ourselves?'"

Director David Nutter admits that he had become a bit nervous tackling the show because it had grown so popular between seasons. "I wanted to avoid the pitfalls of these shows that become phenomenons — really hot — and then fade away really quickly. I, like everybody else, wanted this to be a long-running program. By the end of the first season, it was like a ship pulling away from port: 'There it goes!'

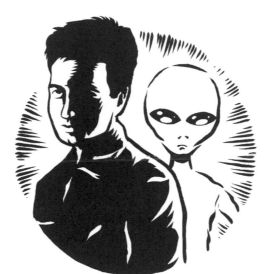

"I thought 'Little Green Men' was a tough show to do. I thought the introduction of the show was wonderful, and I loved the paranoia we were able to generate in that episode,

"I was irked that the government had shut down the SETI project and I wanted to address that."

especially during the first meeting between Mulder and Scully. I thought Mulder was very good in the scene with Senator Matheson.

There was also a lot of action, what with the car chase and all. I also very much liked the bookending of the show, opening with Mulder on a mundane surveillance assignment and closing the same way."

For producer J. P. Finn, perhaps the most difficult aspect of the episode was trying to achieve Puerto Rico in Vancouver. "Which I guess we pulled off, though if you look closely you'll see pine trees in the back." He laughs. "Anyway, a great little show to get going with. A typical *X-Files* show, where more is suggested than you actually see."

Interestingly, actor Darren McGavin (forever known as Carl Kolchak) was approached to play Senator Richard Matheson (whose namesake adapted Jeff Rice's *Night Stalker* novel for TV).

"We tried very hard to get him," says James Wong. "I'm not sure what happened. Our casting director called before we started second season and spoke to McGavin's agent and said, 'We want him for the first show; lock him up, and we're willing to pay the price.' By the time it came down to getting him, suddenly the agent said, 'He doesn't know about the show' or 'He's not available.' It became some kind of weird thing and it just didn't happen."

Rating/Audience Share: 10.3/19

Episode 2.2 (#26)
"The Host"
Original airdate: September 23, 1994
Written by Chris Carter
Directed by Daniel Sackheim
Guest starring: Freddy Andreiuci (Det. Norman), Marc Bauer (Agent Brisentine), Darin Morgan (Flukeman), Mitch Pileggi (Assistant Director Walter S. Skinner), Gabrielle Rose (Dr. Jo Zenzola)

When the decomposed body of a man is found in the sewers of Newark, Mulder is given what seems to be a routine murder case to investigate — punishment, he believes, for his work on the X-Files — but it turns out that the perpetrator is actually a flukeworm mutated into humanoid form by radioactive material being transported on a cargo vessel from Chernobyl.

❈ ❈ ❈

Chris Carter notes, "'The Host' has become a real popular episode. That's one of our traditional monster shows — although we don't do *traditional* monsters, obviously. I was in a funk when I wrote that episode, actually. We were coming back from hiatus and I was trying to find something more interesting than just the Flukeman. I was irritated at the time, and I brought my irritation to Mulder's attitude. Basically he had become fed up with the FBI. They had given him what he felt was a low assignment, which was sending him into the city after a dead body. But lo and behold, he finds that this is a case that for all intents and purposes is an X-File. It's been given to him by a man he's never looked at as an ally, Skinner. So it's an interesting establishing of the relationship between them."

"A Carter script, but a bit of a departure for a Carter script," says J. P. Finn. "Chris's scripts tend to deal with alien subject matter. Although we had done some creature parts the first year, this time we got to see more of the creatures than we had before. That was a departure. Graeme Murray did a great job building those sewers. It was very cleverly designed. On one of our stages we have a pit, which is about ten feet deep, sixteen by sixteen wide. He basically built two sewers, with one main sewer that he renovated to a central area. At one point, we actually went into a real sewage plant for those exterior shots. That was the real McCoy. It was also a hot summer day — about ninety degrees — and it was a pretty difficult and smelly day for the cast and crew."

Emmy-winning director Daniel Sackheim enjoyed the episode as much as anyone. "It's classic Chris Carter," he says. "I remember when I read the script I said, 'You've got to be kidding me.' It has elements of *Creature from the Black Lagoon.* It's what makes the show the show. Nobody else would attempt to do something like that. It has to be done with a fine touch so that you wouldn't be laughed off of the screen. The concept is fairly preposterous, and the subject matter is a little stomach-churning. I think he wrote a terrific script, and I would like to think it was handled adeptly.

"You know, there was one thing that was a great thing Chris taught me, and I think it is the signature of the show. I don't know what he would call it, but I call it event writing. What I mean by that is two or three times during the course of an act, he would have an event transpire that would always get the audience's attention. A lot of the show is expository, with Mulder talking about how this project happened, and Scully responding. In 'The Host,' the event is when the guy is brushing his teeth and he starts to choke. Blood starts to

come out of his mouth, he goes into the shower, and this fluke comes out of his mouth. It's

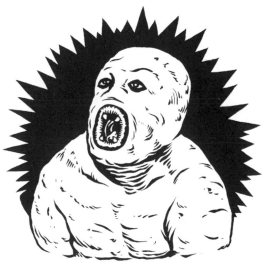

"I remember when I read the script I said, 'You've got to be kidding me.' It has elements from *Creature from the Black Lagoon.*"

such a testament to what is great about the writing of the show: these events that don't require any dialogue."

"I will *never* forget that toothpaste scene," adds James Wong. "I thought that was the grossest piece of television ever put on the air, so that was cool."

Glen Morgan proclaims, "My brother the Flukeman! My brother Darin wore the costume of Flukie. At one point, I saw Darin getting made up at five o'clock in the afternoon. After dinner and a few drinks, I went back to Darin's trailer at like one in the morning, and there's this thing in a rubber suit with my brother's voice. I said, 'I really can't deal with this; I've got to go.'"

During the shooting of "The Host," David

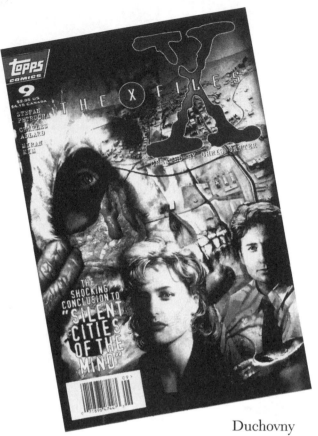

said, 'I'm Flukeman!' Duchovny was quite impressed that Darin was willing to wait a half hour into the flight before he pulled the joke."

For his part, Darin Morgan doesn't remember his actual work as Flukeman with such levity. "It was hell! The suit required a very long makeup job. It was very uncomfortable, I couldn't breathe, and it smelled bad. I couldn't urinate or anything else. It was just sort of generally unpleasant being in that suit. I started suffering from sensory deprivation, where I couldn't really feel anything. It was a very bizarre experience which I hope never to repeat."

But, it's pointed out, Chris Carter has said that they might bring back Flukie. "If they do, it won't be me," Morgan says matter-of-factly.

Rating/Audience Share: 9.8/17

Duchovny never saw Darin Morgan outside of his Flukeman suit. They spoke and got along — in fact, Darin was asked to join the writing staff. When Darin was flying to Vancouver to prep "Humbug," by coincidence he sat next to Duchovny, who didn't know who he was. About a half hour into the flight, Darin leaned over to Duchovny and said, "Could you sign an autograph?"

"David made the best of the situation and said, 'What do you want me to write?'" Glen Morgan recounts. "Darin said, 'I want you to write, "To my nemesis — Fox Mulder."'" Duchovny is like, 'What nut am I next to?' and he said, 'Why am I your nemesis?' And Darin

Episode 2.3 (#27)
"Blood"

Original airdate: September 30, 1994
Story by Darin Morgan
Teleplay by Glen Morgan and James Wong
Directed by David Nutter
Guest starring: Tom Braidwood (Frohike), John Cygan (Sheriff Spencer), Andre Daniels (Harry McNally), Kimberly Ashlyn Gere (Bonnie McRoberts), Dean Haglund (Langly), Bruce Harwood (Byers), John Harris (Gary Taber), William Sanderson (Ed Funsch), Diana Stevan (Mrs. Adams), George Touliatos (County Supervisor Larry Winter)

A string of seemingly random killings occur in a small Pennsylvania town, which brings Mulder in to profile the murderers. He discovers that not one of them had a history of violence, and all died at the end of their sprees. The only clues available are destroyed electronic devices — whose LCDs triggered the murders — and an unknown organic substance.

❈ ❈ ❈

"Darin was supposed to write that one," Glen Morgan recalls, "but scheduling wouldn't allow it. We wanted to do something about postal workers and paranoia about pesticides and decided to merge the two ideas. We worked with Darin on the story, but we needed a script really fast, so Jim and I did it. We took some heat for the ending when William Sanderson climbs a tower and starts shooting people. On the Internet people would say, 'Couldn't they come up with something more original?' But that was the point. It's almost like the joke that people at work who are stressed say: 'I'm going to go up in a tower with a gun.' That's what everyone points to when they're going to flip out. We really lucked out getting William Sanderson."

According to Glen Morgan, director David Nutter and Sanderson were working so well together that Nutter was seemingly reaching out to him personally for the ending sequences in the tower. "Almost all of that stuff that's in the end was pre-slate; it wasn't in the take. Jim and I had read a lot about the beginning of *Apocalypse Now* when Martin Sheen puts his hand through the mirror. He had cut himself in reality and the camera operator stopped. [Director Francis Ford] Coppola said, 'No, no, keep going.' Which is why they put jump cuts in that scene, because they had a moment where the camera stopped. So Nutter said, 'Why don't we cut the best psychotic moments that this actor is

Playing the Flukeman, Darin Morgan said, "I was suffering from sensory deprivation, where I couldn't really feel anything."

feeling and we'll put them all together like that?' That's why this act is cut like that. We spent a lot of time on it, and that's something I was very happy with. None of that stuff is between 'Action' and 'Cut.'"

Nutter explains, "I always love to get a hold of an actor like William Sanderson. At the ending, what I tried to do was allow him to get into it and let the camera roll while he did so.

Different actors you treat in different ways. He was the kind of actor that wanted to, emotionally, get into it. I let him get pumped up

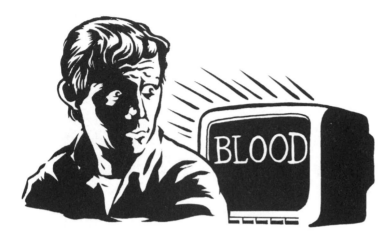

for it, and filmed what he was doing. Most of the stuff you see in the episode came during the prep."

Chris Carter offers that the genesis of the story came "from films Darin Morgan had seen of pesticides being sprayed on unknowing populations by a government who said this was good for you, and what the effect of our government spraying may be now on some level. I think it works because it feels like it can happen in your own backyard." David Nutter notes, "Glen, Jim, and I had talked about doing shows that were very different from each other. I thought 'Blood' was a real throwback to *The Twilight Zone*. It was a show shot in a standard way, where a lot of editing was involved."

"When we did that show, we were of the opinion that it should feel different in style than the other episodes," says James Wong. "We wanted a more sterile, static kind of feel to it. I'm not sure if we were able to get that with the direction. We missed communication with David in terms of what we felt it should look like. I liked the idea of the show, and I really liked William Sanderson. I don't think it was the most successful, but it wasn't the worst."

Controversy arose when Morgan and Wong cast former porn star Kimberly Ashlyn Gere as a suburban housewife.

"She was trying to go legitimate, and we were trying to be punks and ruffle feathers," recalls Glen Morgan, who later cast her in several episodes of his series *Space: Above and Beyond*. "She said, 'What's the sex thing I have to do in it?' and I said, 'We wouldn't be that obvious. You play a housewife.' I was very proud of her and scared to death, because Bob Goodwin said, 'Why are we casting this girl?' I think people suspected monkey business, but I said, 'We're casting her for the same reason *Miami Vice* cast Gordon Liddy — it's a weird, cool thing to do, and she's a better actress than Gordon was.'"

Rating/Audience Share: 9.1/16

Episode 2.4 (#28)
"Sleepless"

Original airdate: October 7, 1994
Written by Howard Gordon
Directed by Rob Bowman
Guest starring: William B. Davis (Cigarette-Smoking Man), Jonathan Gries (Salvatore Matola), Nicholas Lea (Agent Alex Krycek), Mitch Pileggi (Assistant Director Walter S. Skinner), Don Thompson (Henry Willig), Tony Todd (Augustus Cole), Steven Williams (Mr. X)

Mulder and Agent Krycek, the new partner who has been foisted on him, investigate a series of bizarre deaths that don't make sense: for instance, a scientist whose demise is consistent with burning, although there is no evidence of fire or burns. Ultimately, it is discovered that a series of Army experiments to create a better soldier during the Vietnam War induced permanent insomnia in some soldiers. None of them have slept in twenty-four years, and one of them, Augustus Cole, has moved to a higher plane, where he can make dream and reality one. His goal is to bring salvation — through some fairly violent means — to his comrades.

✧ ✧ ✧

For supervising producer Howard Gordon, "Sleepless" was significant in that it represent-ed the first time in nine years he was writing without a partner.

"I had some insecurity in the beginning," he admits. "I was now on my own and had to investigate all new processes. I did a story on agricultural engineering. It was a good idea, but a very oblique script. I did the outline with Chris, but as I wrote the story I knew something was wrong. I spent an undue amount of time on it, really stressed out over it, and gave it to Jim Wong to read and said, 'This isn't very good, is it?' He read it and said, 'No, it's not.' Meanwhile, I was two weeks away from prepping on my first episode as a solo person, and I had a script that sucked. I basically couldn't fall asleep for two nights straight, I was so anxious. I figured that my career was over, I figured I was done, I had no talent, and I was history. Not being able to sleep for two nights, I began to think, 'Gee, what if somebody couldn't ever sleep?' So I went to Chris and said, 'I'm putting a pin on that other script and I'm writing this story.' Chris could have thought, 'Oh man, we're dead.' Not only was I insecure about my solo act, but Chris might have been as well. But he had this really great confidence in me and said, 'Whatever you want, just do it. I trust you're going to do it.' It's that kind of trust that just gave me the confidence to do it. I beat out the whole story in twenty-four hours and it came out well."

"I really love that show," Christ Carter enthuses. "It's a great idea, well executed. I guess the hardest part was that it required a lot of night shooting, and of course we were shooting in the middle of the summer in Vancouver, where it's the land of the midnight sun. That was a challenge for the cast and crew. We had a good cast; Tony Todd was wonderful. Production-wise, I think there's a lot of suggestion of violence there rather than what you see. You're shown what's going to happen, but you don't actually see it."

"He's out killing people, but the reason he's killing people is well supported. His victims *want* to die."

For director Rob Bowman, an enjoyable aspect of "Sleepless" was the ambiguity of the drama. "You couldn't tell who the good guy was and who the bad guy was. The apparent antagonist, played by Tony Todd, was on a mercy mission. You could absolutely endorse this guy's point of view. He's out killing people, but the reason he's killing people is well supported. His victims *want* to die. We even added something to the first killing, the soldier in the apartment. Just at the moment he realizes he's going to be killed, he closes his eyes, rolls his head back, and thinks to himself, 'It's over. Finally, relief. I can sleep.' That was something I put in there because Howard Gordon had talked a lot about how these guys have been suffering for twenty-four years. If they know they're going to be killed, there should be a moment of release there. I found that very interesting, and it made the audience think for a second as to who was right and who was wrong."

In one particularly memorable scene, a soldier is greeted by armed Vietnamese men, women, and children who seem ready to exact revenge.

"None of the people could speak English," Bowman recalls. "I think it was the first time any of them had been on a set, so they were looking at the camera, the people, and the hardware. I had to reshoot it another day, and it was an exercise in blank expressions and nonresponsive looks from all of them. But the little boy right in the foreground of the shot seemed to understand through an interpreter what the scene was about. The direction was along the lines of, 'This man has hurt your family and you've come to make him pay his debt.' This boy gave one of these steely-eyed, dagger-filled stares. He did it every time. I remember saying to all of them, 'Hold court with your eyes, by looking very final in your conclusion that he has to pay his debt.' A little smoke, a little crosslight, a little blood and some prosthetics, and you have it. The other thing is to put so many people in the room that they could only have appeared magically. I think originally there were like three people on the set and it looked like they could have walked in there. We put nine people in there, literally in the blink of an eye, and there's no way they just walked in."

James Wong says, "Stylistically, it had some very strong shots. We also introduced Mr. X in that episode. Mr. X, originally, was a woman. But when we watched the dailies, we realized that it wasn't going to work."

Glen Morgan adds, "Chris didn't like her, and I said, 'How about Steve Williams? He's a great guy and an intense actor.' As a result, X's scene with Mulder was actually David playing against an actress, but then we went back, shot Steven Williams, and inserted the footage."

Rating/Audience Share: 8.6/15

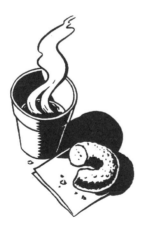

Episode 2.5 (#29)
"Duane Barry"

Original airdate: October 14, 1994
Written and directed by Chris Carter
Guest starring: William B. Davis (Cigarette-Smoking Man), Nicholas Lea (Agent Alex Krycek), CCH Pounder (Agent Lucy Kazdin), Steve Railsback (Duane Barry), Frank C. Turner (Dr. Del Hakkie)

Episode 2.6 (#30)
"Ascension"

Original airdate: October 21, 1994
Written by Paul Brown
Directed by Michael Lange
Guest starring: William B. Davis (Cigarette-Smoking Man), Sheila Larken (Margaret Scully), Nicholas Lea (Agent Alex Krycek), Mitch Pileggi (Assistant Director Walter S. Skinner), Steve Railsback (Duane Barry), Steven Williams (Mr. X)

In part one, Former FBI agent Duane Barry escapes from the mental hospital where he's being held, and takes several people hostage. Blaming his erratic behavior on the fact that he was abducted by aliens, Barry is convinced he must find someone else to sacrifice to the aliens to save himself, and he finds that someone in Dana Scully.

In the second part, Mulder pursues Duane Barry and the captured Scully, a chase that leads him to the mountains and near-death on a tram car. It is revealed that Agent Krycek is

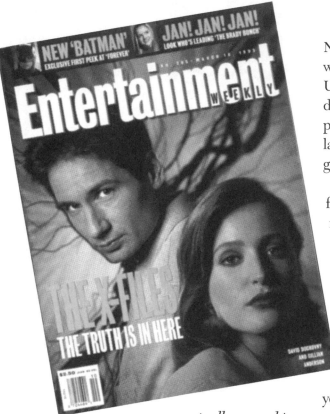

actually working for the Cigarette-Smoking Man, who seems to be pulling everybody's strings. At episode's end, Scully is gone, Barry claims she's been taken by a UFO, and Skinner reopens the X-Files.

❊ ❊ ❊

Chris Carter, who directed "Duane Barry" as well as wrote it, says he's very proud of the episode. "It was a chance for me to show people what I thought the show could be and should be, and I think I was very successful. I had a lot of help from a very dedicated crew and really nice technical help from David

Nutter as far as the economy of direction and where to put cameras at certain times. Ultimately, though, it was me on the set directing. No one can do it for you. I was very pleased that when I first said 'Action,' no one laughed. From that point on, I knew I was going to be okay."

"Directing for the first time is a nightmare for anyone," says Robert Goodwin. "So to make your first time an episode of *The X-Files* is crazy. We have sent so many directors home in body bags, but Chris came in and did a very good job."

Carter did find some significant differences between just writing and both writing and directing a show. "There are so many different problems to solve," he notes matter-of-factly. "As a director, you have to solve them practically. As a writer, you have to solve them creatively. When you're a writer, you put everything on the page and hope that everybody does exactly what you've asked them to do. But when you're a director, you take it to the set and discover that some things written on the page just won't work and you have to be able to rework them."

J. P. Finn admits, "We were all pretty nervous doing that one, because Chris Carter was a new director and not so much because he's the boss. It turned out that he directed very well. In fact, that's the episode that won the Golden Globe. It was a great script, a great cast, and he ended up directing a home run. One of the charming things about it was the end, where we had these alien heads placed on young children. It was so endearing to see them on the set between takes, playing with Chris and everyone. They were more like lep-

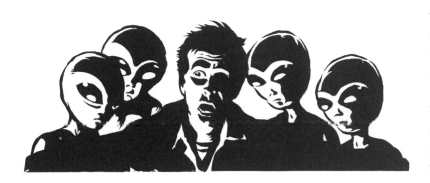

rechauns than aliens; they were the most charming aliens you've ever met, because they were just a great bunch of kids that we adopted for three or four days of the show. A big highlight of the year."

"The difficult part of the episode ['Ascension']," reflects J. P. Finn, "was to get the stunt gag on the cable car. At first we had written the scene for night, which would have been impossible, given our schedule. So we went for a transition period over late afternoon to twilight. Production-wise, given that we couldn't light a whole mountaintop and shoot the cable car at night — besides, you wouldn't be able to see the mountain at night anyway — there wouldn't be any sense of jeopardy. The production point of view was timing it all out so that you were right on the money as far as finishing

each segment by the beginning of twilight. There was a bit of a stopwatch there. A pretty good two-parter, though the first part might have been a little better than the second."

"I think Duchovny is a very brave and dedicated actor to hang off of that tram car," muses Glen Morgan. "Jim Wong made that scene work because he's a really good editor. It was missing a lot of stuff. If you go back, you see all kinds of little insert things. Jim said, 'You've got to show the dial, you've got to see the other car' — that kind of thing. And that ending is the kind of thing I wish I had done. A guy just standing at a point where he

"Duchovny is a very brave and dedicated actor to hang off that tram car."

feels he's completely lost. Let's face it, Mulder loves Scully. It's the same thing he felt for his sister, and now he's just looking into the abyss. I thought that was wonderful."

Says Wong, "I thought 'Duane Barry' and 'Ascension' worked together relatively well. 'Ascension' was kind of an ambitious show to do. We had sky-tram stuff, and that made it difficult. But Steve Railsback was really good. It was interesting, because that was one of the few times that we really see aliens, so we didn't know whether or not it was going to work. Ultimately I think it's okay, because you don't know whether it's reality or not. What I really remember is the nightmare of post[production]. We were doing the sound dub on 'Ascension' and running late and the guy from Twentieth kept saying, 'I'm going to shut you down at twelve! You better be done!' It's that kind of stuff I remember more than anything."

**Rating/Audience Share ("Duane Barry"): 8.9/16
Rating/Audience Share ("Ascension"): 9.6/16**

Episode 2.7 (#31)
"3"
Original airdate: November 4, 1994
Story by Chris Ruppenthal
Teleplay by Glen Morgan and James Wong
Directed by David Nutter
Guest starring: Frank Ferrucci (Det. Nettles), Tom McBeath (Det. Munson), Frank Military (The Son/John), Gustavo Moreno (The Father), Perrey Reeves (Kristen Kilar), Justina Vail (The Unholy Spirit)

To keep his sanity after Scully's disappearance, Mulder continues his work on the X-Files. He recognizes that a series of murders follow the patterns of the Trinity Murderers, a trio of killers with a fetish for drinking blood. While investigating, he finds himself drawn into their circle by the mysterious Kristen Kilar.

❋ ❋ ❋

"Several mistakes took place," says Glen Morgan. "Howard Gordon was supposed to do episode seven, but it wasn't going to happen. There was a script by Chris Ruppenthal that was sitting around, and we said, 'Look, we'll do number seven and eight back to back.' Howard agreed, and then I read the script and said, 'Oh my God!' It was a lot of work to do. That was mistake number one. I think mistake number two was to just do a vampire show, which to me shouldn't be a mistake. If there's one thing that's kind of a letdown about the *X-Files* audience, it's that even though it's a show that should be able to do anything, the Internet and feedback tells me, 'You just shouldn't do vampires.' My feeling is, Why not? We did the manitou last year, which was essentially a werewolf, and they hated that too.

"My feeling," he elaborates, "is that it's a legend that's been around since the eleventh century. In starting to do research, I began to find out about these people who felt it was a sexual fetish to ingest blood. Obviously the [Broadcast] Standards people say, 'Huh? What the . . .' I think we caved in on too many points to the Standards people. In the first draft it was a really kinky, erotic episode. It lost that because we didn't battle hard enough with the Standards people. Then we took heat for Mulder falling for this woman. People said, 'How could he sexually accept someone so soon after he lost Scully?' but to me that would be the perfect time. Another problem is that Perrey Reeves is David's real-life girl-friend. I think because the two of them have a sexual relationship offscreen, there's a tension that's missing that you'd have with two people who *haven't* messed around. The whole thing is that she should have been so alluring and there would be a chemistry between them, and there wasn't at all. That's why I think it wasn't successful."

James Wong admits that the episode was disappointing in the sense that "the script was much better than the show. The problem is twofold. Broadcast Standards really had lots of problems with that show. We had the blood fetish stuff going on. When you took away all that stuff, it really didn't make any sense any-more. Also, the blood kinkiness really helped the vampire aspect of it work as well as made the show a lot more interesting, because it's not something you normally see. We had to take that away and by doing that, it really less-ened any impact that might have been there."

Notes David Nutter, "A very different show, because it's the first one without Scully. She's been away for quite some time. It's a sit-uation where Mulder is in a dark place, doesn't know which way to turn, and is really very much on his own. The whole vampire thing happened because he went to a dark place that he normally wouldn't have gone to. For some people it worked, for a lot of people it didn't. I thought it worked pretty well."

Rating/Audience Share: 9.4/16

Episode 2.8 (#32)
"One Breath"

Original airdate: November 11, 1994
Written by Glen Morgan and James Wong
Directed by Robert Goodwin
Guest starring: Tom Braidwood (Frohike), Jay Brazeau (Dr. Daly), Nicola Cavendish (Nurse G. Owens), Don Davis (Capt. William Scully), William B. Davis (Cigarette-Smoking Man), Dean Haglund (Langly), Bruce Harwood (Byers), Sheila Larken (Margaret Scully), Melinda McGraw (Melissa Scully), Mitch Pileggi (Assistant Director Walter S. Skinner), Steven Williams (Mr. X)

Scully mysteriously appears in a Washington, D.C., hospital, where she is being kept alive by life support devices. Relieved that she's back but frustrated that he doesn't know what hap-pened to her, Mulder begins trying to uncover the truth, leading him to a confrontation with the Cigarette-Smoking Man that could take Mulder down the path of darkness and make him resemble those he despises. In the end,

Scully's spirit is visited by her late father, who nudges her back to the world of the living.

❋ ❋ ❋

"One of our most popular episodes," says Chris Carter. "I guess that's really the third episode of the 'Duane Barry'–'Ascension' trilogy. It's the return of Gillian, and it has very little paranormal stuff in it. I think there were some people at Fox who didn't like it for that reason, but on the Internet it was received as one of our best."

Glen Morgan explains, "Duchovny challenged us to do a 'Beyond the Sea' for him. The show had been so dark and bleak, and Jim [Wong] and I feel that there is a side to the paranormal that's very hopeful — the phenomena of angels and hope and peace. We wanted to do that side of it. I had read a book called *Raising the Dead,* about a guy who was a surgeon and a writer. He was in his study and the next thing he knows, he's lying on the floor, there's a paramedic over him, and his wife is freaking out. What happened is that it was Legionnaire's disease. He had gone into a coma. The guy wrote a diary of his time in that state of consciousness, which is fascinating. The original intent was that was what the whole episode was going to be. I had wanted to do this from the beginning of the year. I thought it would

be a great opportunity for Duchovny, but then the situation came up with Gillian's pregnancy. We needed to get her off her feet anyway. There's a line in there where Scully's sister says, 'Just because the belief is positive and good doesn't make it silly or trite.' It was the whole theme of the show."

"I really love that show," says James Wong. "I thought David did a wonderful acting job. The biggest problem we had was in postproduction when we saw Gillian just lying on the table. I want to put this tactfully, but she had just had a baby and her breasts were enormous, and she was wearing a tight hospital gown. There was nothing we could do about it, but it was *very* noticeable."

"Bill Davis was hired to smoke a cigarette. That's what his job was."

"One Breath" also marked a significant development of the Mr. X character, as he executes — in front of Mulder — two men who have seen him.

Morgan explains, "At first, Steve [Williams] wasn't going over too well, and they were unhappy with him. I said, 'Jerry Hardin brought so much to Deep Throat, and we're kind of giving Mr. X Jerry's lines.' That's why they didn't use X for a while. But Steve is a good actor, which is why we could do the scene in this episode where he performs an execution. Deep Throat was a guy willing to lose his life for letting out the secret, whereas X is a guy who's still scared. He's somewhere between Mulder and Deep Throat."

"What's so unusual about 'One Breath' is that it had very little to do with our usual X-File stuff," says Robert Goodwin, who directed the episode. "It was more about human emotions, drama, relationships."

A real highlight of the episode is when Mulder confronts the Cigarette-Smoking Man. Ironically, for quite some time Glen Morgan and James Wong were told not to give the actor, Bill Davis, much to do. "They thought he might not be a good actor," says Morgan. "I said, 'He's great. He's an acting teacher,' but that's how they felt. When it came time to do 'One Breath,' Bob Goodwin said, 'Cut down his scene,' and I said, 'No, he can pull it off,' and he did."

Goodwin explains, "Bill Davis was hired to smoke a cigarette. That's what his job was. He was hired for the pilot and told to stand there and smoke a cigarette. He didn't even say a word. Gradually, over the course of the show, we gave him a scene here or there, but he was never expected to do very much. Frequently when you hire an actor for a part where he has to smoke a cigarette, you find out that that's basically all he can do. We had no idea if this guy was going to be able to come up to the plate and handle this kind of stuff. But he's just fabulous. He evolved over the course of

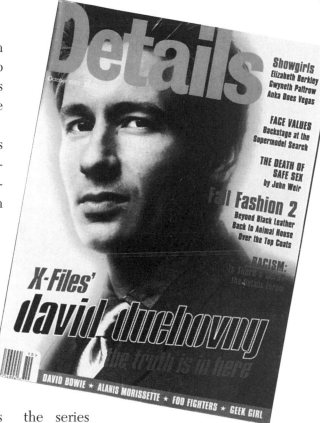

the series as this sort of Nazi figure.

The easy thing to do in that kind of role is twist your mustache, arch your eyebrows, and overplay it. He and I talked about it, we talked about the kind of power this guy has, and he just gave us an incredible performance in 'One Breath.' And he continues to do it."

Rating/Audience Share: 9.5/16

Episode 2.9 (#33)

"Firewalker"

Original airdate: November 18, 1994
Written by Howard Gordon
Directed by David Nutter
Guest starring: Hiro Kanagawa (Peter Tanaka),
David Kaye (Eric Parker), David Lewis
(Vosberg), Tuck Milligan (Dr. Adam Pierce),
Leland Orser (Jason Ludwig), Torben Rolfsen
(Technician), Shawnee Smith (Jesse O'Neil),
Bradley Whitford (Dr. Daniel Trepkos)

*When a robot designed for volcanic explo-
ration yields evidence of a life-form living
within the caves of a volcano, Mulder and
Scully — reunited at last — begin an investigation to see whether they can discover the
identity of this life-form. Once there, they
begin working with the remnants of the
research team, who all seem delusional.*

❈ ❈ ❈

"A very successful episode," notes Chris
Carter. "David Nutter added a nice directorial touch; the guest performances were very
good. We had a cool interior of a volcano set.
When I walked on that set, I had no idea how
the hell they were going to shoot it, but they
utilized a special crane to do it. I think that's
the first time in our second season that we
were telling what's one of our serial stories
rather than our mythological stories. In other

words, it was an X-File rather than one of the
cosmology shows that explore the characters."

"It was a tough shoot at the beginning,"
says David Nutter, "because it was a situation
where they were trying to redo 'Ice.' What
happened, though, is we got a terrific group of
actors who pulled it out for us, and I thought
the volcano stuff was real interesting and different. I think it all worked out pretty well. It
was not a painfully bad show, but if there had
not been an 'Ice,' it would have been wonderful."

Says J. P. Finn, "That was a big production
number. We built the volcano, and there was
another great job of makeup done. The cave
was the biggest part of the job. Whenever you
do any special effects or visual effects, it takes
more time. So from a production point of
view, it's not easy to pull off the building of a
cave that size on a TV schedule."

While "irked" at the similarities to "Ice,"
Glen Morgan nonetheless enjoyed the parasitic creature the episode presented. "A nearby museum said there is an ant in Africa that
once it ingests this virus, it climbs up to a tree,
hangs from it, and this spike juts out of its
head. Howard and I talked about that, and he
put it out through the neck, which is gorier."

About the similarities to "Ice," James
Wong says the primary problem is "if the show
starts to cannibalize itself, there's going to be
trouble."

"I know there are some similarities to
'Ice,'" says Howard Gordon, "but I think once
you get beyond the similarities of a group of

people in a confined space going up against a creature, there are enough differences to separate the two."

Rating/Audience Share: 9.0/16

Episode 2.10 (#34)
"Red Museum"
Original airdate: December 9, 1994
Written by Chris Carter
Directed by Win Phelps
Guest starring: Gillian Barber (Beth Kane), Steve Eastin (Sheriff Mazeroski), Lindsey Ginter (Crew-Cut Man), Mark Rolston (Richard Odin), Paul Sand (Gerd Thomas)

Reports of cows being injected with alien DNA lead Mulder and Scully to a Wisconsin town, where several teens are found wandering outside in their underwear, with the words "HE IS ONE" or "SHE IS ONE" scrawled on their backs. What the duo encounter is a strange vegetarian cult in a meat-producing township.

✾ ✾ ✾

"Red Museum" brings back the Crew-Cut Man, the guy with the gun who blew away Deep Throat at the end of season one. According to Glen Morgan, however, this wasn't exploited as effectively as it could have been.

"My feeling, and Chris knows this, is that to bring this guy back, his presence should have been better developed," Morgan says, "and he's shot offscreen. I thought, 'Geez, this is the guy who killed Deep Throat, who the audience loved, and it's kind of tossed away.' The episode just seems like half of one thing for a while, then half of something else. I think that was a curious choice for Chris. He wanted to take a real left turn, but I'd rather have seen a whole episode about that guy showing up and Mulder getting back at him."

"A pretty straightforward show," says J. P. Finn. "I think the meat plant was the hardest part for the cast and crew. We went to a real meat plant to shoot that, and it was tough for David and Gillian. We learned our lesson: when we did 'Our Town' later in the season and needed a poultry factory, we created our own."

Adds James Wong, "I think that was one of the most confusing episodes I've ever seen. It had some really neat ideas in it, but I don't think it pulled together finally."

This episode was at least partially designed to serve as a crossover with David Kelley's CBS series *Picket Fences*. The episode for that show, "Away in the Manger," had cows giving birth to human children — which is actually par for the course for life in Rome, Wisconsin. Kelley's concept was for Mulder to come to Rome to investigate the situation, believing it would provide information on the "Red Museum" case. The search is fruitless, however, when the cow phenomenon turns out to be human embryos placed in the cows' wombs by a wannabe-mother. Both episodes were ultimately produced, but without Mulder on the CBS show.

"I spent days on the phone with a producer of *Picket Fences*," says Robert Goodwin. "We spent days organizing our schedules. Then at the very last minute, of course, we found out that no one had told CBS, and they said, 'Forget it. We're having enough trouble on Friday nights without publicizing *The X-Files.*' It's too bad."

Chris Carter was disappointed as well. "I'm sorry it didn't happen," he says. "But I still like to think the crossover happened. We just didn't see Mulder in Rome, Wisconsin."

Rating/Audience Share: 10.4/18

Episode 2.11 (#35)
"Excelsis Dei"

Original airdate: December 16, 1994
Written by Paul Brown
Directed by Stephen Surjik
Guest starring: Frances Bay (Dorothy), Eric Christmas (Stan Phillips), David Fresco (Hal Arden), Teryl Rothery (Nurse Michelle Charters), Sab Shimono (Gung Bituen)

Mulder and Scully proceed to a Massachusetts convalescent home, where a nurse claims she was raped and beaten by an invisible force. They learn that a mystical drug is allowing one of the residents to unleash his psychic desires as well as the spirits of former residents.

❊ ❊ ❊

"Kind of a troublesome episode," says Chris Carter. "The original script came in and I didn't like it. It was completely unproducable. It was just too big and all over the map. During the week of prep there were changes made in the script, and I actually think that, in the end, it turned out to be an interesting and touching episode that had some pretty good effects in it. The story also had a nice resonance to it."

James Wong offers, "It was one of the hardest shows we've put on, because the script came in in really bad shape and Chris was rewriting it until the last minute, even while we were shooting it. Again, I think that show had some neat stuff in it, but I don't think it came together at the end either."

One feature of the episode that J. P. Finn points out is that most of the guest actors were more "senior than I think the audience is used to. I don't think they're used to seeing older people act. Everything was different and odd.

"I guess the hardest part of the production was when David was in a room that was flooded with water. On location we had a tank dressed as the room, which we lowered into a pit of water to give the impression of flooding.

When the door is opened and the water comes flooding into the hallway, that was shot on location. The overall image worked really well."

Rating/Audience Share: 8.9/15

Episode 2.12 (#36)
"Aubrey"
Original airdate: January 6, 1995
Written by Sara B. Charno
Directed by Rob Bowman
Guest starring: Joy Coghill (Ruby Thibodeaux), Terry O'Quinn (Lt. Brian Tillman), Deborah Strang (Det. B. J. Morrow), Morgan Woodward (Old Harry Cokely)

While dreaming, a policewoman experiences the memory of a serial killing and discovers the body of an FBI agent who was assigned to investigate it nearly fifty years earlier. Then the serial killer strikes again, drawing Mulder and Scully into the investigation and raising the issue of a killer's genes being handed down to his descendant.

✤ ✤ ✤

"Sara Charno's first effort, something she had been working on for several months," Chris Carter recalls. "By the time we got to produce it, it was a finely honed script. There was a lot of help given to Sara by Glen

Morgan and James Wong, who helped shepherd that script along. I think it came out great, and the casting was terrific. Deborah Strang, who played B. J., was top-notch, and we put her in for an Emmy nomination. Morgan Woodward was excellent as well. Rob Bowman came through for us and gave us an excellent job, following on 'Sleepless,' which was wonderful as well."

Says Bowman, "'Aubrey' was set in the Midwest. My father's family is all in Kansas, so I knew the look this episode had to have. I knew what these people needed to be like, these smalltown people. I also thought that it was the most horrorlike

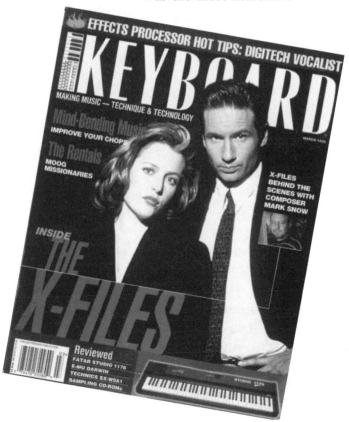

episode I had done. I thought, 'Okay, let's make a good slasher episode.'

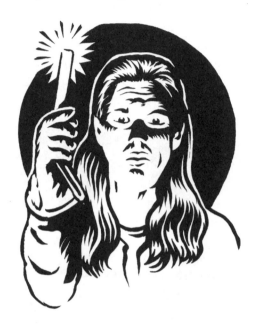

"With that episode," he continues, "I felt more confident and freer to experiment. Some of that experimentation I blew, and I managed to learn a lot from that episode about what Chris Carter wants, how his taste had evolved, how to do a slasher episode that was truly scary. I'm proud of the sequence that begins when B. J. is in her bedroom and she wakes up, there's blood on her chest, she goes to the bathroom and sees that she's slashed herself. She comes out, closes the door, and there's Harry Cokely. The script girl couldn't watch us shoot the scene because it was too scary."

Bowman has high praise for guest star Deborah Strang, who he feels tracked herself

through a very complex storyline that originally was *too* complicated for a one-hour TV show.

"We had to simplify it just a little," says Bowman. "She was always very careful about making sure one scene went into another logically. I remember the character was always in some kind of state, so at some point in the script I felt she had to be a totally ordinary person. So when she's in the hospital after finding a dead body, I wanted the scene to be totally normal, absolutely believable, no great storytelling techniques. There was a lot of nice shading of her character and peeling away of different sides of her. I just thought she did a great job of coloring the character and making her believable."

Rating/Audience Share: 10.2/16

Episode 2.13 (#37)
"Irresistible"

Original airdate: January 13, 1995
Written by Chris Carter
Directed by David Nutter
Guest starring: Nick Chinlund (Donald Eddie Pfaster), Robert Thurston (Jackson Toews), Bruce Weitz (Agent Moe Bocks), Christine Willes (Agent Karen E. Kosseff), Denalda Williams (Marilyn)

Mulder and Scully are called to Minnesota by an agent who believes that a mutilated body might have been ravaged by a paranormal phenomenon. What they find instead is that they're up against a necrophiliac — Donald Pfaster — who has begun a killing spree, with a captured Scully one of his intended victims. The only paranormal aspect of the story is that Pfaster sometimes appears as a demonlike creature for an instant, which could be Scully's subconscious mind dealing with her supposed abduction by aliens.

✿ ✿ ✿

"My first chance to work with David Nutter in a long time, and I wanted to give him something he could sink his teeth into," Chris Carter recalls. "It's a little bit different for us. It doesn't really have a paranormal aspect, except for Scully's perceptions of her deepest fears. I felt that I had to figure out what she is most afraid of, and she is most afraid of those things that most of us are afraid of. The idea of dying at the hands of someone — creature or not — and she is helpless to do anything about it. I thought it was a very good way to explore Scully's character. I thought it was a wonderfully creepy villain, played by Nick Chinlund. The casting of that show was very difficult. We saw many actors, but there was a quality I was looking for and I couldn't put a name on that quality. I finally figured out what it was when Nick came in and he had a kind of androgynous quality that worked. I thought he looked like Joe College, but he could scare the hell out of you."

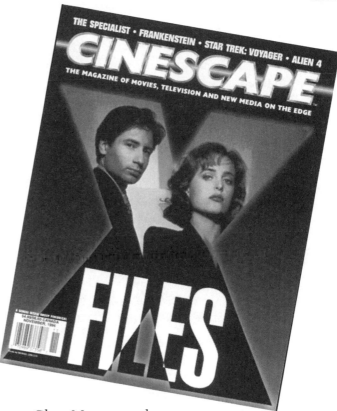

Glen Morgan enthuses, "I think that's David Nutter's best episode in that when you read the script you said, 'Yeah, that's okay,' but he just gave it the whole atmosphere it needed. And the actor — Nick Chinlund — was outstanding. They just made it work."

"I was leaving the show," says Nutter, who departed to direct the pilot of *Space: Above and Beyond,* "and I didn't know if I would ever be coming back. I was hoping that it was a good script, because I wanted to go out with, as they say, a bang. The script was very good, but a lot of it depended on the actor. Chris was adamant about getting the right guy for the role. Well, Nick Chinlund was wonderful to work with; the guy was like putty in my hands. He was great. If you're looking for someone to underline the weirdness and strangeness of the character, he did that.

"I really worked hard to make a special show, because I thought it *was* special. It was Gillian's post-traumatic-stress episode, because she had not really had the opportunity to vent her feelings about the whole Duane Barry situation. This was an opportunity to sit back and let all that happen."

Some criticism was leveled against the show in terms of Pfaster appearing as a demon to someone besides Scully, thus negating the possibility of its being a purely psychological reaction on her part.

"In many ways," says Nutter, "Chris wanted to sell the idea that, as established in Mulder's closing dialogue in the show, not all terror comes from the paranormal. It could

"The idea [behind 'Irresistible'] is that sometimes our deepest fears are collective fears."

come from the person next door. The other part of that is, obviously, the pressure to show something different and paranormalish about

the demon. I thought it was really a matter of perspective."

Carter supports the aired version, stating, "The idea is that sometimes our deepest fears are collective fears."

Rating/Audience Share: 9.2/15

Episode 2.14 (#38)
"Die Hand Die Verletzt" (The Hand That Wounds)
Original airdate: January 27, 1995
Written by Glen Morgan and James Wong
Directed by Kim Manners
Guest starring: Susan Blommaert (Phyllis H. Paddock), Dan Butler (Jim Ausbury), Shawn Johnston (Pete Calcagni), Heather McComb (Shannon Ausbury)

Some teenagers pretend to perform an occult ritual in an effort to impress some of their classmates, when they inadvertently cause the death of one of the group. Mulder and Scully discover that members of the PTA are actually practicing Satan worship.

❅ ❅ ❅

"We were leaving the show," says Glen Morgan of his and James Wong's departure, "and ever since *21 Jump Street* we had wanted to do a script about Satanic cults kidnapping people and burying them. I wanted that to be the hoax episode — that Mulder was so sure it was going to be something and it became something else. Jim and I felt the things people liked out of the two of us were the Tooms episodes ['Squeeze' and 'Tooms']. It just seemed like the time for a scary episode. I don't know if it was the mood we were in, but except for the situation with the girl who confesses how she was molested, it was almost a comedy. A comedic premise that PTA members are Satan worshipers. I like that. Of course we had fights with Standards on that as well.

"We had to let the leader get away at the end," he continues. "How are you going to catch the Devil? The self-indulgent part of the episode comes from the fact that we love the crew and the show so much, we wanted a message, so at the end when Mulder reads the note Blommaert's left on the blackboard that says, 'It's been nice working with you, see you soon,' that's really from Jim and me to the crew. I remember there was one take where David and Gillian come up to the blackboard, they're looking at it, and David says, 'Goodbye, it's been nice working with you. Thanks for using us to get our own show.' Gillian says, 'Fuck off — the Wongs.' Then David says, 'I'm going to miss those guys,' and she says, 'Me too,' and they both start laughing."

Says Chris Carter, "It was a fun script that turned this big corner when the girl had the emotional breakdown. It suddenly became a very creepy, dark, disturbing episode. It was vintage Glen and Jim, and we had a great, great performance by the guest stars. A really good, solid episode that actually veered a little more toward the horror genre. But it worked because of Mulder and Scully."

For J. P. Finn, a couple of snakes used in the episode stick out in his mind more than anything. "John Bartley, our wonderful director of photography, was shooting at really low light levels," says Finn. "We had this twenty-foot, two-hundred-fifty-pound snake coming down the stairs. We had two cameras on it. The dolly grip, who was underneath the stairs, said, 'Can't see it, can't see it.' He turned around and the snake was about six inches from his face. The crew just cleared out of there."

Rating/Audience Share: 10.7/18

Episode 2.15 (#39)
"Fresh Bones"

Original airdate: February 3, 1995
Written by Howard Gordon
Directed by Rob Bowman
Guest starring: Roger Cross (Pvt. Kittel), Katya Gardner (Robin McAlpin), Matt Hill (Pvt. Harry Dunham), Peter Kelamis (Lt. Foyle), Adrian Malebranche (Skinny Man), Callum Keith Rennie (Groundskeeper), Jamil Walker Smith (Chester Bonaparte), Steven Williams (Mr. X), Bruce Young (Pierre Bauvais)

After a soldier stationed at a North Carolina resettlement camp for Haitians drives himself into a tree, Mulder and Scully are called in when the man's widow contacts the agency. The duo investigate and find themselves immersed in the world of voodoo, practiced by local residents and the colonel commanding the refugee area.

✵ ✵ ✵

Chris Carter says, "I would say that ranks as one of the best of our series episodes — not the mythology episodes. They're stand-alone episodes that don't push forward the mythology of the Mulder–Scully search for the truth against the wishes of those who don't want them to know it. 'Fresh Bones' is one of the episodes I'm most proud of this season. I thought Howard did a good job with the script and Rob did a great job with the directing. I just love the darkness of the episode."

"The story came very much out of the newspaper," Howard Gordon explains. "During the invasion of Haiti, several servicemen died at their own hands in a very short period of time. It was a tragic event, but also an interesting speculation: Could there have been something unsavory, more centered on a cultural phenomenon, at work here too? Since we couldn't shoot it in Haiti, we thought about the refugee situation with the Cubans and Haitians. These were all real stories happening on the front pages, and we approached it from a voodoo angle, because voodoo is an

obvious area for an X-File. The trick was to do it with some kind of fidelity."

"Agony," moans Rob Bowman, "because it was such an enormous episode. There were lots of extras, and it was difficult to shoot. First of all, find two hundred black people in Vancouver. We did it, but it felt like an impossibility. Make an internment camp in Vancouver that looks anything like Virginia or the Carolinas.

"The goal was to create believability in this voodoo storyline and not to make it silly, filled with bloody chickens and all of the things we've seen before. We wanted to create a very believable scenario."

One of the most frightening sequences in the episode is when Scully suffers a vision in which she's looking at her hand and another hand bursts through the skin and begins choking her, with blood pouring out of her mouth.

"Our editors are wonderful cutting things together," comments makeup maestro Toby Lindala. "We had a mechanical hand and had a guy doubling the actor's hand stuff his fingers up through it. There was gelatin skin on the hands, which I thought played very well and was believable and fleshy. The hand double had tubes attached to his fingers, so as he pushed up it tore it open a little bit and you see the plasma and the skin rips. They played that so well in the final cut."

Robert Goodwin says, laughing, "Gillian loves doing those scenes. We've got her in the car at one in the morning, it's sixteen degrees, and she has to have blood gushing out her mouth over and over again. She just thought that was great."

Rating/Audience Share: 11.3/19

Episode 2.16 (#40)
"Colony"

Original airdate: February 10, 1995
Teleplay by Chris Carter
Story by Chris Carter and David Duchovny
Directed by Nick Marck
Guest starring: Tom Butler (CIA Agent Ambrose Chapel), Peter Donat (Mulder's Father), Dana Gladstone (Dr. Landon Prince/Gregor), David L. Gordon (FBI Agent), Bonnie Hay (Field Doctor), Tim Henry (Federal Marshal), Andrew Johnston (Agent Barrett Weiss), Megan Leitch (Samantha Mulder), Michael McDonald (Military Policeman), Capper McIntyre (First Jailer), Mitch Pileggi (Assistant Director Walter S. Skinner), Rebecca Toolan (Mulder's Mother), Brian Thompson (Pilot)

Episode 2.17 (#41)
"End Game"

Original airdate: February 17, 1995
Written by Frank Spotnitz
Directed by Rob Bowman
Guest starring: Colin Cunningham (Lt. Terry Wilmer), Peter Donat (Mulder's Father), Tim Henry (Federal Marshal), Megan Leitch (Samantha Mulder), Mitch Pileggi (Assistant Director Walter S. Skinner), Brian Thompson (Pilot), Steven Williams (Mr. X)

In part one, a series of murders occur after an ad is placed in a newspaper seeking out a particular doctor. Especially unusual about the deaths is that all of the victims have the same face! Mulder and Scully start looking for yet another clone in order to get some answers, when Mulder is contacted by his father and told that his sister, Samantha, has come home.

Part two has an alien bounty hunter determined to get Samantha Mulder — a clone — back. To gain the upper hand with Mulder, he abducts Scully and will return her only in exchange for Samantha. When Mulder learns that the hunter knows where the real Samantha is, he travels to the North Pole for a final battle with this extraterrestrial.

❉   ❉   ❉

"I think the two-parter of 'Colony' and 'End Game' was extremely ambitious," says Chris Carter. "It encompassed a couple of desires from the first year which I couldn't fulfill. In 'Ice' I wanted to be in the North Pole, which is something we couldn't do. Nick Marck did the first episode, which had some cool effects.

"I also thought it was an interesting exploration of Scully and Mulder's different perspectives as well. I wanted to reestablish what their points of view were; to reaffirm her belief in science and his belief in the paranormal.

"It was a different way to tell a story. I've always wanted to tell a story backwards like that, an inspiration I took from the original *Frankenstein,* which is told the same way."

Producer–director Rob Bowman notes, "It was around this time that *The X-Files* finally exploded into bigger than life. These were the sweeps episodes, and the scripts became enormous, requiring several units to shoot them."

For most of the staff, "End Game" was the ultimate *X-Files* episode because of its incredible production values.

"We rented a submarine that was being decommissioned from the Canadian Navy," says J. P. Finn. "We used it on three different episodes: as an icebreaker in 'Colony,' the submarine in 'End Game,' and as a ship in 'Dod Kalm.' It was just an incredible set piece that we were able to use."

Robert Goodwin points out that in many cases — particularly in this two-parter — there is no need for special effects on the show because the crew physi-

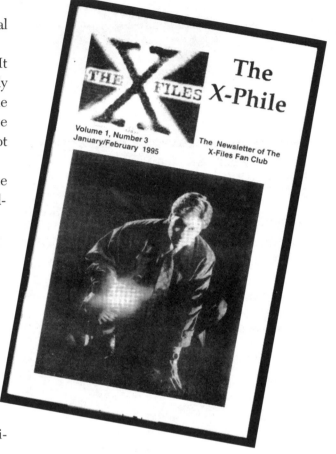

"*The X-Files* finally exploded into bigger than life. These were the sweeps episodes, and the scripts became enormous, requiring several units to shoot them."

cally does what is seen on film. "In 'End Game,' there was a nuclear submarine coming up through the polar ice cap. In the last act, Mulder and this alien hit man are having a vicious fight and Mulder is dangling off the top of this conning tower when the thing starts to submerge. He drops to the ice and is nearly crushed to death. I swear to God, it was like something out of *Die Hard,* and we did it on a stage."

Adds Bowman, "'End Game' really is an example of what *The X-Files* can do best, because it was a huge, huge production. We had a hundred and fifty tons of snow shipped in to us down to a stage that was refrigerated. We had built a full-scale mock-up of a conning tower with articulated wings!"

Writer Frank Spotnitz explains that shortly after he was hired, he went to Chris Carter and said, "'It's been so many years since Mulder has seen his sister — what if someone shows up and says she's his sister? What would he make of this?' Chris saw how that could immediately fit in to what he and David had already been talking about for the two-parter — the bounty hunter and the alien clones — and I was brought on to do the second part.

"As big as the episode was," Spotnitz adds, "my initial draft was even bigger. There were two scenes that I had to cut out because there wasn't time to shoot them. One was going to take place very early in the story, after Mulder bursts into the motel room and Scully has already been taken. He walks out into the breezeway and he sees the federal marshal we had seen at the end of 'Colony,' and he's very paranoid that this could be the bounty

"'It's been so many years since Mulder has seen his sister — what if someone shows up and says that she's his sister?'"

hunter, because he could be anyone. So there's this big thing where he draws his gun on a federal marshal and there's a showdown between the two of them. Ultimately it turns out to be the marshal and not the bounty hunter. The other sequence that was going to be really big is at the top of act two. It's the morning after the hostage trade (when Mulder has traded his sister for Scully). I was going to have him meet his father at the bridge and as he's driving he sees his sister, wet and cold on the side of the road. He pulls over, she gets in, and he's driving, when he suddenly realizes it's *not* her, it's the bounty hunter. She morphs into the bounty hunter right before his eyes, they struggle for the wheel of the car, they end up jumping out of the car, the car crashes, and then he rushes to the abortion clinic where the other clones are, and the bounty hunter is right after him. We ended up cutting all of that. Great stuff, but the story really didn't *need* either of those scenes. I didn't realize it when I was writing that you *can't* do a show of that size in eight days."

**Rating/Audience Share ("Colony"): 10.3/17
Rating/Audience Share ("End Game"): 11.2/19**

**Episode 2.18 (#42)
"Fearful Symmetry"**
Original airdate: February 24, 1995
Written by Steve DeJarnatt
Directed by James Whitmore, Jr.
Guest starring: Charles Andre (Ray Floyd), Jayne Atkinson (Willa Ambrose), Tom Braidwood (Frohike), Lance Guest (Kyle Lang), Bruce Harwood (Byers), Jack Rader (Ed Meecham)

A series of animals, ranging from elephants to tigers to gorillas, are blamed for a string of murders, though witnesses claim not to have seen any animals. Investigations seem to indicate that aliens are involved, abducting animals to perhaps create their own version of Noah's ark.

❁ ❁ ❁

"A quirky little episode for us," Chris Carter recalls with a smile. "It had kind of a cool teaser, which featured an elephant running down the highway. I thought it was a touching episode and a very original idea. Right now I'm reading this book about the paranormal, and there's this idea that aliens are working like Noah with his ark to collect us. I thought it was, by and large, a successful episode, and a little bit of a diversion for us after coming off of 'Colony' and 'End Game.' A lot of people really responded to it."

Says J. P. Finn, "A tough show schedule-wise. We had to shoot everything second unit because of the animals. The hardest part was getting the elephant here. I started working on getting a permit for the elephant to come across the border to Vancouver way back at the first of December. Right up until the day it had to leave Los Angeles to be here, we finally got the permits from the proper government agencies. Once she got here — her name was Bubbles — she was fantastic to work with."

Rating/Audience Share: 10.1/17

Episode 2.19 (#43)
"Dod Kalm" (Dead Calm)
Original airdate: March 10, 1995
Teleplay by Howard Gordon and Alex Gansa
Story by Howard Gordon
Directed by Rob Bowman
Guest starring: Mar Anderson (Halverson),
Dmitry Chepovetsky (Lt. Richard Harper),
David Cubitt (Capt. Barclay), Stephen
Dimopoulos (Ionesco), Vladimir Kulich
(Olafsson), John McConnach (Sailor), Bob
Metcalfe (Nurse), Claire Riley (Dr. Laskos),
John Savage (Henry Trondheim)

*The U.S.S. Argent's last position was in the
Norwegian Sea, and a boatload of survivors
are discovered — all of them apparently having aged decades in only a few days. Mulder
and Scully board the vessel and suffer the
same fate, desperately searching for a cure
before they die.*

❉ ❉ ❉

"Back on the ship again," says Rob Bowman.
"The episode from hell, because it was seven
or eight days straight on that battleship. On
'End Game' the ship had been white, the
color the ship actually is. For 'Dod Kalm' we
painted it rust brown. It was dark and depressing every day. The work was very slow in coming because David and Gillian both had hours
of makeup every day. They're tired by this
time of the season anyway, but to put a pound

of makeup on their face and then act had to be
too much. I was pretty tired too, because the
prep of 'Dod Kalm' was completely filled with
shooting second unit for 'Fearful Symmetry.'

"Ultimately it ended up being one of my
favorite episodes, filled with atmosphere. John
Savage proved to be a very interesting man to
work with. He is very intelligent, but he's used
to a feature schedule. I've had that before,
when people who aren't used to a TV schedule are forced to learn so much dialogue for a
single day. But I think he did the show proud.
His being slightly uncomfortable helped in
the playing of the character."

Of the makeup task, Toby Lindala
explains: "There's kind of a standard when
you're aging someone, but this was a little different. It was supposed to be caused by dehydration rather than actual aging, so you don't
have the effect of the hair graying. You don't
have a lot of form change, so we tried to focus
more on texture. We didn't want a cheesy
aging effect, although we still tried to cheat a
little bit while keeping it stylized where we
didn't age their noses. Both David and Gillian
have quite distinctive noses, so their characters are identifiable through that, and then we
stylized it, and we didn't age their ears either.
Just to keep the idea of the textural age rather
than the form age. You're not getting that big
wattle under the neck, but rather more a wrin-
kling of the skin."

Says Chris Carter, "Although we had used
that ship for 'Colony' and 'End Game,' what I
had planned to use it for all along was an

episode like 'Dod Kalm.' I didn't want to do a Bermuda Triangle episode per se, because I thought that was an obvious way to go with it. So what looks like a Bermuda Triangle story turns out to be something else. I thought it would be a great money saver, and production value would be built in, but it ended up being very expensive, very costly time-wise. For one thing, the makeup for David and Gillian took a long time to put on, and they were miserable. The boat was cold inside; it was cramped, tight quarters. It's one of those situations where you think you're brilliant, but things don't go exactly like you planned."

Rating/Audience Share: 10.7/18

Episode 2.20 (#44)
"Humbug"
Original airdate: March 31, 1995
Written by Darin Morgan
Directed by Kim Manners
Guest starring: Michael Anderson (Mr. Nutt), Alex Diakun (Curator), The Enigma (The Conundrum), Wayne Grace (Sheriff Hamilton), John Payne (Jerald Glazebrook), Jim Rose (Dr. Blockhead, a.k.a. Jeffrey Swaim), Vincent Schiavelli (Lanny), Debis Simpson (Walter), Blair Slater (Glazebrook, older), Gordon Tipple (Hepcat Helm), Devin Walker (Glazebrook, younger)

Investigating a long series of ritualistic killings that follow no particular pattern, Mulder and *Scully proceed to Gibsonton, Florida, a town built around a carnival and its sideshow acts. Mulder suspects the paranormal — particularly when he watches the bizarre Crocodile Man — but he is completely off base this time.*

❀ ❀ ❀

"Darin Morgan writes with a very comedic voice," Chris Carter explains. "When he handed me this script, he didn't know how I was going to respond to it, because it is so whacked. But I read it and I laughed out loud. I thought it was wonderful, but I thought to try and do it any time sooner would have been too big a risk, because its tone was so different from what has become a traditional *X-Files* script. But I figured that by the forty-fourth episode, we had earned that right, so I stood behind it, despite head-scratching and resistance from the studio. What you get from Darin's scripts are pretty offbeat shows. I think it's a nice ingredient to add to the show."

Darin Morgan explains, "One of the reasons I was uncomfortable joining the staff is that I'm a comedy writer and this *isn't* a comedy show, so I was trying more or less to have an episode with a little bit of humor, without telling anybody what I was doing. They asked me to do something about freaks and gave me a tape of one of Jim Rose's stage performances. I watched the tape and started doing research on sideshows, and that's where the script developed."

"I love 'Humbug,'" says Robert Goodwin.

"Talk about offbeat. It's very theatrical and grandiose. The trick was being careful that it

> **"The trick [with 'Humbug'] was being careful that it didn't become like a bad Vincent Price movie, but it really worked."**

didn't become like a bad Vincent Price movie, but it really worked out well."

Producer–director Kim Manners thought "Humbug," as the first *X-Files* that was a comedy, was particularly challenging. "A bizarre show," he recalls with a laugh. "Chris said he was throwing the audience a curveball. Well, he threw a whole lot more than a curveball. There I am, I'm a new producer and I'm directing my second episode, and it's a comedy. I'm working with Jim Rose, who's an entertainer, not an actor, and he's got five pages of dialogue, exterior, days. He's outside in just a pair of pants, hanging upside down over a boiling cauldron, and it was like fifty degrees out. At night, the Enigma, who plays the Conundrum, is running around literally in a loincloth and it's thirty-three degrees. These

were the challenges of 'Humbug,' and I've got to tell you, I was scared to death. The sun was going down and Jim Rose couldn't remember his dialogue and I had to give him a hug and say, 'It's okay,' and literally give him off-camera line readings in order to get the show done. We got it done and Jim Rose came off terrific. Everyone was great."

Rating/Audience Share: 10.3/18

Episode 2.21 (#45)
"The Calusari"
Original airdate: April 14, 1995
Written by Sara B. Charno
Directed by Michael Vejar
Guest starring: Lilyan Chauvin (Golda), Helene Clarkson (Maggie Holvey), Jacqueline Dandenau (Nurse Castor), Bill Dow (Dr. Charles Burk), Kay E. Kuter (Head Calusari), Joel Palmer (Charlie/Michael Holvey), Ric Reid (Steve Holvey), Oliver and Jeremy Isaac Wildsmith (Teddy Holvey), Christine Willes (Agent Karen E. Kosseff)

When a child is killed under mysterious circumstances, Mulder and Scully discover that the boy's older brother is possessed by an evil spirit. The parents contact a group of Romanian ritualists to perform an exorcism, in which Mulder participates.

❋ ❋ ❋

"Accomplishing this episode was really arduous," says Robert Goodwin. "There were *so* many special effects to be coordinated, and we had a teaser involving a toddler wandering onto a railroad track in an amusement park. In making that a believable sequence, you have to work from the framework that kids are restricted by child-labor laws in terms of how much time they can work. A good episode, but a tough one to make happen."

Adds Chris Carter, "Sara Charno and I had gone to lunch and she hit on the evil-twin idea and how best to approach that. We worked on that idea, she wrote the story and came back, and I felt that it wasn't quite scary enough. I wanted her to add the Calusari, and their addition really upped the stakes. I think the episode came out to be one of the best of the season. It's funny sometimes how some of the most difficult episodes turn out to be some of the best. It felt like it should have been a very contained episode, but it didn't work out that way. During the exorcism — if you want to call it that — there were so many elements to it. It's a show that never let up."

Rating/Audience Share: 8.3/16

Episode 2.22 (#46)
"F. Emasculata"
Original airdate: April 28, 1995
Written by Chris Carter and Howard Gordon
Directed by Rob Bowman
Guest starring: William B. Davis (Cigarette-Smoking Man), Kim Kondrashoff (Bobby Torrence), Dean Norris (U.S. Marshal Tapia), Morris Paynch (Dr. Simon Auerbach), Mitch Pileggi (Assistant Director Walter S. Skinner), John Pyper-Ferguson (Paul), Bill Rowat (Dr. Robert Torrence), Charles Martin Smith (Dr. Osborne), John Tench (Steve), Angelo Vacco (Angelo Garza)

Mulder and Scully are sent into a prison from which two prisoners have escaped. At first they're completely confused as to why they're involved in this situation, until it's revealed that a highly contagious and deadly disease has infected many of the inmates and, quite possibly, the escapees as well.

❅ ❅ ❅

"Howard Gordon and I teamed up again after having not teamed up for a while," says Chris Carter. "I think we work well together, and having Rob Bowman as director made it delightful. Rob loved directing it, saying that it came to him easily. He and Kim Manners are producer–directors on the show and both are top-notch and they'll give you everything they've got. Anyway, I think it was a very successful show, very creepy. One thing I'm astounded at is what we pull off in an hour of television. The look of that episode was wonderful."

Rob Bowman notes, "I had begun to change my diet and working out, because after 'Dod Kalm' I was in such bad shape that I

"I knew I was working on *The X-Files* when I heard myself say, 'I need the pus to go from left to right.'"

needed to do *something*. I kind of got my legs beneath me again when it came time to do this episode. Not a particularly emotional show, but it's a great X-File because there are some things in it that are just about as disgusting as anything you could imagine. It's about cover-ups, viruses; it's a chase. Basically it was a cops-and-robbers show with an *X-Files* twist. It was one of those episodes that seemed to go easy for Chris when he wrote it, it was easy for me to shoot, and Chris and I were absolutely in sync. I think we needed an episode at that time that didn't kill everybody in production or editing. It just came together and was a gift for everyone."

For Toby Lindala, "F. Emasculata" was a "fun" episode. "Bladder effects had become a standard for us." He smiles. "But the idea of actually using a bladder and a virus as a weapon while holding a hostage is wonderful.

We had actors rigged with bladder boil pieces on their faces, going through up to three different phases each. The boils just keep getting larger until they blow pus. We rigged each of the pieces with two different tubes so that they could spew different distances."

Speaking of pus, Robert Goodwin has one particular memory of the making of this episode. "Rob Bowman was doing shots of the boils exploding on one of the dead victims. He said, 'I knew I was working on *The X-Files* when I heard myself say, "I need the pus to go from left to right."' I love that show. It was disgusting, but so well done. Toby really outdid himself. He loves to do things that seem like they're impossible, especially impossible given the time frame. These guys who work on films have months to set themselves up. We usually have a week or two at the most. The thing with Toby is sometimes he really grosses me out and I tell him so, and his response is, 'Thank you.'"

Rating/Audience Share: 8.9/16

Episode 2.23 (#47)
"Soft Light"
Original airdate: May 5, 1995
Written by Vince Gilligan
Directed by James Contner
Guest starring: Forbes Angus (Government Scientist), Steve Bacic (Second Officer), Nathaniel Deveaux (Det. Bradley Baron), Guyle Frazier (Barney), Kevin McNulty (Dr. Christopher Davey), Robert Rozen (Doctor), Tony Shalhoub (Dr. Chester Ray Banton), Kate Twa (Det. Kelly Ryan), Steven Williams (Mr. X), Donna Yamamoto (Night Nurse)

Scully is asked by a former student to investigate a series of mysterious disappearances in which the only thing that remains from each victim is a black spot on the ground. Mulder suspects spontaneous human combustion, but the truth is that a scientist finds himself trapped in his own experiment, resulting in his shadow drawing in anything that gets in its way — essentially a mini–black hole.

❀ ❀ ❀

"A tough show from the point of view of visual effects," says J. P. Finn. "That was the technical challenge there. It's very tough to light a show in an interesting way, while not having the actor cast a shadow."

Explains Graeme Murray, "A fair amount of work for us on that one. We did some work on a nuclear research facility, a particle accelerator, and the necessary computers. It was a good high-tech set, and as contrast we had to build a hospital and government facility where the investigations took place. A good show for us in terms of contrast."

"This show was written by a writer whose work I admired before I even began working on *The X-Files*," says Chris Carter. "I think 'Soft Light' is a real popular episode. Maybe a little more science fiction than our other episodes, but I think there's some really good scientific principles involved that helped to make it believable. The lighting problems were difficult to work out, but luckily the director we had was a former DP [director of photography], so he could solve them."

Rating/Audience Share: 8.5/15

Episode 2.24 (#48)
"Our Town"
Original airdate: May 12, 1995
Written by Frank Spotnitz
Directed by Rob Bowman
Guest starring: Gary Grubbs (Sheriff Tom Arens), Caroline Kava (Doris Kearns), John MacLaren (George Kearns), Hrothgar Mathews (Creighton Jones), John Milford (Walter "Chic" Chaco), Gabrielle Miller (Paula Gray), Robin Mossley (Dr. Vance Randolph), Timothy Webber (Jess Harold)

When they are informed of a missing poultry inspector, Mulder and Scully come to Dudley, Arkansas, where — they eventually learn — cannibalism is a way of life.

❀ ❀ ❀

"Frank Spotnitz wanted to do a cannibalism episode, and I guess this is it." Chris Carter laughs. "He had done some research on chicken processing plants and discovered that they were perhaps the most despicable and vile things you could imagine — therefore perfect *X-Files* material. This idea of a town protecting its deepest, darkest secret and Mulder and Scully getting involved while we were making our move toward the season finale was wonderful. Standards was a little concerned, but I think our handling of cannibalism was tastefully done."

Spotnitz explains, "I knew I wanted to do something about cannibalism, because it was something we hadn't done and I think it's one of those things people are naturally morbidly fascinated by. I was reading articles trying to think of a way into this story, when I came across something about salamanders eating other salamanders. There are very few cannibals in nature, but there sometimes are, and they get sick when they consume sick members of their species. That was it for me. What if you're a cannibal and you get food poisoning? That was my way into the story, and the

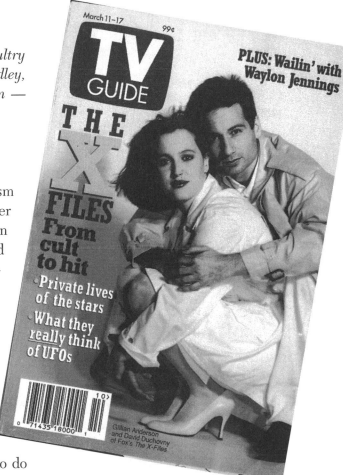

rest was figuring out how cannibalism got to the United States and who would be an interesting person to give them food poisoning. The story sprang from there. The only supernatural aspect to the story was the idea that if you ate other people and performed this magic ritual, it would prolong your life, which is sort of stretching real beliefs from cannibal tribes.

"I was very pleased with the way it was executed, and I think it was a good mystery," he adds. "Some people have complained about seeing Scully in jeopardy again, and I've got to say that they have a good point. After having seen her abducted twice, beaten up, and all the things she had been through, I could understand why some fans didn't want to see that again. If I had that to think over, I'd probably come up with another way to get out of that story."

Rob Bowman terms "Our Town" "a sick little episode. I have to classify this as a classic X-File where Mulder and Scully are handed a case and they search out the creepy aspect of whatever the situation is and solve the crime. I must admit to being very tired and not very inspired. I felt my job on this one was to do the best I could with a tired crew. We didn't want to create too many waves; we just wanted to get it done. It ended up taking a lot of extra time to finish because we were all so brain-dead. And it took us a while to figure out how to make it end. A fastball-down-the-middle kind of X-Files; no skew to it."

Rating/Audience Share: 9.4/17

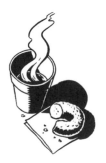

Episode 2.25 (#49)
"Anasazi"

Original airdate: May 19, 1995
Teleplay by Chris Carter
Story by David Duchovny and Chris Carter
Directed by Robert Goodwin
Guest starring: Tom Braidwood (Frohike), Bernie Coulson (The Thinker, a.k.a. Kenneth Soona), William B. Davis (Cigarette-Smoking Man), Aurelio Dinunzio (Antonio), Peter Donat (Mulder's Father), Dean Haglund (Langly), Bruce Harwood (Byers), Nicholas Lea (Agent Alex Krycek), Paul McLean (Agent Kautz), Byron Chief Moon (Father), Renae Morriseau (Josephine Doane), Mitch Pileggi (Assistant Director Walter S. Skinner), Michael David Simms (Senior Agent), Floyd "Red Crow" Westerman (Albert Hosteen)

At first Mulder is overjoyed when he is given a computer disk that supposedly contains classified government information on UFOs, but the fact that it's encrypted begins a downward spiral for him: he starts behaving erratically, culminating in his punching out Skinner. Scully eventually learns that Mulder has been drugged. Upon recovering from its effects, he proceeds to the Nevada desert, where he finds a buried boxcar that seemingly contains the bodies of numerous extraterrestrials — although further examination indicates that they could conceivably be humans who had undergone government experimentation. The Cigarette-Smoking Man shows up and orches-

trates what could be Mulder's death in the boxcar.

❊ ❊ ❊

Robert Goodwin, who directed this season's finale and the first year's, finds that whereas season one's "Erlenmeyer Flask" was a locomotive that couldn't be stopped in terms of its pacing and the physical action it presented, "Anasazi" was more dramatic, focusing intensely on the characters. "From the moment you see Mulder, you get the feeling that something is wrong," he says. "When he hits Skinner, it's a genuine shock for the audience. I thought David and Gillian were both great. While Mulder is going through what he's going through, Scully is really caught between a rock and a hard place. She's trying to protect him, but at the same time she knows there's something wrong with this guy and she's got to figure out what it is, or she's going to go down with him. I just thought there were a lot of personal things happening for both of them."

In reflecting on this episode, Glen Morgan brings up the interesting notion that, after all she's seen and been through, Scully could — if Mulder were actually dead — step into his shoes. "It's almost as though she's in the position where she would have that cynicism, that

darkness, yet she would now have the hopeful, believing edge," he muses. "To me, Scully's in a position to become Mulder. I just don't believe she's a skeptic anymore. I thought there was a possibility after 'One Breath' for her to be thrown back to her skeptical state, her really hardcore position, because she was in such denial over what had happened to her. But it didn't come out that way."

But Chris Carter, holding fast to the believer-versus-skeptic relationship that underpins the show, doesn't agree with Morgan. "My feeling is that she acknowledges there is definitely someone trying to keep certain things from us," he says. "But her bias is a scientific one. She admits there is a conspira-

"'Anasazi' was the culmination of a lot of ideas. Darin Morgan called this the kitchen sink episode."

cy afoot, but is she able to take Mulder's place? I would say no. She's not willing to take his place as a believer. She's still a skeptic."

Of "Anasazi" itself, Carter observes: "This episode was the culmination of a lot of ideas. Generally, when we pitch stories to the staff everyone comments on them, and Darin Morgan called this the kitchen sink episode, because it had so much in it, he didn't know how we would pull it off. But I'm very proud of the script. David Duchovny and I worked quite closely on the story and he had a lot of input, and then I sat down and wrote the script, which is always tough. You write the words 'fade in' and realize that you have *not* asked yourself so many questions. But I'm proud of the way it came together, what it did for the series, and the overwhelmingly posi-tive response it has gotten. I'm very pleased beginning season three with where this episode put us — which is that it posed more questions than it answered."

Rating/Audience Share: 10.1/18

The X-Files

**CHAPTER SIX
Year Three: The
Mythology**

Now that *The X-Files* has established a secure foothold for Fox on Friday nights — a prime-time slot when audiences have historically been difficult to pin down — the young network is looking for its big show to do some more heavy lifting in the 1996–97 season. With NBC's *Mad About You,* CBS's *60 Minutes,* ABC's *Lois & Clark: The New Adventures of Superman,* and a regular lineup of high-profile movies and miniseries, the Big Three networks

haven't allowed Fox to lure a regular viewership on Sundays. So Fox is throwing its best at the competition — a risky move that surprised many industry watchers, including Chris Carter.

"I had heard rumors about the move [before it happened]," says Carter. "Fox had mentioned it to me and I was not pleased with the suggestion. Now that it's happened, of course, I've got to live with it. But it's not something that I had anticipated or welcomed. I just love that Friday-night slot for *The X-Files.* Once a show proves that it works somewhere, I'm loath to [move it around]. Maybe it's a part of me that's resistant to change, but I just hate to see *X-Files* leave its Friday slot."

Lessening the sense of dislocation for Carter, the network has put his new show, *Millennium,* in *The X-Files'* Friday slot. "*Millennium* is a scary show too," he says, "so I believe it will work there."

What Fox execs are banking on is their belief that *The X-Files* will work anywhere. After all, it has worked not only on Friday nights, but in retail shops, bookstores, and Blockbuster Video. The comic book series that's based on the show more or less saved the hemorrhaging Topps comic line, HarperCollins has scored big with hardcover *X-Files* novels, videocassettes of the series's early episodes are also hot sellers (even more so overseas), and merchandise inspired by the show has become ubiquitous. "I'm always nervous about merchandising the show," Carter says. "I don't want the show to be perceived as shameless commerce, but there's a demand for mer-

Millennium

Chris Carter is attempting to capture lightning in a bottle a second time with the creation of a new Fox series, *Millennium*, which will be assuming *The X-Files'* Friday-night time slot as that show shifts to Sunday.

"It's about a former FBI agent who is working with a kind of mysterious group of men," Carter says. "He is using his expertise, which he gained in the FBI and which has actually evolved into a kind of intuition where he can get into a criminal's head, to solve cases."

As Fox's official press release notes, many prophecies have predicted that the approach of the millennium will coincide with the demise of humanity, a fact apparent each night on the evening news. In *Millennium*, a force is at work to reverse the seemingly inevitable. Lance Henriksen (*Near Dark; Aliens; The Terminator*) stars as Frank Black, whose uncanny ability to enter the minds of criminals and capture them has led him to leave the FBI out of fear that something could happen to his wife or daughter. As a result, he leads an enigmatic — and secret — task force to strike back at those who would prey on society's fears. At the same time, the series will contrast its darkness with Black's suburban Seattle home life, and look at the relationship between him and his wife, Catherine (Megan Gallagher), and daughter, Jordan (Brittany Tiplady). Catherine is a social psychologist who has to help Black in his struggle to retain his humanity by overcoming his inner demons.

David Nutter, who directed the pilot episode of the series, believes *Millennium* owes a tip of its hat to such features as *Manhunter* and *Silence of the Lambs*, as well as the *X-Files* episode "Grotesque."

"We have gone for a compelling reality in the creation of this show," Nutter explains. "The characters are people who have seen things; people who have lived a life and have so much to offer from their experience. Lance is an actor with caliber and strength who could really portray a character burdened by his expe-

rience in many ways, but who can offer us hope and is fighting for right. We needed someone who would be able to go in and out of characters and make them believable. You can trace the idea to the notion 'When you want to study Picasso, study his paintings.' To study serial killers, you need to study victims. So basically, what happens is that Frank Black is the kind of character who looks into the grotesque — the things you and I would turn away from — in order to find an MO, find that signature, find that *something* you can track the serial killer down with. He basically gets into their head by being able to retrace their steps, put on their shoes, and live in their environment. These killers don't see the world as we do. They don't hear the world as we do. It's a situation where he really immerses himself until he finds them."

"I've just always been a fan of his work," adds Carter of Henriksen, who seems like an odd choice for the lead of a prime-time series, given his offbeat, eclectic film roles. "He brings to the role, for me, a clarity, maturity, and a centered quality I was looking for. A very reserved and masculine heroic quality that I felt was really the character I wanted to create."

Both Carter and Nutter agreed that *Millennium* needed to have its own signature, much as *The X-Files* did when it began. To this end, they spent a great deal of time putting together a production crew and creating a look the show could call its own.

"My attitude is that whenever you turn on *The X-Files*, you know what you're watching before you see a title or before you see a main character," says Nutter. "This show has to have the same attitude, and I'm really happy that it does. People are very, very excited by the look and the style of it."

Carter notes that there is, nonetheless, a certain sense of kinship between the two series. "It's going to be scary," he says matter-of-factly. "It's going to deal with some elements of psychological terror that *The X-Files* sometimes delves into. I think the associations will be made, but the differences are greater than the similarities."

chandise based on the show. I guess we're just satisfying that demand."

"What's amazing to me," offers co-producer Paul Rabwin, "is that in its third year *The X-Files* clearly became a part of the cultural lexicon. You cannot get an issue of *TV Guide* or *Entertainment Weekly* or *People* without someone referring to the show. There have been political cartoons, references in the funnies, and newspaper headlines. It's no longer something that needs explanation."

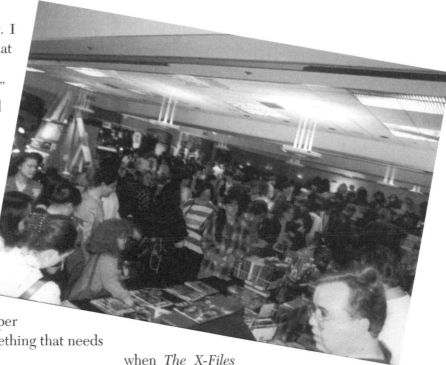

Story editor Frank Spotnitz muses that the enormous popularity of the show is, in some ways, a little bit painful for longtime fans. "I think there's a nostalgia for the first season, when *The X-Files* was their own little discovery and there was a very small but intensely loyal audience for the show. Now I think a lot of people feel it's not just their private 'find' anymore. They are sharing it with a mass audience and seeing it on magazine covers everywhere."

To Carter, all this attention isn't simply momentum, but a reward for discipline. "I think it's all because we are still doing what we set out to do, which is to tell very good stories. I think that's what

"What's amazing is that in its third year *The X-Files* clearly became a part of the cultural lexicon. It's no longer something that needs explanation."

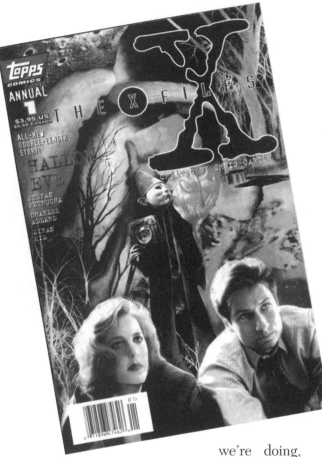

series's moral compass. And yet, paradoxically, it is the remarkable popularity of these conspiracy-themed episodes — what Carter calls *The X-Files'* mythology — that threatens to undermine the show's original premise: the believer, Mulder, and the skeptic, Scully, investigating individual cases of the paranormal each week from their very different vantage points.

The mythology episodes, which feature the enigmatic Cigarette-Smoking Man, were originally designed to be just one of many thematic arcs in the series. But by the latter part of the second season, it was clear that the mythology had become the show's guiding force, leading some of the *X-Files* writers to puzzle over how to handle it. With all that Scully has seen and experienced (see "Duane Barry," "Colony," "End Game," and "Paper Clip"), how does she remain a skeptic? And how do the duo return to individual cases after some of their astonishing discoveries in pursuit of the conspiracy? The official line out of the *X-Files* office rejects such concerns. "If you look at the series in a linear fashion, I agree that it's a problem," producer–director Rob Bowman says. "But God only knows when these things occur in terms of chronology; who knows in what order of the fictional lives of Mulder and Scully these events take place? If you look at this in terms of a person's life, in the end it doesn't make sense. You go from Scully seeing aliens in the tunnel in 'Paper Clip' to rock-

we're doing, and now a lot of talented people have come to work on the show and the cumulative power of that talent has made the show better and better. All that I do, to be honest, is try and make this TV show as good as it can possibly be. All of these other things that have come from it are the rather improbable offspring of a good idea well realized."

In the third season, Carter continued to embroider on his good idea, ratcheting up the pressure on Mulder and Scully to face down the government conspiracy that serves as the and-roll boy in 'D.P.O.' How come there is no carryover? Well, because we never said that that was week two and this is week three in their lives. We are just saying that that was episode two and this is episode three and it happened *whenever.*"

Carter, meanwhile, points to the tidy voiceover at the close of "End Game" as a defining moment, where he "reaffirms [Scully's] belief in science and [Mulder's] belief in the paranormal."

Not everyone on the creative staff, however, can dismiss the contradiction so easily. Says co–executive producer Howard Gordon, who wrote "D.P.O.," the first stand-alone episode of the season, "The third year really gave rise to the mythology episodes in a more concerted fashion. I think we started building a much more sustained narrative, a kind of ladder that Chris describes as the scaffolding from which the rest of the series is hung. We don't have the isolated abduction stories anymore. In fact, I think that's why [the stand-alone episodes sometimes can be] disappointing, because the mythology episodes are not only dealing with the broad conspiracies, they are also the stories in which we weave in the main characters' families. The mythology shows have an emotional power

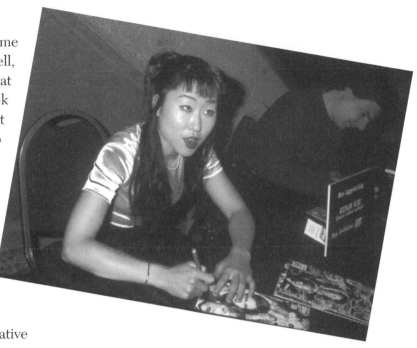

Miran Kim, illustrator for Topps' X-*Files* comic books series.

that the stand-alones simply cannot have. I think some of the stand-alone episodes that are the best are the ones that involve one of the characters in a very deep way, where you find an 'in' that can exploit some emotional adrenaline for our main players. But it is definitely difficult to compete with those [mythology] episodes, there's no doubt about it.

"That being said," he adds, "in some ways I think the stand-alones are going to be the ones that survive in syndication. Ultimately, when people rediscover the show in syndication, a lot of the mythology episodes will be a prob-

The Triumph of Evil

"The world isn't safe at all," Chris Carter says. "Good doesn't necessarily win. In fact, it wins a surprisingly paltry amount of the time — and we often live in denial of that."

Not anymore. If you watch television, the presence of evil is undeniable. Just as Carter found seeds of inspiration in such '60s and '70s scare fare as *The Invaders* and *The Night Stalker*, his colleagues are now trying to imitate the dark cynicism of *The X-Files* with their own sinister offerings in prime time. Among the recent launches — some of them limited to a single season — designed to provoke paranoia and fear are *American Gothic; Nowhere Man; Poltergeist: The Legacy; Strange Luck;* and *Dark Skies*. All were born from the success of *The X-Files* and viciously play upon our feelings of helplessness against a power structure that is increasingly faceless, remote, and unaccountable.

"We never say that evil is more interesting than good," Carter asserts. "We don't try to make a statement about evil and good per se; we just try to do scary stories each week." And Carter understands that the best way to scare people is to hit them where it already hurts: the very real fears — about crime, money, technology, officialdom — that keep them up at night.

And thanks to Carter and his admirers in the television industry, this many Americans haven't been wide awake at night since Johnny Carson was in his prime.

Karl Schaefer, creator of the Fox series *Strange Luck*, calls Carter's legacy the "new noir," which he says is driven by "the ambiguity of our times. There are no clear-cut bad guys anymore. The Soviet Union is gone, and it's a big mess. Things used to be pretty simple, and now it's a little bit like when the original noir came along at the end of World War Two. Women were in the workplace, we were rebuilding Germany and Japan, and nobody knew exactly what shape the world was going to take. Even though it was ostensibly a happy, peaceful time, there was this undercurrent of darkness and fear beneath that. I think that's similar to the times we live in now. There's not one big enemy to focus our energies on, so we're turning on each other."

The original film noir was indeed a by-product of the Second World War and the birth of the nuclear age. The movement was tethered to the notion of a civilization in decline and gave rise to the antihero. In the 1960s, TV shows like *The Invaders* and *The Prisoner* could connect with viewers as Cold War or even apocalyptic metaphors. But now, in the wake of Watergate, Iran-Contra, Whitewater, even Ruby Ridge (to name just a few prominent examples), Americans fear that the threat to their security doesn't come only from outside the country, it also comes from within their own government. The government, many people believe, is no longer just unresponsive, it is playing an active part in the subversion of our values and way of life.

"The government is really hurting in terms of public relations," says Stuart Fischoff, professor of media psychology at California State University, Los Angeles. "It's come to the point where if you make the argument that the government is behind a conspiracy or is covering up something, people are immediately ready to believe you. Government conspiracies seem much more likely today — at least that's what people believe. When you had Patrick McGoohan and

The Prisoner, you didn't have the pervasiveness of electronic surveillance capability. Today the big thing is that government, corporations, computer hackers, and everybody else can get access to your private life. Their reach is far more pervasive now than it was back in the sixties and seventies when people who were good didn't really have to worry. Today it doesn't matter if you're good or not. People want a big uncle to look out for them, but they feel that all they're getting is Big Brother."

Leo Braudy, professor of English at the University of Southern California and the author of *The World in a Frame: What We See in Films*, concurs, adding that the idea of Big Brother has taken on dimensions above and beyond government and technology. "People are more apt to believe in conspiracies now because of the information superhighway," he says, "because the technology seems so powerful and there are so many organizations out there that seem to be coercive and repressive." But the true source of this fear is not the government, he adds. "It's the all-powerful eye of God — but it's some malevolent God who not only has his eye on the sparrow but wants to squash the sparrow."

The show's ongoing thematic arc — or mythology, as Carter refers to it — has revealed a government conspiracy involving alien corpses recovered by the U.S. military from Roswell, New Mexico, the location of an alleged UFO crash in 1947. Mulder's personal crusade to obtain proof of both the crash and government experiments involving human and alien DNA gives the show its driving force.

"Mulder represents the current seeker of the American dream," says *X-Files* producer–director Rob Bowman. "And he can only achieve it by finding the truth. There's something very classic and American about Mulder. If you strip away the obsession with the paranormal, he's a very ordinary person who is kicked about by a big, dark overseer that doesn't necessarily have the best interests of the people in mind. It's hard for him to handle. 'I thought you were supposed to represent the people,' he says to them. 'Why do I find constant cover-up? I'm really confused by this.' I identify with him completely, and I think the audience does as well."

Professor Braudy suggests that Mulder's appeal comes from his willingness to battle insurmountable opposition, his willingness to continue to fight evil even though he knows he cannot obliterate it. "The genie is going to get out of the bottle again," Braudy says. "The whole approach [of the show] is to stanch the flow but not stop the seepage. *The X-Files*, in that regard, is the most realistic show on the air right now, because it understands that evil is a multiheaded hydra. If you chop off one head, another one is going to appear somewhere else."

And so Mulder's battle continues.

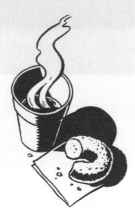

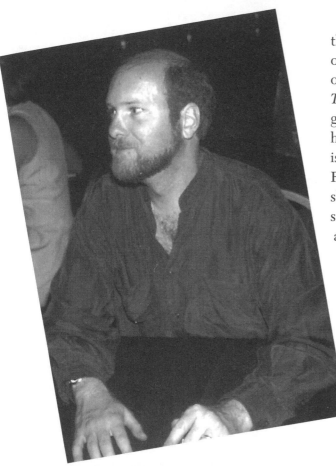

Kevin Anderson, author of a number of *Star Wars* and *X-Files* books.

the simple reason that they've begun to figure out how the series operates. At the beginning of the first season, he says, viewers thought of *The X-Files* solely as a UFO series. "Then we got 'Squeeze,' which made it a monster show," he says with a laugh. "Then we got 'Ice,' which is really a suspense thriller; and 'Erlenmeyer Flask,' which was a government paranoia show. Then Darin Morgan came along and suddenly we have humorous, ironic episodes, and so it has really gotten so that you turn on the show and it could be one of five different genres. People don't know what to expect, so the mythology episodes are the core [of the series] that people have been able to pin down."

Former story editor Jeff Vlaming adds, "Next year will be a tough nut to crack, because it's getting to the point where you almost can't believe that Mulder is doing anything but pursuing these monumental discoveries he is making in search of the conspiracy. Why is he worrying about fat-sucking vampires when he knows that his father was involved in his sister's disappearance?"

lem, because they rely too much on what came before. For die-hard fans it's great, but, ultimately, when people watch these shows chopped up, I think the stand-alones are the ones that are going to have a longer shelf life."

Spotnitz believes that the tension between the two types of episodes has become more noticeable to viewers in the third season for

And yet Carter is determined to prevent *The X-Files* from becoming *The Conspiracy Show*. It's the thematic and narrative variety of the series, he believes, that keeps it creatively fresh.

"The truth is, you can't have Mulder and Scully pursuing the conspiracy forever. Those episodes, even though they're very popular, have to come along only occasionally in order to give the show its breadth, its life, and its longevity. From the beginning, the search for

Carter is determined to prevent *The X-Files* from becoming *The Conspiracy Show*. It's the thematic and narrative variety of the series that keeps it creatively fresh.

the truth about what the government may or may not know about the existence of extraterrestrials has been the backbone of the series. The stand-alone episodes have become the all-important search for other truths that may in fact impact on those larger truths. I think the audience has to be forgiving and is — wonderfully so — because if we just made this a mythology show, it wouldn't be as good a show as it is."

None of which means he doesn't like the twists and turns of the mythology any less than the next guy. "I think from the beginning to the end [of the third season], we brought things to an interesting point," Carter says. "We learned more about the Cigarette-Smoking Man, what Mulder's past is — his personal history is now seemingly quite intertwined with some early government stuff. We know now that Mulder's father had connections to these men. We know there's an international cabal of sorts, a syndicate, that has spread the conspiracy beyond the borders of the U.S., and I think we see that there are improbable alliances between people in the scientific community who in fact may be conducting a much larger conspiracy than what was once imagined."

And such labyrinthine intrigues, of course, go to the heart of what *The X-Files* is all about. "As we know," Carter says with a smile, "the truth is very difficult to arrive at. In fact, there are *many* truths. I think that what we're playing with here is the complexity of what the truth is."

The X-Files

Episode 3.1 (#50)
"The Blessing Way"

Original airdate: September 22, 1995
Written by Chris Carter
Directed by R. W. Goodwin
Guest starring: Forbes Angus (MD), Tom Braidwood (Frohike), Lenno Britos (Luis Cardinal), Mitch Davies (Camouflage Man), William B. Davis (Cigarette-Smoking Man), Peter Donat (William Mulder), Ernie Foort (Security Guard), Benita Ha (Tour Guide), Jerry Hardin (Deep Throat), Dakota House (Eric Hosteen), Alf Humphreys (Dr. Mark Pomerantz), Sheila Larken (Margaret Scully), Nicholas Lea (Agent Alex Krycek), Melinda McGraw (Melissa Scully), Tim Michael (Albert's Son), John Moore (3rd Elder), John Neville (Well-Manicured Man), Mitch Pileggi (Assistant Director Walter S. Skinner), Michael David Simms (Senior Agent), Rebecca Toolan (Mrs. Mulder), Ian Victor (Minister), Stanley Walsh (2nd Elder), Floyd "Red Crow" Westerman (Albert Hosteen), Don Williams (1st Elder)

While Mulder lies somewhere between life and death as his spirit undergoes a Navajo healing ceremony conducted by Albert Hosteen (during which Mulder is visited by the spirits of his father and Deep Throat), Scully finds herself pitted against her superiors as the search for the MJ documents DAT intensifies. Later, she is warned by the Well-Manicured Man, part of an international group of conspirators, that her life is in danger. Indeed, Agent Krycek assassinates her sister, Melissa, by mistake when he breaks into Scully's apartment. At the same time, Skinner has obtained the DAT and comes to Scully with it, but she believes he's attempting to kill her, and it ends in a standoff with the two of them aiming guns at each other's head.

❖ ❖ ❖

According to story editor Frank Spotnitz, "The Blessing Way" represented a difficult challenge due to the fact that it was the middle chapter in a trilogy of episodes.

"The expectations were very high coming after a summer's worth of anticipation to see how Mulder got out of the boxcar," he says. "We knew that we had to answer that question and still leave an intriguing enough dilemma at the end of the show to bring viewers back for the third and final part. I also thought it was a big gamble to do all of that Indian mysticism stuff. It was very spiritual, which is not something the show is usually about. I thought a lot of people would not necessarily respond to that. There is nothing cynical about spiritualism. There is nothing dark about it. It appeals to a different part of our nature. So I was nervous about that, but very excited about the Scully storyline and the way all of that played out with Mulder and Skinner."

Co-producer Paul Rabwin notes that for the Blessing Way ceremony, a sand painter was brought on location and spent a full day creating two paintings. "One of them was preserved so that it wouldn't move, and then he had to create another one that could be wiped out at the end. But there were two intricately designed sand paintings utilized."

For co–executive producer Robert Goodwin, who also directed the episode, a disappointing aspect of production was the sequence in which Mulder is floating in a netherworld and encouraged in his search for the truth by his late father and Deep Throat.

"On a technical level," he explains, "it is the kind of thing that is basically a monologue. To make it interesting, I wanted to keep the camera moving. I wanted to be circling around and floating and all of that, but because of the technical difficulties they had with the special effects, I was forced to make it much more static than I wanted. That's just a minor thing, though. That is a case where a technical aspect overrides the creative aspect. Nobody's fault; that's just life. Frankly, I thought the third part of the story, 'Paper Clip,' was just sensational. Rob Bowman did a great job with that."

Rating/Audience Share: 12.3/22

Episode 3.2 (#51)
"Paper Clip"
Original airdate: September 29, 1995
Written by Chris Carter
Directed by Rob Bowman
Guest starring: Tom Braidwood (Frohike), Lenno Britos (Luis Cardinal), Peta Brookstone (ICU Nurse), William B. Davis (Cigarette-Smoking Man), Martin Evans (SM), Walter Gotell (Victor Klemper), Dean Haglund (Langly), Bruce Harwood (Byers), Sheila Larken (Margaret Scully), Nicholas Lea (Agent Alex Krycek), Robert Lewis (ER Doctor), Melinda McGraw (Melissa Scully), John Moore (3rd Elder), John Neville (Well-Manicured Man), Mitch Pileggi (Assistant Director Walter S. Skinner), Rebecca Toolan (Mrs. Mulder), Stanley Walsh (2nd Elder), Floyd "Red Crow" Westerman (Albert Hosteen), Don Williams (1st Elder)

The standoff between Scully and Skinner comes to an end when Mulder enters the scene, returned to health by the Navajo. As Skinner attempts to negotiate the DAT for Mulder and Scully's reinstatement with the Cigarette-Smoking Man, the duo make their way to a mine in West Virginia, where they make a number of incredible discoveries. First off, Mulder sees what can only be described as a UFO taking off, Scully catches sight of what appears to be a group of aliens running by her, and the two of them find a series of filing cabinets. Within the innumerable cabinets are folders containing medical information, including DNA samples. Among the files are ones for Scully (dating back to her abduction by Duane Barry in season two) and Samantha Mulder, though Fox's name was on the folder first. Later, Mulder confronts his mother and learns that his father had been a part of the government conspiracy and had been forced to give up one of his children to ensure his silence about "the project" known as Operation Paper Clip, inviting scientists from Nazi Germany and Japan.

Meanwhile, agent Alex Krycek manages to beat the hell out of Skinner and obtains the DAT, and Krycek in turn barely avoids being killed by agents of the Cigarette-Smoking Man. Then, when Skinner tries to make his deal with the CSM, his bluff is called — until Skinner informs him that Albert Hosteen has decoded the tapes and, "in the oral tradition of his people," has shared its contents with many other Navajo. Should anything happen to him, Mulder, or Scully, all of that information will be available with a simple phone call.

✿ ✿ ✿

Frank Spotnitz enthuses, "I love 'Paper Clip.' I was thrilled with the plot. I know it moved very fast for some people, but I actually think that for some of these shows you don't need to

understand everything. I think it is more exciting to go at rocket speed. Everybody was on the mark in that one: David and Gillian's performances, Rob Bowman's direction, Chris Carter's writing — everything was just terrific in that show."

Says Bowman, "I was disappointed that my

"We have done several aliens in the past, where we used a bunch of little girls, like nine or ten years old. Because we had so much fighting and struggling in the mine scene, we used boys."

first episode of the season wasn't going to be a mythology episode, then Chris Carter writes 'Paper Clip.'" He laughs. "There were elements of that show that really stretched the boundaries of the series, what with the spaceship, the shooting we did in the mine, and so on. First of all, I think the episode gave the audience something they have waited for, which is 'Let's watch Mulder have a protracted encounter.' Several of the other episodes have had brief, fleeting glances and it's over.

Let's get a long, drawn-out orgasm and we'll make it glorious, but we will do it in the style that we usually do it. We will tease the hell out of the audience. There is proof. It is theory no more. It is not hypothesis. There is the ship. Mulder runs upstairs and he comes outside and our challenge was showing the ship without actually showing the ship.

"Then there's Scully's little encounter. How does she react to this? It was up to me to provide these different points of view. The aliens are whipping around and we just see body parts and pieces. It sure looks like something there, but it's kind of like a deer in a headlight because they are just charging. I think that opened the season with something very cinematic. When I finished 'Paper Clip,' I thought, 'I don't know what else I am going to do this year to top this.'"

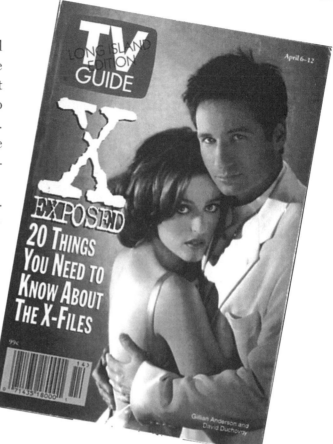

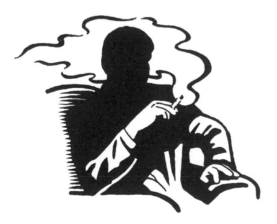

Another highlight for Bowman was a sequence in a small diner where Skinner is meeting with Mulder and Scully to discuss the deal he will try to arrange with the Cigarette-Smoking Man.

"I just think Mulder is a very calm person in there," he explains, "not screaming and yelling. There is this quality in the scene. People are expressing their heartfelt emotions. Scully is saying she thinks they should take the deal because, damn it, she wants to see her sister. Well, what human being in that situation wouldn't say the same thing? There was a certain rhythm to that scene that was not rushed or skipped through that I liked, and David had a lot to do with that.

"'Paper Clip' had all the big characters in it," Bowman continues, almost giddily. "And the storyline was almost *Godfather*-like, with Krycek and Skinner, Skinner getting beaten up, and then the attempt made on Krycek in his car. It was a big, sweeping show with many locations, interesting people, and full of great drama. There were a lot of beautiful things in the episode too. Even the scene with Scully in the hospital. I have to tell you, I hate hospital scenes. Every time I see one I just cry, because they're so dull; somebody is going to one day tally up how many times Mulder and Scully did a hospital scene. So every time I see one I say, 'Do we have to do this in a hospital room?' And they'll say yes or no, and then I'll take it from there. But I feel the hospital scenes in 'Paper Clip' are probably the only hospital scenes I have directed in this whole series that I liked just because of the emotion of the scene."

"One other thing that comes to mind about that episode," Robert Goodwin adds, "is the little aliens in the mine. We have done several aliens in the past; the first group we did was in 'Duane Barry,' where we used a bunch of little girls, like nine or ten years old. Because we had so much fighting and struggling in the mine scene, we used boys. I'll tell you something, and I hate to say it, but girls are a hell of a lot smarter than boys. They were born smarter and they always stay smarter. Girls are just a lot easier to direct, especially the younger ones. We just kept shooting and shooting and shooting. Next time we need a bunch of aliens, you can count on them being played by girls."

Of the mine itself, production designer Graeme Murray says it was actually an old mine in Vancouver that has become a museum. "We got into some of the old tunnels and built all of those filing cabinets and the doors that led into it. When we started in there, we were actually going to bring in real filing cabinets and line them up against the wall there. On the survey day, Chris looked at it and thought, 'It would be way better if they were built into the mine itself.' They were kind of false fronts for the whole thing built into the rock, and I thought it looked pretty interesting.

"We also put together a spaceship — really just a framework with a bazillion lights on it. Those were quite huge kinds of effects — or rather, on other shows they would be huge, but on this show they seem to have become pretty standard."

Rating/Audience Share: 11.1/20

Episode 3.3 (#52)
"D.P.O."
Original airdate: October 6, 1995
Written by Howard Gordon
Directed by Kim Manners
Guest starring: Peter Anderson (Stan Buxton),
Mar Andersons (Jack Hammond), Jack Black
(Bart "Zero" Liquori), Brent Chapman (Traffic
Cop), Cavan Cunningham (2nd Paramedic),
Jason Anthony Griffith (1st Paramedic),
Bonnie Hay (Night Nurse), Ernie Lively
(Sheriff John Teller), Steve Makaj (Frank
Kiveat), Giovanni Ribisi (Darin Peter Oswald),
Kate Robbins (Darin's Mom), Karen Witter
(Sharon Kiveat)

Mulder and Scully investigate a series of deaths by lightning, and are led to Connerville, Oklahoma, where a teenager, Darin Peter Oswald (hence the title "D.P.O."), seems to have acquired the ability to control lightning and is using it to seek retribution against anyone who crosses him.

✵　✵　✵

"This was an idea floating around the office for some time," Howard Gordon explains. "There was literally an index card that said 'Lightning Boy,' but no one had come up with a way to crack the story. I wanted to use the idea of lightning as a metaphor for the collision of boredom and hormonal anxiety. That's what it felt like, and lightning seemed like the perfect analog for that kind of thing. The idea was Beavis and Butt-head electrified. That was really the germ of the idea. It was a way to investigate with a tragic and comic lens what it's like to be numb from television and video games, and it dealt with illiteracy and single parenthood and everything else."

Story editor Frank Spotnitz admits there was some discussion among the staff as to how "D.P.O." could possibly follow the trilogy of mythology episodes in which so much had happened to Mulder and Scully. "Originally," he explains, "we said we should try to incorporate those events into the story of 'D.P.O.,' but then we decided it didn't make sense for a variety of reasons, because, ultimately, each episode has its own integrity and has to stand alone.

"I also thought it was a risky show for us to do, which is something I feel whenever we go to a high school setting. This is an adult show, and you need to find a way to make it interesting to adults. The storyline was really about adolescence and the violent impulses you have when you're a kid. But if you take it a step further and imagine yourself having the powers this kid did, it suddenly becomes an X-File. I thought the actor, Giovanni Ribisi, was really, really good. We also used the music differently in that show than we ever had before."

Director Kim Manners notes that the episode was an incredibly emotional experience for him because on the third day of shooting, his best friend and that man's son were killed in a drowning accident.

"He was my best friend for thirty-one years and he died and I was stuck in Vancouver," he says. "I couldn't leave the show, though I did leave it in the sense that my body was there while my mind was elsewhere. I hardly remember the shoot, but the show worked, miraculously. My wife came up and kind of babysat me so that I could get through it, and I learned a great lesson in life. I should have left the show and let somebody else take over and dealt with my emotions. I guess that's the 'show-must-go-on' attitude. I think 'D.P.O.' could have been much better than it was, though the fans liked it."

Co–executive producer Robert Goodwin opines, "An interesting show, though a little difficult to do all of the effects work that was required. They were done through physical effects of sparks and explosions and stuff that we shot right on film with the actors, combined with individual lightning effects that were put in after the fact. It was a real coordination between the two departments. One without the other would be nothing. I think the best thing about it was the lead and his sidekick, both of whom were great. One interesting thing is that it took us forever, but we finally got permission to use a real dead cow for a scene where a cow had been struck by lightning. All these animal rights people are very, very watchful. We had a phony cow originally, but it *really* looked phony, so we got permission from a slaughterhouse to use a real cow."

Graeme Murray offers, "It was a 'small-town America' type of show. Probably the biggest construction event for us was the crossroads where the traffic lights were. The kids are sitting there and triggering the lights to cause accidents. That was a big setup for us. We had to plant telephone poles and build this billboard. The road was there; it had been married people's quarters during the war, but all the houses had been torn down. We've used it for a couple of shows. It was just an overgrown vacant lot, basically, with three or four roads crisscrossing through it. We also used it in 'Apocrypha' for the exteriors of the missile silo."

Rating/Audience Share: 10.9/20

Episode 3.4 (#53)
"Clyde Bruckman's Final Repose"
Original airdate: October 13, 1995
Written by Darin Morgan
Directed by David Nutter
Guest starring: Greg Anderson (Photographer), Peter Boyle (Clyde Bruckman), Jaap Broeker (Yappi), Frank Casini (Det. Cline), Stu Charno (The Puppet), Alex Diakun (Tarot Dealer), Karin Konoval (Madame Zelma), Dwight McFee (Det. Havez), David Mackay (Mr. Gordon [Young Husband]), Doris Rands (Mrs. Lowe), Ken Roberts (Clerk)

A serial killer is stalking fortune tellers in Minneapolis. When an insurance salesman named Clyde Bruckman comes across one of the bodies, he gets in touch with Mulder and Scully and ultimately reveals that he himself has the ability to foresee how people will die. When Bruckman leads them to two additional bodies, Scully becomes convinced that he just might be the man they're seeking, but Mulder doesn't accept that theory, believing instead that Bruckman can lead them to the real killer.

✵ ✵ ✵

"A show that worked on every level," says story editor Frank Spotnitz. "Actually, that's my favorite of Darin Morgan's shows, because there are so many levels to it. He is really literate in the way he constructs things, and it also just has so much heart. Peter Boyle was a great success, particularly after we agonized over who we should cast in that role. Darin had originally written the part with Bob Newhart in mind, which probably would have been great, but we ended up going with Peter Boyle. In the end, everybody thought that show was just thrilling.

"One thing about Darin," he continues, "especially since 'Clyde Bruckman,' is that he's always tried to do something the show would never think of doing and he's pulled it off. I think he really helped people see that this show was even more versatile than they imagined it could be."

Amazingly, the person most disappointed with the episode is Morgan himself. "I wanted to do an episode that was more serious and more depressing and more along the lines of [season one's] 'Beyond the Sea,'" he explains. "My original idea was to do one without any jokes. I was just so depressed over the whole writing of the script. It was so painful I didn't even bother to watch it when it first aired. Some of the script really works, but I just felt it didn't come out as good as it should have.

"I just wanted it to be the most depressing thing ever. I guess part of it comes from the fact that when I was writing [season two's] 'Humbug,' the feeling was that it was going to be funny and a lot of the fans would have a problem with the comedy — which they did. They were worried it was going to ruin the show and I felt, after it was done, that maybe they were right. So after it aired, I went back and watched 'Beyond the Sea' and said this is *really* what the show should be like. So I wanted to do something that was much more serious. Of course I ended up putting jokes in it anyway. The thing is, I got away with it on this one because the story was much more similar to a standard X-File, so people didn't have any problems with it. The difference between the two seasons I've been involved with the show is that when I turned in 'Humbug,' everyone said, 'This is funny; we can't do this.' When I turned in 'Clyde Bruckman,' everyone said, 'I love this. This is so funny.' It was the difference between before and after.

"The other main gist of 'Clyde Bruckman' was the research," he continues. "We have these books on homicide investigations and they have these crime scene photos of dead bodies and how you are supposed to conduct an investigation. The book is so disturbing that when people look through it they say, 'Oh, that doesn't bother me,' then they come back a day or two later and say, 'You know, there is a picture in that book that I just can't get out of my head.' I really can't describe how disturbing some of these photos are. So I was just thinking about psychics, people claiming to see other people's future. If they really could, they should be able to see a person's ultimate future, which is their death. If they could see exactly how people will die, just like these crime photos, they would just go insane. They would be depressed to the point of suicide. So that was really what that whole show was about."

The finished product, however, once he finally did see it, is something he's proud of. "That was totally my favorite episode that I wrote, and Peter Boyle was great. I guess another reason for writing it was we had been going over budget and I wanted to see if I could write something that could be done very, very simply. So a lot of the scenes take place in Bruckman's apartment or a hotel room. It came in under budget and on schedule. It was just a very easy show to do."

For director David Nutter, the script was definitely the thing. "The writing was so tight and so crisp and so fresh that I think, as a director, the only thing you have to do is create the atmosphere, set up the characters, set up the shots, and you are basically invisible," he says. "Then you step back and just let it happen. Find the moment, know how you are going to cut it; know how you are going to outline the sequences, and so forth. Know all that before you do it, of course, but when you do it, let it happen and use a very free hand on it, because it is a situation where some of it is really created on the set with respect to the attitude and the characters."

"Clyde Bruckman" was fairly character-intensive, which Nutter feels provided him the opportunity to take a slightly different directorial approach. "A lot of time people in Hollywood classify you and categorize you. He does drama. He does horror. She does comedy. Whatever. With this show, you definitely get to see that I can handle all aspects. I'm very, very proud of it."

In designing Clyde Bruckman's apartment, Graeme Murray notes, the idea was to "keep things as bland as possible. He's kind of hiding in this little bland place, whereas everything else around him is strange and brightly colored, with odd stuff going on. One of the more meaningful shows for me; it had some real depth to it."

For Robert Goodwin, the most interesting aspect of the episode was Peter Boyle, particularly given the fact that Boyle didn't really want to do the show.

"Peter is not interested in episodic television," he explains. "He is more interested in theater and features, but somehow he did it. I don't know whether it was a combination of coercion and bribery or what, but when he first arrived, you could tell that he didn't want to be there. But he melted and thawed out very quickly, and by the end of the show he was very exuberantly thanking me for the wonderful experience and asking for T-shirts. Peter's been telling people that he's gotten more response from that show than anything he had done in his entire career."

Rating/Audience Share: 10.2/18

Episode 3.5 (#54)
"The List"
Original airdate: October 20, 1995
Written and directed by Chris Carter
Guest starring: Michael Andaluz (Tattooed Prisoner), Denny Arnold (Key Guard), Craig Brunanski (Guard), Badja Djola ("Neech" Manley), Ken Foree (Parmelly), April Grace (Danielle Manley), Mitch Kosterman (Fornier), Don Mackay (Oates), Bruce Pinard (Executioner), Paul Raskin (Dr. Jim Ullrich), Greg Rogers (Daniel Charez), J. T. Walsh (Warden Leo Brodeur)

Immediately before his execution, prisoner Napoleon "Neech" Manley swears he will seek vengeance beyond the grave against his enemies — a very personal hit list of those who he feels have wronged him. Naturally the warden and everyone else dismiss this, but then guards begin dying under mysterious circumstances. Mulder and Scully are called in to investigate before the so-called list expands.

❈ ❈ ❈

Story editor Frank Spotnitz opines, "I think this is a vastly underrated episode. I also think it was a very brave and different show to do and that it will weather the test of time very well. I think it was brave because there is not a single likable character — nobody you can root for. Mulder and Scully do not solve the case, and that is something I had been interested in doing for some time. I originally wanted [season two's] 'Our Town' to end with them not solving the case, but we changed that at the last minute.

"'The List' is not scary in a big flashy way. It is more sneaky and ominous. It also had a look to it that was unlike any other show we had done, using greens — which is a very hard color to work with, especially in television. On the level of performance, writing, the way it was shot and directed, I think it was a stand-out episode. I was initially surprised that more people didn't just flock to it because of all the qualities, but I think because Mulder and Scully didn't solve the case and because there was nobody to root for, it made it harder for some fans to jump up and down about it."

"The hardest part about 'The List,'" says co–executive producer Robert Goodwin, "was the set design, because we built this big, expensive two-story prison, and it was a major undertaking. And once it was built, it was very tough to work in, because you've got to deal with these tiny cells. Physically, it was a nightmare, and extremely difficult to work in. I

"How do you make a prison sound unlike a typical prison?"

sympathize with Chris. But I thought there was a great performance from J. T. Walsh as the warden."

The episode marked Chris Carter's second writing-directing effort, following season two's "Duane Barry."

"I wanted to give it a look like no other X-File," Carter says. "First of all, the color palette is green. John Bartley and I lit it with pink light, and then in the postproduction process that pink was taken out, which saturated the green, giving it a submarine quality. In the sound of the show, too, I added a submarine quality. I wanted it to feel like you were compressed at the bottom of the sea. There were just things I wanted to do that were different from other episodes we'd done. I feel very proud of the results. I felt more assured as a director this time, but it's extremely hard and demanding physically."

According to co-producer Paul Rabwin, particular attention was paid to sounds in this prison. "There were tons of levels of sounds," he says. "How do you make a prison sound unlike a typical prison? We wanted to get lit-

tle subtle sounds from these prisoners, but we didn't want it to sound like a James Cagney picture. Throughout the prison there was a deep, dark, rumbly kind of an effect that we put in. You could never really put your finger on it, but there was something uneasy and cavernous about the sound on that show. If you listen to it very carefully, you would notice that if you turned the bass up a little bit it was almost like the inside of a submarine. We just permeated the whole soundtrack with that, and that was kind of interesting."

Rating/Audience Share: 10.8/19

Episode 3.6 (#55)
"2Shy"
Original airdate: November 3, 1995
Written by Jeffrey Vlaming
Directed by David Nutter
Guest starring: Lindsay Bourne (Hooker's John), Timothy Carhart (Virgil Incanto), Glynis Davies (Monica Landis), Beverly Elliot (Raven), James Hardy (Det. Alan Cross), Suzy Joachim (Jennifer Workman), Randi Lynne (Lauren Mackalvey), William MacDonald (Agent Dan Kazanjian), Dean McKensie (Lt. Blaine), Aloka McLean (Jesse Landis), Jans Baily Mattia (Hooker), Catherine Paolone (Ellen Kaminski), P. J. Prinsloo (Tagger), Kerry Sandomirsky (Joanne Steffen), Brad Wattum (Patrolman)

148

Mulder makes the connection between the disappearance of a lonely, overweight woman and that of several women before her, who all had made contact with someone over the Internet. The investigation leads Mulder and Scully to a killer who has the unimaginable ability to suck the fat out of his victims' bodies.

❋ ❋ ❋

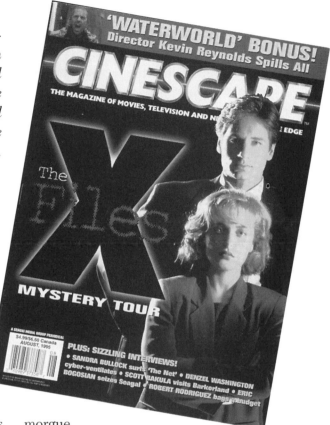

Of the episode's genesis, Jeff Vlaming explains that he had been working at Universal on *Weird Science*, when he got the opportunity to pitch to Chris Carter.

"Originally," he explains, "the guy wasn't sucking fat out of his victims as much as he was sucking the oil from them. Everybody has body oil, and he would suck that. He preferred women, but he wasn't doing fat women. Just who this guy was went through some changes as well. At first he was creepy-looking, wearing a turtleneck up to his chin, sunglasses, and a hat — very much like the Phantom of the Opera — and then we changed him to a good-looking guy who stays behind his computer and only meets these women after he's charmed them with his words and his voice. Finally, we went with a fairly normal-looking guy. Originally he was a butcher, literally working in a butcher shop, so he knew how to get fat out. It went through a number of permutations and just got better and better."

One of the grossest *X-Files* moments occurs in this episode, when Scully opens a morgue drawer and finds that the woman's body that had been there has dissolved to a puddle of muck.

"People like that disgusting stuff," says David Nutter. "They liked Flukeman [in season two's 'The Host']. They are into this stuff, so I definitely wanted to give the audience what they wanted with this episode. I also really love the teasers of the show. When I read the script and it was so soft and wonderful and warm at the outset, I knew I just wanted to really hit the audience with *something* by the time the teaser ended."

Story editor Frank Spotnitz reflects,

"When Jeff Vlaming initially came up with the idea of a fat-sucking vampire, I had my reservations, because the idea of somebody preying on fat women can be very offensive. But one thing I've got to say for Chris is that he never

"One thing I've got to say for Chris is that he never worries about whether something is going to be politically correct."

worries about whether something is going to be politically correct. He just trusts in his ability to tell a good story and, the truth is, if you tell a good story, you don't need to worry about [being offensive] because the story has its own integrity. In the end, I thought that was a fun, old-fashioned sort of X-File."

The notion of the killer getting his victims from the Internet was an inventive one. "Chris's approach to the show is to base everything in reality," says Spotnitz, "and it just seemed so believable that somebody would pick victims that way. It was also topical."

"I think the idea of using the Internet was Chris's," adds Vlaming. "He liked the vulnerability of it. Anybody could be on the other end of the computer, which really freaked out a lot of people who were on-line."

Co–executive producer Robert Goodwin

remembers the woman the vampire is kissing in the teaser pulls back in horror and there is slime covering her mouth. "That poor girl," he says. "She almost lost it. All of that slime was Jell-O, but it was disgusting, and she had to do this thing where she could barely breathe and see the slime coming in and out. We felt bad for her, and even sent her flowers. I thought the guy who played the lead, Timothy Carhart, was terrific. A very nice guy, extremely gentle. Every time I saw him I said, 'You are the most disgusting human being I have ever seen.' 'Well, thank you. Thank you.'"

"That was an episode," says co-producer Paul Rabwin, "where you had to ask, 'What is the sound of sucking fat and wrapping people up in mucous membrane?' How stretchy do you want to make it? It was a fun sound show for us."

He also notes that this episode, which on a surface level reminded many people of season two's "Irresistible," actually had more than a few things in common with that episode. "Besides being directed by David Nutter again, there were two blatant 'Irresistible' moments. One was the hooker scene, where this guy is trying to pick up a hooker and your reaction is, 'My God, it's the same scene that was in "Irresistible."' Number two is that the woman who is the landlady in this episode was

150

the same actress who made the cookies and invited Donnie in in 'Irresistible.' The truth is, when you have the limited talent pool of actors in Vancouver, you tend to use the same ones periodically. On very small parts we have used an actor more than once in a season. But in the end, '2Shy' was quite different."

Rating/Audience Share: 10.1/17

Episode 3.7 (#56)
"The Walk"
Original airdate: November 10, 1995
Written by John Shiban
Directed by Rob Bowman
Guest starring: Andrea Barclay (Frances Callahan), Pat Bermel (Therapist), D. Harlan Cutshall (Guard), Paul Dickson (Uniformed Guard), William Garson (Quinton "Roach" Freely), Deryl Hayes (Army Doctor), Thomas Kopache (Gen. Thomas Callahan), Brennan Kotowich (Trevor Callahan), Rob Lew (Amputee), Paula Shaw (Ward Nurse), Nancy Sorel (Capt. Janet Draper), Don Thompson (Lt. Col. Victor Stans), Ian Tracey (Sgt. Leonard "Rappo" Trimble), Beatrice Zeilinger (Burly Nurse)

Mulder and Scully are drawn into the investigation of a number of Gulf War veterans who have tried to commit suicide but have, strangely, been unable to do so because of an invisible presence. They are inescapably drawn to a quadruple amputee, whose physi-cal limitations seem only to have enhanced his psychic powers of astral projection.

❊   ❊   ❊

This episode was somewhat rushed due to the fact that "731" was originally scheduled for this production slot but was pushed off when the producers decided to turn it into a two-part episode.

"The last thing to happen is the director gets to sit down and figure out a scene," Rob Bowman reflects. "He is so busy putting out fires for the various departments before he can sit down and say, 'Okay, go shoot it.' Now that I have everybody else taken care of, what about me? How about the tone of the take? We kind of rushed into this episode, but I felt that we made the most of it and got some very good performances.

"Graeme Murray really performed way above the call of duty. We were ripping ceilings out of hospitals to get more pipes, and painting walls metal gray, coming up with scenes of reflection. Every time you turned around there was a mirror, so Graeme suggested that we paint everything high gloss and play lots of reflections. I thought about it and then I put it in every shot that I could. I just kept putting in reflections. If you watch that episode, and if you look for reflections, you will see they are in windows, they are here and there, and it's done to keep the audience wondering when this guy is going to show up."

Graeme Murray elaborates, "We wanted to

make everything shiny and see if we could get odd reflections everywhere to give off the idea of ghostly reflections all around these guys who had ghost pains and the one guy who was able to astral project. The result, hopefully, is that you weren't quite sure what was real and what wasn't, who was real and who was a reflection."

"There was only one element of that episode that I didn't agree with," says Bowman. "A friend of mine lost his son in a beach accident where the boy was accidentally buried in the sand — he dug a hole and it caved in. There was a scene in the script that was very similar. I called the writers and said, 'Hey, listen, I can't shoot this scene.' 'Why?' I told the story and said I didn't want my friend to think I was using that tragedy for creative material. I was very averse to doing it and asked, 'Why do we have to kill kids anyway? Can't we think of a story that doesn't involve killing a kid?' I was opposed to it but had to shoot the scene, so I tried to be as oblique about it as I could."

Conversely, Bowman is pleased with a sequence in which a woman is swimming in a pool when the spirit attacks her. It's a moment that suggests the opening scene of Steven Spielberg's *Jaws*.

"It was a challenge to create tension with somebody swimming around in a pool," he admits. "That script needed help visually, because it is all interior, and when you get interior you get claustrophobic. So I just felt that it was my job to breathe life into it visually, create a show that would be uncomfortable

> "I had trouble watching the dailies of that episode because the armless and legless guy was so realistic, it was very upsetting."

for people to watch. In the end, I was very proud of the episode."

Co–executive producer Robert Goodwin admits, "I had trouble watching the dailies of that episode because the armless and legless guy was so realistic, it was very upsetting. That was really an incredible piece of work by Toby Lindala. You make the beds so that the arms and legs go through holes and are hidden underneath, but, man, was it realistic. The guy who played him, Ian Tracey, is someone we've been trying to cast for three years. He's a local guy out of Canada who could probably be the star of a series or something, but he refuses to move to Los Angeles. The episode was also a tricky combination of physical and visual effects, but Rob Bowman really pulled it off."

Rating/Audience Share: 10.4/18

Episode 3.8 (#57)
"Oubliette"
Original airdate: November 17, 1995
Written by Charles Grant Craig
Directed by Kim Manners
Guest starring: Sidonie Boll (Daphne Jacobs),
Michael Chieffo (John Wade), Tracey Ellis
(Lucy Householder), David Fredericks
(Photographer), Jaques LaLonde (Henry),
Alexa Mardon (Sadie Jacobs), Ken Ryan
(Banks), Dollie Scarr (Supervisor), Jewel Staite
(Amy Jacobs), Dean Wray (Tow-Truck Driver)

Scully believes Mulder is allowing his obsession with his sister's abduction to cloud his thinking, but he is convinced there is a psychic connection between a woman named Lucy Householder, who had been kidnapped and held prisoner by a madman for five years as a child, and a little girl who was recently abducted. Lucy seems to be feeling the girl's pain and bleeding her blood. Given that situation, she is their only hope of locating the kidnapper and his victim.

❋   ❋   ❋

By the time "Oubliette" came along, Kim Manners had had the opportunity to deal with his emotions following the death of his best friend (see "D.P.O.").

"I was very much in touch with my emotions, very sensitive," he says,

"and here we have a story about a woman who gives her life so that another young girl might live. The actress, Tracey Ellis, was phenomenal. She was very fragile, very sensitive, and really got into the role. David responded beautifully to her acting, and in the scenes they did together, he got down as an actor. Just a fabulous experience. It was the first *X-Files* in a long while that was based strictly on an emotional level, and it worked like gangbusters.

"With the mythology shows," he

adds, "when Mulder's father was killed, he broke down; the scenes where he dealt with his sister being kidnapped, he broke down. Here he breaks down over a complete stranger; a girl who is basically a drug addict and whore, but he is so touched by her giving her life for this little girl, and he played such a big part in her decision to do so. I thought that was a special moment for *The X-Files,* and David just did a great job. But he's always wonderful when he's not doing one of those — as I call them — Joe Friday scripts, 'Just the facts, ma'am.' And David makes no bones about it, either. We did an episode [later in season three] called 'Quagmire' and in the entire third act it's just David and Gillian stranded on a rock together and they have a conversation for about nine and a half pages. After we shot it I told him that he and Gillian had kicked the shit out of that scene. David looked at me and said, 'Well, Mulder finally had a conversation.'"

Says Robert Goodwin, "'Oubliette' was terrifying because it was a little more reality-based than most of our shows. The abduction of a young girl and holding her hostage in the basement and all of that stuff just touched on reality. A terrible thing had happened two weeks earlier up in Vancouver to a little girl who was a friend of our construction coordinator's daughter: She was abducted and killed, so it hit very close to home. I remember that being a somber experience.

"The biggest problem, physically, with that episode is in the last act where they find the kidnapper in the river, drowning her, and they come on, shoot him, and she comes back to life. I think we shot that in October. The rivers up in Vancouver are glacially fed, so they are all very, very cold. As a consequence, it is difficult for actors to work in them for any length of time, but this particular spot was a shallow part of the river, about eighteen inches deep. In sunlight it would warm up a bit. Anyway, the bottom line is that it started raining like hell. We got up there on the day they were supposed to shoot and it was suddenly like the Colorado River. It was completely impossible to put anybody in that water. It went on for weeks — we kept trying to find a time when the water would drop so we could shoot it. We barely got the damn thing done before we went on the air. We were shooting that river sequence up to the very last minute. In the end, though, I think it looks great."

Rating/Audience Share: 10.2/17

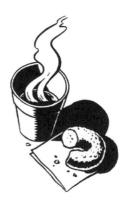

Episode 3.9 (#58)
"Nisei"

Original airdate: November 24, 1995
Written by Chris Carter, Howard Gordon, and Frank Spotnitz
Directed by David Nutter
Guest starring: Roger Allford (Harbormaster), Gillian Barber (Penny Northern), Raymond J. Barry (Sen. Richard Matheson), Brendan Beiser (Agent Comox), Tom Braidwood (Frohike), Dean Haglund (Langly), Bruce Harwood (Byers), Robert Ito (Dr. Ishimaru), Corrine Koslo (Lottie Holloway), Paul McLean (Coast Guard Officer), Yasuo Sakurai (Kazuo Takeo), Carrie Cain Sparks (Train Station Clerk), Warren Takeuchi (Japanese Escort), Lori Triolo (Diane), Bob Wilde (Limo Driver), Steven Williams (Mr. X)

A mail-order alien autopsy tape leads Mulder and Scully to investigate a salvage ship that may have raised an alien ship from the ocean floor. Separating as a means of furthering their investigation, Scully checks out a woman involved with the salvage company but, instead, finds a group of women who claim to know her, who have all had computer chips implanted in their necks, and who have been abducted on numerous occasions. Mulder, meanwhile, finds himself on a train that may very well be carrying a living alien.

❊ ❊ ❊

As Frank Spotnitz explains it, the "Nisei" follow-up, "731," was originally intended to be a one-part episode.

"The script was written that way," he says, "and we discovered that it was just impossible to do all the stuff we wanted to do with the train, in terms of both logistics and expenses, as a one-part show. Chris made the decision to expand it to a two-parter and push it back until we had time to prepare. So we ended up working backwards, taking elements from that single-episode script and spreading them out over two parts, then adding new elements. The idea of the alien autopsy video came in late, as well as adding these other women who have had the same experience Scully had. These were things we did to expand the story, and so we ended up writing episode nine very quickly; it became a group effort for me, Chris, and Howard."

Howard Gordon became involved with the writing of this episode when he complained a bit to Chris Carter that he wanted to participate in the mythology episodes. Carter's response was for Gordon to simply join in on this script. "I think 'Nisei' and '731' knocked the audience off balance," Gordon says. "It allowed us to retrench and ultimately answer questions from Scully's point of view. She had it her way, basically, proving that the aliens are not coming down and that they are genetic experiments. That science is responsible."

David Nutter admits, "This was the first of the mythology shows that I directed, and I was nervous about it, believe it or not.

Fortunately, it turned out very well, I thought. I just wanted to do the best job I could, because of the mythology episodes directed by people like Rob Bowman, Kim Manners, and Bob Goodwin, which I think really brought scope to these shows and made them, in a sense, mini-features."

For Robert Goodwin, the guy supervising physical production of the series, the real challenge of "Nisei" was the fact that the episode involved a train, and a climactic moment when Mulder has to leap on top of it.

"We had to use three different train cars," he recounts. "We had a freight car, a car that had the laboratory in it, and a sleeper car. They had to be built on great big inflated inner tubes so that we could rock it. You have to rock it to feel like it was really moving. So we shot a portion of it, including the portion in the passenger car, on a real train. The real train is a nightmare because it is a train. You do take one and the train comes around the bend and [a stuntman] jumps on top of it and it's 'Okay. Cut. Let's go to take two.' Well, that means you have to stop the train, roll it two miles or however far it is to get it back around the bend, and start it up again. In between takes it could be an hour and a half, and we have to shoot thirty takes a day to get the show done. That was difficult, plus I was very nervous about the stunt with Mulder jumping on the train. David, if you would let him, would do everything himself. So it was a combination of safety and visual effectiveness. I insisted on a number of tests, and I'm glad I did, because we found out that the manner in which we were going to shoot this, which was basically have the camera mounted on top of the train shooting straight back, was very ineffective. Even a train going sixty miles an hour, if you are shooting straight back it doesn't appear to be going that fast. In reality, you can't get it going much more than twenty to twenty-five miles an hour in order to do the stunt. It would almost look like he was standing still, whereas if you come around on a side angle, say somebody standing on top of the train and you shoot him from the side, you are seeing the trees and houses and everything on the side whisk past. They sort of blur and you could be going fifteen miles an hour, but it looks as though you are going much faster.

"The one place where it worked," Goodwin elaborates, "was just after Mulder does his jump and he sees the overhead footbridge go by and disappear behind him. At that moment, looking straight back, you have a sense of speed, because you have that bridge just suddenly going backward, but as soon as it was gone it became nothing. So I designed a shot where we had a crane mounted on top of the train, we were shooting back initially, and as soon as Mulder landed at the end of the shot (David actually was standing and just dropped to the top of the train, because we did the stuntman part of the jump prior to that), the crane swung out around the side of the train so you were shooting over to the side of it. If you look at it again, it's a very effective shot. Timing-wise it was perfect. He lands, you see the bridge go by, and then you swing around to the side. In the end, it worked out great."

Rating/Audience Share: 9.8/17

Episode 3.10 (#59)
"731"

Original airdate: December 1, 1995
Written by Frank Spotnitz
Directed by Rob Bowman
Guest starring: Brendan Beiser (Agent Pendrell), Sean Campbell (Soldier), Colin Cunningham (Escalante), Robert Ito (Dr. Shiro Zama), Stephen McHattie (Red-Haired Man), Victoria Maxwell (Mother), Mike Puttonen (Conductor), Don S. Williams (Elder), Steven Williams (Mr. X)

Mulder finds himself trapped in a bomb-rigged train car with an apparent assassin who, he assumes, has been sent to kill an apparent alien locked in a compartment of the area they're in. Scully calls Mulder on her cell phone and provides him with what she feels is convincing proof that alien beings do not exist; that the government has been performing genetic experiments with human beings and has used the notion of aliens as a smokescreen. Trying to piece it all together in his mind, Mulder suggests to the assassin — though he is never told for sure — that the creature locked in the compartment was created to be a test subject that would survive the fallout of any weapon known to man. Nothing is ever proved, however, when X arrives, kills the assassin, and removes Mulder from the train just before it explodes.

❖ ❖ ❖

In reflecting on his inspiration for the episode, Frank Spotnitz notes: "I read an article in the *New York Times* a year earlier about these Chinese war crimes that I had never even heard of before. I was just shocked, first of all, that I had never heard of them, and then by the details. Prisoners of war were exposed to bacterial agents; experiments were done on children. Just unbelievably cruel and horrible experiments. So there was something new there to be dealt with. I ended up reading books on it, and part of the aftermath was that our government basically pardoned these people in exchange for their science. One of the leaders of this unit — called 731 — that conducted this experiment was spotted in the United States at an Army base in the 1950s, presumably to share this information with our military. Anyway, I thought there was something in there, and that is where the character in 'Nisei' came from. Also, I love train movies, particularly *North by Northwest* and *The Train*, an old John Frankenheimer film. So I just loved the idea of Mulder on a train.

"What ended up particularly interesting about the episode," he continues, "is that it really gave us a chance to set the counter back.

"I read an article in the *New York Times* a year earlier about these Chinese war crimes that I had never heard of before . . . so there was something new there to be dealt with."

I think after 'Paper Clip' people thought, 'That's it. Scully saw aliens and both of them are going to be believers now,' and this gave us a chance to say, 'Wait a minute. You can't be sure of that. What did she, in fact, see? Were they aliens, or were they people who were disfigured, subjects in an experiment?' I think we concluded the two-parter with Scully believing that alien abduction is all a hoax, a sham, a cover-up for government experiments which our government has actually admitted to, as Scully referred to when she was talking about the president admitting that we were doing experiments on innocent civilians. That was in the news a few months prior to that. So it is a credible alternative theory for Scully to have and an opportunity to say, No, she has not been corrupted into being a believer like Mulder. She has a very compelling real-world alternative explanation for what she has seen."

When shooting the episode, Rob Bowman took two different approaches to a significant scene, when Mulder is on the train and Scully is telling him over the cell phone that there are no aliens, just a government conspiracy.

"I shot Mulder with a Steadicam, which is a kind of handheld camera but it floats a bit," says Bowman. "And I shot him off center. He is kind of paranoid because the assassin may come in the room and jump him. I wanted a completely different feeling with Scully. I wanted Scully to feel like the Rock of Gibraltar. I wanted her to feel symmetrical, balanced, confident, strong — how do I do that? Well, all of her shots are on the dolly and are very graphically balanced."

Rating/Audience Share: 11.9/20

Episode 3.11 (#60)
"Revelations"
Original airdate: December 15, 1995
Written by Kim Newton
Directed by David Nutter
Guest starring: R. Lee Ermey (Rev. Patrick Finley), Nicole Roberts (Mrs. Tynes), Hayley Tyson (Susan Kryder), Kenneth Welsh (Millennium Man/Simon Gates), Selina Williams (School Nurse), Kevin Zegers (Kevin Kryder)

A bit of role swapping for Mulder and Scully, with Scully believing that their current case involves religious phenomena, while Mulder thinks there is a more earthly explanation. Eleven reported stigmatics are stalked and killed by a religious zealot, and the FBI duo find themselves protecting a twelfth, a young boy who just may be the real thing, exhibiting blood from the same kinds of wounds that were inflicted upon Jesus Christ when he was crucified.

❉   ❉   ❉

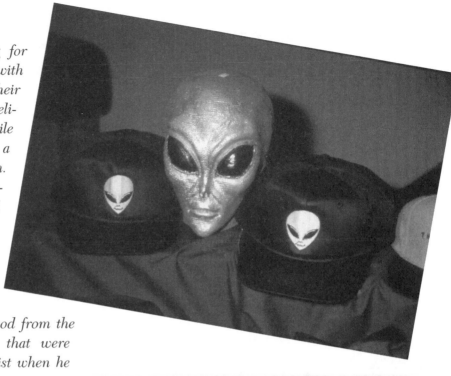

Official alien wear.

"'Revelations' was tough at first because it was kind of a softer show, and you have to be really careful with the softer shows so that they don't lose the overall *X-Files* edge," says David Nutter. "There always has to be a taste of horror in there somewhere.

"The relationship between the boy and Gillian was very strong, with much of it not actually being stated. There was just a connection between them. I also love the performance of R. Lee Ermey, who was the drill sergeant in *Full Metal Jacket.* He was also in the pilot of *Space: Above and Beyond,* and he

has always wanted to do an *X-Files,* so it was wonderful to get him."

Offers co-producer Paul Rabwin, "A show with script problems. It's difficult to sell the concept of religious magic and people appearing in two places at one time. It was a very emotional show, because it got into an important area of Scully's background, but trying to pull off the mystical parts was problematic. The script went through several rewrites and was still being worked on until the time of production. We figured, 'Nutter is a strong guy; he'll bring that in okay.' It did come off

"Some of us thought ['Revelations'] was DOA. We were on the operating table with that show and had it on life support."

very well, but there were some inconsistencies and pieces in it that just didn't seem to make sense to me. We went into a very detailed editing marathon, and we ended up with a show that just didn't work on a number of different levels. At one point, we couldn't sell the idea of this kid being in two places at the same time. There were some things missing that really tied together the kid and Owen, who's this mystical bald-headed character — just a number of things that weren't satisfactory about it. Some of us thought that show was DOA. We were on the operating table with that show and had it on life support.

"But I think it's one of the better examples of what happens when all of the creative forces come together. The kid had already gone home to Toronto. We flew him back to Vancouver, wrote some detailed lines for the Millennium Man. We had people writing new sequences; our second-unit crew was set up to shoot some stuff. We went back in and recut and restructured and the show started to make sense. By the time that show came out,

we were in awe because it played well. It amazed us. The response on-line was, 'Great show,' 'Meaningful show,' and people just loved it. We thought it was going to be one of the dogs of the season, and it turned out to be a very popular episode."

Rating/Audience Share: 10.1/17

Episode 3.12 (#61)
"War of the Coprophages"
Original airdate: January 5, 1996
Written by Darin Morgan
Directed by Kim Manners
Guest starring: Dion Anderson (Sheriff Frass), Raye Birk (Dr. Jeff Eckerle), Alex Bruhanski (Dr. Bugger), Alan Buckley (Dude), Bill Dow (Dr. Rick Newton), Tom Heaton (Resident #1), Ken Kramer (Dr. Alexander Ivanov), Tyler Labine (Stoner), Tony Marr (Motel Manager), Nicole Parker (Chick), Bobbie Phillips (Dr. Bambi Berendaum), Wren Robertz (Orderly), Bobby Stewart (Resident #2), Norma Wick (Reporter)

Mulder and Scully are drawn to Miller's Grove, Massachusetts, responding to reports of a town being overrun by cockroaches. Upon further investigation the question arises: Are these insects man-made robotic creatures, or alien probes sent to Earth as a means of terrifying us?

✾ ✾ ✾

"I came across a picture on the cover of an old magazine of a robotist named Rodney Brooks who was creating these robots that looked like insects, and he was giving them artificial intelligence that tried to duplicate the way the brain works," says Darin Morgan. "He decided to give the machine the most simple of programs, almost buglike, and these creatures actually appeared to be thinking. They appeared to be living, because they were reacting to things in the environment, which gave them a sort of lifelike quality. So you look at that and you say, 'There's a story in there somewhere.' An interesting science that somehow got crossed with cockroaches only because the place I was living in for a while had cockroaches.

"Even though I do funny shows, there always has to be a certain scare element," he adds. "The cockroaches are the built-in scare factor. So there was that, and I also wanted to do something like *War of the Worlds,* in a sense. Not a hoax, but people having mass hysteria. I don't know how I made the connection, but humans often think they have a highly developed brain and always think things out clearly and rationally. Yet in the case of mass hysteria, they really react like insects, swarming around. Somehow I made the connection between that and this artificial intelligence research. Robots and thought patterns — somehow that all came together to make the episode what it was."

Kim Manners deems this episode incredible due to the luck they had with the required cockroaches.

"You can't imagine how lucky we were. Debbie Cove, who is our animal trainer, has got around four hundred cockroaches. Two hundred from one school and two hundred from another, and we can never intermingle them. We also have to be careful not to hurt them. There were some shots where I wanted to tie cockroaches into the scene with actors, and every time we set up to do what I wanted to do, we were unsuccessful.

"There is one story I have to share because it's a classic," Manners continues. "We did a shot where I had Bill Dow, a local Vancouver actor, sitting on a toilet and the camera was outside the stall doors. We dollied into his face and he is sitting there reading a magazine. We went up and over his head and tilted the camera down to the back of the toilet tank. At that point on cue I needed about a half dozen cockroaches scurrying up on top of the tank. The minute I cleared Bill's head, they had to be there. Well, we were releasing them through a hole in the back of the set and so they had about a one-inch gap between the set and the toilet. Anyway, we did the shot four or five times and the trainers were releasing the cockroaches when I called 'Action,' but they weren't there. So, after five takes, we gathered them all back up and put them in a plastic bucket. Debbie Cove walked out of the set to go behind the wall. I said, 'Just come here a minute.' I stuck my head in the bucket and said, 'Listen, you sons of bitches. There are two cues. The first one is for camera. The second one is for you. When I say "Action," you guys run your asses to the top of the toilet

"The sounds of cockroaches were also great fun. Since these were alien mechanical cockroaches, we ended up taking a combination of something organic and something metallic."

tank. Do you hear me?' Now, the crew got a big kick out of that. Well, the next take, I said, 'Camera action' and 'Action,' and the little bastards did exactly what I told them to do."

Co-producer Paul Rabwin recalls with a laugh, "A Darin Morgan show — what can I say? It had at the same time among the funniest material in *The X-Files* as well as the most horrific sequences ever. I think the scene in which the cockroach crawls *into* someone's arm affected more adult professional people I work with than any other sequence we've ever done. When we see things happen to other people, usually we don't relate them to something that could happen to us. One of the things *The X-Files* tries to do is get into every-

body's psyche. Well, everyone has bug nightmares. Spielberg knew this when he did *Raiders of the Lost Ark*. So cockroaches are something near and dear to everyone's heart, and we all get freaked out by them. To relate to one crawling up our arm — and then into the arm — is unbelievable, and people went nuts. It was well done.

"The sounds of cockroaches were also great fun," he continues. "Since these were alien mechanical cockroaches, we ended up taking a combination of something organic and something metallic. We took a cicada sound and then we took some metallic scrape sounds and combined them and played them up about three octaves and got a little echo to it. We did about five or six different versions of this combination of organic and metallic sounds. We tried different pitches and speeds and came up with one we thought was really cool. That became the signature. Then we had to run it through the multiplier and create thirty or forty different sounds working simultaneously. It worked well and had a nice feel to it. And then we wanted to make sure it had a sound that was reminiscent of a cell phone, because of the big joke at the end where Mulder's cell phone goes off and the doctor thinks he's a cockroach. So we used an element of the cell phone blended in with the cockroach chirp."

Rating/Audience Share: 10.1/16

Episode 3.13 (#62)
"Syzygy"

Original airdate: January 26, 1996
Written by Chris Carter
Directed by Rob Bowman
Guest starring: Wendy Benson (Margi Kleinjan), Richard Brown (Minister), Garry Davey (Bob Spitz), Tim Dixon (Dr. Richard Godfrey), Lisa Robin Kelly (Terri Roberts), Gabrielle Miller (Brenda J. Summerfield), Russell Porter (Scott Simmons), Ryan Reynolds (Jay "Boom" DeBoom), Dana Wheeler-Nicholson (Det. Angela White), Denalda Williams (Zirinka)

Fears arise in a small town that a Satanic cult has taken root in the local high school, particularly in a pair of teenage girls. Mulder and Scully become convinced of this as well, although a local astronomer seems to answer some questions by explaining that once every eighty-four years a planetary alignment — a syzygy — occurs and that this town's location makes it a "cosmic G-spot" for the repercussions.

❊ ❊ ❊

Rob Bowman is not a fan of this particular episode. "The show proved to be much more difficult than I anticipated, and there wasn't enough time to shoot the show properly, because we were so close to the Christmas break. I felt extremely pressured and frustrated, although there are things in it I love, particularly the banter between Mulder and Scully. But overall, I thought the show was very oblique. I don't feel that the characters ever knew what was going on, and I don't think it is all that cool that kids are murdering people. I didn't feel like I was shooting an episode of *The X-Files*, and I think I let Chris down a little bit. Truth is, I don't like doing episodes I don't want to watch. I don't like doing episodes I don't feel like I can do a great job on, and I didn't do a great job on it. I don't think it is representative of me or the show.

"When you go too fast, you make mistakes," he continues. "Like in movies, you do half a page a day and you do it right. Here is a storyline where at one point the girls split off and at the same pace of shooting — one page of shooting is credited as one page of production time. Well, unfortunately, we had parallel action. I had to shoot two scenes in two separate locations. I had to go out in the countryside and shoot the people on the road, and that is counted as one page. Unfortunately, I also had to go back to the garage for Mulder and the other girl telling the other side of the story. So instead of shooting one scene and completing that page, I wound up shooting many pages twice. The result is that what appears to be a fifty-page script is actually closer to seventy-five or eighty pages. Well, I'm sorry, we can't shoot eighty pages. I am responsible for my own goofs on that episode, and I just couldn't enjoy it."

Co–executive producer Robert Goodwin reflects, "The hardest part of the show was the whole sequence at the police station where the girls go against each other psychically and all of the guns are going off. It was just a combination of physical effects and special effects, and it all worked really well."

Rating/Audience Share: 10.8/17

Episode 3.14 (#63)
"Grotesque"

Original airdate: February 2, 1996
Written by Howard Gordon
Directed by Kim Manners
Guest starring: Paul J. Anderson (Paramedic), Susan Bain (Agent Sarah Sheherlie), John Milton Brandon (Rudy Aguirre), James McDonnell (Glass Blower), Kasper Michaels (Young Agent), Amanda O'Leary (Doctor), Levani Outchaneichvili (John Mostow), Mitch Pileggi (Assistant Director Walter S. Skinner), Kurtwood Smith (Agent Bill Patterson), Greg Thirloway (Agent Greg Nemhauser), Zoran Vukelic (Peter [Artists' Model])

Mulder and Scully find themselves working with Mulder's former mentor, agent Bill Patterson of the behavioral sciences unit, when Patterson arrests a serial killer obsessed with gargoyles. But the killings nonetheless continue. What they need to know is whether the confessed killer, John Mostow, had an accomplice or has inspired someone to pick up where he left off. Using an expertise not often demonstrated in the series, Mulder essentially allows himself to get into the killer's mind, thinking as he would think and beginning to act in a peculiar manner. The descent into madness gives hints of possible demonic possession.

❋ ❋ ❋

For Howard Gordon, "Grotesque" was a personal crowning achievement of the season. "I had spent the better part of a month writing a story that really involved a possession, about the spirit of one particular gargoyle. I wrote a whole draft and literally three days before prep I said to Chris, 'This episode just is not working.' He sat with me on a Saturday, and we retrenched. It occurred to me on that morning and at the eleventh hour that this was not a story about an actual demon, but the demon of one man's mind. It was roughly the same structure I had done before, but with a completely different and much more internal and psychological story. On *The X-Files* we have often decided that the psychological is less interesting than the paranormal or external phenomena, but in this case the internal was really the way the story needed to be told, about the duality of people. It's a story that's been done before, but I think we added a really unique twist to it.

"This being *The X-Files*," Gordon continues, "I was looking for something visual, something that would ground you in the episode. I was walking the streets of New York and was looking up, noticing these gargoyles at every corner staring down at me. I was just fascinated by that. That's really where the episode was born. I also thought that in many ways, getting into the mind of a criminal is a kind of sculpture, so the idea of a sculptor came to me. I also thought people really enjoyed the fact that the episode told something about Mulder before Scully, which is always interesting. We also saw some of what made Mulder the man we know."

"David Duchovny drove himself, and he was brilliant in that show," adds Kim Manners. "I also think 'Grotesque' may have been the template for Chris Carter's new show, *Millennium,* because it is quite the same storyline, with someone becoming the person he's hunting; driving himself into the darkest, deepest corner of his mind. Asking the question, What is evil? And then experiencing evil so that he can recognize it and therefore capture it. I think 'Grotesque' is a frightening show. I think it is a disturbing show, and I think that's why — for me — it's such a good show. We pulled off making the viewer feel uneasy. *I* even found it a difficult show to watch. Yeah, it was a pretty dark hour

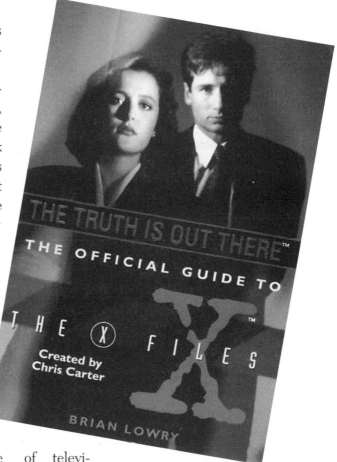

of television, and I would like to do more of those."

Co-producer Paul Rabwin recalls, "In one of the last scenes, when we pan up to see a gargoyle on top of a building, it happened to be shot on a particularly windy evening in Vancouver. The gargoyle was flopping around in the wind because there was no way to secure it. So optically we had to basically freeze the gargoyle itself and keep it in the shot because the camera was moving. It's supposed to be a big stone gargoyle attached to the building, and it was moving around like the papier-mâché that it was."

Rating/Audience Share: 11.6/18

Episode 3.15 (#64)
"Piper Maru"

Original airdate: February 9, 1996
Written by Chris Carter and Frank Spotnitz
Directed by Rob Bowman
Guest starring: Jo Bates (Jeraldine Kallenchuk), Paul Batten (Joan Gauthier), Lenno Britos (Luis Cardinal), Robert Clothier (Commander Chris Johansen), Russell Ferrier (Medic), Rochelle Greenwood (Waitress), Richard Hersley (Capt. Kyle Sanford), Darcy Laurie (2nd Engineer), Nicholas Lea (Agent Alex Krycek), Robbie Maieri (World War II Pilot), Tegan Moss (Young Dana), David Neale (Guard), Morris Paynch (Gray-Haired Man), Mitch Pileggi (Assistant Director Walter S. Skinner), Tom Scholte (Young Johansen), Peter Scoular (Sick Crewman), Joel Silverstone (1st Engineer), Ari Solomon (Gauthier), Christine Viner (Young Melissa)

A French salvage ship discovers a World War II plane at the bottom of the ocean, its pilot somehow still alive. However, a transfer takes place, with an alien force going from the pilot to the diver, eventually to the diver's wife, and then to agent Alex Krycek, who is in Hong Kong. That is where Mulder finds Krycek and

brings him back to the United States to turn over the DAT. Unbeknownst to Mulder, however, the alien has taken possession of Krycek's body.

❋   ❋   ❋

"'Piper Maru' began with two things that Chris had known for a while he wanted to do," says Frank Spotnitz. "One, he knew he wanted a diver to go down in one of these deep-diving suits and find a World War II plane with the pilot alive in the cockpit. He hadn't thought about how that would work, like what the explanation was, whether this was a real thing the diver was seeing or an illusion. He just knew he wanted that image. Two, he wanted to have a flashback in black and white aboard a submarine.

"That was it. That was my assignment, and I had a number of false starts. I started working on it immediately after we finished '731,' and, finally, flying back from a convention in Minneapolis, I realized I didn't have any paper with me. I just had a pen and a magazine that was on the plane. During the flight it occurred to me that Scully's sister had been dead for many months and we hadn't dealt with it. Death — that was what the show should be about. Death and dealing with the dead. So I started thinking about Mulder and Scully, and then Krycek came to mind, and very quickly I started writing all over the white spaces in the magazine. 'Piper Maru' came together very quickly, as dealing with the dead behind you seemed to tie in nicely with the idea of this buried secret at the bottom of the ocean. Something terrible had happened there and the people who knew about it had to live with it the rest of their lives. That became a theme through both episodes ['Piper Maru' and 'Apocrypha']. Krycek in the missile silo, still alive, at the end of 'Apocrypha' was a nice period on that thought.

"Rob Bowman directed the first part, and it was a big, big deal shooting underwater," Spotnitz continues. "It was a very complicated sequence — actually having a tank, a P-51 the art director had designed, and having a diver go down there. We shot water and smoke and used every trick in the book, which was great. What's amazing to me is that we write these things in Los Angeles and then we go to Vancouver and in a matter of eight days — eight working days — the crew has turned the scripts into the episodes you see. It never ceases to amaze me. It is this huge operation; they build these sets and find these props and locations. They not only do good work, but they do it week in and week out and in such a short time period."

Rob Bowman enthuses, "'Piper Maru' was sent from heaven. Part of the story was based on my very first night scuba dive. Everything

was pitch black except for the little glow lights on the tanks and the bright flashlights used to light the water. I thought it was cool, and that we should do an episode where they go down into the ocean and discover something creepy. I mentioned that to Chris. He took it and said, 'Let's put a P-51 Mustang in there with a guy in the cockpit.' That is basically 'Piper Maru.' The rest of the script was generated from that. Here is a show where we got great mythological scenes with Mulder, and then a wonderful

> **"What's amazing to me is that we write these things in Los Angeles and then we go to Vancouver and in a matter of eight days — eight working days — the crew has turned the scripts into the episodes you see."**

balance of the emotional storyline for Scully. And, again, great performances by all."

An interesting moment for Bowman was a Scully flashback when she's visiting the place where she grew up, and remembers playing with her late sister.

"These little girls playing were not there that day. We're driving up the street; the sun is gone. We're waiting for our light to get this shot. I'm in the back seat of the car, operating the camera that shoots over her shoulders, and I'm directing Gillian while we're driving, and I say, 'Okay, here we go. Here come the kids. Up there on your right is a tree — make that tree you and your sister.' The idea was that the close-up of Gillian would be reflective and loving toward her sister — and she was acting to a tree! I saw the dailies of that and called her up and said, 'You are my hero. No one will ever know what you did, and I'm going to tell everybody I can that you just did that great reaction to a tree.' Two weeks later, our second unit went out and shot the girls and then put it together and you say, 'Oh, my God.'

"In terms of the mythology," says Bowman, "once again we're going forward and it feels natural. At the end of '731' you're confused because of everything Scully has told Mulder, but with 'Piper Maru' you feel that it's the truth; that there are aliens. I also love the end of it with Krycek coming out of the bathroom and he and Mulder are walking along. You always have to be ready to fix something that's not right. They are walking along and David says, 'You feel better?' Nick [Lea] says, 'Like a new man,' they walk past the camera, and that's the end of the episode. *I don't think so.* What am I going to do? I jump on the camera and, of course, we're behind schedule and everybody is looking at me like, 'Rob, we don't have time for you to fix this.' But we did it again, and I remembered a moment in a film

I had seen that was the same kind of long walking shot and I thought, Well, this is really going on too long. There has to be something going on here. I told Nick to plant his face right in the camera. Nick will jump in front of a truck if he thinks it will make a scene better. So he walked right up to the camera; he shot his head forward into the camera and I came off the camera after rehearsal and said, 'Now we have an ending,' and then it was a matter of asking Mat Beck if we could make his eyes go with the moving camera, filled with that black oil stuff that represented the alien presence. All of a sudden we went from, 'Oh shit, we can't end the episode this way,' to one of my favorite endings ever."

Rating/Audience Share: 10.6/18

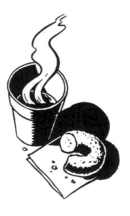

168

Episode 3.16 (#65)
"Apocrypha"

Original airdate: February 16, 1996
Written by Frank Spotnitz and Chris Carter
Directed by Kim Manners
Guest starring: Brendan Beiser (Agent Pendrell), Tom Braidwood (Frohike), Eric Breker (Ambulance Driver), Lenno Britos (Luis Cardinal), Jeff Chivers (Armed Man #1), Harrison R. Coe (3rd Government Man), William B. Davis (Cigarette-Smoking Man), Martin Evans (Major Domo), Francis Flanagan (Nurse), Dean Haglund (Langly), Bruce Harwood (Byers), Richard Hersley (Capt. Kyle Sanford), David Kaye (Doctor), Nicholas Lea (Agent Alex Krycek), Brian Levy (Navy Doctor), Kevin McNulty (Agent Brian Fuller), Sue Mathew (Agent Linda Caleca), John Neville (Well-Manicured Man), Mitch Pileggi (Assistant Director Walter S. Skinner), Peter Scoular (Sick Crewman), Stanley Walsh (2nd Elder), Craig Warkenten (Young Cigarette-Smoking Man), Don Williams (1st Elder)

Skinner is wounded in what appears to be a random shooting, but as Scully investigates, she learns that the shooter, Luis Cardinal, is the same man who was working with Krycek and who pulled the trigger on her sister, Melissa. Meanwhile, Mulder and the alien-possessed Krycek return to America from Hong Kong to retrieve the DAT, but their car is run off the road by agents of the Cigarette-Smoking Man. While Mulder is unconscious, Krycek irradiates the agents, retrieves the tape on his own, and strikes a deal with CSM: The alien will be told where its spacecraft is in return for the tape. Eventually, Mulder and Scully proceed to a missile silo in North Dakota in pursuit of Krycek, but they are restrained by CSM's men and taken away. Unbeknownst to them (though Mulder suspects it), the silo actually contains an alien spacecraft and now the completely mortal Krycek, who will apparently be trapped for the rest of his life.

✿ ✿ ✿

"I actually think you didn't learn a lot more about the conspiracy in these two episodes ['Piper Maru' and 'Apocrypha']," says Frank Spotnitz, "but, emotionally, I think they were really good episodes. 'Nisei' and '731' were good for advancing Mulder and Scully's attitude toward what is really going on, but these shows were much more emotional, focusing on the consequences of the quest they are on. It is really easy to go through a lot of these action things with people dying and never addressing them. So I thought it was very interesting to do so."

Kim Manners was intrigued by the episode because it was his first mythology. "Rob Bowman had done 'Piper Maru.' I read the script, and I said, 'Well, Robbie's got this bitchin' underwater sequence where they find the monster and we see the monster transfer from body to body.' Then I got Krycek, and now I had to put the whole thing to rest. That was a show I really directed from instinct alone."

He notes that he approaches the mythology shows differently from the stand-alones. "Each stand-alone has to have, for me, a different means of presenting the story to the audience. With the mythology shows, you don't have to find an approach. What you need to do as a director is to be sure that the performances are there and the camera is working well and that the yarn is presented in its cleanest and most interesting fashion. It is not as creative a thing for us, but we've got to make sure that it is a damn good quality hour of television, whereas with the monsters of the week there is some individual creative contribution from the directors. The mythology shows are spooky or disturbing or interesting on their own. They really are, I think, easier to direct, and there is something about them that's of a better quality."

Rating/Audience Share: 10.7/18

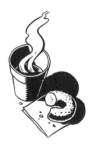

**Episode 3.17 (#66)
"Pusher"**
Written by Vince Gilligan
Directed by Rob Bowman
Guest starring: Julia Arkos (Holly), Steve Bacic (Agent Collins), Meredith Bain-Woodward (Defense Attorney Brent), Roger R. Cross (SWAT Lieutenant), Ernie Foot (Lobby Guard), Janyse Jaud (Nurse), Darren Lucas (Lead SWAT Cop), Don Mackay (Judge), D. Neil Mark (Deputy Scott Kerber), Mitch Pileggi (Assistant Director Walter S. Skinner), Vic Polizos (Agent Frank Burst), J. D. Sheppard (Prosecutor), Henry Watson (Bailiff), Robert Wisden (Pusher/Robert Modell)

Mulder and Scully go up against a man named Robert Modell, who refers to himself as "Pusher" and has the ability to control people's minds with the sound of his voice (for example, inducing a police officer to drive his squad car into the path of a truck; giving an FBI agent a heart attack over the phone simply by describing arteries shutting down and his heartbeat slowing). The stakes become personal when Pusher uses his power to turn Mulder and Scully against each other.

❊ ❊ ❊

"This was, I believe, a pure *X-Files* script," says Rob Bowman. "What if we don't have a train? What if we don't throw all the money in Fort Knox into an episode? How well can we do it? So Vince Gilligan sat down and arced out an episode about this character. Directorially, this was a time for me to step out of the way. It's the opposite of many other shows, where it is about embellishment. This was one where I just had to make sure that the performances were well timed. Also, I was just so tired. 'Piper Maru' was a killer, just brutal, and thank God 'Pusher' came along, because I had just enough energy to walk up and talk to the actors but not enough energy to create a visual palette of colors and light and everything else. I was really challenged by the idea of fulfilling the expectations for an *X-Files* episode but without any hardware — no aliens, no spaceships. I also thought Robert Wisden was great as Pusher. He is a very energized kind of confident actor with lots of ideas of his own. It took me about a day and a half to get him into it, and then I never had to speak to him again, because he had that look in his eyes. I would walk up to talk to him about the scene and I could see that he was already there."

Rating/Audience Share: 10.8/18

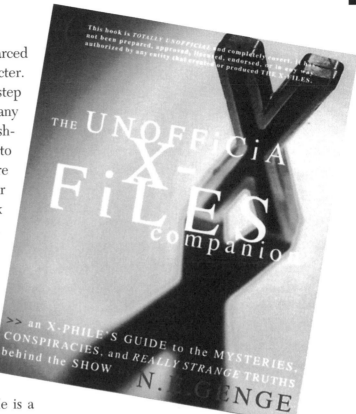

Episode 3.18 (#67)
"Teso dos Bichos"
Original airdate: March 8, 1996
Written by John Shiban
Directed by Kim Manners
Guest starring: Garrison Chrisjohn (Dr. Winters), Tom McBeath (Dr. Jerrold Lewton), Janne Morth (Mona Wustner), Alan Robertson (Dr. Carl Roosevelt), Ron Sauve (Mr. Decker), Gordon Tootoosis (Shaman), Vic Trevino (Dr. Alonso Bilac)

When ancient archaeological items are removed from a sacred burial ground in Teso dos Bichos, Ecuador, those involved in the expedition begin to disappear, leaving a trail of blood. Mulder and Scully are sent in to investigate, and find themselves up against spirits, rats, and multitudes of savage cats.

✻ ✻ ✻

An episode, according to Kim Manners, marred by one distinct problem: cats. Although the ending sequence involving hundreds of them seems quite effective, he suggests that viewers turn off the sound to see how tame it really is.

"Do you know what's scary about that scene?" he asks rhetorically. "One full day on the dubbing stage mixing act four. What is scary, what is frightening, is the sound you hear, not at all what you see. It's ridiculous. I thought the first three acts were terrific, though. I pulled out all the horror stops and I thought it worked rather well until the fourth act."

Co–executive producer Robert Goodwin concurs, noting that it is extremely difficult to make domestic cats look dangerous.

"If you thought cockroaches were tough to shoot, cats are forty times harder," he says. "First of all, they don't look that scary. They look like cats, and you can never get all of those cats to do the same thing at once. I mean, if you have eighteen cats in a scene, it would take you half a day just to get them all in one place and roll the camera. You get ready to go, and three of them disappear on you. One of the things that was pointed out to me is that they all looked fluffy and clean. I wanted to go back and reshoot the cats, but I wanted them greased down and dirty. No more white cats, only gray cats and black cats and brown cats. I wanted them really scruffy and greasy. So we've got twelve cats in a scene, all greasy and scruffy but, like I said, it takes forever to get them all in place so that we can shoot. While we're taking forever to get them in place, what do cats do? They clean themselves. So we have these scruffy, dirty cats, but by the time we get to shoot, they've

"If you thought cockroaches were tough to shoot, cats are forty times harder."

cleaned themselves up and look absolutely beautiful. We had to build a little cat puppet that I thought was marginal, but it actually did work. But it was something I thought we would never be able to pull off."

Co-producer Paul Rabwin elaborates, "We probably spent twenty hours just filming cats, trying to get them to react and behave a certain way. Trying to get cats milling around, looking evil, which is difficult, because cats are basically domesticated. We ended up having Mat Beck take a certain group of cats that were holding still and multiply them optically. So one of the cat shots we saw looking down through a grate was something Mat had to create."

Rating/Audience Share: 10.7/18

Episode 3.19 (#68)
"Hell Money"

Original airdate: March 29, 1996
Written by Jeffrey Vlaming
Directed by Tucker Gates
Guest starring: Doug Abrahams (Lt. Neary), Stephen Chang (Large Man), Donald Fong (Vase Man), Dina Ha (Dr. Wu), James Hong (Hard-Faced Man), Ed Hong-Louie (Money Man), Lucy Liu (Kim Hsin), Graham Shiels (Night Watchman), B. D. Wong (Det. Glen Chao), Paul Wong (Wiry Man), Michael Yama (Shuyang Hsin)

Mulder and Scully are called in to a situation where a Chinese immigrant has been burned alive in a crematorium and another dead man has a living frog inside his body. What seems to be a Chinese spirit at work turns out to be an ancient secret cult that holds a lottery in which participants wager parts of their body against the financial jackpot.

❊ ❊ ❊

"I had two different ideas," says writer Jeff Vlaming. "One dealt with a lottery in a small town — you know, Nowhere, USA — and the

At the end of this episode one is left wondering just what the hell that show was about.

other was about the goings-on in Chinatown where a corporate being assembles the destitute. It was all very mystical, and Chris just combined the two ideas, turning it into a lottery story involving organs. I thought this would be the episode the audience has been waiting for, where Scully is right. But in the end, Mulder came out to be the guy who put it all together."

Co-producer Paul Rabwin admits to not being a fan of this episode, primarily because he feels it was never really an X-File. "If you can take Mulder and Scully out of the show and it doesn't change anything, it's not an X-File. They weren't affected personally, and the other characters weren't affected by them. That's what makes the series unique: it's got great interaction."

Like season two's "Irresistible" and "Grotesque" earlier in season three, "Hell

Money" represented a show that suggests the paranormal without completely filling that bill.

"I think the paranormal is a great big all-encompassing label," offers Chris Carter. "I still feel that 'Grotesque' and 'Hell Money' in fact were paranormal. Though they may not have been directly or high conceptually paranormal, they both have elements of the paranormal. I like those episodes very much, much like I'm very fond of 'Irresistible,' which other people have cited as a non-paranormal X-File. But I still think those are, for me, certainly another way to look at the show, just as Darin Morgan has found a unique way of looking at the show."

Rating/Audience Share: 9.8/17

Episode 3.20 (#69)
"Jose Chung's *From Outer Space*"
Original airdate: April 12, 1996
Written by Darin Morgan
Directed by Rob Bowman
Guest starring: Terry Arrowsmith (Air Force Man), Jaap Broekar (Yappi), Alex Diakun (Dr. Fingers), Michael Dobson (Lt. Jack Sheaffer), Jason Gaffney (Harold Lamb), William Lucking (Roky Crikenson), Mina Mina (Dr. Hand), Larry Musser (Det. Manners), Charles Nelson Reilly (Jose Chung), Sarah Sawatsky (Chrissy Giorgio), Andrew Turner (CIA Man), Jesse Venture (Man in Black #1), Allan Zynyk (Blaine Faulkner)

174

Alien abductions or a government campaign of disinformation? That is the question addressed in what is undoubtedly the most bizarre and surreal episode of The X-Files *ever produced. Scully is interviewed by famed author Jose Chung, who is trying to expose the truth about alien abductions. A variety of conflicting stories unfold and grow more strange as they go on, leaving the viewer with just one question when the episode concludes: What the hell was that show about?*

✣ ✣ ✣

"I had the pieces for that script for a really long time," says Darin Morgan. "Where Gillian's abductors get abducted — I really thought that was neat. I had done research on hypnosis, and I'd read a book about government cover-ups of UFOs. The author believes UFOs exist, but doesn't think there are alien craft or beings from some other planet. He believes it's a phenomenon that somehow manipulates time and space. His point is that our government doesn't know what to believe or what to do about it, so they try to use it for their own purposes. Talking about whether or not it is true is something I found interesting.

"Some people like the show, some people hate it. I really like the show. For whatever reason, this one required me to watch it. I had to watch it so many times before it was finished that I got sick of it, but I think it turned out good. It was jam-packed with stuff. You usually don't see that on an hour television show. I actually learned a great deal about production, which you can't really learn as a writer until you do it. Writing is one thing and production is another. Overall, I learned that some of my stuff will work. When you are writing scripts you have no idea whether or not it is going to work or whether people will understand it. So this show provided me with a chance to see that people will understand my stuff."

One person who barely "understood his stuff" was director Rob Bowman. "A difficult show," he says, "because I had to speak to the writer and say, 'What was your intention here?' I can honestly tell you that there was probably not one person in Vancouver and probably one or two in Los Angeles who knew what the hell was up with that script. Darin Morgan has his own voice, and maybe his scripts are not quintessential *X-Files*, but they are certainly entertaining. After reading the script fifteen times, and then having about an eight-hour session with Darin in my hotel room, I was into this script deep. I did a great deal of storyboarding and whatnot, because this was a puzzle. This was an episode that was not 'follow-the-bouncing-ball.' We were going to present different pictures to you. It would be up to you to line them up. So it is my job to make sure each one of those pictures is perfect and that the transition from scene to scene propels you

forward or backward clearly, and to get the tone of every actor and every line perfectly, because it affects the overall concept. So it was a mind-blowing episode. It was a ball-buster, but that is not to say this script is a better or worse script than 'Pusher.' It's a

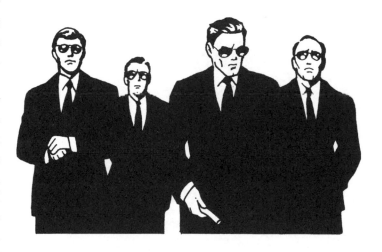

different script. This is more of a mosaic, and it is so thick and complicated that it is up to me, the storyteller, to be as simple and direct as I can. A very difficult show to do, but a very satisfying one as well.

"As wacky as the episode was," Bowman continues, "it still had the *X-Files* creepiness and truthfulness to it, and I think it could have easily been screwed up and become a comedy. I was hellbent on making sure that Mulder and Scully were true to themselves. They were not going to be funny, they were going to be real. They were on a case. Mulder and Scully had to drive us to this thing, so they had to be themselves so we could trust them. Then

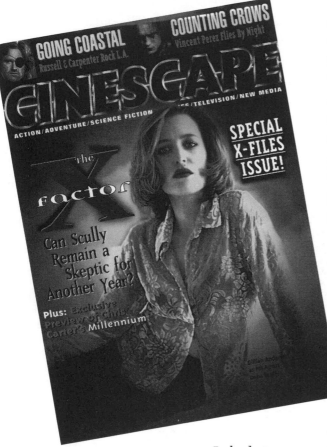

I had to see how I could color it. It was just a fun bit of orchestration, and it was very expensive. But it is an episode that really puts a spin on the expectations of an *X-Files* viewer. They turn on the show on Friday night and they see that episode and think, 'Boy, you can never predict what you are going to get on this show.'"

Another member of the totally confused "Jose Chung" fan club is Robert Goodwin. "I must have read that script a dozen times and never understood it," the co–executive pro-

ducer says sheepishly. "Even Darin Morgan, who wrote it, didn't understand it. In reality, it is one of those shows you have to see to get. You can't get it by reading it. It is extremely confusing, because so much of it is flashbacks told from one character's point of view or another character's point of view. Until you put it all together and can visually follow what is happening, it doesn't make any sense. So the biggest problem we had was understanding what the hell they were talking about. What was going on, who was doing what to who, is this scene real or someone's point of view? It became a true challenge, I think, directorially more than anything else, because the director had to keep all these lines going as to which was the flashback and which was real.

"The most fun on that episode," Goodwin adds, "was the casting of Charles Nelson Reilly. I couldn't wait to watch dailies, because he is hysterical when he is doing the dialogue, but even funnier when he goes off it. He forgets his lines. If you saw the dailies, you would die. I don't know how Gillian could continue to act because it was so funny. As opposed to Peter Boyle, who arrived not wanting to do the show, Charles definitely wanted to do it, was thrilled doing it, and could not thank me enough."

Of Darin Morgan's overall contribution to the series, Chris Carter notes, "It's been a wonderful coincidence of timing, talent, and the success of the show, allowing it to stretch in a direction it would never have been able to if it had been less successful or if it had been a younger show. Darin is a truly original comic mind. I don't know anybody in the world working in film, and that's what we work in here even though it appears on television, who has the voice Darin has. He is one in many million."

Co-producer Paul Rabwin proclaims, "An instant classic. One of those seminal episodes. You know, when people talk about *The Twilight Zone*, they say 'Remember "Eye of the Beholder"?' Or 'Trouble With Tribbles' on the original *Star Trek*. 'Jose Chung' is going to be one of those episodes that is immediately revered."

Rabwin also remembers a particular post-production challenge of the episode. "There's a sequence where this guy is found wandering naked on the streets. Mulder passes by him. We had this very long shot of this naked man coming out of the bushes. In fact, he was really in a body suit, so it didn't show anything anyone might care about, but he appeared to be without clothes. Standards and Practices came down and scrutinized it. We couldn't see anything, but as far as they were concerned it was the *impression* of a naked person, and they didn't want to show that. So we had Mat Beck, our visual effects producer, take the headlight beam from Mulder's car from the distance and put one of these big left-to-right horizontal beams that totally wiped out the whole center of the screen. So we had this headlight beam covering the man's body between his belly button and his knees. It

looks okay, but that's about as big a stretch that they've had us go."

Rating/Audience Share: 10.5/19

Episode 3.21 (#70) "Avatar"

Original airdate: April 26, 1996
Teleplay by Howard Gordon
Story by David Duchovny and Howard Gordon
Directed by James Charleston
Guest starring: Brendan Beiser (Dr. Rick Newton), William B. Davis (Cigarette-Smoking Man), Stacy Grant (Judy Fairly), Jennifer Hetrick (Sharon Skinner), Tom Mason (Det. Waltos), Morris Paynch (Gray-Haired Man), Mitch Pileggi (Assistant Director Walter S. Skinner), Bethoe Shirkoff (Old Woman), Michael David Simms (Senior Agent), Tasha Simms (Jay Cassal), Malcolm Stewart (Special Agent Bonnecaze), Amanda Tapping (Carina Sayles), Cal Traversy (Young Detective), Janie Woods-Morris (Lorraine Kelleher)

Walter Skinner is accused of murder when he awakens in a hotel room next to the corpse of a slain prostitute. Suspicion of him mounts when it's revealed that he doesn't remember what happened to the woman, his marriage is about to end in divorce, and he is seeing a psychiatrist for a severe sleep disorder. Mulder and Scully try their best to clear him of these charges, but things don't look good. Skinner's salvation lies in the apparition of an elderly woman who continues to materialize before him.

❈   ❈   ❈

"This began as a germ of an idea that David Duchovny came up with," says Howard Gordon. "It came from David saying, 'Mitch [Pileggi] is a great guy and Skinner is a great character; we don't use him enough.' He and I had been talking about doing another episode entirely, but we felt it was a good time in the season to deal a little more with Skinner rather than his just being a curmudgeonly foil for them.

"The story evolved and, again, I think it became more psychological than supernatural. I think in the best *X-Files* fashion it left to the imagination whether these apparitions Skinner was seeing were for real or not. What's interesting is that it examined this character in some depth. We saw what work meant to him and how this closed-off part of him had forced his marriage to end, even though this apparition came to him begging him to open himself up to the possibility of love, basically. In a very broadstroke way it attached the idea of a conspiracy to him. It then of course touched on Skinner's function in the *X-Files*. He served as Mulder and Scully's patron, sort of, and knocking him out was one way to weaken the power of Mulder and Scully."

Robert Goodwin notes that the episode introduced a new director to the series, James Charleston. "He came in and worked very hard during prep and he had great ideas," says Goodwin. "He shot it very visually and right on schedule. The funny part about that show is that the whole episode was written for rain. It was about how the constant rain was driving people to madness and depression. Every day we shot, it was bright and sunny and we had to keep making our own rain — in Vancouver! People always talk about how the rain always helps with the mood of the show. It is true, but we're fighting sunlight just as often as we fight the rain."

Rating/Audience Share: 9.3/16

Episode 3.22 (#71)
"Quagmire"
Original airdate: May 3, 1996
Written by Kim Newton
Directed by Kim Manners
Guest starring: Mark Acheson (Ted Bertram), R. Nelson Brown (Ansel Bray), Chris Ellis (Sheriff Lance Hindt), Peter Hanlon (Dr. William Bailey), Terrance Leigh (Snorkel Dude), Murray Lowry (Fisherman), Nicole Parker (Chick), Timothy Webber (Dr. Paul Farraday)

A "frog holocaust" in Georgia draws Mulder and Scully in, particularly after reports of a

Loch Ness Monster type of creature in the waters. Scully is more skeptical than ever, though that skepticism is put to the test when body parts start appearing, and she and Mulder witness actual attacks.

✵ ✵ ✵

"Not a great show, but a good one," opines Kim Manners. "It's a lighter show. There is a lot of humor in it, but I think it's a hit with fans because there is some wonderful Mulder and Scully relationship stuff. The entire third act is just the two of them talking, which is actually kind of interesting.

"The episode was a challenge to me because it is what I call a 'blue sky' show. There are very few interiors. It is all outside on a lake, and that is tough. One of the reasons *The X-Files* works is that it's dark and we're in tight, cramped, scary places. Now suddenly you are under a canopy — how do you make that scary? I just had to do my best to make the attack scenes scary with this secret monster. It actually does chew up quite a few people, so that part of it worked nicely. Overall, though, it is not the way I would have chosen to go out of the season. I would have liked to have another 'Grotesque.'"

Notes Robert Goodwin, "It's always difficult working with water, on water, around water — anything to do with water, especially up here because, as I've said, everything is glacially fed so it's freezing cold. Everyone has to have wetsuits, and you can only be in the water for a certain amount of time. So that was the big challenge. I also happen to like the very last shot of the show: Mulder kills this creature that has been killing off these people and it's a huge fourteen-foot alligator, and the last shot as he walks by, you hold on the water and see this sea monster go by."

Rating/Audience Share: 10.2/18

Episode 3.23 (#72)
"Wetwired"
Original airdate: May 10, 1996
Written by Mat Beck
Directed by Rob Bowman
Guest starring: Linden Banks (Joseph Patnik), Tom Braidwood (Frohike), Colin Cunningham (Dr. Henry Stroman), William B. Davis (Cigarette-Smoking Man), Dean Haglund (Langly), Bruce Harwood (Byers), Sheila Larken (Margaret Scully), Zinaid Memisevic (Lladoslav Miriskovic), Mitch Pileggi (Assistant Director Walter S. Skinner), Sandy Tucker (Helene Riddock), Steven Williams (Mr. X)

A wide variety of sudden homicides in Maryland attracts the attention of Mulder and Scully. They learn that everyone involved watched an awful lot of televison. When Scully begins acting erratically and, eventually, psychotically, Mulder comes to the conclusion that somehow the populace is being manipulated by their television signals.

❄ ❄ ❄

"I dug the script," says Rob Bowman. "I felt it was a good old-fashioned show, and people who didn't like 'Jose Chung' would like 'Wetwired' because all the bad boys are back. Again, the objective was to guide the performances so that Scully proceeds into her state of paranoid delusion naturally. A good clean steak-and-potatoes type of episode."

Interestingly, the episode ends with X getting into a car with the Cigarette-Smoking Man, adding further layers to this enigmatic character.

"Wetwired" was written by special-effects producer Mat Beck, whose imagination was obviously piqued from working on the series.

Rating/Audience Share: 9.7/17

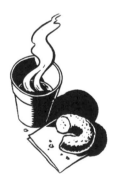

Episode 3.24 (#73)
"Talitha Cumi"

Original airdate: May 17, 1996
Teleplay by Chris Carter
Story by David Duchovny and Chris Carter
Directed by R. W. Goodwin
Guest starring: Brian Barry (Last Man), Ross Clarke (Pleasant Man), William B. Davis (Cigarette-Smoking Man), Stephen Dimopoulos (Detective), Bonnie Hay (Night Nurse), Hrothgar Mathews (Galen Muntz), Mitch Pileggi (Assistant Director Walter S. Skinner), Roy Thinnes (Jeremiah Smith), Angelo Vacco (Doorman), Steven Williams (Mr. X)

The notion of aliens among us intensifies when Jeremiah Smith heals the wounds of several shooting victims with the palms of his hands. Later, we learn that he is well known to the Cigarette-Smoking Man, and the implication is that CSM is working closely with the aliens in preparation for the day of colonization. Meanwhile, Mulder's mother is hospitalized with a stroke shortly after meeting with CSM (where it's revealed that they knew each other far better than anyone previously suspected), and Mulder sees the healing powers of Smith as her only hope. He never finds out, however, because he and Scully discover themselves about to engage in a deadly tug of war with the Pilot, the alien bounty hunter (from season two's "Colony" and "End Game"), whose mission is to kill Smith.

✿ ✿ ✿

For Robert Goodwin, who directed the episode, the toughest part was the opening sequence in the fast-food restaurant where several people are shot and Jeremiah Smith heals them.

"If you watch it closely," he explains, "you see that the scene is made up of a trillion tiny pieces of film, and in order to get a trillion tiny pieces of film, you have to shoot them all. That's the way I thought it should be shot to be most effective. It's all handheld. I used two cameras. If you look at it, you'll see all these little cuts where it actually jumps and cuts from one position to another. That makes it more scary. The Jeremiah Smith character, who's supposed to be Godlike, was always on Steadicam. Everybody else was jumping, moving, fast, panning, jump to that, and he was always rock steady. In his first appearance I overcranked, which means he was actually in slow motion. The music helped that too. It is very quick and something that is only subliminal, but I think it has a psychological impact on the audience. It makes the Roy Thinnes character something other than real."

Another highlight for Goodwin was a scene between the Cigarette-Smoking Man and Jeremiah Smith, in which the latter morphs into the image of Deep Throat.

"It was hard to do only because when you do those things, you have to use a video splitter and basically do the first half of the morph," he explains. "So you film the first half of the scene with Roy Thinnes. He lowers his head into position, and then you cut. Then you put Jerry Hardin [Deep Throat] in, and you get him into the chair and everything else ready to go. You run a videotape of what you shot with Thinnes, freeze that moment at the end where he has his head down, and then you can have Jerry on a separate scene just to

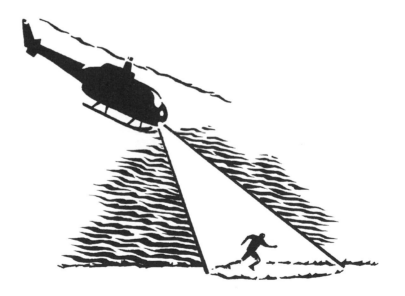

the right of that, getting into position. They are also about to superimpose one over the other on the video, so you are lining them up almost perfectly. The problem was that Jerry had a movie he had to do when we were shooting. We shot all that stuff in the prison on the last day and Jerry couldn't work that day. So Chris had to direct Jerry's part in the scene three days earlier. He videotaped that and I had to do the morph backwards: I had to match Roy to Jerry instead. That was actually quite difficult to match up. I got Jerry on tape and froze him in position. Of course, it's not just a question of position, but you have to have the same lens size, the camera position has to be the same, everything has to line up where it will work seamlessly. So that was difficult.

"The other morph, where Smith changes into Mulder's father and then back again was easier," he adds. "He looks down and he then looks back up and he's the father. That was easy because I had both of them there. In that case you set up the camera, stop, cut, put in the actor, and do it again. The camera is already in the correct position."

There are moments in "Talitha Cumi" that indicate alien colonization is a process that may be starting shortly. Indeed, it's an accusation Mulder actually makes in the episode. Chris Carter, however, just smiles when it's brought to his attention.

"If you go back and look at that episode very carefully, you'll see there were things posited but nothing ever addressed," he says. "I would suggest that anyone who feels they are now zeroing in on what we are doing, make sure they stay tuned for the opener of season four."

Rating/Audience Share: 11.2/21

The X-Phile Encyclopedia
SEASONS ONE—THREE

All entries are based on the original shooting teleplays.

001013: FBI Special Agent Dana Scully's e-mail account number. ["End Game"]

000517: FBI Special Agent Fox Mulder's e-mail account number. ["End Game"]

Note: The pilot episode (episode #1 in the series) is the only one that has no story title.

[A]

ABRAMOWITZ PLUMBING: The name on the side of a panel truck that is actually being used as cover by government agents. ["The Erlenmeyer Flask"]

ADAMS, MRS.: She is working at the blood drive table at a department store in Franklin, Pennsylvania. ["Blood"]

ADULT VIDEO NEWS: The trade magazine of the adult movie industry. Scully catches Mulder reading a copy. ["Beyond the Sea"]

ADVANCED RESEARCH PROJECT AGENCY: The government agency behind the **Arctic Ice Core Project.** ["Ice"]

AHAB: Scully's pet name for her father, taken from the main character of Herman Melville's novel *Moby Dick.* ["Beyond the Sea"]

AIKLEN, STAFF SGT. KEVIN: A soldier whose case is oddly similar to that of **Lt. Col. Victor Stans.** His family died in a fire, and Aiklen tried to commit suicide by throwing himself into a wood chipper. Like Stans, Aiklen claims that someone would not let him die. ["The Walk"]

AIR FORCE: One of the people who interrogates **Chrissy Giorgio.** At first she remembers him as looking like a Gray Alien. ["Jose Chung's *From Outer Space*"]

AGUIRRE, RUDY: The instructor of the art class at **George Washington University.** ["Grotesque"]

AL-HADITHI, MOHAMMED: An Iraqi military officer who sees UFOs on radar which apparently attack a jet. ["E.B.E."]

ALLEGIANCE, USS: The U.S. Navy nuclear submarine on a cartography mission that encounters the **Pilot**'s submerged spacecraft and is disabled by it when the sub tries to follow orders and destroy the UFO. When Mulder reaches the submarine stranded in the ice, he finds all its crew members dead, apparently done in by the Pilot, an alien assassin. The sole survivor, Lt. **Terry Wilmer,** is actually the Pilot, who uses the vessel to get back to his own ship. ["End Game"]

ALIEN AUTOPSY: Captured on videotape, it was conducted inside a train car on a siding in Knoxville, Tennessee. Soldiers dressed in black burst into the train car in the middle of the autopsy, shot the four Japanese doctors, and took the Gray Alien corpse away in a body bag. A satellite dish on the top of the train car had been broadcasting the autopsy at the time of the hit on the doctors, and this broadcast was intercepted by someone in **Allentown, Pennsylvania.** ["Nisei"]

ALIEN BOUNTY HUNTER: An alien who hunts down and kills alien clones. ["Talitha Cumi," "Colony," and "End Game"] He reappears in "Talitha Cumi" and is clearly bent on assassinating the gentle alien clone, **Jeremiah Smith.**

ALLENTOWN POLICE SUB-STATION: Where Mulder and Scully take the Japanese man they catch at the scene of a murder. Not only does the man turn out to supposedly be a diplomat, but Assistant Director **Walter S. Skinner** comes to Allentown himself to secure the man's release (see also **Rat Tail Productions** and **Kazuo Takeo**). ["Nisei"]

ALLENTOWN, PENNSYLVA-NIA: Where a man intercepted the satellite transmission of an alien autopsy. He sells copies of it on videotape for $29.95 plus shipping. ["Nisei"]

ALTA: A Navy icecutter that observed a UFO going down in the Beaufort Sea, north of the Arctic Circle; the crew of the *Alta* rescued the alien **Pilot,** who led them to believe he was the survivor of a Russian plane crash. ["Colony"]

ALT.-FUELS INC.: Runs a **methane research facility.** Their motto is "Waste is a terrible thing to waste." ["War of the Coprophages"]

AMARU: A powerful female shaman, whose remains are discovered in their sacred burial urn in Ecuador by **Dr. Alonso Bilac** and **Dr. Carl Roosevelt.** Roosevelt is killed under mysterious circumstances at the dig where the Amaru Urn was discovered; it is brought to the Boston Museum of Natural History in accordance with his final wishes. His body was never recovered. ["Teso dos Bichos"]

AMBASSADOR HOTEL: Where Walter Skinner picks up a woman, takes her to his room, and wakes up the next morning to find her lying dead next to him. ["Avatar"]

AMBROSE, WILLA: A naturalist brought in by the Board of Supervisors to oversee activities at the **Fairfield Zoo** in Idaho. She's questioned about how **Ganesha,** an elephant, somehow escaped from her locked cage. When Ambrose began working for the zoo, one of the first things she did was to prohibit the use of chains holding elephants in place. ["Fearful Symmetry"]

AMERICAN RONIN: A guns-and-mercenaries magazine Robert Modell used to advertise his talents as a killer. The ads lead Mulder and Scully to a pay phone in Virginia, where Modell calls to taunt them and leave a clue. ["Pusher"]

AMRITH: A viscous, honeylike substance sometimes produced during magical rituals. Amrith oozes from the walls of **Charlie Holvey**'s hospital room when the **Calusari** perform the Ritual of Separation. ["The Calusari"]

AMROLLI, MOHAMMED: A terrorist linked with the radical Iranian group known as Isfahan. He and an accomplice attempted to kill **Lauren Kyte,** only to be killed by the ghost of **Howard Graves.** Mulder identifies the body by covertly getting a fingerprint on his glasses. ["Shadows"]

ANAPHYLACTIC SHOCK: Fatal reaction to an insect bite. ["War of the Coprophages"]

ANASAZI: A Native American tribe that vanished from the New Mexico area some six hundred years ago. Anthropologists have determined that the Anasazi practiced cannibalism. ["Our Town"] According to **Albert Hosteen,** their name means "ancient aliens." Hosteen claims the Anasazi were carried away by aliens. ["Anasazi"]

ANKUSES: Poles used by animal trainers to control elephants. ["Fearful Symmetry"]

ANNAPOLIS SAVINGS AND LOAN: The first bank robbed by **Warren James Dupre** and **Lula Philips,** on May 9, 1993. ["Lazarus"]

ANTHROPOMANCY: The ancient art of predicting the future by studying the entrails of a disemboweled human being. Mulder refers to this practice at the scene of the **Doll Collector**'s murder. The killer (see **Puppet**) has left part of his victim's intestines

184

sitting on a table next to her eyes. ["Clyde Bruckman's Final Repose"]

ANTONIO: A subordinate of a high-ranking Italian diplomat in the United Nations, Antonio informs his superior that the **MJ documents** have been stolen. ["Anasazi"]

ARCTIC ICE CORE PROJECT: A scientific expedition to study the Earth's past climate by drilling for samples of very deep Arctic ice. After several months, the project team, headed by **John Richter,** draws samples from depths of nearly two miles. This unusual depth is due to a meteor strike eons earlier; the samples contain an ancient alien microorganism that infects the team members with a parasite that encourages violent behavior, resulting in their deaths. Two more victims succumb to the virus in the course of the X-Files investigation: **Bear,** a pilot, dies, while **Dr. Nancy Da Silva** is cured. The site is destroyed by the government after the survivors are airlifted out. ["Ice"]

ARDEN, HAL: A seventy-four-year-old Alzheimer's patient at the Excelsis Dei Convalescent Home for eight years. Nurse **Michelle Charters** claims he raped her, only he was invisible at the time of the attack

. . . or so she says. Shortly thereafter, Arden is killed by an unseen force after he threatens to reveal a secret about the capsules of drugs **Gung Bituen** has been giving them. Traces of ibotenic acid, a powerful hallucinogen, are found in his body. ["Excelsis Dei"]

ARGENT, USS: A destroyer escort, commissioned in 1991 by the U.S. Navy and commanded by **Capt. Phillip Barclay,** the *Argent* was reported lost in the North Atlantic. By the time Mulder and Scully reach it, it looks as if it had been there for thirty years. Advanced corrosion has caused the ship to "bleed" rust. Mulder and Scully are rescued by Navy SEALs and taken to Bethesda, where Scully's detailed notes on their experience help save their lives. The ship sinks after its inner hull corrodes away. ["Dod Kalm"]

ARECIBO IONOSPHERIC OBSERVATORY: Site of a radio telescope in Arecibo, Puerto Rico, which is shut down after the project designed to scan the sky for radio transmissions of an intelligent extraterrestrial origin is terminated by **Sen. Richard Bryon.** This dormant station becomes mysteriously reactivated when it receives a trans-

mission recorded from the Voyager spacecraft years after the Voyager left our solar system. ["Little Green Men"]

ARENS, SHERIFF TOM: The seemingly friendly sheriff of **Dudley, Arkansas,** who explains away the scorch marks in a nearby field as illegal trash burning. As the masked executioner in the cannibalistic rituals performed in Dudley, Arens is on the verge of decapitating Scully when he is shot dead by Mulder. ["Our Town"]

ARGOTYPOLINE: A highly flammable rocket fuel that **Cecil L'ively** [a.k.a **Bob**] mixes with paint in order to accelerate fires started with his pyrokinetic powers. ["Fire"]

ARLINGTON, VIRGINIA: The Washington suburb where the **Holvey** family lives at the time of the deaths of Teddy, Steve, and Golda. Scully encounters the malevolent ghost of Michael Holvey in the Holvey house. ["The Calusari"] Also the location of a fast-food restaurant where a robbery and shootings take place. But the victims do not die because **Jeremiah Smith** is there and he heals all the injured. ["Talitha Cumi"]

ARMY: One of the people who interrogates **Chrissy Giorgio.** At first she remembers him as looking like a Gray Alien.

["Jose Chung's *From Outer Space*"]

ASTADOURIAN LIGHTNING OBSERVATORY: A scientific facility located near **Connerville, Oklahoma,** where scientists study lightning, and produce it with hundreds of ionized rods pointed at the sky. ["D.P.O."]

ASTRAL PROJECTION: The psychic ability to leave one's physical body. **Sgt. "Rappo" Trimble** has this power, which he uses to murder the families of his enemies. Mulder carries dental x-ray film to various murder scenes in order to detect radiation traces associated with this phenomenon. ["The Walk"]

ATKINSON, MIKE: Employee of the Mutual UFO Network (MUFON). ["Irresistible"]

ATLANTIC CITY, NEW JERSEY: The police here covered up a series of brutal murders involving the homeless. ["The Jersey Devil"] Bank robbers **Warren James Dupre** and **Lula Philips** were married here in May 1993. ["Lazarus"]

ATSUMI, LEZA: The special agent who explains, with considerable skepticism, that all of the binary figures written down by **Kevin Morris** can be deciphered, including fragments of Shakespeare's sonnets, the Koran, and Bach's Brandenburg Concertos. ["Conduit"]

AUERBACH, DR. SIMON: One of the doctors involved in **Pinck Pharmaceuticals'** unethical test of a newly discovered disease at the **Cumberland State Correctional Facility,** and the ensuing cover-up. ["F. Emasculata"]

925 AUGUST STREET: The address in Dinwiddie County, Virginia, of **Elizabeth,** the girlfriend of the escaped convict **Paul.** Mulder and U.S. marshals arrest her here, and find another escapee dead of *F. Emasculata.* ["F. Emasculata"]

AUSBURY, JIM: A member of a coven in Milford Haven, New Hampshire. His sixteen-year-old stepdaughter, Shannon, accuses him of having abused her when she was a small child. He is eaten by a python and reduced to bones. ["Die Hand Die Verletzt"]

AUSBURY, BARBARA: Jim's wife. She doesn't believe the accusations against him. ["Die Hand Die Verletzt"]

AUSBURY, SHANNON: She complains of witnessing occult rites as a child and claims she had three babies who were killed by the coven, and that her sister was murdered when she was eight. Shannon is later killed by the black magic of the demon in the form of **Phyllis Paddock.** ["Die Hand Die Verletzt"]

AUSTIN, DR.: A physician at the National Institutes of Health who provides Mulder and Scully with information about **Dr. Joe Ridley**'s progeria studies and the unethical activities that led to his dismissal. ["Young at Heart"]

AVALON FOUNDATION: A cryogenics facility where the head of **Dr. Arthur Grable** is preserved in liquid nitrogen. Grable died in a car accident and his body was too badly damaged to be frozen as well. ["Roland"]

[B]

BAILEY, DR. WILLIAM: Member of the U.S. Forestry Service. He rejects **Dr. Paul Farraday**'s request to place the frog known as the *Rana Sphenocephala* on the endangered species list, deeming Farraday's results inconclusive. Moments later, something comes out of the lake and drags him into the water to his doom. ["Quagmire"]

BAKER, DR. AARON: One of the **Gregor** clones, killed by the **Pilot** in his home in Syracuse, New York. ["Colony"]

BALBOA NAVAL HOSPITAL: Military hospital in San Diego where the crewmen of the *Piper Maru* are treated for radiation burns. [*"Piper Maru"*]

BANANA CREAM PIE: The dessert Mulder steps in shortly before being attacked by the **Puppet** in a hotel kitchen, as predicted by **Clyde Bruckman.** ["Clyde Bruckman's Final Repose"]

BANTON, DR. CHESTER RAY: A brilliant scientist who built an incredibly compact particle accelerator for use in his studies of subatomic particles, particularly dark matter, at Polarity Magnetics. While bombarding an alpha target with beta particles, Banton got in the way and received a massive dose of particles, which burned his shadow onto the wall but miraculously did not kill him. Instead, his shadow somehow became a separate entity of dark matter, which can kill people by completely absorbing their mass and energy. Banton suspects that the shadow might be able to survive without him. Abducted by **X,** he is now undergoing top-secret government testing at an undisclosed location. ["Soft Light"]

BARBALA, RUDY: Detective at Buffalo's 14th Precinct. He is killed by the psychic powers of eight-year-old **Michelle Bishop.** We later learn that he was responsible for the murder of a police officer nine years before. ["Born Again"]

BARCLAY, CAPT. PHILLIP: Commander of the *USS Argent.* His alcoholism actually prolongs his life when his ship's crew experiences accelerated aging due to **free radicals** in their drinking water, but it does not keep eighteen crew members from abandoning ship. Found on his ship by Mulder and Scully, he tells them the ship has begun to bleed. Barclay is the last of his crew to die. ["Dod Kalm"]

BARNETT, JOHN EARVIN: A dangerous criminal from New Hampshire whose extremely violent armed robberies have taken the lives of seven people. Barnett, Mulder's first assignment out of the FBI academy in 1989, killed his hostage and FBI agent **Steve Wallenberg** before being apprehended, convicted, and sentenced to 340 years in the Tashmoo Federal Correctional Facility, where he is experimented on by prison doctor **Joe Ridley,** who reverses his aging process and amputates his right arm, replacing it with one grown from salamander cells. Reported dead of cardiac fail-

ure on September 16, 1989, and supposedly cremated and scattered along the Delaware River, Barnett is actually alive — and younger than ever. Several years later he returns to get revenge on Mulder, killing a jewelry store clerk and FBI agent **Reggie Purdue** and shooting Scully before his death. Scully is saved by her bulletproof vest. ["Young at Heart"]

BARNEY: A purple TV dinosaur popular with children, but eight-year-old **Cindy Reardon** prefers to watch congressional investigations on television. ["Eve"] Also the name of one of the Richmond, Virginia, policemen killed by **Chester Ray Banton**'s shadow. ["Soft Light"]

BARON, DET. BRADLEY: A senior detective on the Richmond, Virginia, police force who supervises **Kelly Ryan**'s first (and last) case. He is perplexed to learn of Mulder and Scully's involvement when he comes to arrange **Chester Ray Banton**'s transfer from the Yaloff Psychiatric Hospital to the city jail. ["Soft Light"]

BARRINGTON, DR. LAWRENCE: A doctor at the Avalon Foundation, a cryogenics institute. ["Roland"]

BARRY, DUANE: A former FBI agent with an impeccable

record who left the Bureau in 1982. The official story is that he was shot in the brain with his own weapon while on a drug stakeout in the woods, rendering him a dangerous psychotic with severe delusions. Barry believes himself to have been abducted by aliens on numerous occasions and implanted with various devices. He escapes from the Davis Correctional Treatment Center on August 7, 1994, with his psychiatrist as hostage and holes up in a travel agency, taking other hostages; Mulder negotiates with him until a marksman shoots Barry in the chest. Medical examinations reveal mysterious pieces of metal in his gums, sinuses, and abdomen. The wounded Barry escapes from Jefferson Memorial Hospital in Richmond, Virginia, and kidnaps Scully from her home. ["Duane Barry"] Mulder later finds Barry on top of Skyland Mountain in Virginia, site of his first abduction by aliens; seemingly freed from his mental problems, Barry claims that aliens have taken Scully away in his place. Barry dies shortly afterward, possibly poisoned by **Alex Krycek.** ["Ascension"] Barry's name appears in the most recent entries of the encoded **MJ documents**

passed on to Mulder by the **Thinker,** alongside Scully's name ["Anasazi"]

BAUER, ERIC: A basketball player at Grover Cleveland Alexander High School in Comity. During a practice game he crashes into a table on the sidelines, spilling lemonade all over **Terri Roberts** and **Margi Kleinjan.** When he later goes to retrieve a basketball under the bleachers, the bleachers close on him, crushing him to death. ["Syzygy"]

BAUVAIS, PIERRE: A Haitian witch doctor and voodoo high priest. He's kept imprisoned by **Col. Jacob Wharton,** who is also secretly into voodoo. ["Fresh Bones"]

BAYSIDE FUNERAL HOME: San Francisco mortuary where a Chinese man is murdered in the crematorium. ["Hell Money"]

BEAR: The civilian pilot who flies Mulder, Scully, and their team from **Jimmy Doolittle Airfield** in Nome, Alaska, to Icy Cape. When an infected dog attacks him, Bear becomes infected by the ice worm microorganism, but covers up his symptoms. While he does not harm anyone as a result of his infection, he dies when the ice worm is removed from his

neck, making him its sixth victim. ["Ice"]

BEAR CREEK STATE PARK: Two escaped convicts from the **Cumberland State Correctional Facility** kill a father of two in the men's room at this Virginia park and steal his family's motor home, leaving the widow and orphans stranded. ["F. Emasculata"]

BEATTY, MELVIN: The FBI's arson specialist at the Washington office, he does not believe in spontaneous human combustion and postulates the use of an accelerant, such as argotypoline or other rocket fuel, in a series of arsons and murders later linked with the pyrokinetic **Cecil L'ively.** Beatty helps Scully devise a character profile of the arsonist. ["Fire"]

BEHEMOTH: A.k.a. Lord **Kinbote;** a.k.a. the Behemoth from the Planet Harryhausen. A real alien who kidnaps **Harold Lamb** and **Chrissy Giorgio,** along with two military men disguised as aliens (**Lt. Jack Sheaffer** and **Col. Robert Vallee**). ["Jose Chung's *From Outer Space*"]

BELIEVER: The name of one of the phony Gray Aliens who interrogate people they abduct. ["Jose Chung's *From Outer Space*"]

BELLEFLEUR, OREGON: The site of five mysterious deaths, where Scully and Mulder have their first mission together. [Pilot]

BELT, LT. COL. MARCUS AURELIUS: A former astronaut who went on to become head of the Viking Orbiter project, and eventually headed the space shuttle program. As head of the Viking program, Belt denied that the giant sculpted face reported on Mars was anything more than an optical illusion created by erosion. However, he knows this is not true: while spacewalking as an astronaut, he was possessed by a mysterious space entity, somehow related to the face, that has controlled him ever since. This almost leads him to sabotage a shuttle mission in the 1990s, but he unconsciously alerts communications commander **Michelle Generoo,** who in turn alerts the FBI. Realizing almost too late what he has done, he provides the information needed to save the shuttle flight, then jumps out a thirtieth-floor window in Houston. ["Space"]

BENNETT, DR. M.: Director of the **Luther Stapes Center for Reproductive Medicine.** Explains in vitro fertilization, or egg implantation, to Mulder and Scully and reveals that the **Simmons** family used the same procedure. Also reveals the reasons for **Dr. Sally Kendrick**'s dismissal from the Center. ["Eve"]

BERENDAUM, DR. BAMBI: A beautiful entomologist from the USDA Agricultural Research Service, she is studying what cockroaches respond to in order to better determine how to eliminate them. ["War of the Coprophages"]

BERNSTEIN, DANIEL: A cryptologist at FBI headquarters in Washington. He agrees to examine **Kevin Morris**'s handwriting in exchange for Mulder's tickets to a Redskins–Giants game. ["Conduit"]

BERTRAM, TED: The owner of Ted's Bait & Tackle on Heuvelmans Lake in Georgia. He's a huge **Big Blue** fan, although he's never actually seen it. He sells Big Blue souvenirs in his store and makes fake Big Blue footprints around the lake to maintain interest and lure tourists. One night while he's making the tracks, something snatches him and pulls him into the lake. Was he eaten by his hobby? ["Quagmire"]

BERUBE, DR. TERRENCE ALLEN: Graduated Harvard Med in 1974. Works on the **Human Genome Project** in the Molecular Research Lab at the EmGen Corporation in Gaithersburg, Maryland. He conducts experiments on human beings by injecting them with extraterrestrial DNA. ["The Erlenmeyer Flask"]

BETA TEAM: A military unit involved in **Operation Falcon,** headed by a **Lt. Fraser.** This unit corners the alien pilot, only to be blasted by an intense white light. Team members closest to the blast are obliterated; Fraser and Jackson suffer severe burns. Four members of Beta Team survive and are sent to the Johns Hopkins Burn Unit; they have not been identified. ["Fallen Angel"]

BETHANY MEDICAL CENTER: In Aubrey, Missouri. Where **Det B. J. Morrow** is taken after she claims she was attacked by **Harry Cokely.** ["Aubrey"]

BETHESDA NAVAL HOSPITAL: A renowned hospital in Bethesda, Maryland, where U.S. presidents are often treated. Mulder and Scully are called there to take a look at two corpses whose throats seem to have been crushed from the inside. ["Shadows"] FBI agent **Jack Willis** is revived here after being shot by **Warren James Dupre** in a bank shootout. ["Lazarus"] **Lt. Richard Harper** dies here, apparently of accelerated aging; Scully and Mulder are treated here for the same affliction, but survive, thanks to Scully's field notes and **Dr. Laskos.** ["Dod Kalm"]

BETHESDA SLEEP DISORDER CENTER: Where **Walter Skinner** had been receiving treatment for three months prior to the mysterious murder of **Carina Sayles.** Skinner had been experiencing a recurring dream in which he's confronted by an old woman. ["Avatar"]

"BEYOND THE SEA": A song recorded by Bobby Darin. It was playing on the radio when **William Scully** proposed to his wife in the late 1950s, and was played at his funeral service as well. **Luther Lee Boggs** sings it when he first meets Dana Scully. ["Beyond the Sea"]

BIG BLUE: The name given by locals to a mysterious serpent that lives in **Heuvelmans Lake** in Georgia. Mulder thinks Big Blue might just be a serpent serial killer, after people start vanishing at the lake and some turn up dead. Mulder thinks it might be a prehistoric plesiosaur. The killer in the lake turns out to be an alligator, and Mulder just misses catching a glimpse of Big Blue when he turns away moments before it appears on the surface of the lake under a full moon. ["Quagmire"]

THE BIG BOPPER: Stage name of J. P. Richardson, best known for his 1950s hit "Chantilly Lace." The Bopper was a passenger on the doomed airplane flight that also claimed the life of Buddy Holly. The young **Clyde Bruckman** was a big fan of the Bopper. Believing that the Bopper was on that airplane thanks to a fateful coin toss, he tells Mulder that his obsession with the chance nature of the Bopper's death eventually triggered his own psychic ability to foresee people's deaths. (In reality, it was Ritchie Valens who won his seat through the flip of a coin. The lucky person who lost the coin toss was Waylon Jennings.) ["Clyde Bruckman's Final Repose"]

BIG CITY HOSPITAL: In Providence, Rhode Island, where Mrs. Mulder is taken after she has a stroke. ["Talitha Cumi"]

BILAC, DR. ALONSO: A brilliant and impetuous archaeologist born in Brazil. He opposes **Dr. Carl Roosevelt**'s plans to take sacred Secona artifacts from Ecuador to the United States. He may have killed several people, including Roosevelt, because of his beliefs in this matter . . . or he may have been possessed by an ancient jaguar spirit. His mutilated body is found in the sewers beneath the Boston Museum of Natural History. ["Teso dos Bichos"]

BINGHAMPTON GLOBE & MAIL: A local newspaper in Binghampton, Pennsylvania, upstate from Scranton. It runs an ad featuring the face of the three identical doctors murdered by the **Pilot;** the ad leads Mulder to **Dr. Aaron Baker** in Syracuse, New York, but he arrives too late. The ad may have been placed by the Pilot, masquerading as CIA agent **Ambrose Chapel.** ["Colony"]

BIODIVERSITY PROJECT: The research project that brings **Dr. Robert Torrence** to Costa Rica in search of new biological samples. Presumed to have been sponsored by **Pinck Pharmaceuticals.** ["F. Emasculata"]

BISHOP, JUDY: The mother of **Michelle Bishop.** ["Born Again"]

BISHOP, JIM: Father of Michelle, who is now divorced from Judy. ["Born Again"]

BISHOP, MICHELLE: An eight-year-old girl in whom the

psychic spirit of a murdered policeman has emerged. She lives at 121 Shady Lane, Orchard Park, New York. When she is found alone near the 14th Precinct station in Buffalo, New York, and is taken into the station, she is interviewed by **Rudy Barbala,** whom she kills by using psychic powers to hurl him through a window to the street below. She is terrified of water and refuses to go swimming. ["Born Again"]

BITUEN, GUNG: An Asian orderly at the **Excelsis Dei Convalescent Home.** He's helping the old men who live there by giving them a special drug he extracts from mushrooms in the basement. The drug contains ibotenic acid, a powerful hallucinogen. ["Excelsis Dei"]

BLACK CROW MISSILE COMPLEX: Allegedly abandoned military site in North Dakota where a recovered alien craft is stored. Also the last resting place of **Alex Krycek.** ["Apocrypha"]

BLAINE, LT.: A Cleveland policeman who informs Mulder and Scully of the 911 call that leads to **Virgil Incanto.** ["2Shy"]

BLEDSOE, DR. ELLEN: The Philadelphia county medical examiner, who confirms that

Howard Graves is dead and provides the autopsy report to prove it. ["Shadows"]

THE BLESSING WAY: A Navajo Indian healing ceremony for those who are near death. It is used to save Mulder's life and give him insight into his mission. ["The Blessing Way"]

BLEVINS, SCOTT (SPECIAL AGENT IN CHARGE): Advises Scully that Mulder should not investigate events at **Ellens Air Force Base** in Idaho, as the case has been reclassified as a strictly military affair, but does not interfere, hoping the case will discredit Mulder. ["Deep Throat"] Intends to deny Mulder permission to pursue the disappearance of **Ruby Morris,** but is convinced otherwise by Scully. ["Conduit"] Arranges for Mulder and Scully to assist CIA agents Webster and Saunders. ["Shadows"] Blevins works in the violent-crime division of the FBI training facility at Quantico, Virginia, and assigns Scully to work with Mulder on the X-Files. [Pilot]

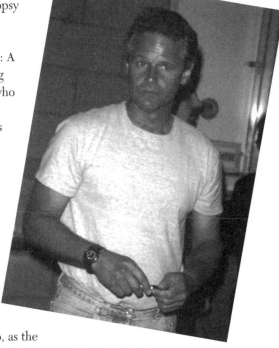

BLOCKHEAD, DR.: An escape artist who emerges from the ground beneath **Jerald Glazebrook**'s coffin at his funeral and proceeds to pound a spike into his own chest. **Sheriff Hamilton** is not amused. Dr. Blockhead claims to be from Yemen. His real name is Jeffrey Swaim and he's from Milwaukee. ["Humbug"]

BLUE BERET UFO RETRIEVAL TEAM: A secret government force dispatched to the site of any detected contact with extraterrestrials where evidence might be found. This team has the authority to kill any unauthorized personnel discovered at the site of a genuine UFO crash. ["Little Green Men"]

BLUE DEVIL BREWERY: In Morrisville, Virginia. **Lucas Jackson Henry** dies there while fleeing the law. As predicted by **Luther Lee Boggs,** he dies under the sign of the devil: the brewery's logo. ["Beyond the Sea"]

BLUE EARTH, IOWA: After Mulder is rescued from the **Quarantine Car** by **X,** an anonymous 911 call is placed from Blue Earth, Iowa, to come and pick up the injured FBI agent. ["731"]

BLUE RIDGE MOUNTAINS: The location of Heuvelmans Lake. ["Quagmire"]

BLUE "SAMANTHA": An alien clone in blue surgical garb whom Mulder meets at the **Women's Health Services Center** in Rockville, Maryland. She, along with the rest of the "Samantha" clones, is killed by the **Pilot.** ["End Game"]

BOAR'S HEAD: A tavern in Sioux City, Iowa, where Mulder goes to look for **Ruby Morris**'s alleged boyfriend, **Greg Randall.** Instead he meets a biker named **Kip,** who has a UFO tattoo. ["Conduit"]

BOB: The name used by **Cecil L'ively** during his activities in the United States. This is probably the name of the caretaker he killed and replaced at Lord and Lady **Marsden**'s Cape Cod retreat. ["Fire"]

BOCKS, MOE: A special agent for the FBI who calls on Mulder and Scully after he finds a grave desecrated in Minneapolis. ["Irresistible"]

BOGGS, LUTHER LEE: A multiple murderer who killed all the animals in his housing complex when he was a child of six; strangled five relatives at a Thanksgiving dinner when he was thirty; and embarked on a serial-killing spree, committing many more murders before being apprehended in 1985. Boggs was about to be executed in 1992 but the execution was stayed; he claims this near-death experience provided him with psychic channeling abilities. Boggs leads lawmen to the fugitive **Lucas Jackson Henry,** but whether this was due to psychic knowledge or to communication with Henry is uncertain. Boggs's second trip to the North Carolina gas chamber, in 1993, is not interrupted. ["Beyond the Sea"]

BOISE STREET: The escaped tiger from the **Fairfield Zoo** turns up near a fast-food restaurant here. **Ed Meecham** is forced to shoot and kill the tiger when the big cat moves to attack **Willa Ambrose.** ["Fearful Symmetry"]

BONAPARTE, CHESTER: A ten-year-old boy who greets Mulder and Scully at the Folkstone Processing Center. He sells Mulder a magic charm of protection. Chester later turns out to be a ghost. ["Fresh Bones"]

BONNECAZE, SPECIAL AGENT: He is going through the material in **Walter Skinner**'s office after the Assistant Director becomes the suspect in a murder. He tells Mulder that Skinner is also being investigated by the FBI in this matter. ["Avatar"]

BOSHAM, ENGLAND: A town seventy miles southwest of London, where **Cecil L'ively** was employed as a gardener on the estate of an aristocrat, whose death by fire he caused. ["Fire"]

BOULLE, PETER: A park ranger who found the body that attracted Mulder to the Atlantic City murders. At first he is tight-lipped, but later admits that he's seen the Devil and his traces. Close to retirement, he doesn't want to jeopardize his retirement benefits, but later goes out on a limb for Mulder and Scully. ["The Jersey Devil"]

BOZOFF, AGENT: Relieves Mulder of his boring surveillance duty so that he can go on his new assignment. ["The Host"]

BRADDOCK HEIGHTS, MARYLAND: A small town where some TV sets have been wired to receive a special signal that drives viewers to kill. ["Wetwired"]

BRAIDWOOD: One of the phony names used by Mulder and Scully to get inside a complex where an E.B.E. (extraterrestrial biological entity) is apparently being held. Braidwood is the name of the actor who played Frohike. ["E.B.E."]

BRAUN, DR. SHEILA: Developmental psychologist at Brylin Psychiatric Hospital who sees **Michelle Bishop** twice a week. ["Born Again"]

BRAY, ANSEL: A photographer who is an expert on **Big Blue,** the mysterious serpent that lives in **Heuvelmans Lake.** He's determined to get a photo of Big Blue that will leave him set for life, but gets swallowed by his ambition. ["Quagmire"]

BREM: FBI agent in charge of the tactical (SWAT) operations aspect of the **Duane Barry** hostage situation. ["Duane Barry"]

BRENMAN: A graduate student whom Scully interviews as a possible suspect in the fat-

sucking-vampire murders. The real perpetrator is **Virgil Incanto.** ["2Shy"]

BREWER, WESLEY: A trucker barreling down Route 7 near Fairfield, Idaho, who suddenly sees a ten-foot-tall elephant in the road in front of him. He's barely able to stop in time, whereupon the elephant turns and runs past the truck. ["Fearful Symmetry"]

BRIGGS, FRANK: A police detective who once hunted **Eugene Tooms,** he now lives at the dilapidated Lynn Acres Retirement Home, where Scully goes to see him to obtain information on one of the earlier crimes committed by Tooms years before. When Briggs was a sheriff investigating the Powhattan Mill murders in 1933, he suspected Tooms but could not indict him; he has collected evidence over the years, however, including photos of Tooms at the time of his 1963 murders. ["Squeeze" and "Tooms"]

BRIGHT WHITE PLACE: Where abductees claim they have been taken, but were they taken there by humans or by aliens? ["Nisei"]

BRISENTINE, AGENT: Tells Mulder that his new assignment is a murder in Newark, New Jersey, and that the reassignment request was made by

Assistant Director **Walter Skinner** himself. ["The Host"]

BRODEUR, LEO: The warden of **Eastpoint State Penitentiary,** who oversees the execution of **"Neech" Manley.** He believes the murders committed after Manley's death are the work of an accomplice, not of a reincarnated spirit. He beats the prisoner **Sammon Roque** in an attempt to find out who's on Manley's revenge list. Brodeur is number five on Manley's list, and dies in a car wreck with Manley's fingers around his throat. ["The List"]

BROTHER AARON: The member of the **Kindred** who collapses during Mulder and Scully's dinner with the religious group. His body is subjected to a strange ritual and placed in a hivelike crypt, where it undergoes an apparent gender transformation and is revived. ["Genderbender"]

BROTHER ANDREW: The member of the **Kindred** who offers to help Scully and Mulder, but then tries to seduce Scully with his pheromonic powers—possibly an attempt to kill her. He was the closest friend of the runaway Kindred named **Marty.** ["Genderbender"]

BROTHER OAKLEY: The member of the **Kindred** who

insists that Mulder and Scully give up their guns. ["Genderbender"]

BROTHER WILTON: The member of the **Kindred** who becomes angry at Mulder's questions but is censured by **Sister Abby** for expressing rage. Mulder suspects that the outbreak was an act intended to put an end to his questions. ["Genderbender"]

BROWN, DEBORAH: Member of a witches' coven. **Calcagni** kills her while he is under the domination of the demon. ["Die Hand Die Verletzt"]

BROWNING: The police pathologist who examines the burned and blackened body of the Son. ["3"]

BRUCKMAN, CLYDE: The first genuine psychic encountered by Mulder, Bruckman is an aging insurance salesman who possesses one paranormal ability: he can see the way people are destined to die. His greatest regret is his inability to guess the winning Lotto numbers. Scully mistakes Bruckman's prediction of his own final moments as a pass at her. After helping Mulder and Scully capture the serial killer known as the **Puppet,** Bruckman commits suicide with sleeping pills and a plastic bag. When Scully discovers his body, she is next to him, fulfill-

ing his prediction that they would wind up in bed together. ["Clyde Bruckman's Final Repose"]

BRUMFIELD, ELLEN: A customer on **Donnie Pfaster**'s frozen food delivery route. He steals some discarded hair from her bathroom wastebasket. ["Irresistible"]

BRUMFIELD, LISA: The sixteen-year-old daughter of Ellen Brumfield. **Donnie Pfaster** steals some discarded hair from her bathroom wastebasket. ["Irresistible"]

BRUNDTLAND, TORK: Norwegian coaster captain who refuses to take Mulder and Scully to their desired coordinates, and acts as if he's afraid to go there. ["Dod Kalm"]

BRUNO: Teenage boy who dies under mysterious circumstances. ["Syzygy"]

BRUSKIN, PHIL: An older FBI agent who has traded in his cigarettes for nicotine gum, which he hates; present at the scene of **Tommy Philips**'s murder when **Jack Willis** reappears. Bruskin tracks Willis and Scully to **Lula Philips**'s apartment, only to discover all three missing, and follows the case to its end with Mulder. ["Lazarus"]

BRYLIN PSYCHIATRIC HOSPITAL: Where **Dr. Sheila Braun** counsels **Michelle**

Bishop, an eight-year-old girl with emotional problems. ["Born Again"]

BRYON, SEN. RICHARD: First-term senator who pulls the plug on the project designed to scan the sky for radio transmissions of an intelligent extraterrestrial origin. ["Little Green Men"]

BUCHANON, DR. HARVEY: A doctor who died in an arson fire at an abortion clinic in Teaneck, New Jersey. His name appears on a list of similar deaths e-mailed to Mulder by an anonymous source. Mulder is baffled upon learning that all three doctors, although apparently unrelated, were identical — and no body was recovered in any of the cases. ["Colony"]

BUDAHAS, ANITA: The wife of Col. Robert Budahas, who reports her husband's incarceration by the military as a kidnapping in the hope that the FBI might be able to secure his release. When her husband is finally returned to her and her children, she refuses to believe that it is actually him, but later — probably as a result of official pressure — accepts the situation and refuses to speak to the FBI. ["Deep Throat"]

BUDAHAS, COL. ROBERT: A test pilot at **Ellens Air Force**

Base in Idaho who is arrested by military police after allegedly violating base security by stealing a military vehicle. This, apparently, is related to a mysterious mental disorientation and a strange rash that affected him two years prior to this; Mulder believes these symptoms were caused by extreme stress induced by flying experimental, UFO-based aircraft at remarkable velocities. Budahas is returned to his family after a lengthy disappearance, but he is so changed that he seems a stranger to them; although he can remember facts as specific as the Green Bay Packers' lineup in the 1968 Super Bowl, he seems to have had all memories of his career as a pilot erased. In fact, Mulder believes this is exactly what happened to him. All told, a very sad fate for an officer who once received a presidential commendation. ["Deep Throat"]

BUFFALO MUTUAL LIFE BUILDING: Where **Leon Felder** works. ["Born Again"]

BUGGER, DR.: A professional bug exterminator in his fifties. He is somehow killed by the cockroaches he comes to exterminate. ["War of the Coprophages"]

BUNDESNACHRICHTEN-DIEST BUILDING: A government building in Pullach, Germany. A German official here phoned the **Cigarette-Smoking Man** to inform him that the **MJ documents** had been stolen, after being informed himself by a Japanese diplomat. The Cigarette-Smoking Man, of course, was already aware of this. ["Anasazi"]

BURKE: A crew member on board the Canadian fishing vessel *Lisette*, which finds Lifeboat 925 from the *Uss Argent* and rescues its survivors. ["Dod Kalm"]

BURK, CHUCK: The digital imaging expert Mulder asks to examine the photos taken of **Teddy Holvey** moments before his death. Burks extracts what appears to be a ghostly image from the photo, and later identifies the ash found in the Holvey home as vibuti, a Sanskrit term meaning "holy ash." ["The Calusari"]

BURST, FRANK: The FBI agent who captures **Robert Modell,** a.k.a. Pusher, only to have him escape when a semi hits his car. Burst survives this encounter and vows to capture Modell again. A bit overwrought, Burst lets Modell talk him into a fatal heart attack over the phone. ["Pusher"]

BUSCH, SPECIAL AGENT: At FBI headquarters in Washington, he works in the latest fingerprint analysis lab. ["Irresistible"]

BUXTON, SARAH: **Kevin Kryder** shoots a spitball at her, which sticks to her hair. ["Revelations"]

BUXTON, STAN: The coroner of Johnston County, Oklahoma, where an unusually high incidence of death by lightning attracts the attention of Mulder and Scully. ["D.P.O."]

BYERS: One of the editors of the magazine *The Lone Gunman*. ["E.B.E." and "Blood"] He informs Mulder that the **Thinker** wants to meet him. ["Anasazi"] Mulder shows him a strange video trap device. He and Frohike determine that it sends another signal in along with the normal cable TV signal, which contains tachistoscopic images designed to influence the person watching the program. ["Wetwired"]

[C]

CABLE MAN: He has been putting strange video traps on certain homes. These emit a signal that causes people to hallucinate and commit murder. The Cable Man is killed, along with **Dr. Stroman,** by **X.** ["Wetwired"]

CALCAGNI, PETE: Member of a witches' coven who commits suicide while under control of a demon. ["Die Hand Die Verletzt"]

CALECA, LINDA: A young agent right out of the FBI academy. Partnered with **Brian Fuller,** she helps guard **Walter Skinner** after he is shot. ["Apocrypha"]

CALIFORNIA INSTITUTE OF TECHNOLOGY: Home of the volcano observatory, in Pasadena. ["Firewalker"]

CALLAHAN, FRANCES: The wife of Gen. Thomas Callahan, killed by **"Rappo" Trimble** after he kills her son, Trevor. ["The Walk"]

CALLAHAN, GEN. THOMAS: Commanding officer of Fort Evanston, Maryland. He resists the FBI's investigation into the Stans case. Like **Lt. Col. Stans,** he is haunted by the ghostly image of a soldier. After his family is killed, he learns the identity of his tormentor from Stans, and confronts **"Rappo" Trimble** in his hospital room. He is saved from Trimble's psychic attack when Stans smothers Trimble. ["The Walk"]

CALLAHAN, TREVOR: Gen. Callahan's eight-year-old son. Fingerprints discovered after Trevor sees an intruder lead to the arrest of **"Roach" Freely,**

but Trevor is killed by **"Rappo" Trimble**'s astral body after Freely's arrest. ["The Walk"]

CALTROP: Spikes left in the road to disable logging trucks. ["Darkness Falls"]

CALVERT STREET: The location of the office building where **Eugene Tooms** extracts the liver of Baltimore businessman **George Usher,** shortly before killing him. ["Squeeze"]

CALUSARI: In Romanian folk culture, elders responsible for the proper performance and observance of sacred rituals. A group of them are called in by **Charlie Holvey**'s grandmother **Golda** to perform a Ritual of Separation, but they encounter numerous obstacles before gaining Mulder as an unexpected ally. ["The Calusari"]

CAMOUFLAGE MAN: Apparent leader of the troop of commandos who burn out the boxcar where Mulder hides. ["Anasazi"] He pulls over Scully's car as she drives through the desert and retrieves the printouts of the secret files (Scully does not have the **MJ** files DAT). For some reason, he and his men do not harm Scully. ["The Blessing Way"]

CAMPBELL: One of the suicides at the **Arctic Ice Core Project.** ["Ice"]

CAMUS COUNTY: Where **Fairfield,** Idaho, is located. ["Fearful Symmetry"]

CANCER MAN: The nickname Mulder gives the **Cigarette-Smoking Man.**

CAPE COD, MASSACHUSETTS: Where Lord and Lady **Marsden** bring their family to avoid death threats. ["Fire"]

CARBOBOOST: An energy drink **Robert Modell** consumes in large quantities. Imposing his will on others drains his energy and leaves him exhausted. ["Pusher"]

CARDINAL, LUIS: One of **Alex Krycek**'s partners in skulduggery, involved in the inadvertent murder of **Melissa Scully.** ["The Blessing Way"] When **Walter Skinner** ignores threats to stay off the Melissa Scully murder case, the **Cigarette-Smoking Man** assigns Cardinal to shoot him. ["Piper Maru"] When Cardinal tries to finish off Skinner, Scully captures him. He tells her where to find Krycek in North Dakota, but is killed in his cell by associates of the Cigarette-Smoking Man, who make the death look like a suicide. ["Apocrypha"]

CARL: A twelve-year old boy, one of the children **Kevin**

Kryder tells a ghost story to at the Linley Temporary Home Shelter. When Kevin is kidnapped by **Owen Lee Jarvis,** Carl gives the police artist a good description of the man. ["Revelations"]

THE CAROLINIAN: A North Carolina newspaper that runs a fake article claiming **Liz Hawley** and **Jim Summers** have been rescued from their kidnapper. Mulder planted the article to trap **Luther Lee Boggs** in a lie, but the plan backfires. ["Beyond the Sea"]

CARPENTER, DR. ANN: Works in the Microbiology Department at Georgetown University. ["The Erlenmeyer Flask"]

CARVER, COMMANDER: Los Angeles Police Department officer overseeing the investigation into the murder of **Garrett Lorre.** ["3"]

CARYL COUNTY SHERIFF'S STATION: Where Scully interviews **Terri Roberts** and Mulder interviews **Margi Kleinjan.** The two teenage girls claim that **Jay DeBoom** was possessed and then killed by Satanic worshipers who were wearing hoods and carrying black candles. ["Syzygy"]

CASCADE VOLCANO RESEARCH TEAM: Using the robot named **Firewalker,** it is exploring the volcano at Mount Avalon. ["Firewalker"]

CASH, JOSEPH: The warden of Central Prison in Raleigh, North Carolina. He refuses Scully's request to postpone **Luther Lee Boggs**'s execution. ["Beyond the Sea"]

CASSAL, JAY: **Walter Skinner**'s divorce lawyer. ["Avatar"]

CASTOR, NURSE: The young nurse assaulted by the ghost of **Michael Holvey** when she tries to give **Charlie Holvey** a shot. ["The Calusari"]

771 CATHERINE STREET: Location, in Washington, D.C., of the **Hotel Catherine,** where the FBI tracks **Marty** of the **Kindred** through credit card use. ["Genderbender"]

CDC: Centers for Disease Control, the federal agencies with jurisdiction over infectious diseases. May have been partly responsible for the destruction of the research base at Icy Cape, Alaska. ["Ice"] **Dr. Auerbach** and **Dr. Osborne** claim to be working for the CDC, but Osborne later reveals that they actually are working for **Pinck Pharmaceuticals.** ["F. Emasculata"]

CELLBLOCK Z: The cell in the **Whiting Institute** basement that holds the extremely dangerous **Eve Six,** as well as the late **Dr. Sally Kendrick**'s two clones. ["Eve"]

CENTRAL PRISON: The state prison in Raleigh, North Carolina, where **Luther Lee Boggs** is imprisoned and executed. ["Beyond the Sea"]

CERULEAN HAULING: One of their trucks smashes the sheriff's car carrying **Robert Modell,** enabling him to escape. Modell had been talking about cerulean blue right before the impact, somehow hypnotizing the sheriff's deputy so he could not see the truck. ["Pusher"]

CHACO CHICKEN: The sole employer operating in **Dudley, Arkansas,** founded by **Walter "Chic" Chaco.** Bodies from local rituals are sometimes disposed of in the chicken feed grinder at the company's processing plant. ["Our Town"]

CHACO, WALTER "CHIC": Founder of **Chaco Chicken** and patron of **Dudley, Arkansas,** Chaco was born in 1902 and died in 1995 but looked like a man in his sixties at the time of his death. Chaco crashed in the Pacific during World War II and spent six months living among the Jalee tribe of New Guinea, where he apparently learned how to prolong human life through cannibalistic rituals. He founded

Chaco Chicken, as well as Dudley's bizarre version of a town picnic, upon his return from the war. Chaco loses his life when the townspeople turn against him, but his body is never found. ["Our Town"]

CHAMBLISS, DET.: Plainclothesman in Hollywood, investigating the murder of **Garrett Lorre.** ["3"]

CHANEY, SAM: An FBI agent who disappeared in 1942. He and his partner **Tim Ledbetter** were early experts on "stranger killings" (now known as serial killings). His body is found in a shallow grave in a vacant lot in 1995. ["Aubrey"]

CHAO, GLEN: A young Chinese-American detective with the San Francisco Police Department. Assigned to help Mulder and Scully investigate mysterious deaths in Chinatown, he is actually providing protection for a very sinister game. Working-class Chinese immigrants pay to enter a lottery to win a large jackpot; the catch is that they could wind up donating their own organs if they lose. Chao breaks up the game in disgust, discovers it was rigged, and rescues a participant, **Shuyang Hsin,** from having his heart removed. In retaliation, Chao

is burned alive. ["Hell Money"]

CHAPEL, AMBROSE: A CIA agent who approaches Mulder and explains that the identical doctors being killed in arson fires are the product of Soviet genetic experiments, planted in the United States to sabotage medical facilities in case of war, and that the Russians were killing them off with help from the U.S. government. He is actually the shape-shifting alien hit man known as the **Pilot.** ["Colony"]

CHAREZ, DANIEL: The court-appointed lawyer who represented **"Neech" Manley** eleven years before his execution. He felt he had been too young and inexperienced to defend Manley competently. He is smothered to death, the fourth victim of Manley's revenge from beyond the grave. ["The List"]

CHARLIE: The plant engineer at the Newark County sewage processing plant. ["The Host"]

CHARLOTTE'S DINER: A roadside restaurant in Craiger, Maryland, where Mulder and Scully meet **Walter Skinner** after their narrow escape from covert government forces at the **Strughold Mine.** They argue over turning over the DATs in order to save their

lives; Scully and Skinner win the argument. ["Paper Clip"]

CHARTERS, MICHELLE: A nurse at the **Excelsis Dei Convalescent Home** who is raped by an unseen force in one of the rooms. ["Excelsis Dei"]

CHARYN, DR. PENELOPE: Works at the **Grissom** Sleep Disorder Center in Stamford, Connecticut. ["Sleepless"]

CHECKPOINT ALPHA: The checkpoint where Mulder bypasses military security, enters a secured crash site in Wisconsin, and observes the remains of an alien spacecraft. ["Fallen Angel"]

CHESAPEAKE LOUNGE: The bar in the Ambassador Hotel in Washington, D.C., where **Walter Skinner** picks up a woman, takes her to his room, and wakes up the next morning to find her lying dead next to him. ["Avatar"]

CHICK: She and her friend **Stoner** witness the cockroach attack on **Dude.** ["War of the Coprophages"] She and Stoner turn up at **Heuvelmans Lake** in time to see **Snorkel Dude** get pulled underwater by a mysterious creature. ["Quagmire"]

CHOC-O-SAURUS: A chocolate treat, shaped like a dinosaur, favored by the unwilling psychic **Clyde Bruckman.**

["Clyde Bruckman's Final Repose"]

CHUNG, JOSE: Author of the novels *The Lonely Buddha* and *The Caligarian Candidate.* His publisher has assigned him the task of writing a nonfiction work about alien abduction. Chung calls it "nonfiction science fiction." He spent three months in Klass County, Washington, investigating an alien abduction case and everyone he spoke to had a different interpretation of what happened. He interviews Scully because she investigated the case (see also **Diana Lesky** and **Reynard Muldrake**). ["Jose Chung's *From Outer Space*"]

CHURCH OF THE RED MUSEUM: A strange religious cult in Delta Glen, Wisconsin. Their leader, **Richard Odin,** came to Wisconsin from California and bought a cattle ranch. They are all vegetarians and have made the five hundred head of cattle their pets. They believe that those who slaughter flesh also slaughter their own souls. They dress in white muslin and look like Sikhs, except that their turbans are red. ["Red Museum"]

CIA: One of the people who interrogate **Chrissy Giorgio.** At first she remembers him as looking like a Gray Alien.

["Jose Chung's *From Outer Space*"]

CIGARETTE-SMOKING MAN: Mulder calls him "Cancer Man." A government insider who does not approve of the X-Files because of the secrets they get close to, even going so far as to hide away evidence of the existence of UFOs [pilot episode]. He apparently pulls **Alex Krycek**'s strings throughout the **Duane Barry** incident, but his motives remain unclear. ["Ascension"] Tries to set up and discredit Mulder in the *F. Emasculata* outbreak, although he claims no knowledge of the disease. If Mulder had gone public with the information on the disease, he would have had no corroboration. ["F. Emasculata"] He is probably behind the contamination of the soft water tanks in Mulder's apartment building, an insidious plan to drive Mulder insane that doesn't work out as planned. He informs **William Mulder** that Fox is in trouble but claims he was "protecting" Fox and later denies any involvement with William's death — but this is a man whose main policy in life is "deny everything." He tells Fox that William had approved "the project," erroneously assuming that William had told Fox the truth before he died,

and tracks Fox to the Navajo reservation through his cellular phone. There he orders the destruction of **"the merchandise."** ["Anasazi"] He orders troops to set fire to the boxcar where Mulder discovers the alien corpses and presumes that Mulder has died in the fire. Unwilling to admit failure to the **Elders,** he tells them that the **MJ** files DAT tape has been recovered, an error in judgment that probably causes him more than a few sleepless nights. ["The Blessing Way"] Krycek's murder of **Melissa Scully** puts him in serious hot water with the Elders. He later claims that the DAT tape was destroyed in the car bomb explosions that "killed" Krycek, even though he knows Krycek is very much alive and has the tape in his possession. Skinner gets the upper hand over him with the help of **Albert Hosteen.** ["Paper Clip"] He retrieves the tape from an alien-possessed Krycek and then has the man sealed in a missile silo with an alien aircraft. ["Apocrypha"] **Mrs. Mulder** (Fox's mother) used to associate with CSM socially at the time that her husband, William, worked for the government, but she hates him now. When he comes to her to try to secure information she still has, she becomes violently angry, and moments after he leaves she suffers a severe and debilitating stroke. Only because **X** had been secretly observing her and made an anonymous call to 911 did she receive immediate paramedic assistance. When X shows Fox photos of CSM visiting Mrs. Mulder, Fox becomes incensed and comes close to killing him. He appears to be working closely with aliens on earth, who are perhaps mapping out colonization of the earth. ["Talitha Cumi"]

CLINE, ANDREA: One of the four teens who uses an occult book that summons a demon. ["Die Hand Die Verletzt"]

CLINE, DET.: One of the police detectives investigating a string of murders whose victims are all professional (or semi-pro) psychics of one sort or another. Cline calls in the Stupendous **Yappi** to help with the case. ["Clyde Bruckman's Final Repose"]

CLUB TEPES: Named after Vlad Tepes — a.k.a. Vlad the Impaler — of fifteenth-century Romania. Most of the people in the after-sunset club are pale-skinned and wear black. ["3"]

CLYDE: A security guard in the Eurisko Building. ["Ghost in the Machine"]

COCKROACH: An insect that is thought to have originated 350 million years ago, in the Silurian period. There are 4,000 known species. Mulder and Scully go up against roaches with artificial intelligence. ["War of the Coprophages"]

COCOON: Used by the prehistoric wood mites to imprison and kill those who disturb a certain area of the forest in the Pacific Northwest. ["Darkness Falls"]

COKELY, HARRY: A seventy-seven-year-old ex-con who went to prison in 1945 for rape and attempted murder. He carved the word "sister" on the chest of his victim, **Ruby Thibodeaux.** His weapon of choice was a strap razor. He served his time in the McCallister Penitentiary until he was released December 5, 1993. He was actually the Slash Killer but couldn't be connected to those crimes at the time. He now lives in Nebraska and needs a portable oxygen tank to get around. ["Aubrey"]

COLE, AUGUSTUS: One of the experimental subjects of **Dr. Saul Grissom**'s Vietnam-era experiments in sleep deprivation, assigned to Special Force and Recon Squad J-7. Of the thirteen original squad members, he is one of only two sur-

vivors. Cole and **Henry Willig** had four thousand confirmed kills while in Vietnam: the highest kill ratio in the Marine Corps. Cole has developed strange powers and kills Grissom with them to exact revenge. Twenty-four years after Phu Bai, the massacre of three hundred children by Recon Squad J-7, Cole decides to avenge the atrocities by murdering those he blames for creating the out-of-control killing machines. ["Sleepless"]

COLLINS: FBI agent on agent **Frank Burst**'s team. **Robert Modell** wills him to set himself on fire, but Scully douses the flames before he can be killed. ["Pusher"]

COLLINS, DR. RICHARD: A witness at the sanity hearing of **Eugene Tooms** in Baltimore. He comments favorably on the mental health of Tooms and claims he was the victim of false arrest by the FBI. ["Tooms"]

COLTON, TOM: FBI agent who trained at Quantico when Scully did. An ambitious rising star in the FBI's violent-crimes section. Asks Scully for help with a series of violent, locked-room murders in Baltimore, possibly because he's too embarrassed to ask "Spooky" Mulder for help directly. Interferes with Mulder's pursuit of the case and is reassigned to the white-collar crimes division in South Dakota. ["Squeeze"]

COMITY: A city of 38,825 which has been experiencing a rash of strange deaths. The town's motto is "The Perfect Harmony City." Astrologically speaking, Comity is in a geological vortex, sort of a cosmic G-spot. All of this culminates on January 12, when the planets come into perfect alignment. ["Syzygy"]

COMMERCIAL TRUST BUILDING: The site of a massacre committed by **Gary Taber** in Franklin, Pennsylvania. ["Blood"]

COMOX, SPECIAL AGENT: A forensics specialist who examines the piece of metal found in **Duane Barry**'s abdomen. He finds inexplicable microscopic etchings on it, resembling a bar code; it triggers a bizarre response when Scully runs it over a supermarket checkout scanner. ["Duane Barry"]

CONDUCTOR: On a train to West Virginia, Mulder gives the Conductor a gun to try to capture **Dr. Zama.** When the red-haired man (see **Malcolm Gerlach**) tries to chase down and kill the Conductor, he is just able to slam a train car door in the assassin's face,

thereby locking him in with Mulder in a car that has a bomb planted in it. ["731"]

CONNERVILLE, OKLA-HOMA: A small town where lightning strikes more people than is statistically feasible. This might be due to the proximity of the **Astadourian Lightning Observatory,** or it might have something to do with an unusual teenager named **Darin Peter Oswald.** ["D.P.O."]

THE CONUNDRUM: A circus freak living in Gibsonton, Florida, who has a jigsaw design tattooed on his entire body. He is a "geek," meaning he can eat anything: rocks, corkscrews, live crickets. Ultimately he eats **Leonard,** the misguided Siamese twin. ["Humbug"]

COOLEY, NURSE: On duty at the VA Medical Center when **Augustus Cole** somehow escapes. She claims **Dr. Pilsson** signed the order for Cole's release, which Pilsson denies. ["Sleepless"]

COUNTY ROAD A7: The main highway running past **Dudley, Arkansas.** Not a good place to stop for a picnic. ["Our Town"]

COUNTY ROAD D7: Location of the fire caused by the UFO crash near **Townsend, Wisconsin,** two miles west of the road's intersection with

Canyon Ridge. ["Fallen Angel"]

CRANDALL, JOE: A prisoner at **Tashmoo Federal Correctional Facility** who befriended **John Barnett.** Crandall was the sole beneficiary of Barnett's will. He confirms to Mulder that Barnett did not have heart problems, and discloses the operation he saw **Dr. Joe Ridley** performing on Barnett. ["Young at Heart"]

CRAZY BEDBUG MOTEL: Where the motel manager dies mysteriously and his body is found covered by cockroaches. ["War of the Coprophages"]

CREUTZFELDT-JAKOB DIS-EASE: A rare disease that eats holes in its victims' brains, reducing them to the consistency of sponges. It can be passed along by eating infected tissue, which leads to an unfortunate turn of events for the people of **Dudley, Arkansas:** twenty-seven citizens contract fatal cases, thanks to their cannibal barbecues. ["Our Town"]

CREW-CUT MAN: A government assassin who is killed by the father of a boy he kills in "Red Museum." Crew-Cut Man killed **Deep Throat** in "The Erlenmeyer Flask" and Mulder wanted to take him alive, but to no avail.

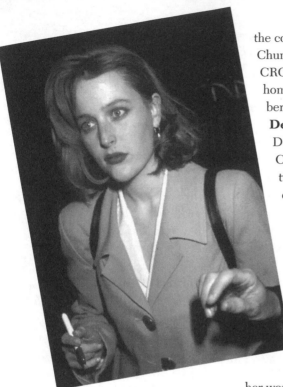

CRIKENSON, ROKY: A blue-collar utility worker in his fifties who is checking on a mysterious power outage in **Klass County, Washington.** Two black-clad men in a black Cadillac drive into his garage and spout anti-UFO gibberish. Crikenson believes they do this because he has written a manuscript called *The Truth About Aliens* in which he claims an alien he calls Lord **Kinbote** is not from outer space at all, but from the Earth's core. He quits his job with the power company and relocates to El Cajon, California, to preach to the converted. ["Jose Chung's *From Outer Space*"]

CROCKETT, ROGER: A homeless man dismembered by the **Jersey Devil.** ["The Jersey Devil"]

CROSS, DET. ALAN: A twenty-five-year veteran of the Cleveland Police Department's homicide squad who calls Mulder and Scully in on the murder of **Lauren Mackalvey.** A bit old-fashioned, he at first does not register Scully as an equal, but is soon content to let her work with her partner when he witnesses their intuitive chemistry. He is fatally slimed by **Virgil Incanto** while canvassing suspects. ["2Shy"]

CRYSTAL CITY, VIRGINIA: Headquarters of the Eurisko Corporation. ["Ghost in the Machine"]

CULVER CITY PLASMA CENTER: Los Angeles–area blood bank investigated by Mulder in his search for the people in the **Trinity** gang of vampiric killers. ["3"]

CUMBERLAND STATE CORRECTIONAL FACILITY: Virginia state prison where **Pinck Pharmaceuticals** and an unknown government agency conduct a controlled outbreak of a newly discovered disease that goes haywire when two infected prisoners escape. ["F. Emasculata"]

CURATOR: An elderly man who has a facial deformity and is in charge of the **Odditorium,** a museum of curiosa in **Gibsonton, Florida.** It's a musty place resembling an antique store. Admission is free to freaks. Among the exhibits are photos of circus freaks from years past. ["Humbug"]

[D]

DALTON, LAURA: Television reporter who covers the evacuation of **Townsend, Wisconsin,** and accepts the government's cover story about a toxic cargo spill. ["Fallen Angel"]

DALY, DR.: Intensive care doctor in charge of Scully at the Northeast Georgetown Medical Center in Washington, D.C. ["One Breath"]

DANIELS, LILLIAN: Wheelchair-bound wife of **Sheriff Maurice Daniels.** He believes **Samuel Hartley** is a fake and won't allow her to go to him to be healed. ["Miracle Man"]

DANIELS, OFFICER: Rookie cop who refuses to let **Jack Willis** enter the scene of **Tommy Philips**'s murder without his ID badge, until Scully identifies him. ["Lazarus"]

DANIELS, SHERIFF MAURICE: He believes the **Rev. Hartley** and his **Miracle Ministry** are running a scam. He ultimately has **Samuel Hartley** beaten to death. ["Miracle Man"]

DARK MATTER: Theoretical subatomic particle whose existence is proved, somewhat disastrously, by **Chester Ray Banton,** whose shadow becomes dark matter after a laboratory mishap. Thereafter, his shadow can reduce human matter into pure energy and absorb it like a black hole — fatal for anyone who touches the shadow. Banton is harmless only in the dark or in even, shadowless soft light. ["Soft Light"]

DARNELL, DET. JOE: Of the Aubrey, Missouri, police. He is the assistant of **Lt. Brian Tillman.** ["Aubrey"]

DA SILVA, DR. NANCY: Attractive but uptight civilian toxicologist who accompanies Mulder and Scully to investigate the **Arctic Ice Core Project** disaster. She is infected by the ice worm but survives after Scully and **Dr. Hodge** determine how to destroy the infection by introducing a second worm into the body. Unfortunately, this happens too late to save **Dr. Denny Murphy,** whom she killed while infected. ["Ice"]

DAT: Digital Audio Tape containing encrypted files of government conspiracy regarding UFOs. ["Paper Clip"]

DAVEY, DR. CHRISTOPHER: **Chester Ray Banton**'s business partner at **Polarity Magnetics.** He closes down the company after Banton's accident. He witnesses Banton's murder of **Det. Kelly Ryan,** and locks Banton in the accelerator chamber where the accident first occurred, intending to hand him over to the government. He is murdered by **X,** who disintegrates Davey's body in the accelerator chamber to make Mulder think Banton is dead. ["Soft Light"]

DAVIS CORRECTIONAL TREATMENT CENTER: The mental hospital in Marion, Virginia, where **Duane Barry** is held until his escape in 1994. He stabs a guard with a fountain pen, steals his gun, and takes **Dr. Del Hakkie** hostage. ["Duane Barry"]

DAWSON, SHARON: Administrator of the **Excelsis Dei Convalescent Home.** ["Excelsis Dei"]

D.C. CORRECTIONAL COMPLEX: Located in Lorton, Virginia. **John Mostow** is taken there after he's arrested for a series of murders. ["Grotesque"]

DEADHORSE, ALASKA: Mulder catches a military plane from Tacoma, Washington, to Deadhorse in his quest to catch up with the **Pilot.** ["End Game"]

DeBOOM, JAY "BOOM": Quarterback of his high school football team in Comity. A friend of **Bruno,** the boy who died under mysterious circumstances. It is believed Bruno was kidnapped and murdered by some unknown Satanic cult. Then the same thing happens to Jay: he is found in the woods, hanging from a rope. Although the verdict is suicide, some suspect foul play because Jay's is the third death of a high school boy in three months. He has actually been killed by **Margi Kleinjan** and **Terri Roberts.** At his funeral his coffin mysteriously catches on fire. When his corpse is examined, there is an image on the chest that some think resembles a horned beast. ["Syzygy"]

DEEP THROAT: Mulder's secret government contact, a

well-placed official who takes an interest in Mulder and the X-Files. When Mulder decides to investigate **Ellens Air Force Base,** Deep Throat reveals himself to warn Mulder off the case. ["Deep Throat"] Advises Mulder on the whereabouts of Eurisko Corporation founder **Brad Wilczek.** ["Ghost in the Machine"] Informs Mulder that a military operation to retrieve a crashed alien vehicle is under way in and around **Townsend, Wisconsin;** countermands FBI section chief **McGrath**'s decision to oust Mulder from the FBI following his insubordination in this case. ["Fallen Angel"] Clues Mulder in to the **Litchfield** cloning experiments and the location of **Eve Six** in the Whiting Institute. ["Eve"] Explains to Mulder that murderer **John Barnett** was negotiating with the federal government for the sale of **Dr. Joe Ridley**'s research, and that the government had known all along that Barnett was at large. ["Young at Heart"] He always tells Mulder, "Trust no one." He appears to Mulder in a vision while Mulder is undergoing the **Blessing Way** ceremony. ["The Blessing Way"] He was probably the third man who interviewed a *Zeus Faber*

crewman with **William Mulder** and the **Cigarette-Smoking Man** in 1953. ["Apocrypha"] After **Jeremiah Smith** is taken to a maximum security prison where he is interrogated by the Cigarette-Smoking Man, he gets into an argument with him and at one point Smith casually alters his appearance so that he looks like the by then deceased informant Mulder knew only as Deep Throat. ["Talitha Cumi"]

DELTA GLEN, WISCONSIN: Home of the **Church of the Red Museum,** a harmless religious cult being unfairly blamed for sinister activity. Incidents being investigated in Delta Glen by Mulder and Scully include a peeping Tom, kidnappings of teenagers, a plane crash, murder, and cattle being injected with alien DNA. ["Red Museum"]

DEN OF THE GREAT UNKNOWN: A special room of the **Odditorium.** Inside is a box that Scully opens to find — nothing! She was humbugged into paying five dollars to see what was in this room. ["Humbug"]

DEPRANIL: An enzyme-inhibiting drug used by **Dr. John Grago** to increase acetylcholine in the brains of his

Alzheimer's patients. ["Excelsis Dei"]

DEPARTMENT OF AGRICULTURE: An installation supposedly operated by this government agency is conducting experiments in Miller's Grove, Massachusetts, to determine what cockroaches respond to in order to better determine how to eliminate them. ["War of the Coprophages"]

DESMOND ARMS RESIDENT HOTEL: The sleazy dive near Washington, D.C., where **Jack Willis** kills **Tommy Philips.** Covering up his identity problems, Willis then shows up at the crime scene and misplaces the fingerprints that would have revealed him as the killer. ["Lazarus"]

DIAMOND, DR. ROGER: Scully's anthropology professor at the University of Maryland, who assists her and Mulder in the pursuit of the female **Jersey Devil.** ["The Jersey Devil"]

DICKENS, DR. JAMES: The fourth identical doctor, whose picture is e-mailed to Scully. He worked in Washington, D.C. He jumps out a second-story window in Germantown, Maryland, when he sees CIA agent **Chapel,** who then assumes his true identity as the **Pilot** and kills Dickens in an alley. Dickens's body is never found, although Scully ruins a pair of new shoes by stepping in the green residue left behind by his disintegration. ["Colony"]

DIE HAND DIE VERLETZT: "His hand is the hand that wounds." ["Die Hand Die Verletzt"]

DINWIDDIE COUNTY, VIRGINIA: Where Mulder tracks the escaped convict **Paul** by tracing the last call from a pay phone near **Angelo Garza**'s gas station. ["F. Emasculata"]

DINWIDDIE COUNTY HOSPITAL: **Paul**'s girlfriend **Elizabeth** is held here after her arrest because of her infection by the parasite that inhabits the insect *F. Emasculata*. ["F. Emasculata"]

DIXON, SGT. AL: A veteran of the Scranton, Pennsylvania, police force who arrests the **Rev. Calvin Sistrunk** as a suspect in the murder of **Dr. Landon Prince,** but the charges won't stick. ["Colony"]

DMITRI: Young Russian seaman who is trying to remove the blockage from inside a ship's sewage tank when he is attacked by a creature that pulls him into the water of the tank, where he disappears. The crew then flush the tanks, emptying them into the ocean. ["The Host"]

DOANE, JOSEPHINE: Administrator at the Washington, D.C., offices of the Navajo Nation who confirm that the documents in Scully's possession are in Navajo, and points out two words: "merchandise" and "vaccination," both modern additions to the Navajo language. She helps Scully contact **Albert Hosteen.** ["Anasazi"]

DOLE, LISA: FBI handwriting expert at the headquarters in Seattle, Washington. ["Roland"]

DOLL COLLECTOR: A victim of the serial killer known as the **Puppet,** who targets psychics. He left her eyes and intestines on the table in her living room, which is filled to the brim with her doll collection. Detectives at first can't see the link between this and the other murders until Mulder notices a cup with tea leaves in it and points out that she practiced tasseography. **Yappi,** a commercial psychic, claims the killer raped her before murdering her; **Clyde Bruckman** says she instigated the sex. ["Clyde Bruckman's Final Repose"]

DOMINION TOBACCO: A North Carolina tobacco company located in the Raleigh–Durham area. One of their executives, **Patrick Newirth,** is reduced to a stain on a carpet after **Chester Ray Banton** knocks on his hotel room door by mistake. ["Soft Light"]

DORLAND, ROBERT: **Howard Graves**'s partner in HTG Industrial Technologies, he set up the company's illegal arms dealings with an Iranian extremist group. When Graves protested, Dorland had him murdered in a way that made it look like suicide. His subsequent attempts to silence **Lauren Kyte** aren't quite as successful. Dorland is eventually indicted for Graves's murder and a large number of federal charges. ["Shadows"]

DOUGHERTY, MRS.: **Michelle Bishop**'s latest nanny, who is mysteriously locked in the wine cellar when Michelle disappears from the house. ["Born Again"]

DRAKE, BENJAMIN: CEO of the Eurisko Corporation, mysteriously murdered by an electrical booby trap in the bathroom of his office. ["Ghost in the Machine"]

DRAPER, CAPT. JANET: Army officer at Fort Evanston, Maryland, who advises Mulder and Scully to drop the **Stans** case at the request of **Gen. Callahan.** She is drowned in a swimming pool by **"Rappo" Trimble.** Scully finds bruises on her neck, indicating a struggle. ["The Walk"]

DRUID HILL SANITARIUM: In Baltimore. **Eugene Tooms** had been housed here until a sanity hearing allowed him to be released. ["Tooms"]

DUDE: A drug user who sees a cockroach burrow into his arm through an open wound. He uses a razor blade to try to get it out and accidentally severs an artery, dying as a result. ["War of the Coprophages"]

DUDLEY, ARKANSAS: Home of **Chaco Chicken,** the town is practically ruled by **Walter Chaco,** who is as much its spiritual as economic leader. The river running through Dudley yields at least nine skeletons, including that of **George Kearns.** All are missing their skulls, and all appear to have been cooked by boiling. At least eighty-seven people disappeared near Dudley between 1944 and 1995. ["Our Town"]

DUKENFIELD, CLAUDE: The late owner of Uranus Unlimited, and a firm believer in astrology. He is killed by the **Puppet** and dumped in the woods around Shove Park, where Mulder and Scully find him with the assistance of **Clyde Bruckman** . . . who had sold him an insurance policy a few months before his

death. ["Clyde Bruckman's Final Repose"]

DUNAWAY'S PUB: A tavern in Washington, D.C., where Mulder often goes. The informant known as **Deep Throat** first approaches Mulder in the men's room here in order to warn him against investigating events at **Ellens Air Force Base** in Idaho. ["Deep Throat"]

DUNHAM, PVT. HARRY: A friend of **Pvt. John McAlpin.** He reveals that **Col. Jacob Wharton** ordered the beating of inmates at the Haitian refugee center. He's later found murdered, and it emerges that he was filing a complaint against Wharton just prior to his death. ["Fresh Bones"]

DUPRE, WARREN JAMES: Born in Klamath Falls, Oregon, Dupre, age thirty, worked as a prison guard until his affair with **Lula Philips** led him to a life of crime. Their bank robberies are marked by extreme violence and seven deaths, including that of a sixty-five-year-old female teller at **Annapolis Savings and Loan.** Dupre shoots **Jack Willis** but is killed by Scully during his last robbery at the Maryland Marine Bank. Dupre has a dragon tattooed on his forearm. If one believes

Willis's apparent delusion to be true, Dupre's spirit took over Willis's body and used it to be reunited with his true love, Lula. ["Lazarus"]

DURAN, DAVE: One of the four teens who uses an occult book that summons a demon. He checked out the book, *Witch Hunt: A History of the Occult in America.* ["Die Hand Die Verletzt"]

DWIGHT: Night watchman at the Skyland Mountain tram when Mulder and **Krycek** arrive there in pursuit of **Duane Barry.** He tells the agents that the tram is closed for the summer, but Mulder persuades him to start it up; Krycek disposes of Dwight while Mulder is riding the tram up the mountain. ["Ascension"]

DYER: One of a group of loggers in the Pacific Northwest who cut into an old tree and unleash ancient wood mites that attack out of self-preservation, becoming active only after sunset and before dawn. ["Darkness Falls"]

[E]

EASTON, WASHINGTON: When the thirteen-year-old **Lucy Householder** escaped from **Carl Wade** after being his prisoner for five years, she was found wandering near this town. This area is also where a tow truck driver has a strange encounter with Wade shortly after the kidnapping of **Amy Jacobs.** When the FBI suddenly arrives on Main Street, by chance Wade is there to see them pull up, and he guesses they are on to him. ["Oubliette"]

EASTPOINT STATE PENITENTIARY: In Florida. **Napoleon "Neech" Manley** is executed there for murder. His death is followed by six others. ["The List"]

E.B.E.: Extraterrestrial biological entity, essentially any creature not originally from Earth. ["E.B.E."]

ECCLESIASTES 3:19: "A man has no preeminence above a beast; for all is vanity." Biblical quote Mulder and Scully see on the marquee of a church following the end of a case involving animals that may be having their fetuses harvested by aliens in order to preserve the species. ["Fearful Symmetry"]

ECKBOM'S SYNDROME: A psychotic disorder suffered by some drug users that causes them to imagine their skin is infested with insects. ["War of the Coprophages"]

ECKERLE, DR. JEFF: President and chief science officer of **Alt.-Fuels Inc.** He

hires **Dr. Bugger** to exterminate cockroaches in his house. He witnesses the strange death of Dr. Bugger. ["War of the Coprophages"]

3243 EDMONTON STREET: The location of the industrial building in Germantown, Maryland, where **Dr. James Dickens** conducted his experiments in merging human and alien DNA. Scully finds the address on Dickens's medical bag and investigates, only to discover CIA agent **Chapel** demolishing the lab. Later investigation reveals the existence of hybrid fetuses there. ["Colony"]

EDWARDS TERMINAL: At this train station in Queensgate, Ohio, the redhaired man (see **Malcolm Gerlach**) who assassinated **Kazuo Takeo** turns up just as **Dr. Ishimaru** arrives. ["Nisei"]

EHMAN, JERRY: In August 1977 this astronomer found a transmission of apparent extraterrestrial origin on a printout and called it a "wow" signal. ["Little Green Men"]

EISENHOWER FIELD: An Air Force base in Siquannke, Alaska; Mulder is taken to the military hospital there for treatment after being found half-frozen on the icefields. ["Colony"] Doctors there treat

him for extreme hypothermia until Scully arrives and convinces them to keep his body cold; this, combined with several transfusions, clears the alien virus from his body. ["End Game"]

THE ELDERS: A group of elderly, powerful men who guard more than a few dark secrets and control the conspiracy that continues to affect the lives of Mulder and Scully. They convene at an office high above 46th Street in New York when the **Thinker** steals the **MJ** data and gives it to Mulder. The **Cigarette-Smoking Man** is apparently one of them, but he is obviously answerable to higher-ranking members such as the **Well-Manicured Man.** ["The Blessing Way"] They are not pleased when the French obtain information about a sensitive site in the North Pacific. Mulder gets the phone number of their office from a package in **Krycek**'s locker, but the number is disconnected after his brief conversation with the Well-Manicured Man. ["Apocrypha"]

ELDRIDGE, USS: U.S. Navy vessel involved in the alleged **Philadelphia Experiment** in 1944. ["Dod Kalm"]

ELIZABETH: Girlfriend of the escaped convict **Paul** (and

mother of his child). She is infected by *F. Emasculata* by Paul's fellow escapee **Steve.** She is arrested by U.S. **marshal Deke Tapia** while Paul is out and remains silent until Mulder convinces her to reveal Paul's destination by explaining the public health risk involved. ["F. Emasculata"]

ELLEN: Scully's best friend, a housewife and mother who tries to set Scully up with a divorced acquaintance, Rob. ["The Jersey Devil"]

ELLENS AIR FORCE BASE: In southwest Idaho. Mulder believes the government has developed top-secret aircraft there that utilize alien UFO flight technology salvaged from the 1947 Roswell crash. This base is so classified, it does not even appear on the U.S. Geographical Survey map of Idaho. Six pilots have been reported missing in action there since 1963. Mulder and Scully investigate the apparent disappearance of test pilot **Robert Budahas** here but encounter serious opposition from the military. Mulder believes he witnessed something incriminating here, but cannot recall anything after his brief incarceration by the military; he suspects they somehow "erased" his memories. Scully's primary recollection of

this investigation is of the extreme measures she resorted to in order to secure Mulder's release. The informant known only as **Deep Throat** first approaches Mulder in relation to this unresolved case. ["Deep Throat"]

ELLICOTT, REGGIE: A member of Parliament who may or may not have been blown up with a car bomb triggered by a car stereo; referred to in a practical joke played on Mulder by his former Oxford classmate, **Phoebe Green.** ["Fire"]

ELLIS, JAMES: The father of Ellis & Sons clothiers. A Memphis murder victim of the vampiric **Trinity.** ["3"]

EMBASSY ROW: In Washington, D.C., where a limo driver picks up **Kazuo Takeo,** the Japanese diplomat Mulder had captured at the scene of a murder. It is a trap: Takeo is murdered in the limo by a red-haired man (see **Malcolm Gerlach**) to cover up Takeo's sloppy work in **Allentown.** ["Nisei"]

EMIL: Teenage boy who sneaks onto **Ellens Air Force Base** to watch mysterious lights in the sky; he and his girlfriend Zoe help Mulder infiltrate the base. ["Deep Throat"]

ERIKSON: Chief seismologist of the **Cascade Volcano**

Research Team, whose body is found by the robot nicknamed **Firewalker.** ["Firewalker"]

ESCALANTE: One of the human–alien hybrids, who escapes execution at the **Hansen's Research Center Compound.** He is found by Scully while she is searching the place. ["731"]

EUBANKS, WALTER: FBI agent from the Seattle office who is investigating the kidnapping of **Amy Jacobs.** ["Oubliette"]

EURISKO BUILDING: Headquarters of the Eurisko Corporation. The building is run by a central operating system (COS) that creator **Brad Wilczek** secretly provided with a prototype artificial intelligence program that develops a mind of its own. ["Ghost in the Machine"]

EVE SIX: An extremely intelligent, psychotic, and dangerous product of the **Litchfield Project,** imprisoned in **Cellblock Z** of the **Whiting Institute** since 1983. She reveals that all the Adams and Eves are dead except her and two others, Eves Seven and Eight, who escaped years earlier. ["Eve"]

EVE EIGHT: The last surviving **Litchfield Project** child at large, she escaped imprisonment in 1985 and has since assumed the identify of a doctor with high military security, **Dr. Alicia Hughes.** ["Eve"]

EXCELSIS DEI CONVALESCENT HOME: In Worcester, Massachusetts. The site of attacks by invisible entities. ["Excelsis Dei"]

66 EXETER STREET: The site of **Eugene Tooms**'s hideout in Baltimore. Tooms has used Apartment 103 in this building at least since 1903, according to the census; the first victim to fit Tooms's murder MO lived in Apartment 203, according to the X-File on this pattern of murders. Mulder and Scully find a strange, slimy nest festooned with Tooms's trophies there. ["Squeeze"]

EXOSKELETON: Mulder finds a cockroach exoskeleton and accidentally crushes it in his hand, which bleeds because the exoskeleton is made out of some kind of metal. ["War of the Coprophages"]

[F]

FACIPHAGA EMASCULATA: An insect of tropical origin, discovered by **Dr. Robert Torrence** in the jungles of Costa Rica. **Pinck Pharmaceuticals** is interested in it because it secretes a dilating enzyme, but the company is unaware that the bug is also

host to a parasite that attacks the human immune system. To further complicate matters, *F. Emasculata* has a complicated reproductive cycle. Its larvae grow in human boils, and spread from host to host after the boils explode when the victim dies. A total of eighteen people, mostly prisoners, died in an outbreak of this unnamed disease, which is covered up by Pinck with government assistance. ["F. Emasculata"]

FAIRFAX MERCY HOSPITAL: The hospital in Washington where **Robert Modell** obtains his prescription for **Tegretol.** ["Pusher"]

FAIRFIELD COUNTY SOCIAL SERVICES HOSTEL: **Teena Simmons** is housed here temporarily after the bizarre death of her father. ["Eve"]

FAIRFIELD, IDAHO: The site of the Fairfield Zoo, where many strange things have been happening. After an elephant escapes and a federal construction worker is killed by an unseen presence, Mulder and Scully are sent to investigate. ["Fearful Symmetry"]

FAIRFIELD ZOO: Ganesha the elephant escapes from here and then dies from exhaustion. Mulder and Scully learn that no animal at this zoo has ever had a successful pregnancy.

There have been other strange escapes and disappearances of animals from the zoo. ["Fearful Symmetry"]

FAIRLY, JUDY: Employee of **Lorraine Kelleher** at an escort service in the Georgetown area of the District of Columbia. When her boss is murdered, Fairly helps Mulder trap the man who did it. ["Avatar"]

FALLEN ANGEL: The code used by **Col. Henderson** to denote a downed alien craft and/or its occupant. ["Fallen Angel"]

FARMINGTON, NEW MEXICO: Where Scully takes Mulder after shooting him, en route to meet **Albert Hosteen.** ["Anasazi"]

FARRADAY, DR. PAUL: A biologist working in Striker's Cove on **Heuvelmans Lake.** He is concerned about the dwindling population of a rare kind of frog. ["Quagmire"]

FAST-FOOD RESTAURANT: Where **Lucy Householder** is working as a trainee when she suffers a strange nosebleed the instant **Amy Jacobs** is kidnapped by **Carl Wade.** ["Oubliette"]

THE FATHER: An older man, one of the vampiric trio of killers. He is killed by **Kristen Kilar,** who then burns his body. ["3"]

FAULKNER, BLAINE: A sci-fi buff in his late twenties, who wears a *Space: Above and Beyond* T-shirt to indicate that he's a real loser. He tells Chung that he wants to be abducted by aliens because he is so bored with life. He describes those who investigated the missing teenagers and their story. He's actually talking about Mulder and Scully, and his description of them is quite bizarre. He says Mulder looked like a "mandroid." He finds a dead alien in a field, who is actually a man wearing a Gray Alien costume. ["Jose Chung's *From Outer Space*"]

FEEJEE MERMAID: The half-man, half-fish creature in an old drawing done by **Hepcat Helm.** The creature is a "genuine fake" P. T. Barnum once exhibited, consisting of a mummified monkey sewn onto the tail of a fish. ["Humbug"]

FELDER, LEON: A thirty-seven-year-old insurance salesman who involves **Tony Fiore** and **Rudy Barbala** in illegal activity. Felder and Barbala kill police officer **Charlie Morris.** Felder is strangled by his scarf when **Michelle Bishop** uses her psychic powers to trap it in the door of a moving bus. ["Born Again"]

FENIG, MAX: A UFO enthusiast Mulder meets while imprisoned by the military during **Operation Falcon.** A member of NICAP (the National Investigative Committee of Aerial Phenomenon). Somewhat paranoid, Fenig is a crackpot version of Mulder who travels the country in an Airstream trailer fitted with all sorts of high-tech equipment. He provides Mulder with information about **Deputy Sheriff Jason Wright,** recorded from his radio scanners. Fenig has a small diamond-shaped scar behind his left ear and claims to have started having epileptic blackouts at the age of ten in South Dakota. Mulder believes that Fenig was a UFO abductee; Fenig himself professes no such belief. He is possibly reabducted by aliens in **Townsend, Wisconsin;** the military's claim that his body was found is probably false. ["Fallen Angel"]

FICICELLO FROZEN FOODS: Where **Donnie Pfaster** gets a job after being fired from the **Janelli-Heller Funeral Home.** He flirts with the receptionist there. ["Irresistible"]

FIEBLING, MR.: Teacher of the night school course "Intro to Mythology and Comparative Religion" that **Donnie Pfaster** attends. ["Irresistible"]

50 GREATEST CONSPIRACIES OF ALL TIME: A book about conspiracies by Vankin and Whelan, a favorite of the **Thinker.** ["Anasazi"]

FINGERS, DR.: A hypnotist who puts **Chrissy Giorgio** under to find out what really happened to her and **Harold Lamb** the night they disappeared for several hours. ["Jose Chung's *From Outer Space*"]

FINLEY, REV. PATRICK: As he is giving a sermon during a worship service, his hands bleed like the wounds of the crucifixion. Afterward he is murdered by the Millennium Man **(Simon Gates).** It is later discovered that the display of **stigmata** was faked. ["Revelations"]

FIORE, TONY: A police detective in his mid thirties who was the partner of **Charlie Morris.** He felt guilty over his connection to Morris's death and so he married Morris's widow. ["Born Again"]

FIORE, ANITA: Wife of Tony Fiore. She is the former wife of murdered policeman **Charlie Morris.** ["Born Again"]

FIREWALKER: A robot survey device invented by **Daniel Trepkos** for working inside a volcano. It looks like a large titanium bug. ["Firewalker"]

FIRST CHURCH OF THE REDEMPTION: In Waynesburg, Pennsylvania, where the **Rev. Finley** gives a sermon right before he's murdered by the Millennium Man. ["Revelations"]

FIRST ELDER: The syndicate leader previously seen in "The Blessing Way" and "Paper Clip." He interrogates Scully when she is captured at the **Hansen's Research Center Compound** in Perkey, West Virginia. In defending the work of **Dr. Ishimaru,** he states, "In a world of madmen, knowledge supersedes morality." He claims Ishimaru experimented on lepers, the homeless, and the insane, and that they were subjected to radiation tests and diseases. Scully believes him because Ishimaru did the same things during World War II. The Elder tells Scully that the man locked in the train car with Mulder has **hemorrhagic fever,** and isn't really a human–alien hybrid. ["731"]

FIRST X-FILE (1946): See **Richard Watkins.** ["Shapes"]

FLOYD, RAY: Construction worker in **Fairfield, Idaho,** who is knocked down and killed by an invisible force moving down the main street. His back is broken and there is an abrasion on his chest the size of an elephant's foot. ["Fearful Symmetry"]

FLUKEMAN: The half-human, half-fluke entity that finds its way to New Jersey from inside a Russian ship. He is cut in half in the climax, but we are led to believe that he may not have died, since the corpse opens its eyes in the final scene — or was that just a reflex muscle spasm? ["The Host"]

FLYING SAUCER DINER: A greasy spoon near **Ellens Air Force Base** in Idaho, which sells hamburgers that look vaguely like UFOs. The diner is owned and operated by a woman named **Ladonna,** who will sell you homemade UFO photos for a price. ["Deep Throat"]

FOLKSTONE INS PROCESSING CENTER: In North Carolina; 12,000 refugees, most of them Haitian, are housed here. It is little more than a collection of crude dormitories and tents. There has been unrest under the command of Marine **Col. Jacob Wharton,** and strange deaths are occurring in and around the town. ["Fresh Bones"]

FORAU: One of the Devil's disciples. This is the name **Simon Gates** uses when he rents a car. ["Revelations"]

FORNIER: A guard at **Eastpoint State Penitentiary** who is skeptical of **"Neech" Manley**'s claims that he'd be reincarnated. Fornier's severed head is discovered, writhing with maggots, inside an empty paint can by a prisoner on work detail. The rest of his body turns up in the office chair of warden **Leo Brodeur.** He is Manley's second victim. ["The List"]

FORT EVANSTON: U.S. Army base in Maryland commanded by **Gen. Thomas Callahan. Sgt. "Rappo" Trimble** is a patient in the base hospital.

FORT MARLENE HIGH CONTAINMENT FACILITY: Site of a secret cryo-lab where experiments with extraterrestrial viruses are conducted on human beings. ["The Erlenmeyer Flask"]

14th PRECINCT HOUSE: In Buffalo, New York. The site of the murder of police detective **Rudy Barbala.** ["Born Again"]

FOX FIRE: A folk legend from the Ozark Mountains. The phosphorescent glow caused by decaying wood was believed by many settlers (and modern-day Southerners) to be the spirits of massacred Indians. Mulder at first suspects such a phenomenon to be involved in a mysterious fire spotted near

Dudley, Arkansas, around the time of **George Kearns**'s disappearance. ["Our Town"]

FOYLE, CAPT.: Military coroner who finds a dog's corpse in the morgue drawer where **Pvt. John McAlpin**'s body is supposed to be. ["Fresh Bones"]

FRANKLIN, PENNSYLVANIA: The site of a spate of mysterious homicides. Seven killers have racked up twenty-two victims in six months by the time Mulder is called in. ["Blood"]

FRASER, LT.: An officer involved in **Operation Falcon,** under the command of **Col. Henderson.** The leader of the **Beta Team** strike force, Fraser is hospitalized with extreme burns, along with the surviving members of his team, after a deadly encounter with an invisible alien presence. ["Fallen Angel"]

FRASS, SHERIFF: Mulder encounters him in Massachusetts and learns from him that there have been an inexplicable series of "roach attacks," one of which the sheriff responds to while talking to Mulder. ["War of the Coprophages"]

FREDDIE: The leader of a group of people holding a UFO party after objects have been sighted two nights in a row. ["E.B.E."]

FREDDIES: Nickname given to employees of the U.S. Forest Service by ecoterrorists. ["Darkness Falls"]

FREDERICK COUNTY MORGUE: In Maryland. Mulder goes there to identify what the police say might be the body of Scully. It turns out not to be. ["Wetwired"]

FREDERICK, MARYLAND: Location of the U.S. Medical Research Institute of Infectious Diseases, where **Dr. Abel Gardner** discovers a mysterious virus in the body of FBI agent **Barrett Weiss.** ["End Game"]

FREELY, QUINTON "ROACH": An Army veteran who works in the mail room of the **Fort Evanston** hospital. He served in the Gulf War with Sgt. **"Rappo" Trimble.** After his fingerprints are found at **Gen. Callahan**'s home, he is arrested. Letters addressed to Trimble's victims are found in Freely's apartment. Freely dies in a locked cell, suffocated by a sheet stuffed down his throat. ["The Walk"]

FREE RADICALS: Chemicals that contain extra electrons and cause human DNA and proteins to oxidize, they are believed to be a primary factor in aging. Scully theorizes that the USS *Argent* and the meteor on the sea floor beneath it are acting as opposite poles of a gigantic magnetic field that is exciting the free radicals in its range, causing massive oxidizing of organic and inorganic matter — in other words, speeding up aging and corrosion. ["Dod Kalm"]

FREEDOM OF INFORMATION ACT: A law passed by Congress allowing American citizens access to formerly classified documents (suitably edited), which include Mulder's travel expenses. According to **Max Fenig,** Mulder's "fans" use these records to follow his activities. ["Fallen Angel"]

FROHIKE: On the staff of the magazine *The Lone Gunman.* He has a buzz cut and wears a Marine Corps watch. He thinks Scully is "hot." About him, Mulder observes, "It's men like you that give perversion a bad name." But his feelings include genuine respect as he goes to visit Scully at the hospital when she is in a coma in "One Breath." He also appears in "Blood," "Anasazi," and "E.B.E." He visits Scully, drunk, after he gets news of Mulder's apparent death, and shows her a newspaper clip about the death of the **Thinker.** ["The Blessing Way"] The last of the Lone Gunmen to see Mulder after his return, Frohike tells Scully of her sister's shooting. ["Paper Clip"] He is shown a strange video trap by Mulder. He and **Byers** determine that it sends another signal in along with the normal cable TV signal, a signal containing tachistoscopic images designed to influence the person watching the program. ["Wetwired"]

FULGURITE: Glass formed by the heat generated when lightning strikes sandy soil. One discovered near **Connerville, Oklahoma,** bears the imprint of a boot (size 8½). Scully also finds traces of antifreeze in the imprint, leading to auto shop employee **Darin Peter Oswald.** ["D.P.O."]

FULLER, AGENT: Head of the FBI's violent-crimes section, he stakes out the Calvert Street office building in the belief that the killer will return to the scene of the crime. Much to Mulder's surprise, **Eugene Tooms** does return, but only because his job with the Baltimore Animal Control Department brings him back to dispose of a dead cat in a ventilation duct. ["Squeeze"]

FULLER, BRIAN: FBI man in his forties who informs Scully that **Walter Skinner** has been shot. ["Apocrypha"]

FULLER, ROLAND: A mentally retarded janitor who works at the **Mahan Propulsion Laboratory.** His ID number is 315. He is actually the twin brother of the late **Arthur Grable.** They were separated at age three and Fuller grew up in an institute for the mentally retarded. After Grable is killed in a car accident and his head is preserved cryogenically, he's able to dominate Roland's mind and take control of his body. ["Roland"]

FUNSCH, ED: A fifty-two-year-old postal worker in Franklin, Pennsylvania, who is laid off due to budget cutbacks. He's a former Navy radio man whose wife died ten years ago. After he cuts himself on his machine, he starts to believe that he sees the machine he works on spelling out commands to "KILL 'EM ALL." It turns out that Funsch is afraid of blood. ["Blood"]

FYLFOT: Another term for the reverse swastika used as a protective charm by the **Calusari.** ["The Calusari"]

[G]

GAFFS: The name circus people give to phony freaks. ["Humbug"]

GALAXY GATEWAY: Mulder's motel in **Atlantic City** (Room 756). He lets **Jack** stay there instead of him. ["The Jersey Devil"]

GAMMADION: Another term for the reverse swastika used as a protective charm by the **Calusari.** ["The Calusari"]

GANESHA: The name of the twelve-year-old female Indian elephant that dies after apparently doing a lot of damage and killing a man in **Fairfield, Idaho.** The only problem is, the elephant was apparently invisible much of the time. ["Fearful Symmetry"]

GARDNER, DR. ABEL: Chief medical officer of the U.S. Medical Research Institute of Infectious Diseases. He discovers a mysterious retrovirus in the body of FBI agent **Barrett Weiss.** Scully had seen this virus before ["The Erlenmeyer Flask"] but is surprised when Gardner reveals that it goes dormant at low temperatures. ["End Game"]

GARNET: According to the **Lone Gunman** named **Byers,** the code name for the black ops (a secret government military outfit) unit dispatched to capture the **Thinker.** ["Anasazi"]

GARZA, ANGELO: A gas station employee who runs afoul of two infected prison escapees. He attempts to assist **Steve** when he finds him in the station's bathroom, but is assaulted by **Paul** for his trouble. Surviving that attack, he becomes infected by *F. Emasculata,* and is carried away via helicopter by **Pinck Pharmaceuticals'** minions. ["F. Emasculata"]

GATES, DAVID: The attorney representing **Jim Parker.** ["Shapes"]

GATES, SIMON: Also known as the Millennium Man. A businessman and CEO of a holding company based in Atlanta. Previous run-in with the law was an arrest on a DUI charge for an accident that paralyzed a young boy. Given a suspended sentence, he left the United States and traveled to Israel. He wears white patent-leather shoes. He exists to murder anyone he detects who has true spiritual power. He himself has supernatural power which he uses when he slays his victims, and leaves a burn mark on the neck of those he strangles. In three years he has murdered eleven people who seemed to be stigmatics, in case they might in fact be among the true twelve stigmatics (see also **stigmata**). ["Revelations"]

GAUTHIER: A French deep sea diver who locates a sunken World War II fighter plane in the Pacific Ocean. When he returns to the surface, he is possessed by an alien entity. By the time his ship, the *Piper Maru,* reaches San Diego, everyone aboard is suffering from extreme exposure to radiation — except him. The alien possessing him exits him in San Francisco and takes over his wife, Joan, leaving him with no memories of his time under its control. When Mulder locates him, Gauthier refuses to speak and demands to see the French consulate. ["Piper Maru"]

GAUTHIER, JOAN: The American wife of the Frenchman Gauthier. The alien that possessed him uses her body to travel to Hong Kong, abandoning her when it finds **Alex Krycek.** ["Piper Maru"] She is found, disoriented, in the men's room at the Hong Kong airport. ["Apocrypha"]

GAYHART, DR. DALE: A doctor who died in an arson fire at an abortion clinic in New York City. His name appears on a list of similar deaths e-mailed to Mulder by an anonymous source. Mulder is baffled upon learning that all three doctors, although apparently unrelated, were identical — and no body was recovered in any of the cases. ["Colony"]

GENERAL MUTUAL INSURANCE: The company where **Clyde Bruckman** was employed as a life insurance salesman. ["Clyde Bruckman's Final Repose"]

GENEROO, MICHELLE: A Mission Control communications commander for NASA in Houston who contacts the FBI when she receives evidence of sabotage from an aborted space shuttle mission. Concerned that the next launch — which her fiancé is flying on — is at risk, she helps Mulder and Scully figure out what is going on in the upper levels of NASA administration. The problem turns out to be **Lt. Col. Belt,** who is possessed by an alien entity of some sort. ["Space"]

GEORGETOWN MEDICAL CENTER: Hospital in Washington, D.C., where **Skinner** is treated after being shot by **Luis Cardinal.** ["Apocrypha"]

GEORGE WASHINGTON HOSPITAL: In Washington, D.C. A glassblower is taken here after he is attacked and his face is badly slashed. ["Grotesque"]

GEORGE WASHINGTON UNIVERSITY: In Washington, D.C. Art students there do sketches of a nude male model; shortly after class ends, the model is killed. One of the students is **John Mostow.** ["Grotesque"]

GERLACH, MALCOLM: The real name of the red-haired man. A professional assassin, his usual method of execution is with a garrote. He is ordered to eliminate **Dr. Zama.** After killing Zama, he attempts to kill Mulder. He claims he works for the National Security Agency. When he beats up Mulder and escapes from the **Quarantine Car,** he is shot and killed by **X.** ["731"]

GERMANTOWN, MARY-LAND: A suburb of Washington, D.C., where Mulder investigates the mysterious death of a businessman; the victim entered his hotel room with a woman, but a man left, tying this in with other cases in Mulder's files. ["Genderbender"] Also where Mulder, Scully, and CIA agent **Chapel** locate **Dr. James Dickens.** Scully later hides out in a motel here as well. ["Colony"]

GIBSONTON, FLORIDA: Where circus freaks live during the winter. It was founded in the 1920s by members of the Barnum & Bailey circus. ["Humbug"]

GILDER, DR.: The doctor who pronounces **Rudy Barbala** dead. ["Born Again"]

GILLNITZ, JOHN: When Helene Riddock imagines she sees her husband, Victor, com-mitting adultery with the woman next door, she grabs a shotgun and kills Gillnitz, her neighbor, whom she mistakes for her husband. ["Wetwired"]

GIORGIO, CHRIS-SY: A beautiful teenage girl who with her date, **Harold Lamb,** is abducted by a UFO one night. When found the next morning she has no memory of what happened, and all of her clothes are on inside out or backward. Mulder believes she is suffering from post-abduction syndrome. ["Jose Chung's *From Outer Space*"]

GIRARDI, DR. FRANCIS: Worked with **Dr. Grissom** on the sleep eradication experiments on Parris Island in 1970. He performed the actual surgery. ["Sleepless"]

GLASS, DR. WILLIAM: Works at the Oregon State Psychiatric Hospital near Bellefleur. **Ray Soames** was his patient. [Pilot]

GLAZEBROOK, JERALD: He has reptilelike skin — hence his circus name, the Crocodile Man. He's married to the

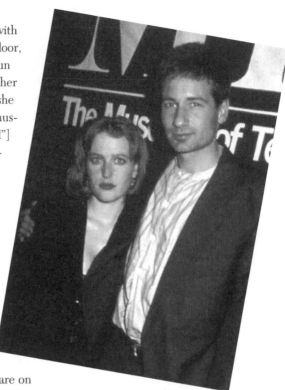

bearded lady, and they have two young boys. He is killed by something that has killed forty-six other people in the previous eight years in Gibsonton, Florida. ["Humbug"]

GLENVIEW LAKE: The body of water where **Clyde Bruckman** correctly predicts the **Doll Collector**'s body would be found. ["Clyde Bruckman's Final Repose"]

GLOSSOLALIA: The religious phenomenon of speaking in tongues (that is, talking unintelligibly). **Lucy Householder** experiences it when **Amy**

Jacobs is kidnapped by **Carl Wade.** The words Lucy speaks are actually the same words spoken by Wade when he kidnapped Amy. ["Oubliette"]

GODFREY, DR. RICHARD: The town pediatrician. He's a cross-dresser. An old surgical bag of his is found buried in a yard with bones in it. It turns out they're animal bones from where someone buried their pet dog, a Mr. Tippy. ["Syzygy"]

GOLDA: The mother of **Maggie Holvey** and grandmother of **Teddy** and **Charlie Holvey.** A Romanian woman who did not approve of her daughter's marriage to an American, **Steve Holvey.** Highly superstitious, Golda brings a bizarre Old World element to the Holvey household when she comes to live there after the death of **Michael Holvey.** Highly superstitious, she performs strange rituals centered on Charlie that lead Scully to suspect her of **Munchausen by proxy.** Golda dies with her eyes pecked out by dead chickens. ["The Calusari"]

GOLDBAUM: A patient at the Bethesda Naval Hospital whose room **Jack Willis** hides in while escaping from the hospital after his near-death experience. ["Lazarus"]

GOODENSNAKE, GWEN: The sister of Joseph Goodensnake. She sees a werewolf kill **Jim Parker** and panics. Did she know that her brother was a shape-shifter? ["Shapes"]

GOODENSNAKE, JOSEPH: A werewolf killed by **Jim Parker.** The examination of his corpse reveals catlike fangs an inch long. His sister refuses to allow an autopsy, which might have revealed internal irregularities. ["Shapes"]

GORDON, MR. AND MRS.: A young couple who resist **Clyde Bruckman**'s pitch for life insurance because the husband would rather spend the money on a nice boat. Exasperated, Bruckman tells him how he will die in a head-on collision with a blue 1987 Mustang two years hence, leaving his wife and as-yet-unborn daughter bereft. ["Clyde Bruckman's Final Repose"]

GRABLE, DR. ARTHUR: An aeronautical scientist who worked at the **Mahan Propulsion Laboratory** until he was killed in a car accident in November 1993. His twin brother is **Roland Fuller,** but because Roland is retarded, the boys were separated at age three and Roland grew up in an institution. ["Roland"]

GRAGO, DR. JOHN: Works three days a week at the

Excelsis Dei Convalescent Home. He has been treating a group of Alzheimer's patients there for seven months. ["Excelsis Dei"]

GRAVENHURST HIGH SCHOOL: Where **Darin Peter Oswald** finishes his education (although not necessarily by completing it). It is here that he develops a serious crush on the remedial English teacher, **Sharon Kiveat.** ["D.P.O."]

GRAVES, HOWARD: Founder of **HTG Industrial Technologies.** When the company began to go under, Graves went along with his partner's plan to illegally sell parts to Iran. After a terrorist attack killed some American servicemen, however, he tried to back out, only to be killed for his trouble. His spirit lingers on for revenge, and to protect **Lauren Kyte,** whom he regarded as the daughter he once had. ["Shadows"]

GRAVES, SARAH LYNN: Howard Graves's daughter, who died at the age of three in a pool accident. Buried with Howard Graves. ["Shadows"]

GRAY, PAULA: A line worker at the **Chaco Chicken** processing plant in **Dudley, Arkansas,** she is the granddaughter of **Walter Chaco.** She flirts with USDA inspector

George Kearns in order to lure him to the community feast off County Road A7 — where he is destined to be the main course. She later attacks her supervisor, **Jess Harold,** with a knife, only to be shot by **Sheriff Tom Arens.** An autopsy reveals that she was suffering from **Creutzfeldt-Jakob disease.** Although born in 1948, she looked like she was only twenty or so when she died in 1995. ["Our Town"]

GREEN, ARLAN AND SUSAN: **Eugene Tooms** rents a room in the house owned by them. ["Tooms"]

GREEN "SAMANTHA": An alien clone in green hospital garb whom Mulder meets at the **Women's Health Services Center** in Rockville, Maryland. She reveals that the "return" of Mulder's sister has been a ruse to gain his assistance. She, along with the rest of the "Samantha" clones, is killed by the **Pilot.** ["End Game"]

GREEN, PHOEBE: A British classmate of Mulder's at Oxford University. They had an affair during their student days. A mover and shaker in Scotland Yard ten years later, she turns to Mulder for help in the **Cecil L'ively** case. Beautiful but prone to play

mind games, she has an affair with Lord **Marsden** while she assists Mulder in the apprehension of L'ively. ["Fire"]

GREENWICH, CONNECTICUT: Wealthy New York suburb where **Joel Simmons** is murdered by his daughter **Teena Simmons,** and Teena is abducted by **Dr. Sally Kendrick.** ["Eve"]

GREGOR: According to CIA agent **Chapel,** the code name for the identical doctors he claims are genetically engineered Soviet spies. In truth, they are alien colonists. Scully finds four more "Gregors" at the warehouse at 3243 **Edmonton Street** and places them in protective custody, but this is not enough to save them from being disposed of by the **Pilot** (see **"Samantha"**). ["Colony"]

GREINER, DEAN: A scientist at the **Astadourian Lightning Observatory** near **Connerville, Oklahoma.** ["D.P.O."]

GRIFFIN, LT.: Officer involved in **Operation Falcon** who reports the movement of the downed alien to **Col. Henderson.** ["Fallen Angel"]

GRISSOM, DR. SAUL: A pioneer in sleep disorders and founder of the Grissom Sleep Disorder Center. He was stationed on Parris Island, where

Marines receive basic training, from 1968 to 1971. In 1970 he conducted sleep eradication experiments there. His two greatest successes were **Willig** and **Cole.** He dies in his apartment when he believes he's trapped by a fire. Even though there is no fire, he suffers all the secondary physiological responses to having been burned, as if his body actually believed it was burning. ["Sleepless"]

GROVER CLEVELAND ALEXANDER HIGH SCHOOL: The school attended by the boys who are murdered by **Terri Roberts** and **Margi Kleinjan.** ["Syzygy"]

GUANACASTE RAIN FOREST: The jungle in Costa Rica where **Dr. Robert Torrence** discovers the insect named **Faciphaga Emasculata,** only to succumb to the parasite that lives in the insect. ["F. Emasculata"]

GUARDIANS OF THE DEAD: Two Indians, Bill and Tom, whose duty is to escort the deceased spirit to the next world as part of the funeral rites. ["Shapes"]

GUTIERREZ, PVT. MANUEL: A Marine who commits suicide. His body is stolen from its grave. ["Fresh Bones"]

[H]

HAGERSTOWN, MARYLAND: Small town where **Lula Philips** robs a drugstore of 200 units of insulin and a box of syringes for **Jack Willis.** ["Lazarus"]

HAGOPIAN, BETSY: Inside a **leather satchel** carried by a Japanese man who flees from a murder scene are high-resolution satellite photos and a list of Mutual UFO Network (MUFON) members in the **Allentown, Pennsylvania,** area. One name circled is Betsy Hagopian. When Scully visits Hagopian's house she finds a gathering in progress of people who claim that they were once abducted and taken to the **bright white place,** and that they recognize Scully as a fellow abductee. Hagopian is in the hospital, at the **Positron Emission Tomography Lab,** due to an undiagnosed cancerous condition. ["Nisei"]

HAKKARI, TURKEY: Where U.S. forces at a NATO surveillance station detect a UFO passing overhead after it is shot down. ["E.B.E."]

HAKKIE, DR. DEL: A psychiatrist at the **Davis Correctional Treatment Center. Duane Barry** takes him hostage, intending to transport him to the site where Barry was once abducted by an alien spacecraft and hand Hakkie over to the aliens. ["Duane Barry"]

HALE, GEORGE: Cover name used by Mulder when he phones Scully at the FBI academy at Quantico. ["Sleepless"]

HALOPERIDOL: An antipsychotic drug given to **Michael Kryder** at the mental hospital where he is imprisoned. ["Revelations"]

HALVORSON: Twenty-one-year-old Norwegian first mate of **Henry Trondheim**'s boat the *Zeal*. He is killed by the pirate whaler **Olafssen** on the USS *Argent*. ["Dod Kalm"]

HAMILTON, SHERIFF: The sheriff of **Gibsonton, Florida.** In 1933 he was a feral child discovered in a forest in Albania. He was exhibited in a Barnum circus as Jim-Jim, the Dog-Faced Boy. He finally escaped to begin a normal life outside the circus. ["Humbug"]

HAMMOND, JACK: A classic small-town character, a former high school football star whose career after graduation never went higher than pizza delivery. His attempt to bully **Darin Peter Oswald** away from his beloved Virtua Fighter 2 leads to his death by electrocution: he is fried to a crisp in his 1968 Oldsmobile 442. ["D.P.O."]

HAND, DR.: One of the people who interrogate **Chrissy Giorgio.** At first she remembers him as looking like a Gray Alien. ["Jose Chung's *From Outer Space*"]

1223 HANOVER STREET: The Georgetown address of the escort service **Carina Sayles** worked for. ["Avatar"]

HANSEN'S RESEARCH CENTER COMPOUND: In Perkey, West Virginia. A group of soldiers arrive there and herd the human–alien hybrids into the forest and shoot them all, Nazi fashion. Only one escapes to bear witness to the crime, although four others also survive the massacre. Scully traces **Dr. Zama** there while trying to track down the manufacturer of the computer chip she finds implanted in her neck. Hansen's disease is the scientific name for leprosy. ["731"]

HARBORMASTER: Visited by Mulder in Newport News, Virginia, when he's searching for the *Talapus*. ["Nisei"]

HAROLD, JESS: The floor manager of the **Chaco Chicken** processing plant in **Dudley, Arkansas.** He is attacked by **Paula Gray** when she succumbs to the effects of **Creutzfeldt-Jakob disease.**

One of the main townspeople to turn against **Walter Chaco,** he is trampled by a panicked crowd after Mulder shoots **Sheriff Tom Arens.** ["Our Town"]

HARPER, LT. RICHARD: A survivor of the USS *Argent* who leads the mutiny of eighteen men, abandoning the *Argent* in Lifeboat 925 over **Capt. Barclay**'s objections. Harper was the last mutineer to die; Scully sees him briefly at Bethesda Naval Hospital, and is stunned to note that he looks ninety years old. He is actually twenty-nine. ["Dod Kalm"]

HARTLEY, REV. CALVIN: The guardian of Samuel, the boy who can raise the dead. Now the owner of the Miracle Ministry, he was once a poor pastor who preached from a soapbox and collected dollar bills in a coffee can. ["Miracle Man"]

HARTLEY, SAMUEL: The adopted son of the Rev. Calvin Hartley. He has the power to bring the recently deceased back to life. In 1983, at the age of eight, he did this at the scene of a horrific car accident. But as an adult of eighteen, he kills people with a touch instead of healing them. He claims his "gift has been corrupted." ["Miracle Man"]

HARVEY MUDD: The college attended by **Dr. Nollette** in the 1970s. His quantum physics professor failed him one semester because he didn't agree with one of Nollette's theories. ["Roland"]

HAVEZ, DET.: The partner of **Det. Cline,** working on the **Puppet** serial killings. A serious chain smoker, he is relieved when **Clyde Bruckman** assures him he won't die of lung cancer. The **Puppet** stabs Havez to death minutes later. ["Clyde Bruckman's Final Repose"]

HAWLEY, LIZ: A nineteen-year-old student at Jackson University in North Carolina. She and her boyfriend **Jim Summers** are kidnapped and tortured by **Lucas Jackson Henry;** Hawley is rescued first, at **Lake Jordan.** ["Beyond the Sea"]

HELL MONEY: Paper currency burned by the Chinese to provide wealth to spirits in the afterlife. ["Hell Money"]

HELM, HEPCAT: A fifty-year-old artist who has lived in **Gibsonton, Florida,** for many years. He is also a mechanic and a carnival operator. He is killed by **Leonard,** the evil Siamese twin. ["Humbug"]

HEMORRHAGIC FEVER: The man imprisoned in **Quarantine Car** has this ail-

ment, and if the bomb in the car detonates, the disease — a deadly, leprosy-like ailment — will be spread to thousands of people nearby. ["731"]

HENDERSON, COL. CALVIN: Air Force officer in charge of **Operation Falcon.** Once assigned to preventing downed U.S. spy planes from falling into enemy hands, he now works in the field of UFO crash retrieval. Advises his prisoner Mulder to forget what he saw near **Townsend, Wisconsin.** ["Fallen Angel"]

HENDERSON, HEATHER: A brilliant FBI lab technician in her late thirties, and a friend of Mulder's. She matches **John Barnett**'s old handwriting to new notes with a 95 percent probability. She seems to have a thing for Mulder. ["Young at Heart"]

HENRY: Halfway house resident who helps **Lucy Householder.** ["Oubliette"]

HENRY, LUCAS JACKSON: A small-time crook, age twenty-eight, with a history of sexual assault and narcotics charges. He kidnaps and tortures **Liz Hawley** and **Jim Summers** in a psychotic attempt to work out his mental problems. An identical kidnapping one year earlier resulted in the deaths of his victims; Hawley and Summers are rescued. Henry may have aided **Luther Lee Boggs** in his last five murders, but this has never been proved. Henry falls to his death in the **Blue Devil Brewery** while fleeing the FBI. ["Beyond the Sea"]

HERITAGE HALFWAY HOUSE: The home of **Roland Fuller.** ["Roland"]

HEUVELMANS LAKE: Located in the Blue Ridge Mountains of Georgia, it has forty-eight miles of coastline. A mysterious creature known as **Big Blue** lives in this lake. ["Quagmire"]

HIGH-RESOLUTION MICROWAVE SURVEY: The project designed to scan the sky for radio transmissions of an intelligent extraterrestrial origin. A radio telescope in this survey is located at **Arecibo,** Puerto Rico. ["Little Green Men"]

HINDT, SHERIFF LANCE: He is investigating the disappearances and deaths at **Heuvelmans Lake** but thinks the deaths are ordinary accidents. ["Quagmire"]

HIRSH, JUDGE: One of the Maryland judges at the sanity hearing for **Eugene Tooms.** ["Tooms"]

HODGE, DR. LAWRENCE: A physician who accompanies Mulder and Scully to investigate the **Arctic Ice Core Project** disaster. Arrogant and suspicious, Hodge erroneously believes that the FBI agents know more than they're letting on. He thinks Mulder is **Murphy**'s murderer until **Nancy Da Silva** is revealed as the real culprit. Hodge and Scully discover a way to defeat the ice worm infestation. ["Ice"]

HOHMAN, MARGARET: A sick woman who goes to be healed at the **Miracle Ministry** tent. When **Samuel Hartley** touches her, however, she dies instead of being healed. But an autopsy reveals that she was poisoned, not killed by Samuel. ["Miracle Man"]

HOLLOWAY, LOTTIE: A Mutual UFO Network (MUFON) member living in the **Allentown, Pennsylvania**, area. She is visited by Scully and is shocked to recognize her, claiming Scully is a fellow abductee. ["Nisei"]

HOLLY: An FBI research librarian, injured in a mugging. Some time after that, **Robert Modell** uses his persuasive powers to get her to provide him information about Mulder. When **Skinner** challenges Modell's presence in the FBI building, Modell makes her think Skinner was the man who mugged her. He escapes when Holly sprays the Assistant Director with Mace. ["Pusher"]

HOLLYWOOD BLOOD BANK: A Los Angeles–area blood bank investigated by Mulder in his search for the people in the **Trinity** gang of vampiric killers. He hits pay dirt: **The Son** is working here as a night watchman and Mulder catches him raiding the blood bank. ["3"]

HOLTZMAN, VICTOR: An agent of the National Security Agency who investigates when Mulder faxes some of **Kevin Morris**'s binary scribblings to an FBI cryptologist. The fax includes top-secret military information, but the rest of Kevin's papers involve nothing classified. Holtzman's handling of the case is less than subtle, and results in the ransacking of the Morris residence. ["Conduit"]

HOLVEY, CHARLIE: The eight-year-old son of Maggie and Steve Holvey, he is a twin whose identical brother Michael died at birth. His grandmother **Golda** has spent years trying to protect him from the spirit of his twin, but these actions have been perceived as destructive superstition by his parents. Charlie knows of Michael's existence even though his parents have never told him about it. ["The Calusari"]

HOLVEY, TEDDY: The two-year-old son of Maggie and Steve Holvey, he is killed when he follows a drifting balloon onto the tracks of the miniature train ride at Lincoln Park in Murray, Virginia. Photo analysis reveals what appears to be a shadowy figure pulling the balloon, prompting Mulder's initial suspicion of poltergeist activity centering around Teddy's older brother Charlie. ["The Calusari"]

HOLVEY, MAGGIE: A Romanian woman who married Steve Holvey, an American diplomat, in 1984. They had three children: Michael, Charlie, and Teddy. Only Charlie has survived. Maggie saw her move to America as a chance to escape from the superstitions of her upbringing, but the events surrounding the untimely deaths of her husband, mother, and son Teddy lead her to reconsider the validity of Romanian folk beliefs. ["The Calusari"]

HOLVEY, MICHAEL: Charlie Holvey's twin brother, who died at birth. His spirit follows Charlie until it is exorcised by a Ritual of Separation; however, the **Calusari** hint that this may not have been Michael's spirit but a more malevolent

demonic force that took his form. This force notices Mulder during the ritual. ["The Calusari"]

HOLVEY, STEVE: An employee of the State Department whose son Teddy dies under unusual circumstances; Holvey's position leads to a routine FBI investigation of the death, which turns out to be anything but routine. Steve Holvey is killed when his necktie is caught in the drive train of an electric garage door opener he is trying to fix, causing death by strangulation while his son Charlie watches. ["The Calusari"]

HOMETOWN TRUST: The bank **Ed Funsch** uses in Franklin, Pennsylvania. The ATM monitor tries to tell Funsch to take the security guard's gun. ["Blood"]

HORNING, CRAIG: A researcher at the Boston Museum of Natural History, murdered by mysterious forces while working on the **Amaru** Urn. ["Teso dos Bichos"]

HORTON, DET. BILL: The investigating officer on the case of the death of **Dr. Saul Grissom.** ["Sleepless"]

HOSTEEN (ALBERT'S SON): Eric Hosteen's father, first name unknown. He takes part in Mulder's **Blessing Way**

ceremony. ["The Blessing Way"]

HOSTEEN, ALBERT: A Navajo code walker who helps translate the original **MJ documents** into Navajo, and later helps Mulder and Scully translate them back. He tells his grandson Eric to take the alien corpse back where he found it. ["Anasazi"] Hosteen and his family are brutalized by the troops controlled by the **Cigarette-Smoking Man,** but do not tell them anything. When Mulder's unconscious body is found in the desert, he conducts the Blessing Way healing ceremony but is unsuccessful. ["The Blessing Way"] By memorizing the information on the MJ files DAT (already encoded in Navajo) and passing it along orally to other members of his tribe, he helps **Skinner** to thwart the Smoking Man's plans for Mulder and Scully. ["Paper Clip"]

HOSTEEN, ERIC: Albert Hosteen's grandson, a Navajo teen who collects rattlesnake skins. He discovers a buried railway refrigeration car in the desert on the Navajo reservation after an earthquake reveals its location, and brings an alien corpse back into town. When Mulder comes to the reservation, Eric drives him to the site on his motocross bike. ["Anasazi"] After the **Cigarette-Smoking Man** interrogates Eric, he is brought back to the Hosteen home. Later, he takes part in Mulder's **Blessing Way** ceremony. ["The Blessing Way"]

HOTEL CATHERINE: The Washington, D.C., hotel where Mulder and Scully track **Marty** of the **Kindred.** They are unable to arrest him/her because he is captured by his own people, who then vanish. ["Genderbender"]

HOTEL GEORGE MASON: The plush Richmond, Virginia, hotel where **Patrick Newirth** is disintegrated. ["Soft Light"]

HOUSEHOLDER, LUCY: A thirty-year-old trainee working in an unnamed **fast-food restaurant.** She has short, dark hair and a pale face with haunted eyes. One night at work she suddenly gets a bloody nose, but this isn't an ordinary bloody nose. It is later determined that the bloodstains on her clothes are of two different types, O-positive and B-positive. Lucy is O-positive and **Amy Jacob**'s blood type is B-positive. When Lucy was eight years old she was kidnapped by an unidentified man (actually **Carl Wade**) and remained his prisoner for five years. When Amy is kid-

napped, Lucy experiences the trauma Amy is feeling. This happens at 10:05 P.M., at the exact moment Amy is kidnapped. Lucy has a variety of lingering emotional problems, including an aversion to being touched. When shown a photo of Wade, she identifies him as the man who kidnapped her years ago. But when the FBI determines that the blood on Lucy's clothes is an exact DNA match for Amy's, they come to arrest Lucy for complicity in the kidnapping. She disappears, only to be found in the basement of Wade's cabin, which she realizes is where she had been held those five years. ["Oubliette"]

HSIN, KIM: A young Chinese woman suffering from leukemia. Her father takes part in a dangerous game to help pay her medical bills. ["Hell Money"]

HSIN, SHUYANG: A carpet layer by trade, he gambles his own organs in an attempt to win money to pay for his daughter Kim's expensive leukemia treatment. He loses an eye in the process, but is rescued by **Glen Chao** before his heart can be removed. ["Hell Money"]

HTG INDUSTRIAL TECHNOLOGIES: A small defense subcontractor in Philadelphia

that becomes the focus of forces from beyond the grave after its founder, **Howard Graves,** is killed. Graves just can't stand to leave any unfinished business behind. ["Shadows"]

HUGHES, DR. ALICIA: The identity assumed by **Eve Eight** after her escape. Hughes has high-level Pentagon clearance. She visits **Teena Simmons** and **Cindy Reardon** after they are incarcerated at the **Whiting Institute.** ["Eve"]

HUMAN GENOME PROJECT: Experiments conducted on human beings with extraterrestrial viruses — the injection of alien DNA into humans. ["The Erlenmeyer Flask"]

HUMPHREYS, STEVE: Head of security for the **Schiff-Immergut Lumber Company.** He accompanies Mulder, Scully, and **Larry Moore.** He's caught inside his pickup truck at night and encased in a **cocoon** by the prehistoric wood mites. ["Darkness Falls"]

HUNSAKER, GEORGE: His son receives an anonymous call from someone who says he knows where a mass grave is located. ["Syzygy"]

HYMAN RICKOVER NAVAL HOSPITAL: In Seattle. Mulder, Scully, and **Larry**

Moore are taken here to be treated after they are cocooned by prehistoric wood mites. Unlike the other victims, they are found and rescued in time. ["Darkness Falls"]

HYNEK, SGT.: He comes to claim the body of Air Force Maj. **Robert Vallee.** His name is an inside joke: Dr. Allen J. Hynek is a UFO investigator who invented the term "close encounters." ["Jose Chung's *From Outer Space*"]

HYPOKALEMIA: A condition in which the blood contains unusually high levels of sodium and a commensurate decrease in potassium. Medical records from the hospital where **Darin Peter Oswald** was treated after being struck by lightning show that he suffered from this condition at the time, prompting Mulder to hypothesize that this unusual concentration of electrolytes enabled Darin to produce electricity with his body. Tests taken after Darin's arrest show no signs of hypokalemia. ["D.P.O."]

[I]

ICARUS PROJECT: The next generation of jet design, capable of doubling current supersonic speeds using half the fuel. Its goal is an engine that can achieve Mach 15 (fifteen

times the speed of sound). ["Roland"]

ICE WORM: An alien parasite brought to Earth by a meteor a quarter of a million years ago that lay dormant under two miles of ice until it is brought to the surface by the **Arctic Ice Core Project.** In its dormant state, it appears to be an ammonia-based microorganism; when it enters the bloodstream of a victim, the single-celled larva develops into a worm approximately one foot long and attaches itself to the hypothalamus gland. At this point it increases that gland's production of acetylcholine, which induces violent behavior in the victim. Removal of the worm by surgical means results in the death of the victim. Introduction of another live worm into the victim, however, causes both worms to kill each other, releasing the victim from the control of the ice worm. ["Ice"]

ICY CAPE, ALASKA: The location of the **Arctic Ice Core Project,** 250 miles north of the Arctic Circle. ["Ice"]

INCANTO, VIRGIL: A man with a rare disease: he has no fatty tissue and must ingest it from others. His body produces a highly acidic slime that allows him to dissolve people's skin.

At first he uses personals ads to find victims, but later moves onto the Internet. His favored victims are lonely, overweight women, but he resorts to prostitutes in a pinch. A scholar of sixteenth-century Italian poetry, he seems able to seduce women with ease. One of his intended victims, **Ellen Kaminski,** kills him with Scully's service revolver. His name was probably a pseudonym drawn from Dante. He killed at least forty-seven women. ["2Shy"]

INDIGO DELTA NINER: The military code used by **Col. Calvin Henderson** to initiate **Operation Falcon.** ["Fallen Angel"]

IONESCO: A crew member on board the Canadian fishing vessel *Lisette* who throws a line to Lifeboat 925 from the USS *Argent.* ["Dod Kalm"]

ISH: An old Indian man with one blind eye and shoulder-length gray hair. He wears a necklace made of animal claws and teeth. He has a scar down his face and was at Wounded Knee in 1973. His son is an Indian manitou, who attacks a rancher. His profession is mechanic. ["Shapes"]

ISHIMARU, DR.: Japanese scientist in his late sixties, with a silver streak in his hair. He is part of a mysterious experiment conducted in a train car. He has supposedly been dead since 1965, but he is still alive in the 1990s. He was in charge of a Japanese medical unit that experimented on living human beings. This included performing vivisections without anesthesia, testing frostbite tolerance levels on babies, and deliberately exposing people to diseases to chart their progress. Mulder believes Ishimaru has been trying to create a human–alien hybrid. Scully recognizes him as having been a part of whatever happened to her during the time she was missing after her abduction (see also **Dr. Zama**). ["Nisei"]

I-10: The interstate highway that runs through **Dudley, Arkansas.** A passing motorist sees a mysterious fire in a field off this highway the night USDA poultry inspector **George Kearns** disappears. ["Our Town"]

IVANOV, DR. ALEXANDER: An artificial-intelligence researcher who designs robots that look like insects. ["War of the Coprophages"]

[J]

JACK: A homeless man in his thirties who gives Mulder information about the activities of the **Jersey Devil** and the **Atlantic City** police. Mulder swaps his motel room for Jack's cardboard box in an alley, which he uses as a lookout point. ["The Jersey Devil"]

JACKSON: A member of **Operation Falcon**'s **Beta Team.** ["Fallen Angel"]

JACKSON: **Capt. Foyle**'s assistant. ["Fresh Bones"]

JACKSON UNIVERSITY: A college in Raleigh, North Carolina, where **Lucas Jackson Henry** kidnapped **Liz Hawley** and **Jim Summers.** ["Beyond the Sea"]

JACOBS, AGENT: She is following Scully when Scully goes to the Miami airport to catch a flight to Puerto Rico to search for Mulder. ["Little Green Men"]

JACOBS, AMY: Fifteen-year-old student at Valley Woods High in Seattle. At 10:05 P.M. one night she is kidnapped from her home by **Carl Wade.** As she is being carried out of her window by Wade, he puts his hand over her mouth and causes a nosebleed (see **Lucy Householder**). Wade keeps her locked up in the basement of his cabin, where there is no light, except for when Wade takes flash pictures of her. At one point she escapes, but Wade recaptures her. ["Oubliette"]

JACOBS, DAPHNE: The mother of Amy Jacobs. ["Oubliette"]

JACOBS, DR.: The Los Angeles Police Department's forensic dentist. ["3"]

JACOBS, SADIE: The five-year-old sister of Amy Jacobs. She shares a bedroom with Amy and witnesses her abduction, but all she sees is the back of the man who is carrying Amy out the open window. ["Oubliette"]

JALEE: Headhunting tribe of New Guinea long suspected of cannibalistic practices, which they taught to **Walter Chaco** when he was shot down near their Pacific island during World War II. ["Our Town"]

JANADI, SADOUN: Iraqi jet pilot who encounters a UFO and is attacked. ["E.B.E."]

JANELLI-HELLER FUNERAL HOME: Where **Donnie Pfaster** works until he is caught desecrating the corpse of a young woman. ["Irresistible"]

JANUS: FBI agent with medical training who goes into the **Travel Time Travel Agency** to assist the wounded hostage, **Bob Riley.** ["Duane Barry"]

JARVIS, OWEN LEE: Hired by **Susan Kryder** to do yard work after her husband is institutionalized, he is the defender of her son Kevin against the Forces of Darkness. When accused of kidnapping Kevin, Jarvis leaps out a second-story window, breaks free of the handcuffs on his wrists, and runs away. He successfully defends Kevin and dies doing so, killed by the Millennium Man **(Simon Gates).** After death his body doesn't decompose and emits the smell of flowers. ["Revelations"]

J.A.S.D. BEEF PACKING PLANT: In **Delta Glen, Wisconsin.** The "beef" it processes turns out to be human. ["Red Museum"]

JASON: The twelve-year-old boy unlucky enough to be headed to Toronto on the same bus as the escaped convict **Paul,** who takes him hostage until Mulder convinces Paul to let him go. ["F. Emasculata"]

J. EDGAR HOOVER BUILD-ING: The FBI's national head-quarters in Washington, named after the Bureau's original director.

JEFFERSON MEMORIAL HOSPITAL: In Richmond, Virginia. **Duane Barry** is hospitalized here after being shot by an FBI marksman at the **Travel Time Travel Agency.** ["Duane Barry"]

JENKINS: Maryland state's attorney at the sanity hearing held for **Eugene Tooms.** ["Tooms"]

JENSEN, DIANE: Secretary to **Assistant Director Walter S. Skinner** of the FBI. ["The Host"]

JERSEY DEVIL: The East Coast version of Bigfoot or the Abominable Snowman, it proves to be more than a legend when Mulder meets one face to face. In this case, it is a female, its mate apparently having died six months earlier, according to park ranger **Peter Boulle.** She is killed by the **Atlantic City** police, but her child survives in the wilds. ["The Jersey Devil"]

JERUSALEM, OHIO: Site of the **Twenty-First Century Recycling Plant,** owned by the holding company of which **Simon Gates** is CEO. ["Revelations"]

JERUSALEM SYNDROME: Affects some people who visit the Holy Land of Israel, leading from religious delusions to irrational religious fanaticism. ["Revelations"]

JIM-JIM, THE DOG-FACED BOY: An exhibit in the 1930s circus of P. T. Barnum. He fled the circus and became **Sheriff Hamilton** in **Gibsonton, Florida.** ["Humbug"]

JIMMY DOOLITTLE AIR-FIELD: A small airstrip in Nome, Alaska, where Mulder and Scully meet **Drs. Denny Murphy, Nancy Da Silva,** and **Lawrence Hodge** on their way to the **Arctic Ice Core Project** base. The pilot known as **Bear** flies them from here. ["Ice"]

JOAN: **Sen. Richard Matheson**'s secretary, who threatens to call security when Mulder, deranged by drugs in his drinking water, barges into Matheson's office. ["Anasazi"]

JOHANSEN, COMMANDER CHRISTOPHER: During World War II, Johansen served as the executive officer on the submarine *Zeus Faber.* He locked the alien-possessed **Capt. Kyle Sanford** below decks with the sick crewman when he realized the captain was a threat. Johansen was one of the seven men who survived the mission without radiation sickness. Later in his career he was a friend of **William Scully,** Dana's father. He tells Dana the true story of the *Zeus Faber*'s mission. ["Piper Maru"]

JOHN 52:54: The Biblical verse that reads "He who eats my flesh and drinks my blood has eternal life, and I will raise him up on the last day." The citation is found written in blood on the wall next to the body of **Garrett Lorre.** ["3"]

JOHNSON, DET.: A Baltimore cop at the scene of the

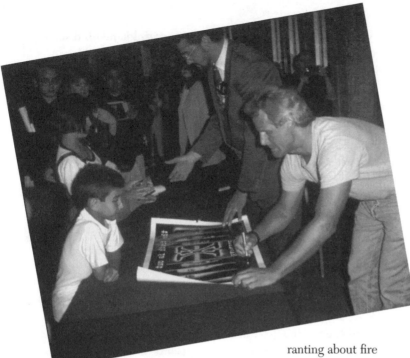

Werner murder. Johnson later informs Mulder that **Tooms** is missing from work. ["Squeeze"]

JOHNSON, VERNA: A murder victim. She was a teacher of high school drama. ["Aubrey"]

JOHNSTON COUNTY, OKLA-HOMA: Location of the town of **Connerville,** site of unusual electrical activity centered on one **Darin Peter Oswald.** ["D.P.O."]

JONES, CREIGHTON: A mental patient who had an unknown traumatic experience in or near **Dudley, Arkansas**, between May 17 and May 20, 1961. He lost an arm as well as his mind, and was later filmed ranting about fire demons hungry for flesh. This film gave Mulder nightmares in college, causing him to remember it vividly when the **George Kearns** case brings him and Scully to Dudley. ["Our Town"]

JORGE: The frightened Puerto Rican man Mulder finds hiding in the bathroom inside the radio telescope building at **Arecibo,** Puerto Rico. The old man, who speaks no English, draws a crude but unmistakable image of an alien with large eyes and a triangular head. Mulder later finds the old man, who apparently died of fright. ["Little Green Men"]

JOSEPHS, DR.: Works at the hospital in Browning, Montana. He finds that **Lyle Parker** has ingested some of his father's blood, which could only have happened had Lyle eaten some of his father's flesh. ["Shapes"]

JOSH: A student and the lab partner of **Shannon Asbury.** ["Die Hand Die Verletzt"]

JTT0111471: Fox Mulder's FBI badge number. ["F. Emasculata"]

[K]

KALLENCHUK, JERAL-DINE: Operator of a salvage company in San Francisco. When she travels to Hong Kong to buy government secrets from **Alex Krycek,** she is killed by agents of the **Cigarette-Smoking Man.** ["Piper Maru"]

KALLENCHUK SALVAGE BROKERS: The salvage company operated by Jeraldine Kallenchuk. Mulder mistakenly assumes there is a Mr. Kallenchuk. ["Piper Maru"]

KAMINSKI, ELLEN: An intended victim of **Virgil Incanto,** she stands him up on their first date but later gives him a second chance that turns fatal not for her, but for him. She kills Incanto with Scully's gun after he has slimed her and is going after Scully. ["2Shy"]

KANE, BETH: A forty-year-old worker at the **J.A.S.D. Beef Packing Plant** in Wisconsin. She and her family have been the targets of a peeping Tom for several years. ["Red Museum"]

KANE, GARY: The sixteen-year-old son of Beth Kane. First string on the varsity football team and member of the 4-H club. He disappears one night and the next morning is found with the words "HE IS ONE" written on his back in black magic marker. He doesn't remember what happened to him, but he thinks a spirit entered him. ["Red Museum"]

KANE, STEVIE: The nine-year-old son of Beth Kane. ["Red Museum"]

KANN, JUDGE: Maryland state judge who presides over the sanity hearing for **Eugene Tooms.** ["Tooms"]

KARETZKY, DR.: A witness at the sanity hearing held for **Eugene Tooms** in Baltimore. She examined him for any physiological dysfunction and couldn't find anything. ["Tooms"]

KAUTZ: FBI ballistics expert who tests Mulder's gun for Scully when she needs to make certain that Mulder didn't shoot his own father. ["Anasazi"]

KAZANJIAN, DAN: A young agent who works in the FBI's computer crime section. He restores **Virgil Incanto**'s computer files and provides Scully and Mulder with a list of the killer's past and intended victims. ["2Shy"]

KAZDIN, LUCY: FBI agent in charge of hostage negotiations with **Duane Barry.** At first skeptical about Mulder, she later tells him about the strange metal objects discovered in Barry's body. ["Duane Barry"]

KEARNS, DORIS: The widow of George Kearns. She knew of her husband's fate but was promised protection by **Walter Chaco** — protection he was unable to provide to her. She became part of the community the **Dudley** way, by ingestion. ["Our Town"]

KEARNS, GEORGE: USDA poultry inspector stationed in **Dudley, Arkansas,** who displayed odd mental problems prior to his disappearance. Sent to investigate the disappearance of this federal employee, Mulder and Scully find his headless skeleton when the local river is dragged, and discover that he had been eaten by the locals. Unfortunately for the citizens of Dudley, Kearns's mental problems had been caused by

Creutzfeldt-Jakob disease, which was passed along to them when they ingested his brain tissue. ["Our Town"]

KEATS: An aeronautical scientist who works at the **Mahan Propulsion Laboratory.** ["Roland"]

KELLEHER, LORRAINE: A woman in her late sixties who runs an escort service in Washington, D.C. She says **Walter Skinner** paid for the services of **Carina Sayles** the night Sayles died. Kelleher is later found dead, a supposed suicide, but her demise conveniently occurs just as Mulder is coming to interview her about who might be trying to frame Skinner. ["Avatar"]

KELLY, LAURA: The daughter of Stan Phillips. He has been living at the **Excelsis Dei Convalescent Home** and doesn't want to leave there to move in with her. ["Excelsis Dei"]

KELLY, LUCY: A woman with cancer who dies after **Samuel Hartley** fails to heal her. ["Miracle Man"]

KELOID SCAR: The surgical scar found on the back of the neck of the subjects in **Dr. Grissom**'s sleep eradication experiments. The operation involves cutting part of the brain stem in the midpontine region. ["Sleepless"]

KENDRICK, DR. SALLY: A product of the **Litchfield Project.** First in her class at Yale Medical School, this biogenetics specialist interned at the **Luther Stapes Center** until she was suspected of tampering with genetic material. In fact, she was implanting her own clones in fertility patients. She disappeared for years after her dismissal. Her clones **Cindy Reardon** and **Teena Simmons** murder her with a lethal dose of digitalis in a cup of soda. Kendrick was Eve Seven. ["Eve"]

KENNEDY: An FBI agent who staked out **Eugene Tooms**'s Exeter Street apartment for Mulder until Agent **Colton** called him off, resulting in unnecessary danger for Scully and Mulder. ["Squeeze"]

KENNEDY CENTER: A performing-arts complex in Washington, D.C.; Mulder meets **X** here and drags him away from a performance of Wagner's "Ring" cycle in order to find out more about the **Pilot.** X reveals where the Pilot's craft is located. ["End Game"]

KENWOOD, TENNESSEE: In 1983, **Samuel Hartley** brings a man back from the dead there at the scene of a horrible accident where the man had burned to death. The local

sheriff believes that the **Rev. Hartley** and his adopted son Samuel are running a scam. ["Miracle Man"]

KERBER, SCOTT: The Loudon County sheriff's deputy killed when a semi hits his car, freeing **Robert Modell** and injuring FBI agent **Frank Burst.** ["Pusher"]

KILAR, KRISTEN: The woman Mulder meets in the **Club Tepes,** where she orders Jordeen — red wine. The vampire trio are hunting her because she was once associated with the **Son.** She is ultimately responsible for the destruction of the Trinity. ["3"]

KINBOTE, LORD: A.k.a. the **Behemoth** from the Planet Harryhausen. A real alien who kidnaps **Harold Lamb** and **Chrissy Giorgio,** along with two military men disguised as aliens (**Lt. Jack Sheaffer** and **Maj. Robert Vallee**). This is the name given the alien in a manuscript written by **Roky Crikenson** called *The Truth About Aliens.* Crikenson claims Lord Kinbote is an alien from the Earth's core. ["Jose Chung's *From Outer Space*"]

THE KINDRED: An Amish-like isolationist religious group that have lived near **Steveston, Massachusetts,** for generations and are known for their distinctive white clay pottery.

The gender-shifting killer known as **Marty** runs away from them but is eventually taken back. The Kindred welcome Mulder and Scully into their community, but only after taking their guns. They seem to have some strange regenerative abilities, but the nature of them is unclear. The entire Kindred community disappears overnight, leaving behind a mysterious crop circle. ["Genderbender"]

KINKERY, MR.: The teacher who is replaced by **Phyllis Paddock.** ["Die Hand Die Verletzt"]

KIP: A biker with a UFO tattoo whom Mulder meets at the **Boar's Head** tavern in Sioux City, Iowa; Kip hints there are strange things out at **Lake Okobogee** at night. Mulder later encounters a biker gang that probably included Kip as one of its members. ["Conduit"]

KISSELL, COL. BLAIN: The director of communications at **Ellens Air Force Base** in Idaho. He refuses to talk to Mulder and Scully when they investigate the case of **Col. Robert Budahas.** ["Deep Throat"]

KITTEL, PVT.: **Col. Wharton**'s assistant. Mulder reveals to him that **Dunham** and **Gutierrez** had both filed complaints against Wharton just prior to their mysterious deaths. ["Fresh Bones"]

KIVEAT AUTO BODY: Where **Darin Peter Oswald** was employed. ["D.P.O."]

KIVEAT, FRANK: Proprietor of Kiveat Auto Body, and husband of Sharon Kiveat. In an attempt to impress Sharon, **Darin Peter Oswald** causes Frank to undergo cardiac arrest, interferes with the paramedics' equipment, and "saves" Frank with his own remarkable electrical powers. ["D.P.O."]

KIVEAT, SHARON: She teaches the remedial reading class at **Gravenhurst High School,** where **Darin Peter Oswald** develops a crush on her. Frightened by Darin's powers, she nevertheless risks her own safety to draw him away from others. ["D.P.O."]

KLAMATH FALLS, OREGON: Birthplace of bank robber and murderer **Warren James Dupre.** ["Lazarus"]

KLASS COUNTY, WASHINGTON: Site of a close encounter of the third kind that is investigated by Mulder and Scully. "Klass County" is an inside joke: Philip Klass is a UFO debunker. ["Jose Chung's *From Outer Space*"]

KLEINJAN, MARGI: A friend of **Bruno,** a boy who dies under mysterious circumstances. She and her best friend, **Terri Roberts,** together have strange powers due to a peculiar alignment of the planets. She's a senior at Grover Cleveland Alexander High School in **Comity.** She has a grade point average of 3.75, and she's on the cheerleading squad with Terri. Astrologically speaking, Comity is in a geological vortex. On January 12 the planets come into perfect alignment. Since January 12 is Margi and Terri's birthday, and they were born in 1979, this gives them a Jupiter–Uranus opposition, which creates a grand square where the planets are aligned in a cross. This causes all the energy of the cosmos to be focused on them. ["Syzygy"]

KLEMPER, VICTOR: A Nazi scientist who escaped punishment at Nuremberg through **Operation Paper Clip.** The **Lone Gunmen** recognize him in the picture that Mulder finds of his father and other associates (including **Deep Throat,** the **Cigarette-Smoking Man,** and the **Well-Manicured Man**). Mulder and Scully track him down, still alive at American taxpayer expense, tending his orchids. He refuses to tell them anything but where the photo was taken: the **Strughold** Mining Company in West Virginia, and a clue to the entry code. His taunting call to the Well-Manicured Man tips off the **Elders** that Mulder and Scully are headed to the mine. He dies soon after, perhaps of a real heart attack, perhaps of one staged by his former associates. ["Paper Clip"]

KNOXVILLE, TENNESSEE: Site where a mysterious train car is detached from a passenger train. The car is marked on top with the numbers 82594, and there is a satellite dish on the roof. ["Nisei"]

KORETZ, CREW CHIEF KAREN: One of the military personnel at the U.S. Space Surveillance Center who tracks a UFO to **Townsend, Wisconsin. Col. Henderson** orders her to report the object as a meteor despite all evidence to the contrary. She spots another, larger craft several days later in the same area. ["Fallen Angel"]

KOSSEFF, KAREN E.: An FBI social worker assigned to file a report on the Holvey family. Arriving at the home slightly before Mulder and Scully, she witnesses a strange ritual performed by the **Calusari** and finds what she thinks is **Charlie Holvey** having an unexplained seizure. When she questions Charlie at her office, however, he claims she had seen Michael — the dead twin brother his parents never told him about. ["The Calusari"] Scully goes to her for counseling because she is disturbed by aspects of the case she's working on involving a fetishist and grave desecrations. ["Irresistible"]

KOTCHIK, MISS: A patron of the **Provincetown Pub** who witnesses **Cecil L'ively** burst into flames. She experiences burns on both her hands from the ensuing bar fire, but is otherwise unhurt; she helps a police artist create a composite sketch of L'ively. ["Fire"]

KRAMER: FBI agent involved in the initial capture of **Eugene Tooms.** He is assigned by Mulder to stake out **Exeter Street** but is called off by Agent **Colton.** ["Squeeze"]

KRESKI: One of the FBI agents searching for **Carl Wade** and his kidnap victim, **Amy Jacobs.** He is with **Lucy Householder** when she starts having a strange attack. ["Oubliette"]

KREUTZER, LEO: A resident at the **Excelsis Dei Convalescent Home.** During the 1930s he was an artist who worked for the WPA. In the rest home he does some drawings, one of which is of a

woman with figures floating above her. ["Excelsis Dei"]

KRYCEK, ALEX: FBI agent assigned to work with Mulder. Mulder comes to trust him, but actually the man is trying to undermine Mulder's credibility. He is secretly reporting to the **Cigarette-Smoking Man.** ["Sleepless"] Krycek accompanies Mulder to the **Duane Barry** hostage situation but does little beyond getting coffee for Agent **Lucy Kazdin.** ["Duane Barry"] Subsequent events reveal the depth of his involvement: He may have provided Barry with Scully's address. Acting under the Smoking Man's orders, he stalls Mulder by stopping the tram up the mountain, and may have poisoned Barry and tried to frame Mulder for his death. A surprisingly inept operative, he doesn't seem to pull off his treachery as effectively as his superiors might have wanted him to. After the Duane Barry case ends, Krycek mysteriously disappears from view, his work apparently completed. ["Ascension"] Krycek crawls back out of the woodwork and murders **William Mulder** after the **MJ documents** are stolen. He may also have been involved in the poisoning of Fox Mulder's water supply with the mind-

altering drug that produced Mulder's psychotic behavior. Krycek then makes several attempts on Mulder's life, one of which almost kills Scully, and another that results in Mulder beating the living daylights out of him. He would probably be dead by now if Scully hadn't shot Mulder in the shoulder; it seems as if Krycek's superiors were setting up Mulder to kill Krycek with Krycek's gun, which would have conveniently framed Mulder for the murder of his own father as well. ["Anasazi"] Assigned to kill Scully by the Smoking Man, Krycek botches the job and kills her sister Melissa instead. ["The Blessing Way"] With his accomplices the **Suited Man** and **Luis Cardinal,** he assaults **Walter Skinner** and steals back the **MJ** files' DAT. He narrowly escapes being killed by his cohorts when they blow up his car; he flees with the tape and makes a threatening call to the Smoking Man. ["Paper Clip"] Escaping to Hong Kong, Krycek manages to break the code of the MJ files on the DAT and begins a lucrative career peddling government secrets. He sells the French the location where a UFO has been recovered, and is about to sell more secrets to

Jeraldine Kallenchuk when he is recaptured by Mulder. Before leaving Hong Kong he is possessed by the alien entity that occupied **Joan Gauthier.** ["Piper Maru"] Back in the USA, he escapes from Mulder and returns the DAT to the Smoking Man. In return, the Smoking Man takes Krycek and the alien to the decommissioned **Black Crow missile complex** in North Dakota, where the aliens' craft is stored. When Krycek regains control of his body, he discovers himself trapped in an abandoned missile silo with the UFO. ["Apocrypha"]

KRYDER, KEVIN: A ten-year-old student in the fifth-grade class of Mrs. Tynes at Ridgeway Elementary School in Loveland, Ohio. While writing on the blackboard in class, his palms start to bleed. He had been temporarily removed from his parents' custody a year before when he bled from his hands and feet. His mother was given custody after his father was arrested and institutionalized after a standoff with the police during which he claimed Kevin was the son of God (see also **stigmata.**) ["Revelations"]

KRYDER, MICHAEL: The father of Kevin Kryder. He knows his son is in danger from the Forces of Darkness who want to bring about Armageddon prematurely. ["Revelations"]

KRYDER, SUSAN: The mother of Kevin Kryder. She is angry at the suggestion that her son be placed in a shelter until the mystery of his bleeding palms can be investigated. She is later killed in a car accident while trying to protect her son from **Simon Gates.** ["Revelations"]

KYTE, LAUREN: **Howard Graves**'s secretary at **HTG Industrial Technologies**. After Graves dies, Kyte decides to leave Philadelphia, frightened that her life is in danger — a fear confirmed after two men attempt to kill her at her ATM machine. She knows why Graves was killed, and by whom, but remains silent out of fear. With a little help from Mulder and Scully — and a lot from the late Mr. Graves — she turns the tables on the treacherous **Robert Dorland.** ["Shadows"]

[L]

LABERGE, DR: He is caring for **Mrs. Mulder** in the hospital and tells Fox that her stroke was serious and she may never regain consciousness. ["Talitha Cumi"]

LACERIO, CAPT. ROY: The police officer in charge of the search for the fugitive who has escaped after an intense chase. The fugitive was shot and has left drops of green blood behind. ["The Erlenmeyer Flask"]

LADONNA: A robust woman in her fifties who runs the **Flying Saucer Diner** near **Ellens Air Force Base.** Claims to have seen UFOs and has a picture to prove it: a grainy shot of a triangular craft nearly identical to the one that allegedly crashed near Roswell, New Mexico, in 1947. She sells Mulder the photo for twenty dollars and draws a map to the air base on a napkin. ["Deep Throat"]

LAKE JORDAN: In North Carolina. Acting on information from **Luther Lee Boggs,** the FBI rescues **Liz Hawley** from **Lucas Jackson Henry** there. Henry shoots Mulder with a shotgun and escapes by boat with **Jim Summers** still his prisoner. ["Beyond the Sea"]

LAKE OKOBOGEE: Near Sioux City, Iowa. Known for its trout fishing and high incidence of UFO sightings, including one in 1967 by **Darlene Morris** and her Girl Scout troop. **Ruby Morris** disappears while camping here. ["Conduit"]

LAKEVIEW CABINS: On Flicker Road near **Heuvelmans Lake** in Georgia. Mulder and Scully stay here when they come to investigate some mysterious disappearances. ["Quagmire"]

LAMANA, JERRY: Mulder's former partner in the violent-crimes division. His career has not been exemplary since they split up, but rather marked by a number of high-profile foulups. Turning to Mulder for help with the murder of Eurisko CEO **Benjamin Drake,** Lamana steals Mulder's notes to make himself look better to their superiors, realizing Mulder was always the brains of their partnership. Killed in a mysterious elevator "malfunction." ["Ghost in the Machine"]

LAMB, HAROLD: A teenage boy who is abducted with his date, **Chrissy Giorgio,** by a UFO one night. ["Jose Chung's *From Outer Space*"]

LAMBERT, GAIL ANNE: A scientist employed at **Polarity Magnetics** who is the first of several unexplainable disappearances in the Richmond, Virginia, area. Her death is caused by a visit from **Chester Ray Banton,** who has yet to realize how deadly his shadow is. ["Soft Light"]

LANDIS, JESSE: Monica Landis's blind twelve-year-old daughter. She realizes that **Virgil Incanto** has done something bad to her mother when she smells Monica's perfume in his apartment. She makes the 911 call that leads Mulder and Scully to Incanto's home. ["2Shy"]

LANDIS, MONICA: **Virgil Incanto**'s landlady, and a would-be poet. She is interested in him, but he is oblivious to her. A slender woman, she's not his type. He kills her only after she discovers Det. **Alan Cross**'s body in his bathtub. ["2Shy"]

LANG, KYLE: An animal rights activist in his late forties, with the W.A.O. (Wild Again Organization). He goes to the **Fairfield Zoo** late one night and is killed by **Ed Meecham.** ["Fearful Symmetry"]

LANGE, MS.: **Lauren Kyte**'s new boss at the Monroe Mutual Insurance Company in Omaha, Nebraska, who doesn't know how lucky she is that **Howard Graves**'s spirit is finally at rest . . . if it really is. ["Shadows"]

LANGLY: The member of the Lone Gunmen who wears glasses with thick lenses. He tells Mulder that the **Thinker**'s real name might be Kenneth Soona. ["Anasazi"]

Helps identify one person in Mulder's mysterious photo of his father and associates: **Victor Klemper.** ["Paper Clip"] He also appears in "Blood" and "E.B.E."

LANNY: A circus freak in his fifties. He has a twin, **Leonard,** whose conjoining body is attached to his stomach. Unbeknownst to everyone else, Lanny's twin can separate himself from his body, and he wants to conjoin with a new brother. ["Humbug"]

LARAMIE TOBACCO: The company that employed **Margaret Wysnecki** until her retirement. The similarity between her disappearance and that of Dominion Tobacco executive **Patrick Newirth** leads Mulder to briefly consider a link based on their professional environment. ["Soft Light"]

LARKEN SCHOLASTIC: The photography company that took the student pictures at **Valley Woods High School.** ["Oubliette"]

LARSON, DR. JERROLD: When he's killed in a plane crash near **Delta Glen, Wisconsin,** it is revealed that he's been injecting local children with a strange substance and then tracking them over the years. The doctor claimed he was giving the children vitamin shots. He was carrying a briefcase filled with hundred-dollar bills. ["Red Museum"]

LASKOS, DR.: The physician in charge of the **Bethesda Naval Hospital**'s intensive care unit when **Lt. Richard Harper** is admitted. Laskos kicks Scully out of the ICU for having an invalid clearance code. She later saves Scully's and Mulder's lives, using Scully's field notes ["Dod Kalm"]

LAZARD, DET. SHARON: A twenty-eight-year-old police detective who works at the **14th Precinct** in Buffalo, New York. She finds a lost eight-year-old girl named **Michelle Bishop** and takes her back to the police station. ["Born Again"]

LEADER: One of the phony Gray Aliens, who interrogate people they abduct. ["Jose Chung's *From Outer Space*"]

LEATHER SATCHEL: Found at the scene of a murder in the possession of **Kazuo Takeo.** Inside the bag are high-resolution satellite photos and a list of Mutual UFO Network (MUFON) members in the **Allentown** area. One name circled is **Betsy Hagopian.** ["Nisei"]

LEDBETTER, TIM: The partner in 1940 of FBI agent **Sam Chaney.** They were early experts on "stranger killings"

(now called serial killings), and both of them disappeared in 1942. Ledbetter's body is found in 1995 beneath a house **Harry Cokely** had rented in 1942. ["Aubrey"]

LEE, MR.: The manager of the apartment building where **Eugene Tooms** claims to live in 1993. Mulder and Scully find no signs of habitation there; Tooms was using it as a front address, preferring his nest in Apartment 103 of 66 **Exeter Street,** Baltimore. ["Squeeze"]

LEONARD: The name **Lanny** gave his Siamese twin. This twin is sentient, and it can separate itself from Lanny's body. ["Humbug"]

LESKY, DIANA: The pseudonym given to Scully in **Jose Chung's** book titled *From Outer Space.* ["Jose Chung's *From Outer Space*"]

LEWIN: One of the agents who has Mulder's residence under surveillance, and who confronts Scully when she goes there. ["Little Green Men"]

LEWTON, DR. JERROLD: Curator of the Boston Museum of Natural History. He is killed shortly after the disappearance of **Craig Horning.** ["Teso dos Bichos"]

LIFEBOAT 925: The lifeboat commandeered by **Lt. Richard Harper** and seven-

teen other mutineers when they defy Capt. **Phillip Barclay** and abandon the *USS Argent* in the Norwegian Sea. ["Dod Kalm"]

LIGHTHOUSE BUNGALOWS MOTEL: North of San Francisco. **Dr. Sally Kendrick** takes **Cindy Reardon** and **Teena Simmons** there. The manager tips off the FBI to their presence, but not soon enough to keep the two young clones from murdering Kendrick. ["Eve"]

LIMO DRIVER: On Embassy Row in Washington, D.C., he picks up **Kazuo Takeo,** the Japanese diplomat whom Mulder had captured at the scene of a murder. It is a trap, and Takeo is murdered in the limo to cover up his sloppy work in **Allentown.** ["Nisei"]

LINCOLN PARK: The amusement park in Murray, Virginia, where **Teddy Holvey** escapes from his baby harness, wanders out of a public bathroom, and is killed by a miniature train. ["The Calusari"]

LINHART, HARRY: FBI composite artist. ["Born Again"]

LINLEY TEMPORARY HOME SHELTER: **Kevin Kryder** is temporarily placed here. ["Revelations"]

LIQUID: One of the phony Gray Aliens, who interrogate people they abduct. ["Jose Chung's *From Outer Space*"]

LIQUORI, BART "ZERO": **Darin Peter Oswald**'s only friend. Zero dispenses change at the local video arcade in **Connerville, Oklahoma.** Believing that Zero has told Mulder and Scully about his powers, Darin kills him with a powerful electric discharge. ["D.P.O."]

LISETTE: The Canadian fishing vessel (ID number CV233) that rescues the mutineers who escape from the USS *Argent.* ["Dod Kalm"]

LITCHFIELD PROJECT: A highly classified eugenics experiment, sponsored by the U.S. government, in which identical, genetically engineered children are raised in a controlled environment in a town called Litchfield. The boys are called Adam, the girls Eve; all are assigned numbers. These children have fifty-six chromosomes instead of the usual forty-six; this allows them to develop superhuman attributes, including enhanced strength, intelligence, and extrasensory abilities. They also suffer from extreme psychosis. Many commit suicide. **Eve Six** has been incarcerated for years; **Eve Eight** is still at large. Eve Seven, a.k.a. **Dr. Sally Kendrick,** has created

clones of herself (**Cindy Reardon** and **Teena Simmons**) who eventually kill her with a poisoned soda. ["Eve"]

L'IVELY, CECIL: A Briton with pyrokinetic, or fire-starting powers. His normal body temperature is 111 degrees. He was employed on the estates of several British aristocrats who died by fire. The name L'ively may be a pseudonym: Lively is the name of a child murdered by a cult in 1963 *and* a solid British citizen who died in 1971. Cecil L'ively murders and replaces the caretaker at the Cape Cod residence where the **Marsden** family has sought refuge, then stages a rescue of their children in order to gain their confidence. Stopped before he can kill again, L'ively, known in the U.S. as **Bob,** suffers severe burns but heals remarkably fast. Finally incarcerated in a high-security federal medical facility, he is confined to a hyperbaric chamber to prevent fires. ["Fire"]

LLOYD P. WHARTON COUNTY BUILDING: The county administrative building of Johnston County, Oklahoma, located in the town of **Connerville.** Scully autopsies **Jack Hammond**'s body in the

postmortem facilities here. ["D.P.O."]

LO, JOHNNY: A Chinese man whose charred body is found in the crematorium at the Bayside Funeral Home. He has been burned alive. ["Hell Money"]

LOCKER 101356: The locker in an airport near Washington, D.C., where **John Barnett** places **Dr. Joe Ridley**'s research. ["Young at Heart"]

LOFOTEN BASIN: Norwegian ships are forbidden to sail beyond this point unless they are classified as ice class vessels. **Henry Trondheim** doesn't have a problem with this: his fifty-ton trawler, the *Zeal,* is completely seaworthy, until it reaches 58° N, 8° E. ["Dod Kalm"]

LONE GUNMAN: A magazine specializing in conspiracy theories. The April 1994 edition has an article on the CCDTH7321 fiberoptic lens micro video camera used by the CIA. ["Blood" and "E.B.E."]

LONE GUNMEN: A group of fringe conspiracy buffs whom Mulder consults on occasion. Three of them come to Mulder's apartment after the **Thinker,** a.k.a. Kenneth Soona, steals the **MJ documents.** A woman in Mulder's apartment building apparently goes crazy and shoots her husband while they are there. ["Anasazi"] They help Mulder locate **Krycek**'s locker, but the **MJ** files DAT is missing. ["Apocrypha"]

LONE GUNMEN'S OFFICE: Mulder goes there to show some high-resolution satellite photos to the guys to see what they can make of them. **Langly** tells Mulder that one of them is of a ship named the **Talapus. Byers** states that he believes the photo is from a Japanese surveillance satellite. **Frohike** states that he believes the Japanese launched it from a secret site in South America. ["Nisei"]

LORRE, GARRETT: A forty-eight-year-old, gray-haired businessman who is killed by a vampiric triumvirate. On the wall near his body, written in his blood, is **"JOHN 52:54."** ["3"]

LORTON, VIRGINIA: Location of the D.C. Correctional Complex. ["Grotesque"]

LOS ALAMOS, NEW MEXICO: The closest city to the Navajo reservation where Mulder is presumed dead by the **Cigarette-Smoking Man** but is rescued by **Albert Hosteen** and his family. ["Anasazi"; "The Blessing Way"] Also where the Manhattan Project scientists tested the first atomic bomb. What other as yet uncovered secret projects has the U.S. government undertaken here?

LOVELAND, OHIO: Location of Ridgeway Elementary School, where **Kevin Kryder** attends fifth grade. ["Revelations"]

LOWE, MRS.: **Clyde Bruckman**'s elderly neighbor. He foresees her death when he takes out her trash for her. Due to the lack of dog food in her apartment, Mrs. Lowe's remains were subjected to certain indignities by her small dog. ["Clyde Bruckman's Final Repose"]

LUDER, M. F.: A pseudonym used by Mulder when he published an article on the Gulf Breeze Sightings in *Omni* magazine. According to **Max Fenig,** UFOlogists following Mulder's career had no problem unscrambling the anagram. ["Fallen Angel"]

LUDWIG, JASON: Robotics engineer for the descent team on the **Cascade Volcano Research Project.** He's killed by **Trepkos** with a flare gun. ["Firewalker"]

LUTHER STAPES CENTER FOR REPRODUCTIVE MEDICINE: A fertility clinic in San Francisco where **Dr. Sally Kendrick** had her residency in 1985. The **Simmons** family and the **Reardon** family both came here while trying to conceive, only to have clones of Kendrick, a.k.a. Eve Seven, implanted instead. ["Eve"]

LYNN ACRES RETIREMENT HOME: A residence for the elderly that is not in very good repair. **Frank Briggs,** a police detective who once hunted **Tooms,** now lives here. ["Tooms"]

LYSERGIC DIMETHRIN: The substance similar in structure and effect to LSD. It is found in the bodies of the killers who went on a rampage in **Franklin, Pennsylvania.** It reacts with adrenaline to cause the person to become psychotic. A secret, experimental insecticide, it is sprayed on plants to cause a fear response in insects that touch them. ["Blood"]

[M]

McALPIN, JOHN "JACK": A twenty-three-year-old U.S. Marine private who dies when his car hits a tree near his home. A strange symbol is painted on the tree. Later his body vanishes and he's found alive. ["Fresh Bones"]

McALPIN, LUKE: Eighteen-month-old son of Robin and Jack. ["Fresh Bones"]

McALPIN, ROBIN: Wife of Pvt. John McAlpin. ["Fresh Bones"]

McCALL, DOROTHY: A resident at the **Excelsis Dei Convalescent Home.** She's able to see the disembodied spirits of the old men who are taking the secret drug. ["Excelsis Dei"]

McCALLISTER, DOREEN: A member of the Girl Scout troop that witnessed and photographed a UFO near **Lake Okobogee** in 1967. ["Conduit"]

McCALLISTER PENITENTIARY: Where **Harry Cokely** served his prison time from 1945 to 1993 for the rape and attempted murder of **Linda Thibodeaux.** ["Aubrey"]

McCLENNEN, JIM: A test pilot at **Ellens Air Force Base** who suffers from a stress-related syndrome called stereotypy (Scully's diagnosis). Disoriented and prone to compulsive, repetitious behavior like picking at his hair, he probably underwent the same stresses that affected **Col. Robert Budahas.** ["Deep Throat"]

McCLENNEN, VERLA: The wife of Jim McClennen. She accepts her husband's problems more readily than **Anita Budahas** accepts hers. ["Deep Throat"]

McGRATH, JOSEPH: FBI section chief who wants Mulder expelled from the Bureau and the X-Files unit disbanded. He almost gets his wish after certain events in **Townsend, Wisconsin,** but **Deep Throat** overrides his decision. ["Fallen Angel"]

MACKALVEY, LAUREN: A lonely, overweight woman whose bizarre murder brings Mulder and Scully to Cleveland, Ohio. Her skin and fatty tissue have been dissolved by a slimelike substance that reduces her body to mere bones a few hours later. She was killed by **Virgil Incanto.** ["2Shy"]

McNALLY, HARRY: **Ed Funsch**'s supervisor at the post office in **Franklin, Pennsylvania.** ["Blood"]

McROBERTS, BONNIE: She goes to pick up her Volvo at the garage in **Franklin, Pennsylvania,** where it's being worked on. The engine analyzer monitor starts telling her that the mechanic is lying to her, then tells her to kill him, which she does, with an oil can spout. When Mulder and Sheriff Spencer go to question her, she attacks Mulder with a knife and is shot and killed by Spencer. Her autopsy reveals that her adrenaline levels were two hundred times the norm. Also, an unknown chemical — later identified as lysergic dimethrin — found in her body has properties that would cause it to react with adrenaline to produce a substance similar in structure and effect to LSD. ["Blood"]

MADISON: A street in **Hagerstown, Maryland. Lula Philips** robs a drugstore at the intersection of Madison and Forge Road. ["Lazarus"]

MAHAN PROPULSION LABORATORY: Located at the Washington Institute of Technology in Colson, Washington, where **Roland Fuller** commits a series of murders. ["Roland"]

MAIN STREET: In Easton, Washington, where the FBI arrive to search for kidnapping suspect **Carl Wade.** ["Oubliette"]

MAJESTIC: The name of a top-secret report that **Deep Throat** gives Mulder. ["E.B.E."]

MALAWI: The African nation from which **Willa Ambrose** rescued **Sophie** the gorilla. The government there wants the gorilla back. ["Fearful Symmetry"]

MALLARD, DENNIS: A classmate of **Amy Jacob**'s at Valley Woods High in Seattle. ["Oubliette"]

MANDAS, MARILYN: She works for **Ficicello Frozen Foods,** which is where **Donnie Pfaster** gets a job after he's fired by the **Janelli-Heller Funeral Home.** ["Irresistible"]

MANDROID: A male android. An artificial person. **Blaine Faulkner** claims this is what he thinks Mulder is. ["Jose Chung's *From Outer Space*"]

MAN IN BLACK #1: He and his partner drive their silent black Cadillac into the garage of **Roky Crikenson** and spout strange anti-UFO gibberish. They try to convince Crikenson that he didn't see a UFO at all, just the planet Venus. ["Jose Chung's *From Outer Space*"]

MAN IN BLACK #2: A.k.a. Alex Trebek. ["Jose Chung's *From Outer Space*"]

MANITOU: An evil spirit that can change a man into a beast. One attacked **Richard Watkins** and began his shape-shifting and murders. ["Shapes"]

MANLEY, DANIELLE: The wife of "Neech" Manley. She has frequent dreams that her husband survived the electric chair. Believing that his soul has passed into the body of her lover, the prison guard **Parmelly,** she shoots him. ["The List"]

MANLEY, NAPOLEON ("NEECH"): A prisoner executed at **Eastpoint State Penitentiary** for a double homicide. Manley did not actually kill anyone, but as the driver of the getaway car he was charged with murder. He vows to be reincarnated and to avenge himself by killing five men. Two days after the execution, a guard is found dead of suffocation in Neech's empty cell. ["The List"]

MANNERS, DET.: He interviews **Harold Lamb,** who is believed guilty of date rape. Lamb's alien abduction story is found a bit preposterous by this hard-bitten detective. He speaks in sentences laced with expletives, but instead of the expletive we hear the words "bleeped" and "blankety-blank." ["Jose Chung's *From Outer Space*"]

MARIO: A new employee at the **Culver City Plasma Center.** Mulder considers him a possible suspect, but he's not the right one. ["3"]

MARION, VIRGINIA: Location of the **Davis Correctional Treatment Center,** where **Duane Barry** is held until his final escape in 1994. ["Duane Barry"]

MARSDEN, LADY: The wife of Lord Malcolm Marsden, she becomes the object of **Cecil L'ively**'s warm attentions; he sends her deranged love letters prior to his attempt on her children's lives. ["Fire"]

MARSDEN, LORD MALCOLM: **Cecil L'ively**'s intended victim, Marsden escaped death by fire in his garage in England and came to the United States for safety. L'ively's attention then shifts from this Member of Parliament to his children. Marsden avoids L'ively's deadly intentions but is unable to resist the more agreeable charms of Scotland Yard investigator **Phoebe Green**. ["Fire"]

MARSDEN, JIMMIE AND MICHAEL: The young sons of Lord and Lady Marsden. ["Fire"]

MARTINGALE: A tie-down chain that pulls an elephant's tusk to the ground. This forces the elephant to its knees, hobbling it. ["Fearful Symmetry"]

MARTY: Formerly Brother Martin of the **Kindred,** he ventures into the outside world to pursue sex with what he refers to as "human men and women." He can change genders at will. Death is an unfortunate side effect of sex with a Kindred, due to the incredibly high amount of **pheromones** they possess. Marty is taken away by the Kindred the night they seemingly disappeared from the face of the Earth. ["Genderbender"]

MARYLAND MARINE BANK: Site of the last robbery committed by **Warren James Dupre** and **Lula Philips.** The FBI is there, thanks to an anonymous tip; Dupre shoots agent **Jack Willis,** but is killed by Scully. Philips, the getaway driver, escapes. ["Lazarus"]

MASSACHUSETTS INSTITUTE OF ROBOTICS: Where an artificial-intelligence researcher designs robots that look like insects. ["War of the Coprophages"]

MATHESON, SEN. RICHARD: One of Mulder's occasional friends in high places, Matheson drops out of the picture when the going gets tough. **X** hints that the government has some incriminating information it uses to keep Matheson in line. ["Ascension"] Matheson takes a convenient vacation to the Caribbean after the **MJ documents** are stolen. ["Anasazi"; see also "Little Green Men"] Mulder goes to see him after a Japanese murder suspect is found dead and Mulder's apartment is ransacked by people trying to locate a briefcase Mulder appropriated from the murder suspect. Matheson advises Mulder to return the

satellite photos, which Mulder is reluctant to do. The senator gives Mulder the names of the four scientists who were murdered during an alien autopsy. ["Nisei"]

MATOLA, SALVATORE: A previously unknown survivor of **Dr. Grissom**'s sleep deprivation experiments at Parris Island. He is located at 2 Jay's Diner, Roslyn, New York. ["Sleepless"]

MAXWELL, MR.: Janitor at the **Hollywood Blood Bank.** ["3"]

MAYWALD, CARINA: A Social Services worker who comes to investigate when **Kevin Kryder** suffers from bleeding palms at school. ["Revelations"]

MAZEROSKI, RICK: The sixteen-year-old son of the sheriff of **Delta Glen, Wisconsin.** He is kidnapped and found with the words "HE IS ONE" written on his back. But he has also been murdered, shot in the head. ["Red Museum"]

MEECHAM, ED: Chief of operations for the **Fairfield Zoo** in Idaho. He has no explanation for how the elephant, **Ganesha,** escaped from her locked cage. He isn't asked whether Ganesha knew how to become invisible or not. The Wild Again Organization believe that Meecham has

been mistreating animals at the zoo, including elephants. ["Fearful Symmetry"]

MEN IN BLACK: Two men in dark suits, present during **Duane Barry**'s 1985 alien abduction ["Duane Barry"] and briefly present with **Alex Krycek** after Barry's capture at Skyland Mountain. ["Ascension"]

"THE MERCHANDISE": A veiled, perhaps coded, reference to the bodies Mulder found in a railroad car buried on the Navajo reservation near **Farmington, New Mexico. William Mulder** uses this term, which also appears in **MJ documents** about experiments conducted by Axis Powers scientists working for the U.S. government after World War II. It is unclear whether these bodies are human, alien, or some sort of hybrid, but Mulder notices smallpox vaccination scars on some of them before they are destroyed. ["Anasazi"]

MERCY MISSION: The soup kitchen in **Atlantic City** where Mulder meets the homeless man named **Jack,** who assists him with his investigation. ["The Jersey Devil"]

METHANE RESEARCH FACILITY: Run by **Alt.-Fuels Inc.** Their motto is "Waste is a terrible thing to waste." It gets blown up when **Dr. Eckerle** goes crazy and starts shooting at cockroaches in the plant. ["War of the Coprophages"]

MICHAEL: A man picked up by the female Marty who narrowly escapes death when the police mistake Marty for a prostitute and try to intervene. He describes Marty to Mulder, who convinces him to reveal that Marty seemed to be changing into a man when she escaped from the police. ["Genderbender"]

MIDNIGHT INQUISITOR: A tacky tabloid newspaper purchased by **Clyde Bruckman** at a liquor store shortly before his first encounter with the **Puppet.** The Stupendous **Yappi** offers celebrity predictions in the issue in question, including a romantic liaison between Madonna and Kato Kaelin. ["Clyde Bruckman's Final Repose"]

MIHAI: A Romanian form of the name Michael, used by **Golda** during the performance of an unsuccessful Ritual of Separation. ["The Calusari"]

MILES, BILLY: A friend of the victims of the mysterious killings in Bellefleur, Oregon, who were members of the high school class of '89. He was in an auto accident with **Peggy O'Dell** and became comatose — except during those times

when he is controlled by a mysterious outside force. [Pilot]

MILES, DET.: The father of Billy Miles. He doesn't want Mulder and Scully talking to his son. [Pilot]

MILFORD HAVEN, NEW HAMPSHIRE: Town where "Die Hand Die Verletzt" takes place.

MILLENNIUM MAN: See **Simon Gates.** ["Revelations"]

MILLER'S GROVE, MASSA-CHUSETTS: The site of some strange "roach attacks." ["War of the Coprophages"]

MINETTE, ETHAN: Scully's boyfriend in the pilot episode. She has to cancel a long-planned vacation with him in order to go to Oregon with Mulder on their first mission together. [Pilot]

MINNEAPOLIS COUNTY MORGUE: Where Scully does the autopsy on **Satin.** ["Irresistible"]

MIRACLE MINISTRY: Run by the **Rev. Hartley** and his son, **Samuel Hartley,** who once brought a man back from the dead. ["Miracle Man"]

MIRAMAR NAVY AIR BASE: North of San Diego, former home of the Top Gun fighter training program. Scully goes there to visit **Commander Christopher Johansen,** an old friend of her father's who

served on the submarine *Zeus Faber.* ["Piper Maru"]

MIRISKOVIC, LLADOSLAV: A Bosnian war criminal. **Joseph Patnik** believed that each of the five people he killed was Miriskovic. When Patnik is incarcerated in the Frederick County Psychiatric Hospital, he is watching TV and sees a news report about Miriskovic, whereupon Patnik becomes hysterical with fear and terror and has to be restrained. ["Wetwired"]

MR. X: See **X.**

M.J.: The roommate of **Michelle Charters.** ["Excelsis Dei"]

MJ DOCUMENTS: The complete Defense Department files on every UFO case from Roswell and after, stolen by the hacker called the **Thinker** and passed along to Mulder. These top-secret files are encoded in Navajo and contain many facts that have yet to be fully translated, including an explanation of Scully's disappearance, the truth about **Duane Barry,** and the story of **William Mulder**'s involvement in certain undisclosed government projects. ["Anasazi"]

MKULTRA: Pronounced M-K-Ultra. Refers to the CIA's mind-control experiments conducted in the 1950s. ["Jose Chung's *From Outer Space*"]

MODELL, ROBERT: A killer with psychic powers of persuasion, whose hits were all written off as suicides until he called up FBI agent **Frank Burst** and bragged about them. He allows himself to be captured twice. The second time, he gets off scot free because the murders have already been ruled suicides — and because he uses his willpower on the judge. Scully discovers that Modell had applied to the FBI for a job but was turned down. An all-too-average guy who never excelled at anything, Modell knows his powers are a direct result of a brain tumor. His condition is treatable, but he prefers to risk death and keep the powers that make him superior to other people for the first time in his life. ["Pusher"]

MOLITCH, HARVEY: When the son of **George Hunsaker** receives an anonymous call from someone who says he knows where a mass grave is located, **Bob Spitz** shows up with a backhoe wanting to dig up Molitch's yard. ["Syzygy"]

MONITORING CHIP: After Scully finds and removes this tiny chip from her neck in "Nisei," she takes it to FBI agent **Pendrell,** who scans it and discovers that it records

memories to the degree that whoever monitors the chip could even monitor a person's thoughts. He discovers that it was manufactured in Japan. It is traced to a **Dr. Shiro Zama** at a facility in Perkey, West Virginia. ["731"]

MONKEY WRENCHERS: Radical environmentalists who drive spikes into trees and sabotage logging equipment. ["Darkness Falls"]

MONROE, KIMBERLY: An employee of the **Travel Time Travel Agency** taken hostage by **Duane Barry.** Mulder persuades Barry to set Monroe and Gwen Norris free. She tells Barry that she believes his alien abduction story. ["Duane Barry"]

MONTE, DR. AARON: The doctor in charge of **Eugene Tooms** at the **Druid Hill Sanitarium** in Baltimore. After Tooms is released, Monte is supposed to supervise him. Tooms later kills him and eats his liver. ["Tooms"]

MONTIFIORE CEMETERY: In Minneapolis. A fresh grave there is desecrated and some of the hair and fingernails are cut from the corpse of Catherine Ann Terle. ["Irresistible"]

MOORE, LARRY: A U.S. Forest Service employee. He goes with Mulder, Scully, and

Humphreys to search for thirty missing loggers. ["Darkness Falls"]

MORGAN, WAYNE: A Navy investigator who accompanies Mulder and Scully when they take a look at the *Piper Maru.* ["Piper Maru"]

MORLEYS CIGARETTES: The brand smoked by the **Cigarette-Smoking Man.** ["One Breath"]

MORRIS, AGENT: He is following Scully when she goes to the Miami airport to catch a flight to Puerto Rico to search for Mulder. ["Little Green Men"]

MORRIS, CHARLIE: Police officer who worked narcotics in the 27th Precinct. He was killed gangland style in Chinatown. When he possesses eight-year-old **Michelle Bishop,** he displays his origami skills. ["Born Again"]

MORRIS, DARLENE: In 1967, she and members of her Girl Scout troop witnessed and photographed a UFO over **Lake Okobogee,** Iowa. In 1993, her daughter Ruby is abducted by a UFO at the same lake. At first cooperative, Darlene refuses to help Mulder and Scully after NSA agents ransack her home; when her daughter is returned, she denies anything unusual ever happened to either of her children (see **Kevin Morris**). ["Conduit"]

MORRIS, JANE: A secretary at **HTG Industrial Technologies** who comforts **Lauren Kyte** after **Howard Graves**'s apparent suicide. ["Shadows"]

MORRIS, KEVIN: The eight-year-old son of **Darlene Morris,** present when his sister Ruby is abducted. Kevin's own exposure to an alien presence enables him to somehow pick up binary transmissions that include some top-secret military satellite information, which he scribbles on pieces of paper. A valuable lead for Mulder, until Darlene blocks all access to her family. ["Conduit"]

MORRIS, RUBY: The sixteen-year-old daughter of **Darlene Morris.** Some believe she spent the month of her disappearance partying with a motorcycle gang, but Mulder suspects otherwise: she exhibits the same physical symptoms experienced by astronauts after prolonged weightlessness. Unfortunately, Darlene will not allow Mulder to talk to either of her children after the incidents around **Lake Okobogee.** ["Conduit"]

MORRISVILLE: A town in Virginia, location of the **Blue Devil Brewery** where **Jim**

Summers is rescued. ["Beyond the Sea"]

MORROW, DET. B. J.: Of the Aubrey, Missouri, police. Her father was also a policeman. She is having an affair with Lt. Brian Tillman and becomes pregnant. She goes to the **Motel Black** and later awakens from a trance to discover that she has uncovered a grave in a vacant field. In the grave is an old FBI badge. She is actually the granddaughter of **Harry Cokely.** Her father was the child **Ruby Thibodeaux** gave up for adoption in 1946. She has become a murderer just like her grandfather was. ["Aubrey"]

MORROW, RAYMOND: The father of B. J. Morrow, he is the son of **Harry Cokely** as a result of his rape of **Ruby Thibodeaux** in 1945. ["Aubrey"]

MOSIER, GARY: The man the tow-truck driver is looking for when he stops to talk to **Carl Wade.** ["Oubliette"]

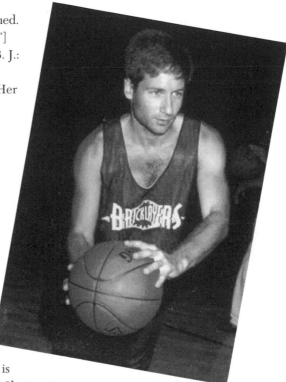

MOSSBERG, BULLPUP: The variety of shotgun with which a soldier strikes Mulder when he intrudes on **Operation Falcon.** ["Fallen Angel"]

MOSSINGER, PAUL: A military agent masquerading as a local journalist, he tries to divert Mulder and Scully from investigating **Ellens Air Force Base** by directing them to local crackpots — not realizing Mulder will turn up a real lead or two that way. When things get serious, "Mossinger" tries to overpower Scully, but she turns the tables and uses him as a hostage to secure Mulder's release from the air base. ["Deep Throat"]

MOSTOW, JOHN: An art student and unemployed house painter, divorced, no children. Emigrated to the U.S. from Uzbekistan, where he'd spent much of his life confined in an insane asylum. In class, the model, Peter, is a nude man, but the drawing he makes is of a gargoyle. He is arrested for the murder of Peter, and is suspected of the serial murders of six other men over three years. The victims were all males ages seventeen to twenty-five. He claims he was possessed by a demon during the times he committed the murders. In his home is a secret room containing the bodies of more murdered men, but they have been covered with clay and made to appear to be statues of gargoyles. ["Grotesque"]

MOTEL BLACK: Where **B. J. Morrow** goes to meet **Brian Tillman** to talk after she tells him she's pregnant. ["Aubrey"]

MOTEL MANAGER: At the 2400 Motel he and Mulder are shot at by Scully. ["Wetwired"]

MOUNT AVALON: Where Mulder and Scully are flown to investigate the **Cascade Volcano Research Project,** which has encountered a serious problem. ["Firewalker"]

MOUNT FOODMORE SUPERMARKET: Site of **Robert Modell**'s premeditated apprehension by FBI agent **Frank Burst.** ["Pusher"]

MOUNTAIN HOME AIR BASE: The **Lone Gunmen** claim that this is a major hotspot in Idaho for UFO activity. ["Fearful Symmetry"]

MOUNTAIN RAVINE: Where the **Quarantine Car** is uncoupled from the train that had been pulling it. ["731"]

MTA OFFICER: He reveals to Mulder that a car has suddenly appeared on the surveillance video of track 17. ["Sleepless"]

MUGWORT: A ceremonial herb used by the **Calusari** while performing the Ritual of Separation on **Charlie Holvey.** ["The Calusari"]

MULDER, FOX: Oxford-educated psychologist who wrote a monograph on serial killers and the occult which assisted in the capture of Monte Propps (a serial killer) in 1988. Considered the violent-crime section's finest analyst. Worked three years for the FBI's behavioral science unit, profiling serial killers. Nickname "Spooky." Developed an intense fear of fire when a childhood friend's house burned down ["Fire"] While open to unusual and bizarre ideas, he refuses to believe

Luther Lee Boggs's claim of psychic abilities. ["Beyond the Sea"] Suffers simultaneously from exposure to extreme cold and a deadly alien virus during a private mission to the Arctic. ["Colony," "End Game"] Experiences accelerated aging, later reversed, on a mission in the North Atlantic. ["Dod Kalm"] Suffers temporary psychosis when the water supply in his apartment building is drugged; is shot in the shoulder by Scully to prevent him from murdering **Alex Krycek.** ["Anasazi"] Trapped in a boxcar filled with alien bodies, Mulder escapes death by fire by crawling through a narrow tunnel dug decades before by the doomed aliens and is nursed back to health by local Navajo healer **Albert Hosteen.** Mulder is originally suspected of killing his own father but later cleared. When he returns to his father's house, he finds an old photo of his father, **Deep Throat,** the **Cigarette-Smoking Man,** and the **Well-Manicured Man** (whom he does not know yet). ["The Blessing Way"] According to an offhand comment by psychic **Clyde Bruckman,** Mulder will die by autoerotic asphyxiation. ["Clyde Bruckman's Final Repose"] The fact that Mulder is red–green colorblind makes him immune to a signal from a TV broadcasting tachistoscopic images designed to influence the person who is watching the program. ["Wetwired"]

MULDER, MRS.: Fox Mulder's mother. She and her husband, William, were divorced by the time Fox was an adult. She is the first person to see her son alive after his disappearance. ["The Blessing Way"] When he confronts her with a photo of his father with **Deep Throat** and other, more sinister associates, she refuses to deal with the memories it awakens. In complete denial about her family's past, she cannot even recall the associates' names. ["The Blessing Way"] She admits to Fox that her husband asked her to choose which of their children should be taken away by aliens, but that she couldn't choose. When William Mulder made his choice, it destroyed their marriage forever. ["Paper Clip"] She used to associate with the **Cigarette-Smoking Man** socially at the time William worked for the government, but she hates him now. When he comes to her to try to secure information from her, she becomes violently angry, and moments after he leaves she suffers a severe and debilitating stroke. Only

because **X** has been secretly observing her and calls 911 does she receive immediate paramedic assistance. When X shows Fox photos of CSM visiting Mrs. Mulder, Fox becomes incensed and comes close to killing CSM. Mrs. Mulder gives Fox a clue to something she had hidden in her cottage at the lake, and Mulder finds the kind of personal weapon needed to kill aliens. ["Talitha Cumi"]

MULDER, SAMANTHA: The sister of Fox Mulder. She disappeared November 27, 1973, when she was eight years old, the apparent victim of alien abduction. According to Scully, Fox told her there was a bright light and a presence in the room when it happened — a classic UFO abduction story that explains Fox's lifelong obsession with cosmic mysteries of all sorts. Under hypnotic regression, Fox recalls that a voice in his head told him not to be afraid: that Samantha would not be harmed, and that some day she would return. ["Conduit"] First mentioned in the episode "Miracle Man." Also mentioned in "Little Green Men" (see also **"Samantha,"** whose true identity is still in question).

MULDER SUMMER HOME: Located on a lake at

Quonochontaug, Rhode Island. ["Talitha Cumi"]

MULDER, WILLIAM: Fox Mulder's father, a distant man who was not close to his son. He calls Fox at the FBI when his daughter Samantha appears to have returned after twenty-two years. ["Colony"] He becomes very angry with Fox when he receives the news that Samantha is lost again; this is before Fox learns that "Samantha" was really an alien clone. He also gave Fox a note from the false Samantha, which led to the abortion clinic at 1235 91st Street, Rockville, Maryland. ["End Game"] William Mulder is somehow associated with past UFO cover-ups, along with the **Cigarette-Smoking Man,** who advises him to deny his past to Fox. William instead decides to tell his son everything, but is murdered by **Alex Krycek** before he can do so, leaving Fox with nothing more than a tantalizing reference to **"the merchandise."** His name appears in the encoded **MJ documents.** ["Anasazi"] He worked on a secret government project years before, and he is assassinated by an agency concerned that he might reveal what he knows to his son. He appears to Fox in a vision during the **Blessing Way** ceremony. ["The Blessing Way"] According to the **Well-Manicured Man,** in the 1950s William Mulder was involved in collecting genetic samples from the general population — the files Fox found at the **Strughold Mine.** When William Mulder realized the true purpose of this activity, he threatened to expose it — so one of his own children was abducted as insurance. He was forced to choose which one. ["Paper Clip"] In 1953 he interviewed one of the surviving sailors who had been exposed to radiation on the submarine *Zeus Faber.* ["Apocrypha"]

MULDRAKE, REYNARD: The pseudonym given to Fox Mulder in Jose Chung's book titled *From Outer Space.* ["Jose Chung's *From Outer Space*"]

MULTREVICH: The manager of the apartment building where **Lula Philips** moves after the death of **Warren Dupre.** He calls the FBI to turn her in for a $10,000 reward, but his call is answered by **Jack Willis** and Scully, with unusual results. ["Lazarus"]

MUNCHAUSEN BY PROXY: A form of child abuse in which a parent or caretaker induces medical symptoms in a child in order to enhance his or her

status as the child's "protector." **Teddy** and **Charlie Holvey** both suffered from frequent and inexplicable childhood maladies, which leads Scully to suspect their grandmother **Golda** was committing Munchausen by proxy. **Steve Holvey** had already suspected as much, but had feared to admit this to his wife. ["The Calusari"]

MUNTZ, GALEN: A disturbed man who starts shooting people in a fast-food restaurant. But when he is shot by the police, **Jeremiah Smith** heals the gunman and the victims of all their wounds with just the touch of his hands. ["Talitha Cumi"]

MURPHY, DR. DENNY: A professor of geology at the University of California, San Diego. He accompanies Mulder and Scully to investigate the **Arctic Ice Core Project** disaster. A devoted football fan who listens to audiotapes of old playoff games. He is murdered at the Ice Core Project camp by **Dr. Nancy Da Silva** while she is under the influence of the alien **ice worm,** making him indirectly its seventh casualty. ["Ice"]

MURRAY, VIRGINIA: The location of **Lincoln Park,** where

Teddy Holvey dies. ["The Calusari"]

[N]

NAPIER'S CONSTANT: The numerical base (27828) for all natural logarithms. **Victor Klemper** mentions it to Mulder and Scully; it turns out to be the entry code to the secret information repository at the **Strughold Mine.** ["Paper Clip"]

NATIONAL COMET: The tabloid paper in which Mulder learns of the abduction of **Ruby Morris.** ["Conduit"]

NATIONAL SECURITY AGENCY: The red-haired man (**Malcolm Gerlach**) claims he works for the NSA. ["731"]

NAVAJO CODE TALKERS: During World War II, the U.S. military used Navajo servicemen to relay sensitive messages in their native language, which was impervious to Japanese code-breaking techniques. The top-secret UFO documents passed on to Mulder by the **Thinker** are encoded in this fashion. ["Anasazi"]

NEARY, LT.: A member of the San Francisco Police Department's homicide squad who investigates the premature cremation of several Chinese men. ["Hell Money"]

NEIL, MARTY: An overzealous classmate of Scully's at Quantico, nicknamed "J. Edgar Junior" by other agents. Mentioned in passing by agent **Tom Colton.** ["Squeeze"]

NELSON: The attorney representing **Eugene Tooms** at his sanity hearing. ["Tooms"]

NEMHAUSER, AGENT GREG: Arrests **John Mostow** for the murder of Peter, an artist's model. He is bitten by Mostow during the arrest. ["Grotesque"]

NEMMAN, THERESA: Daughter of the county medical examiner in **Bellefleur, Oregon.** Fearing for her life, she comes to Mulder for help. She was friends with the other members of the class of '89 who have died. [Pilot]

NEMMAN, DR. JAY: County medical examiner in **Bellefleur, Oregon.** [Pilot]

NETTLES, DET.: Plainclothes detective in Hollywood, California, investigating the murder of **Garrett Lorre.** ["3"]

NEW AGE: The time that will come after **Kevin Kryder** is killed, or so says the Millennium Man (**Simon Gates**). ["Revelations"]

NEWIRTH, PATRICK: An executive of the **Morley Tobacco** company who goes missing from Room 606 of the Hotel George Mason in Richmond, Virginia, leaving behind his luggage, a half-finished glass of Scotch, and a mysterious burn mark on the carpet. Mulder suspects spontaneous human combustion, but the truth is far stranger. ["Soft Light"]

NEWPORT NEWS, VIRGINIA: At the **harbormaster**'s office here, Mulder inquires after the salvage ship *Talapus.* ["Nisei"]

NEWTON, DR. RICK: Medical examiner for Miller's Grove, Massachusetts. ["War of the Coprophages"] He had an article published in the *Journal of Forensic Sciences.* In the FBI Sci-Crime lab Mulder has him test an air bag to see whether the pattern of a face can be picked up from it. The bag is from **Walter Skinner**'s car, which someone borrowed to frame Skinner for attempted murder. ["Avatar"]

THE NIAGARA: An old bar in Raleigh, North Carolina, with a neon sign of a waterfall. This fits a description given by **Luther Lee Boggs,** and leads Scully to find a nearby warehouse where **Lucas Henry** has hidden his victims **Liz Hawley** and **Jim Summers.** This may have been set up by Boggs, unless he really possesses psychic powers. ["Beyond the Sea"]

NICAP: The National Investigative Committee of Aerial Phenomena, a UFO fringe group. **Max Fenig** is a member. ["Fallen Angel"]

NIH: The National Institutes of Health. **Dr. Joe Ridley** worked there on progeria research in the 1970s, until his dismissal for unethical practices. ["Young at Heart"]

"NOBODY'S GOING TO SPOIL US": The words spoken by **Carl Wade** when he kidnaps **Amy Jacobs.** ["Oubliette"]

NOLLETTE, FRANK: A scientist who works at the **Mahan Propulsion Laboratory.** ["Roland"]

NORMAN, DET.: Policeman at the crime scene in Newark, New Jersey, when Mulder arrives. He hands Mulder a pair of yellow boots to put on because the crime scene is inside a sewer. ["The Host"]

NORRIS, GWEN: An employee of the **Travel Time Travel Agency** taken hostage by **Duane Barry.** Mulder persuaded Barry to set her and **Kimberly Monroe** free. ["Duane Barry"]

NORTHEAST GEORGETOWN MEDICAL CENTER: The Washington, D.C., hospital where Scully is brought to the intensive care unit, but no one knows who admitted her.

["One Breath"] Scully is there to recover from the effects of the strange video trap which had caused her to hallucinate that Mulder, the **motel manager,** and even the police were out to kill her. ["Wetwired"]

NORTHERN, PENNY: A Mutual UFO Network (MUFON) member in the **Allentown** area. She claims Scully is a fellow abductee and talks to her about her experience. She reveals to Scully that there is a mark on the back of her neck, which Scully hadn't been aware of before. ["Nisei"]

NUTT, MR.: A midget motel manager in his sixties, in **Gibsonton, Florida.** He owns a pet dog. ["Humbug"]

[O]

OAKES, SHERIFF JOHN: He investigates the murder of sixteen-year-old **Jerry Stevens,** who has been killed by a demon, his heart and eyes cut out. His body is displayed according to the rites of Azazel. ["Die Hand Die Verletzt"]

OATES: The counsel of the governor of Florida. He advises **Daniel Charez** there's little hope that the governor will extend clemency to **"Neech" Manley.** ["The List"]

ODDITORIUM: A museum of curiosa in **Gibsonton, Florida.** It's musty and resembles an antiques store. Admission is free to freaks. Among the exhibits are photos of circus freaks from years past. ["Humbug"]

O'DELL, PEGGY: A friend of the victims of the mysterious killings in **Bellefleur, Oregon,** who were members of the high school class of '89. She was in an auto accident with **Billy Miles.** Confined to a wheelchair in the state hospital for four years, she disappears from there one night and is found dead on the highway. She ran out of the woods and into the path of a truck. [Pilot]

ODIN, RICHARD: The leader of the **Church of the Red Museum** in **Delta Glen, Wisconsin.** Real name Doug Herman. Left the American Medical Association in 1986 over an ethics issue. ["Red Museum"]

OLAFSSEN: A pirate whaler who is rescued by the USS *Argent* when his ship sinks, Olaffsen avoids aging after he discovers that the recycled sewage water on the ship is uncontaminated. He is stranded on the rusting *Argent* when his crew steals **Trondheim**'s boat, the *Zeal.* After he reveals his survival secret to

Trondheim, Olafssen disappears; Trondheim claims he has escaped, but it is more likely that Trondheim has killed him. ["Dod Kalm"]

O'NEIL, JESSE: Member of the **Cascade Volcano Research Team.** She's infected with the silicon-based life form and dies. **Trepkos** takes her body deep into the volcano with him, as they had been lovers. ["Firewalker"]

OPERATION FALCON: Top-secret military mission with the objective of recovering a downed alien craft and any surviving crew. Corollary objectives include evacuating nearby civilians and conducting an intensive disinformation campaign. Mulder walks right into the middle of all this, which is not appreciated by the military. ["Fallen Angel"]

OPERATION PAPER CLIP: A program under which the United States protected Nazi scientists in exchange for their expertise. Werner von Braun and **Victor Klemper** were both beneficiaries of this operation. ["Paper Clip"]

OPPENHEIM, DR. JEFFREY: A physician on duty at the county hospital in **Townsend, Wisconsin,** the night **Jason Wright** is admitted. Angry about the government cover-up, he tells Mulder the truth about Wright, and enlists Scully's aid when soldiers from **Beta Team** are admitted with severe burns, over **Col. Henderson**'s objections. ["Fallen Angel"]

OPTIONS HALFWAY HOUSE: Where **Lucy Householder** lives. ["Oubliette"]

ORIGINAL "SAMANTHA": The original alien visitor from whom many more were cloned, including the one who pretended to be Mulder's lost sister. When Mulder, angry at the trick, refuses to help her and her clones, she claims to have information about the real Samantha, but it is too late: by this time, the **Pilot** has arrived to murder all the clones. It is presumed that he also kills the original "Samantha." ["End Game"]

OSBORNE, DR.: One of the doctors involved in **Pinck Pharmaceuticals'** unethical test of a newly discovered disease at the **Cumberland State Correctional Facility.** Osborne falsely claims to be working for the **Centers for Disease Control,** but reveals to Scully that ten out of fourteen infected prisoners are already dead. Osborne is infected by pus from the body of **Bobby Torrence,** and confides the truth to Scully before he dies: the entire situation is

the work of the Pinck Pharmaceuticals company. His body is incinerated. ["F. Emasculata"]

OSWALD, DARIN PETER: Nineteen years old, barely literate, romantically obsessed with his high school English teacher (who flunked him), Darin would be just another small-town loser in **Connerville, Oklahoma,** if not for his ability to channel powerful electrical currents. This apparently began after he survived being struck by lightning. Several people who annoyed him die of electrocution before his capture, as well as an undetermined number of cattle. He also causes Mulder's cellular phone to melt. After Darin attempts to kidnap **Sharon Kiveat** and kills **Sheriff Teller,** he is held in a special room at the Oklahoma State Psychiatric Hospital. ["D.P.O."]

OSWALD, MRS.: The overweight, TV-addicted mother of the electrified teenager Darin Peter Oswald. ["D.P.O."]

OWENS, G.: An intensive care nurse who watches over Scully, but about whom no one at the hospital knows anything. ["One Breath"]

[P]

PADDOCK, PHYLLIS: The demon who is accidentally summoned by **Jerry Stevens.** She looks like an ordinary fifty-two-year-old schoolteacher, except that she keeps Jerry's eyes and heart in her desk drawer. No one at the school in Milford Haven, New Hampshire, remembers hiring her. ["Die Hand Die Verletzt"]

PALM: The word **Mrs. Mulder** scratches out on a piece of paper. Because of the stroke she has suffered, she scrambles the letters: Fox Mulder later figures out that she had wanted to write the word LAMP. Inside a lamp he finds hidden a device that has a button on it which releases a thin pointed blade, the kind of weapon used to kill alien clones. ["Talitha Cumi"]

PALOMAR OBSERVATORY: Located just north of San Diego; built in 1948 by George Ellery Hale. Mulder claims Hale got the idea from an "elf" that climbed in his window. ["Little Green Men"]

PARKER, JIM: A rancher in his late fifties in Montana who is embroiled in a border dispute with the Trego Indian reservation. One night he shoots and kills an animal that turns out to be an Indian werewolf. Later

Parker is killed by another werewolf. ["Shapes"]

PARKER, LYLE: Jim Parker's son. He's bitten by a werewolf and then becomes one. He kills his father and later is killed by Sheriff **Charley Tskany.** ["Shapes"]

PARMELLY: A prison guard present at the execution of **"Neech" Manley.** He takes Scully aside and tells her that the prisoner named **Roque** has a list of Manley's intended victims. Parmelly is romantically involved with Manley's wife Danielle, making him a suspect. Danielle shoots him because she comes to the conclusion that he is possessed by her husband's spirit. ["The List"]

PATNIK, JOSEPH: A secret TV signal has caused him to hallucinate that everyone he sees is a Bosnian war criminal named **Lladoslav Miriskovic.** He even mistakes his wife for the man and kills her. He also kills four other people before the police arrest him. He is taken to the Frederick County Psychiatric Hospital in Braddock Heights, Maryland. While there, he sees a TV news report about Miriskovic, whereupon he becomes hysterical with terror and has to be restrained. ["Wetwired"]

PATTERSON, BILL: Mulder's former mentor, an FBI agent in his fifties, who runs the investigative support unit at Quantico. He accompanies agent **Greg Nemhauser** when **John Mostow** is arrested for murder. He finds the murder weapon, a bloodstained carpet knife. Patterson becomes possessed by a demon and in gargoyle form is shot and killed by Scully. ["Grotesque"]

PAUL: One of two prisoners at the **Cumberland State Correctional Facility** who use the confusion surrounding the death of **Bobby Torrence** to escape in a laundry cart. He attempts to flee to Toronto by bus, but is tracked down by Mulder, who is on the verge of persuading him to surrender when Paul is shot by unknown government forces covering up the *F. Emasculata* outbreak. With Paul dead, Mulder and Scully are the only witnesses left. ["F. Emasculata"]

PENDRELL: The agent to whom Scully takes the metal implant after she has it removed from her neck. It is just like one she previously came across in "The Blessing Way." Pendrell states that the implant is some kind of microprocessor. ["Nisei"]

PERKEY, WEST VIRGINIA: Site of the **Hansen's Disease**

Research Facility. A mass execution is conducted there. It is also where **Dr. Shiro Zama** (a.k.a. **Dr. Ishimaru**) conducts secret experiments. ["731"]

PERKINS: A logger in the Pacific Northwest, one of a group who cut into an ancient tree and unleash prehistoric wood mites that attack out of self-preservation, becoming active only after sunset and before dawn. He and **Dyer** become imprisoned in **cocoons** by the teeming wood mites. ["Darkness Falls"]

PERKINS: A detective at Buffalo's **14th Precinct.** ["Born Again"]

PERRY, SIMON: The executioner who pulled the switch on **"Neech" Manley.** Mulder and Scully find him tied to a chair in his attic, his body swarming with maggots. He is Manley's third victim. ["The List"]

PETER: An artist's model. He is killed by **John Mostow,** a man possessed by a demon. ["Grotesque"]

PETERSON, CLAUDE: An undercover government agent, probably with the Department of Defense, who infiltrates the Eurisko Corporation as the systems engineer for the building. His real mission is to crack the artificial-intelligence program used in the building security system designed by **Brad Wilczek.** ["Ghost in the Machine"]

PFASTER, DONNIE: Employee of the Janelli-Heller Funeral Home. A fetishist who collects the hair and fingernails of dead young women, he is fired when he's caught cutting off some of the hair of one of the bodies. ["Irresistible"]

PHEROMONES: Hormonal sexual attractants secreted by various animals. Human pheromone production is so minimal that scientists are unsure whether humans actually possess them or not; if **Marty** of the **Kindred** is any indication, his people produce several hundred times more pheromones than any other creature known in nature, raising the question of whether they are actually human. ["Genderbender"]

PHILADELPHIA EXPERIMENT: A top-secret U.S. military project, perhaps mythical, conducted at the Philadelphia Navy Yard on July 8, 1944. The experiment resulted in the disappearance of a battleship, which reappeared hundreds of miles away near Norfolk, Virginia, in a matter of minutes. Mulder suspects that the experiment involved wormholes, and at first believes that

the disappearance of the USS **Argent** has been caused by something similar. ["Dod Kalm"]

PHILIPS, LULA: A career criminal, age twenty-five, she did time at the Maryland Women's Correctional Facility for manslaughter. While there she had a clandestine affair with prison guard **Warren James Dupre;** he was fired when this was discovered. They marry and embark on a short-lived but intense crime career after her release on May 2, 1993, specializing in violent bank robberies. She sets up Dupre by tipping off the FBI to their final bank robbery. When **Jack Willis** claims to be Dupre, she plays along until she can get an advantage by withholding insulin from the diabetic Willis, then demands $1 million from the FBI for the return of the kidnapped Scully. Willis kills Lula shortly before the FBI storms her hideout. ["Lazarus"]

PHILIPS, TOMMY: Lula Philips's brother, a small-time crook so addicted to television that he'll even watch it if the sound isn't working. Killed by **Jack Willis** for finking on **Warren Dupre** and Lula, although Tommy was not actually responsible. ["Lazarus"]

PHILLIPS, DR.: A physician at the University of Pennsylvania Hospital's Bone and Tissue Bank. He confirms that five of **Howard Graves**'s organs were used in transplant surgery shortly after his death, and provides tissue samples which Scully uses to prove that Graves is really dead. ["Shadows"]

PHILLIPS, STAN: A resident at the **Excelsis Dei Convalescent Home.** He's lived there three years and doesn't want to leave. ["Excelsis Dei"]

PIEDMONT, VIRGINIA: Location of **Yaloff Psychiatric Hospital,** where **Chester Ray Banton**'s shadow kills two government operatives out to kidnap him. ["Soft Light"]

PIERCE, ADAM: Member of the **Cascade Volcano Research Team** working at the California Institute of Technology in Pasadena. He accompanies Mulder and Scully to **Mount Avalon** and is killed by **Trepkos** shortly after arrival. ["Firewalker"]

THE PILOT: An alien bounty hunter, according to one of the false Samantha invaders, sent to Earth with a mandate to assassinate the alien colonists involved in human–alien DNA experimentation. He can assume any form at will, and

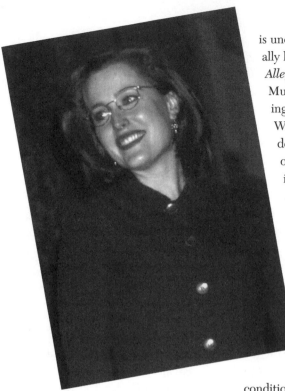

can be killed only by piercing the base of his skull. If shot, he emits a toxic green gas from his wounds, apparently containing an airborne alien virus that kills humans by causing their blood to coagulate. (This same virus was encountered in "The Erlenmeyer Flask.") The virus can be rendered dormant with low temperatures. Although a ruthless assassin, the Pilot seems unwilling to kill humans unless it is absolutely necessary, as is seen in his final confrontation with Mulder on the icebound USS *Allegiance.* In light of this, it is unclear whether he actually killed the crew of the *Allegiance* (as he told Mulder while impersonating Navy Lt. Terry Wilmer) or whether their deaths were caused by other means. The Pilot is last seen taking the *Allegiance* to the location of his own craft. His final words to Mulder are that the real Samantha is still alive. ["Colony," "End Game"]

PILSSON, DR. ERIK: The physician who has been monitoring the condition of **Augustus Cole** for the last twelve years. Cole is kept in an isolation ward because he disrupted the sleep of the other patients. ["Sleepless"]

PINCK PHARMACEUTICALS: One of the largest manufacturers of drugs in the United States, based in Wichita, Kansas. This company was behind the outbreak of contagion at the **Cumberland State Correctional Facility,** apparently during an experiment to test possible treatments of *F. Emasculata*. ["F. Emasculata"]

PIPER MARU: The salvage vessel that takes a group of French scientists, including **Gauthier,** to locate a World War II fighter plane (call numbers JTTO 111470) that contained an alien entity. Its crew, with one exception, later suffered severe radiation burns. When Mulder examines the ship, he detects no radiation, but he does find a videotape of the plane at the bottom of the sea. ["Piper Maru"]

PLAIN-CLOTHED MAN: He meets with Mulder in Washington, D.C., and tells him about **Joseph Patnik** and the five people he killed in **Braddock Heights, Maryland.** He won't say who sent him to give Mulder this information, but apparently it was **X.** ["Wetwired"]

PLITH, DR.: Forensic anthropologist who examines the body found in cement at the **Ruxton chemical plant.** He finds gnawing marks near the ribs. ["Tooms"]

POLARITY MAGNETICS: The company where **Chester Ray Banton** worked prior to his accident. Mulder learns the company name from a patch seen on Banton's jacket in a train station security video. The company's main focus is magnetic levitation design for bullet trains and similar applications, but Banton was pursuing more esoteric research involving subatomic particles. Polarity Magnetics was shut down after the accident. ["Soft Light"]

POMERANTZ, DR. MARK: A psychiatrist who hypnotizes Scully and helps her remember events related to her abduction. She bolts from the procedure, overwhelmed, before anything substantial can be recovered. ["The Blessing Way"]

POSITRON EMISSION TOMOGRAPHY LAB: Where **Betsy Hagopian** is taken due to her undiagnosed cancerous condition. Her body is full of tumors. Scully is told by **Lottie Holloway** that all of the abductees will eventually end up in that condition because of what was done to them when they were abducted. Hagopian, now in her forties, has been abducted many times since she was in her teens. ["Nisei"]

POWERTECH: The facility where an E.B.E. (extraterrestrial biological entity) is being held, and which Mulder and Scully manage to penetrate using phony identification. ["E.B.E."]

POWHATTAN MILL KILLINGS: The 1933 crime spree during which **Eugene Tooms** killed five people and cut out their livers. Only four

of those victims were found; Tooms hid the fifth. ["Tooms"]

PRIEST: After she saves the life of **Kevin Kryder,** a true stigmatic, Scully goes to a Catholic church and inside a confessional she talks to a priest, something she has not done in six years. The priest casually makes a remark that echoes something said to her during this case, about things coming "full circle." Scully has seen things she cannot explain, and that she cannot share with Mulder. ["Revelations"]

PRINCE, DR. LANDON: A physician who died in an arson fire at an abortion clinic in Scranton, Pennsylvania. His name appears in a list of similar deaths e-mailed to Mulder by an anonymous source. Mulder is baffled upon learning that all three doctors, although apparently unrelated, were identical — and no body was recovered in any of the cases. ["Colony"]

PROGERIA: A rare disease that accelerates aging. Some victims may survive to early adulthood, but most die at seven or eight years of age, looking like midget ninety-year-olds. Death is generally due to cardiac arrest or loss of circulation in the brain. **Dr. Joe Ridley** saw progeria as a possible key to slowing or reversing the aging

process, but his methods were too extreme for the National Institutes of Health. ["Young at Heart"]

PROVINCETOWN PUB: A bar burned down by **Cecil L'ively,** probably to taunt the authorities trying to solve his crimes. ["Fire"]

PULASKI, VIRGINIA: Small town where **Duane Barry** lived alone at the time of his alien abduction on June 3, 1985. This was not his first abduction, but it was the one during which he saw humans — government agents — cooperating with the aliens. ["Duane Barry"]

THE PUPPET: A serial killer whose victims are all professional psychics of some sort: astrologers, palm readers, tarot readers, even a tea leaf reader. He possesses a certain limited psychic skill himself, getting glimpses of his crimes before he commits them. He feels as if he has no control over his actions (like a puppet) and hopes that his victims can explain them to him. **Clyde Bruckman** helps clarify matters by pointing out that the Puppet is a homicidal maniac. ["Clyde Bruckman's Final Repose"]

PURDUE, REGGIE: A black FBI agent in his fifties, a widower, who works in the violent-crimes division in Washington, D.C., and is writing a mystery novel in his spare time. He was Mulder's superior on the **John Barnett** case in 1989 and calls his friend Mulder in when evidence suggests that the allegedly dead Barnett is somehow responsible for a new crime. Purdue is killed by Barnett as a warning to Mulder. ["Young at Heart"]

PUSHER: The alias used by **Robert Modell,** the hit man who wills his victims to kill themselves. ["Pusher"]

[Q]

QUANTICO, VIRGINIA: Location of the FBI academy, which is often referred to only as "Quantico" by those who have passed through there.

QUARANTINE CAR: The train car Mulder believes is transporting a human–alien hybrid (see also **Hansen's Research Center Compound).** ["731"]

QUEENSGATE, OHIO: Where **Dr. Shiro Zama** boarded a train that also picked up the inaccessible **Quarantine Car.** (see also **Dr. Ishimaru)** ["731"]

QUEEQUEG: Scully's little dog. Originally the pet of **Clyde Bruckman**'s elderly neighbor **Mrs. Lowe.** When Mrs. Lowe died, the dog had no food and

apparently ate part of its deceased mistress to survive. Bruckman retrieves the dog shortly before his suicide, and suggests that Scully take it. She names it after a character in *Moby Dick,* since she and her father had nicknamed each other after that book's Starbuck and Ahab. ["Clyde Bruckman's Final Repose"] The poor dog meets its end when it's eaten by an alligator. ["Quagmire"]

QUINNIMONT, WEST VIRGINIA: Where Mulder finds a train that he's been looking for, the one with the car where the alien autopsy was interrupted by gunfire that killed four Japanese scientists. He sees some men board the train, including someone in a radiation suit who appears to be an alien. ["Nisei"]

QUONOCHONTAUG, RHODE ISLAND: Where the Mulders have a lakefront house. Mrs. Mulder is met there by the **Cigarette-Smoking Man;** they have an argument. ["Talitha Cumi"]

[R]

RADIO SHACK: A national electronics chain store operated by the Tandy Company. Mulder buys a laser pointer at one of their outlets for $49.95. ["Soft Light"]

RANA SPENOCEPHALA: A type of rare frog on the verge of extinction. It is found in Striker's Cove on **Heuvelmans Lake** in Georgia. The population there of this type of frog has dropped to less than 200. ["Quagmire"]

RAND: One of the agents who has Mulder's residence under surveillance, and who confronts Scully when she goes there. ["Little Green Men"]

RANDALL, GREG: A young man who tended bar at the **Boar's Head** tavern in Sioux City, Iowa, and vanishes around the same time as **Ruby Morris,** but is cleared of any suspicion when he is found dead in a shallow grave near **Lake Okobogee** by Mulder and Scully. He was killed by **Tessa Sears,** who was pregnant with his child. ["Conduit"]

RANDOLPH, DR. VANCE: The staff doctor at the **Chaco Chicken** processing plant who treats **Jess Harold**'s neck wound after he is attacked by **Paula Gray.** ["Our Town"]

RANFORD, CHRISTINE: The wife of Frank Ranford. She discovers that her toilet is blocked and is unaware that **Eugene Tooms** is using the sewer pipe to gain entrance to her house. ["Tooms"]

RANFORD, FRANK: A man in his mid-thirties who is stalked by **Eugene Tooms.** ["Tooms"]

RANHEIM: A truck driver whose vehicle loses power when a UFO comes down nearby. He shoots at what he thinks is an alien, then gets a rash on his face and hands. Scully learns that his real name is Frank Druse and his truck is transporting something secret — possibly an alien or the wreckage of a UFO. ["E.B.E."]

RAT-TAIL PRODUCTIONS: The name of the small company in **Allentown, Pennsylvania,** that sells copies of the **alien autopsy** video. It is located in a private residence, a boarded-up house that appears to be abandoned. Upon entering the house, Mulder and Scully find the still-warm corpse of a man, and Mulder chases a Japanese man, who is carrying a **leather satchel,** and finally catches him. ["Nisei"]

RAVEN: An overweight prostitute attacked and killed by **Virgil Incanto** after a struggle. Scraps of his skin under her fingernails provide an important clue in the case. ["2Shy"]

REARDON, CINDY: An eight-year-old girl, one of **Dr. Sally Kendrick**'s clones. She plotted with **Teena Simmons** to murder their fathers, apparently through a cross-country psychic connection. They later murder Kendricks together, try to divert Mulder's attention, and finally attempt to poison Mulder and Scully when they grow suspicious. ["Eve"]

REARDON, DOUG: A resident of Marin County killed at the exact same time as **Joel Simmons,** in the exact same fashion, right down to the swing. Father of Cindy Reardon. ["Eve"]

REARDON, ELLEN: Wife of Doug and mother of Cindy Reardon. Tells Mulder that Cindy was conceived through in vitro fertilization at the **Luther Stapes Center.** She disowns Cindy after the truth is revealed about the nature of her conception. ["Eve"]

RECYCLING PLANT: Where the Millennium Man **(Simon Gates)** takes ten-year-old **Kevin Kryder** to kill him (see also **Twenty-First Century Recycling.**) ["Revelations"]

RED-HAIRED MAN: See **Malcolm Gerlach.**

RED HEAD: A member of the W.A.O. (Wild Again Organization), he watches with quiet belligerence as Mulder and Scully interrogate **Kyle Lang.** Scully follows him one night when he breaks into the Fairfield Zoo. He is observing a tiger in its cage when it seemingly disappears, then an invisible presence attacks him outside the cage, mauling him to death. ["Fearful Symmetry"]

RED ROCK QUARRY: Location of the buried boxcar containing piles of alien bodies, where Mulder narrowly escapes death. ["The Blessing Way"]

REGAN, LT.: One of the firefighters who finds the dead body of **Dr. Grissom** in his apartment. ["Sleepless"]

REHOBOTH, DELAWARE: The community where the **Thinker,** possibly a.k.a. Kenneth Soona, lived until the authorities' discovery of his access to sensitive government files obliged him to flee. ["Anasazi"]

RETICULANS: Alien beings whom Scully facetiously accuses of being possibly responsible for an experiment involving induced paranoia that seems to be taking place in **Franklin, Pennsylvania.** ["Blood"]

RICH: FBI agent in charge of the complete operation surrounding the **Duane Barry** hostage situation. ["Duane Barry"]

RICHMOND, DR. JANICE: Physician on call when **Eugene Tooms** is brought in to the emergency room. ["Tooms"]

RICHMOND TRAIN STA-TION: **Chester Ray Banton** spends most of his days and nights here after his accident, depending on the waiting room's diffused fluorescent light to keep his shadow from showing. He unintentionally kills two Richmond policemen in an alley outside the station. ["Soft Light"]

RICHTER, JOHN: A top geo-physicist, head of **Arctic Ice Core Project.** A week after retrieving an ice core sample a quarter-million years old, Richter and other members of his team began to show signs of extreme mental disturbance. His last transmission, on November 5, 1993, includes the cryptic words "We're not who we are," and ends when he and his teammate Campbell commit suicide simultaneously. The other three members of the team were already dead. ["Ice"]

RIDDOCK, HELENE: Imagining that she sees her husband, Victor, committing adultery with the woman next door, she grabs a shotgun and kills her neighbor, John Gillnitz, whom she mistakes for her husband. ["Wetwired"]

RIDGEWAY ELEMENTARY SCHOOL: In Loveland, Ohio, where **Kevin Kryder** attends the fifth grade. ["Revelations"]

RIDLEY, DR. JOE: Performed experiments on prisoners at **Tashmoo Federal Correctional Facility** in his efforts to reverse the aging process. Previously he worked at the National Institutes of Health, where he was investi-gating the disease **progeria** until, in violation of NIH poli-cy, he began unapproved human trials. Colleagues secretly nicknamed him "Dr. Mengele" for his Naziesque disregard of his patients as anything but test subjects. The state of Maryland revoked his medical license in 1979 for research malpractice and mis-use of government grant money. After leaving Tashmoo, he disappeared from sight, working in Mexico, Belize, and other Central American coun-tries until **John Barnett** stole his research. Ridley has reversed his own aging, but suffers from cataracts because his "cure" for aging does not work on the eyes for some rea-son; he has a cerebral vascular disease. ["Young at Heart"]

RIGDON, GEORGIA: Mulder drives on County Road 33 through here on his way to **Heuvelmans Lake** to investi-gate the disappearance of a U.S. Forest Service official. ["Quagmire"]

RILEY, BOB: Middle-aged, balding employee of the **Travel Time Travel Agency** taken hostage by **Duane Barry,** who unintentionally shoots Riley during a mysteri-ous blackout. Barry lets him go for medical treatment in exchange for Mulder. ["Duane Barry"]

"RING THE BELLS": A song by the band James, this was the last piece of music heard by **Jack Hammond** before his untimely demise at the age of twenty-one. ["D.P.O."]

RITUAL OF SEPARATION: A Romanian ritual intended to separate the soul of a living child from the soul of a dead twin. When one of her twin sons died at birth, **Maggie Holvey** refused to let her mother **Golda** perform the rite, which led to nothing but trouble for her family. When Mulder helps the **Calusari** finally perform the ritual, he becomes known to the demon-ic entity that had taken the place of the dead twin's soul; according to the Calusari, this is the Devil himself. ["The Calusari"]

RIVERS, POLICE CHIEF: Investigates **Ranheim**'s shoot-ing of what may have been a mountain lion. He doesn't want the FBI investigating it. ["E.B.E."]

ROB: A divorced father who dated Scully once after a mutual friend set them up, but Scully was too involved in her career to see him again. ["The Jersey Devil"]

ROBERTO: A young Latino janitor working at the Idaho Mutual Insurance Trust in **Fairfield, Idaho,** when some invisible force causes the windows at the front of the bank to shatter. ["Fearful Symmetry"]

ROBERTS, TERRI: A friend of **Bruno,** a boy who dies under mysterious circumstances. She and her best friend, **Margi Kleinjan,** together have strange powers due to a peculiar alignment of the planets. A senior at Grover Cleveland Alexander High School in Comity, she has a grade point average of 3.98 and is on the cheerleading squad with Margi. Astrologically speaking, Comity is in a geological vortex. On January 12 the planets come into perfect alignment. Since January 12 is her birthday as well as Margi's, and they were born in 1979, this gives them a Jupiter–Uranus opposition, which creates a grand square where the planets are aligned in a cross. This causes all the energy of the cosmos to be focused on them. ["Syzygy"]

ROCKVILLE, MARYLAND: Location of the Women's Health Services Center, where Mulder meets more alien clones. ["End Game"]

ROOSEVELT, DR. CARL: A respected American archaeologist in his sixties, who disappears from an archaeological site in Ecuador shortly after the discovery of the **Amaru** Urn. ["Teso dos Bichos"]

ROQUE, SAMMON: A prisoner at **Eastpoint State Penitentiary** who taunts **"Neech" Manley** on his way to the electric chair. He supposedly has the list of Manley's intended victims, and tries to get transferred out of Eastpoint. Instead, he is beaten to death by prison guards commanded by warden **Leo Brodeur.** ["The List"]

ROSEN, TRACY: A mentally retarded friend of **Roland Fuller**'s. ["Roland"]

ROSSLYN, VIRGINIA: Location of **Gen. Thomas Callahan**'s family home. ["The Walk"]

ROSWELL, NEW MEXICO: Area where it's believed that a UFO crashed in 1947. The source of much lore on the subject.

ROUTE 44: A highway near the **Kindred** community in Massachusetts, where Brothers Andrew and Martin find the magazines that interest Martin in the outside world. ["Genderbender"]

ROUTE 229: A highway passing through Rixeyville, Virginia, where a highway patrol officer pulls over **Duane Barry** in Scully's car, only to be shot. The officer's car-mounted video camera records the entire incident, and reveals that Scully is in the trunk of the stolen vehicle. ["Ascension"]

RUBES: A term used by circus people to describe outsiders. ["Humbug"]

RUXTON CHEMICAL PLANT: Located in Baltimore. It is where **Eugene Tooms** hid one of his victims in 1933 in the concrete of a then newly poured foundation. In 1994, modern technology is able to locate where the body is entombed. ["Tooms"]

RYAN, DET. KELLY: Newly promoted in the Richmond, Virginia, police force, this former student of Scully's calls in Scully and Mulder for assistance in her first assignment as detective, a missing-persons case that started when **Patrick Newirth** vanished, but she shuts the FBI agents out of the case after two Richmond police officers die and the goings get weird. She dies as a result of contact with **Chester Ray Banton**'s shadow, the only person Banton killed on purpose. ["Soft Light"]

[S]

SAI BABA: An Indian guru whom **Chuck Burk** claims to have witnessed creating an entire feast out of thin air in 1979, a feat accompanied by the production of the holy ash called vibuti. ["The Calusari"]

SAINT IGNATIUS: According to Catholic tradition, he could be in two places at once by creating an illusionary double of himself. **Kevin Kryder** is able to do this. ["Revelations"]

SAINT MATTHEW'S MEDICAL CENTER: Where **Charlie Holvey** is taken after being removed from his family home by FBI social worker **Karen Kosseff.** Mulder and the **Calusari** perform the Ritual of Separation on Charlie there. ["The Calusari"]

SAL: A waitress at a café in **Gibsonton, Florida.** She is half-man, half-woman. ["Humbug"]

SALINGER, BEATRICE: The night nurse on duty at the Siloam County Hospital. She claims she saw **Samuel Hartley** get up and walk out on his own, and his body is missing. ["Miracle Man"]

"SAMANTHA": An alien clone claiming to be Mulder's sister Samantha, she appears at

William Mulder's house during the **Gregor** case. She knows plenty about Fox and his sister, right down to their fondness for the game Stratego, and claims to have been returned to Earth and raised by aliens passing for humans. ["Colony"] According to her, the identical aliens were clones of the two original "visitors" who arrived on Earth in the late 1940s (possibly at Roswell, although she doesn't say). Because their identical appearances made it necessary to disperse across the world, the clones were experimenting to meld alien and human DNA in order to diversify their appearance and increase their numbers. These experiments were unsanctioned, resulting in the arrival of the **Pilot,** whose mission is to destroy the colony. This Samantha is abducted by the Pilot; when her body is recovered, it disintegrates into a green liquid, revealing her to be one of the alien clones. ["End Game"]

SANFORD, CAPT. KYLE: Commander of the submarine **Zeus Faber** during World War II. He was possessed by an alien entity found at the site of a downed UFO. ["Piper Maru"]

SATIN: A hooker in Minneapolis whom **Donnie Pfaster** picks

up and kills. Then he washes her hair. She is his first victim. ["Irresistible"]

SAUNDERS: CIA agent who turns to Mulder and Scully for help when his case, involving illegal arms trading, turns up a potential X-File connection. ["Shadows"]

SAWMILL: The location where everyone meets at the end and there is a question as to who will survive. ["Talitha Cumi"]

SAYLES, CARINA: A former secretary for a Washington, D.C., law firm, she was fired because she was moonlighting for an escort service. Her nude, lifeless body is found in bed with **Walter Skinner,** who remembers picking her up in the Chesapeake Lounge downstairs in the Ambassador Hotel but not how she died. Scully determines that the cause of death was a crushed spinal cord and the cervical vertebrae were fractured. Scully also finds an odd residual phosphorescence covering the dead woman's nose and mouth. ["Avatar"]

SCHIFF-IMMERGUT LUMBER COMPANY: A logging outfit in the Pacific Northwest. Thirty of their loggers have disappeared from a single area virtually overnight. Ecoterrorists are suspected. ["Darkness Falls"]

SCHNABLEGGER, DR.
GLENNA: County pathologist at Atlantic City, she allows Mulder and Scully to observe the examination of a dead homeless man brutally murdered and maimed by human teeth. ["The Jersey Devil"]

SCHOOL NURSE: She treats **Kevin Kryder** after his palms begin to bleed in school, spraying Bactine on the wound. When she takes his temperature, the thermometer in the boy's mouth rises quickly and then pops. ["Revelations"]

SCHUMANN RESONANCE: The radio wave frequency emitted by lightning flashes: eight cycles per second. ["D.P.O."]

SCOPOLAMINE: A drug used for motion sickness, but which in large quantities is an anesthetic with hallucinogenic qualities used to drug those who are to become "victims" of the cult. ["Red Museum"]

SCULLY, BILL JR.: Dana's older brother. ["One Breath"]

SCULLY, CHARLES: Dana's younger brother. ["One Breath"]

SCULLY, DANA: Born February 23, 1960, the daughter of a U.S. Navy captain. She spent part of her childhood living on Miramar Naval Air Base, north of San Diego. ["Apocrypha"] She did her undergraduate work in physics (her thesis was "Einstein's Twin Paradox: A New Interpretation") and took her medical degree at the **University of Maryland,** but then disappointed her parents by joining the FBI. She is assigned by section chief **Scott Blevins** to work with agent Fox Mulder on the X-Files and write field reports and evaluations of their activities. Personal ID number X197735VW3. Her gun is a Smith & Wesson 1056. Initially assigned by her superiors with the intent to debunk Mulder's X-Files investigations, she instead becomes Mulder's greatest ally. Placed on mandatory leave and forced to surrender her badge and weapon in the aftermath of Mulder's disappearance, she is obliged to go through the metal detector at the front of FBI headquarters, whereupon she discovers a small piece of metal, resembling a computer chip, implanted in her neck. ["The Blessing Way"] Disarmed by **Virgil Incanto,** she is saved when **Ellen Kaminski** kills him with Scully's gun. ["2Shy"] Scully captures **Luis Cardinal,** the man who killed her sister and shot **Skinner.** ["Apocrypha"] For six years she has been something of a lapsed Catholic, even though she still wears a crucifix on a chain around her neck. But following the events she witnesses and experiences in "Revelations," she goes to see a **priest** to discuss her concerns and misgivings. For a time she has a little dog named **Queequeg,** which is eaten by an alligator in "Quagmire."

SCULLY, MARGARET: Dana Scully's mother, fifty-eight at the time of her husband's death in 1993. She had four children: Bill Jr., Melissa, Dana, and Charles. ["Beyond the Sea"] She comes to Dana's apartment after **Duane Barry** kidnaps Dana; she had dreamed that someone had taken Dana away, but was embarrassed to tell her about it. Margaret tells Mulder to keep Dana's crucifix necklace until he can give it back to her. ["Ascension"; see also "One Breath"] Dana visits her after Mulder's apparent death. ["The Blessing Way"] When Dana begins to hallucinate that everyone is out to get her, she goes to see her mother. ["Wetwired"]

SCULLY, MELISSA: Dana's older sister. She is apparently psychic, but Margaret doesn't approve of such talk. Melissa says she can feel the emotions of the comatose Dana. ["One Breath"] She tries to comfort

Dana after Mulder's apparent death, and convinces her to undergo hypnosis in order to remember events concerning her own disappearance the previous year. Melissa is erroneously shot in Dana's place by **Krycek** and his associates. ["The Blessing Way"] She dies in a coma after unsuccessful cranial surgery some time later. ["Paper Clip"] Dana becomes consumed with finding her sister's killers.

SCULLY, WILLIAM: Dana Scully's father, a retired Navy captain. He would have been happier if his daughter had stuck with medicine instead of joining the FBI. He dies of a massive coronary at age sixty-three, during the Christmas season in 1993. ["Beyond the Sea"] After his death, he appears to Dana when she is in a coma. ["One Breath"]

SEARS, TESSA: A teenage acquaintance of **Ruby Morris,** who tells Mulder and Scully that Ruby got pregnant by her boyfriend **Greg Randall** and ran away with him. This is a lie: Tessa is pregnant by Greg, but killed him by **Lake Okobogee** because she was jealous of his involvement with Ruby. ["Conduit"]

SEATTLE FBI REGIONAL FIELD OFFICE: Where Mulder and Scully meet with

Agent Eubanks to discuss the status of the case of the kidnapping of **Amy Jacobs.** ["Oubliette"]

SECARE, DR. WILLIAM: The fugitive who has escaped from a government facility involved in alien/human experiments. He has green blood and can breathe underwater. ["The Erlenmeyer Flask"]

SECONA: A tribe that lives in the mountains of Ecuador and still practices ancient shamanistic rituals centered around jaguar worship. ["Teso dos Bichos"]

SEIZER, DR.: Physician at the naval hospital in San Diego who treated the French seamen from the *Piper Maru* for radiation burns. ["Piper Maru"]

SETH COUNTY, ARKANSAS: Location of **Dudley,** home of **Chaco Chicken.** When Mulder and Scully go to the county courthouse to confirm that **Paula Gray** was born in 1948, they discover that all the county records have been burned to ashes. ["Our Town"]

SHAMROCK WOMEN'S PRISON FACILITY: Where **B. J. Morrow** is sent to the psychiatric ward. ["Aubrey"]

SHEAFFER, LT. JACK: Phony Gray Alien #2. He is planning to abduct and interrogate **Harold Lamb** and **Chrissy**

Giorgio when all of them are abducted by real aliens from space. Mulder finds Sheaffer wandering naked down a road saying "This is not happening!" Sheaffer says he has flown a flying saucer and observes, "Afterwards sex seems trite." **Sgt. Hynek** takes him into custody, and shortly thereafter Sheaffer's body is found in a crashed Air Force jet. ["Jose Chung's *From Outer Space*"]

SHEHERLIE, SARAH: An agent in the FBI Sci-Crime Lab. ["Grotesque"]

SHERMAN CRATER: Part of the volcano at **Mount Avalon.** ["Firewalker"]

SHOVE PARK: The wooded region near Minneapolis where **Claude Dukenfield**'s body is dumped. ["Clyde Bruckman's Final Repose"]

SILICON-BASED LIFE FORM: Previously unknown, it is discovered inside the **Mount Avalon** volcano. The robot probe **Firewalker** brings the new life-form to the surface, where it proceeds to infect the research team. ["Firewalker"]

SILOAM COUNTY HOSPITAL: Where the body of **Samuel Hartley** is being kept until it disappears. The night nurse, Beatrice Salinger, claims she saw Samuel walk out under his own power. ["Miracle Man"]

SILOAM COUNTY JAIL HOUSE: Where **Samuel Hartley** is beaten to death in a cell while Deputy Tyson looks on approvingly. ["Miracle Man"]

SIMMONS, JENNIFER: A young woman with long, blond hair who has recently died. Her body is at the **Janelli-Heller Funeral Home** and **Donnie Pfaster** is caught cutting off some of her hair. ["Irresistible"]

SIMMONS, JOEL: Father of Teena Simmons. He dies of hypovolemia: 75 percent of his blood has been drained from his body. His lips have also been surgically removed. Mulder at first thinks this is linked to cattle mutilations. ["Eve"]

SIMMONS, SCOTT: A basketball player at Grover Cleveland Alexander High School in Comity. He's described by **Terri Roberts** as "babe-alicious in overtime." His girlfriend, **Brenda Jaycee Summerfield,** is killed purposely by **Margi Kleinjan** and Terri, and then Scott is killed accidentally by the same blonde duo. ["Syzygy"]

SIMMONS, TEENA: Eight-year-old girl orphaned when her father is killed; her mother died of ovarian cancer some years earlier. Psychic in some fashion, Teena plays in to Mulder's desire to link the murder with aliens, but actually committed the crime herself. In fact, she is a clone of **Dr. Sally Kendrick,** who abducts her. ["Eve"]

SIMPSON, HOMER J.: A yellow-skinned resident of Springfield, Illinois, who is mowing his lawn on the screen saver on the computer in the **Thinker**'s office when the black ops unit break in looking for the **MJ documents.** ["Anasazi"]

SIQUANNKE, ALASKA: Location of Eisenhower Field, where Mulder is taken for medical treatment after his encounter with the **Pilot.** ["Colony," "End Game"]

SISTER ABBY: The member of the **Kindred** who acts as their main spokesperson when Mulder and Scully visit them in Massachusetts. ["Genderbender"]

SISTRUNK, REV. CALVIN: A right-wing fundamentalist originally suspected in the arson fires at several abortion clinics in the eastern United States. He was arrested in Scranton, Pennsylvania, carrying a copy of the newspaper ad with **Dr. Landon Prince**'s picture, but was released when he provided an alibi for the other arsons out of state. ["Colony"]

SIOUX CITY PUBLIC LIBRARY: Mulder and Scully receive a note directing them here, where they receive misinformation from a teenage girl later revealed to be **Tessa Sears** about the disappearance of **Ruby Morris.** ["Conduit"]

65TH PARALLEL: The meteor or alien object that caused the USS *Argent*'s accelerated corrosion was located along this parallel, 8 degrees east longitude, in the North Atlantic. Other ships that vanished there are listed in the X-Files, including a British battleship in 1949 and an entire fleet of six Soviet mine sweepers in 1963. Mulder plots this location by overlapping his X-Files notes with the *Argent*'s course. ["Dod Kalm"]

SKEPTICAL: One of the phony Gray Aliens, who interrogate people they abduct. ["Jose Chung's *From Outer Space*"]

SKINNER, SHARON: Walter Skinner's soon-to-be ex-wife. She visits him one night and shortly thereafter someone runs her off the road; Walter is the prime suspect. Actually someone "borrowed" his car to frame him. She is seriously injured in the accident, but recovers. Her husband takes a leave of absence from the FBI to spend some time with her. ["Avatar"]

SKINNER, ASSISTANT DIRECTOR WALTER S.: Introduced in "Little Green Men." Mulder's immediate superior in the FBI, he is sympathetic to Mulder but walks a fine line between helping him and obeying those superiors who want Mulder out of the picture permanently. After Agent **Krycek** disappears in the wake of the **Duane Barry** incident, Skinner is angry enough to defy his superiors and reopen the X-Files. ["Ascension"] Notifies Mulder that Agent **Weiss** is dead and terminates Mulder's investigation of the abortion clinic murders. Also informs Mulder that there is a family emergency. ["Colony"] Helps Mulder organize a rescue team to free Scully from the **Pilot.** Skinner at first refuses to help Scully find Mulder, but later confronts **X** and extracts the information. ["End Game"] Advises Mulder to forget about the *F. Emasculata* outbreak, and hints that Mulder's enemies are about to speed up their efforts to discredit or destroy him. ["F. Emasculata"] Skinner finds his patience pushed to the limit when Mulder physically attacks him, not realizing that Mulder has been poisoned by the forces out to discredit him.

["Anasazi"] Skinner secretly assists Scully by taking the DAT tape into his own custody, while publicly joining in the FBI's censure of her. When he admits this to Scully, she has a hard time accepting his sincerity. ["The Blessing Way"] He refuses to give up the tape when Mulder reappears, as uncertain as Mulder about who to trust. Krycek and his accomplices (including **Luis Cardinal**) later take the tape from Skinner by force. ["Paper Clip"] Personally intervenes to free **Kazuo Takeo** after Mulder arrests the Japanese man at the scene of a murder in **Allentown, Pennsylvania.** Skinner states that Takeo is a high-ranking diplomat, and it is obvious that someone is pulling Skinner's strings on this one. ["Nisei"] Skinner contests the decision to drop the investigation into **Melissa Scully**'s murder, only to be shot by Cardinal while dining at his favorite coffee shop. ["Piper Maru"] He wakes up next to the nude, lifeless body of a woman he picked up in a bar the previous night, and becomes the chief suspect in her murder. He had been experiencing a recurring dream in which he's confronted by an old woman, but now he is starting to see her when

he is awake as well. She is the same apparition he saw once before, when he was the only survivor of an attack on his unit in Vietnam. Sharon Skinner, Walter's estranged wife, visits him one night and shortly thereafter someone runs her off the road; Walter is the prime suspect. Actually someone "borrowed" his car to frame him. He is cleared and takes a leave of absence to spend some time with his wife and try to put his marriage back together. ["Avatar"]

SKYLAND GRILL: The restaurant, closed for the summer, at Skyland Mountain, used as an interrogation room and holding cell after the apprehension of **Duane Barry. Alex Krycek** may have poisoned Barry there. ["Ascension"]

SKYLAND MOUNTAIN: A tourist attraction near Rixeyville, Virginia, off the Blue Ridge Parkway. Mulder tracks **Duane Barry** to this location, where, Barry claims, he experienced his first abduction by aliens. Mulder does not locate Scully there, but he does find her car and her gold crucifix necklace, and witnesses what may have been an alien craft departing. Agent **Alex Krycek** was last officially seen here. ["Ascension"]

SLASH KILLER: Serial killer in the early 1940s whose three victims were young women between twenty-five and thirty; he carved the word "sister" on their chests. His name was **Harry Cokely.** ["Aubrey"]

SLAUGHTER, DR. RUTH: Navy pathologist who performs the autopsy on **Duane Barry.** Her report does not address Mulder's suspicion that Barry may have been poisoned by **Alex Krycek,** part of a military cover-up. ["Ascension"]

SMALLPOX: An infectious disease that was the focus of an extensive inoculation campaign in the U.S. during the 1950s and 1960s. According to the **Well-Manicured Man,** this was a front to collect genetic materials from the general populace, to be used in alien–human hybridization experiments. ["Paper Clip"]

SMITH, JEREMIAH: A mysterious man (an alien clone?) living in Suitland, Virginia, who can heal people with his touch. He is able to slip away from the scene by changing his appearance in the blink of an eye. He is imprisoned and interrogated by the **Cigarette-Smoking Man,** until Smith tells him that he has cancer. Smith is one of several identical clones all named Jeremiah Smith. ["Talitha Cumi"]

SNORKEL DUDE: At **Heuvelmans Lake** he gets pulled underwater by a mysterious creature while **Chick** and **Stoner** look on dumbfounded. All that floats to the surface is Snorkle Dude's head. ["Quagmire"]

SOAMES, RAY: Third victim of the mysterious killer in **Bellefleur, Oregon.** Upon exhuming his grave, Mulder and Scully find a small, nonhuman corpse, which is later stolen from the coroner's office. [Pilot]

SOCIAL SECURITY OFFICES: Where **Jeremiah Smith** works. ["Talitha Cumi"]

SODIUM CHLORIDE: Ordinary salt. Blood tests conducted aboard the USS *Argent* reveal that Mulder, Scully, and **Trondheim** have impossibly concentrated levels of salt in their bloodstream, causing serious cellular damage. ["Dod Kalm"]

THE SON: One of the vampiric trio of killers known as the Trinity. He is a violent sociopath who firmly believes that he is one of the undead who will live forever so long as he drinks human blood. He has bloodshot eyes, unwashed hair, and cuts and scratches on his face and arms. (One wonders how he ever got hired as a security guard.) When he is exposed to sunlight in his jail cell, he shrivels up and dies horribly from severe epidermal burns. But later he turns up alive in the final confrontation with the Trinity. His real name is John, and **Kristen Kilar** originally met him in Chicago. When she left him, John and the other members of the Trinity began searching for her, committing murders along the way. ["3"]

SOONA, KENNETH: This may have been the real name of the hacker known as the **Thinker,** who stole the **MJ documents.** ["Anasazi"]

SOPHIE: A lowland gorilla at the **Fairfield Zoo** in Idaho. **Willa Ambrose** is fighting a lawsuit with the **Malawi** government, which wants the gorilla back. Ambrose rescued Sophie from a North American customs house ten years earlier and raised the ape herself, teaching her sign language. Sophie can "speak" six hundred words in sign language and understands a thousand. ["Fearful Symmetry"]

658 SOUTH HUDSON AVENUE #23: The Cleveland address of **Ellen Kaminski,** where **Virgil Incanto** meets his fate. ["2Shy"]

SPENCER, JIM: Venango County sheriff investigating the sudden spate of homicides in **Franklin, Pennsylvania.** ["Blood"]

SPERANZA, JOHN: A prisoner at **Eastpoint State Penitentiary.** He believes **"Neech" Manley** was reincarnated, and claims to have seen him after his death. ["The List"]

SPILLER, NANCY: A forensics instructor at the FBI academy, secretly nicknamed "The Iron Maiden" by her students. Organizes the team to investigate the murder of **Benjamin Drake,** which includes the ill-fated special agent **Jerry Lamana.** ["Ghost in the Machine"]

SPINNEY, DOUG: A "monkey wrencher," a radical environmentalist who drives spikes into trees and sabotages logging equipment. ["Darkness Falls"]

SPITZ, BOB: The high school principal in Comity. He shows up at the funeral of **Jay DeBoom** ranting and raving about how they all have to put a stop to these Satanic murders. ["Syzygy"]

SPITZ, DR. JOEL: Hypnotist who regresses **Michelle Bishop.** ["Born Again"]

SPONTANEOUS HUMAN COMBUSTION: A rare phenomenon in which a human body is quickly oxidized without any heat, leaving a pile of ashes without burning anything else in the vicinity. Mulder has a dozen or more case files on this phenomenon, but has never encountered an instance of it himself, although he considers it a possibility in the case of **Patrick Newirth.** ["Soft Light"]

SPREE KILLING: The type of murder committed in a public place in which the killer has a complete disregard for personal safety or anonymity. A number of such killings occur in a short period of time in **Franklin, Pennsylvania.** ["Blood"]

51 STANHOPE: FBI agent **Jack Willis**'s address in Washington, D.C. ["Lazarus"]

STANS, LT. COL. VICTOR: A veteran of recent wars with an exemplary record who tries repeatedly to kill himself in order to escape the psychic torment inflicted on him by **Sgt. "Rappo" Trimble.** He almost succeeds by scalding himself to death in an overheated hydrotherapy tub. Although horribly burned, he later manages to kill Trimble in his hospital bed. ["The Walk"]

STARBUCK: **William Scully**'s pet name for his daughter Dana, taken from a character in Herman Melville's *Moby Dick.*

STATE FORENSIC LABORATORY, HAMILTON COUNTY, OHIO: When **Owen Lee Jarvis** is murdered, the burn marks on his neck are in the form of a hand, and fingerprints are lifted from that mark here. The fingerprints are of **Simon Gates.** ["Revelations"]

STEFFEN, JOANNE: A friend and neighbor of **Ellen Kaminski**'s who advises her not to go out with her Internet pen pal after she receives an FBI alert on her computer screen. ["2Shy"]

STEFOFF: One of the phony names used by Mulder and Scully to get inside a complex where an E.B.E. (extraterrestrial biological entity) is apparently being held. ["E.B.E."]

STEVE: One of two prisoners at the **Cumberland State Correctional Facility** who use the confusion surrounding the death of **Bobby Torrence** to escape in a laundry cart. They hijack a family's motorhome to make their getaway, killing the father in the process. Steve dies of *F. Emasculata* infection at the home of his cellmate **Paul**'s girlfriend, **Elizabeth,** but not before infecting her as well. ["F. Emasculata"]

STEVENS, JERRY: One of the four teens who uses an occult book that summons a demon,

Azazel, which kills him and cuts his heart and eyes out. His body is displayed according to the rites of Azazel. ["Die Hand Die Verletzt"]

STEVESTON, MASSACHU-SETTS: Mulder traces the first of a series of murders here, where a labor organizer is found dead. The case leads him to investigate a religious group called the **Kindred** who live nearby. ["Genderbender"]

STIGMATA: Bleeding wounds that mimic those of Christ when his hands and feet were nailed to the cross, considered a sign from God bestowed upon the righteous. The **Rev. Finley** displays stigmata shortly before he is murdered, but in his case they were fake. According to Christian mythology, there are twelve true stigmatics in the world at any one time, representing the original twelve apostles. ["Revelations"]

STODIE, MRS.: The social worker who runs the Heritage Halfway House for the mentally retarded where **Roland Fuller** lives. ["Roland"]

STONER: He and his friend **Chick** witness the cockroach attack on **Dude.** ["War of the Coprophages"] He and Chick also turn up at **Heuvelmans Lake** in time to see the man called **Snorkel Dude** get pulled underwater by a myste-rious creature. All Stoner wanted to do was find the kind of toad that produces a hallucinogen that you can lick off its back. ["Quagmire"]

STRIKER'S COVE: In **Heuvelmans Lake.** ["Quagmire"]

STROMAN, DR. HENRY: A psychiatrist called down from the District of Columbia to observe the case of **Joseph Patnik** at the Frederick County Psychiatric Hospital in **Braddock Heights, Maryland.** He's actually part of the conspiracy that is causing people to act insanely. Mulder traces Stroman to a local house, where he finds him and the Cable Man dead — killed by **X.** It turns out that the name the man was using isn't his own, as the real Dr. Henry Stroman died in 1978 in Falls Church, Virginia. ["Wetwired"]

STRUGHOLD MINE: The location of ultra-secret government files dealing with alien experiments. The files for 1964 include one for Dana Katherine Scully, complete with a recent tissue sample. The file for **Samantha Mulder** was originally in Fox Mulder's name, but his name has been covered by a label bearing hers. Aliens inhabit some areas of this vast under-ground complex, but may have been evacuated by the UFO Mulder sighted there. The files may have been relocated since Mulder and Scully visited there. ["Paper Clip"]

SUCCUBUS: A female spirit that visits men in the night, sometimes in the form of an old woman. **Walter Skinner** has been experiencing a recurring dream in which he's confronted by an old woman. ["Avatar"]

SUITED MAN: One of **Alex Krycek**'s accomplices, seen lurking around **Melissa Scully**'s hospital room. ["Paper Clip"]

SUITLAND, VIRGINIA: Where **Jeremiah Smith** lives. ["Talitha Cumi"]

SULLIVAN, JUDGE: One of the judges at the sanity hearing for **Eugene Tooms.** ["Tooms"]

SUMMERFIELD, BRENDA JAYCEE: A student at Grover Cleveland Alexander High School in Comity and the girlfriend of **Scott Simmons.** At the birthday party for **Terri Roberts** and **Margi Kleinjan,** she is killed by flying glass from a broken mirror. ["Syzygy"]

SUMMERS, JIM: A nineteen-year-old student at Jackson University in North Carolina. He and his girlfriend **Liz Hawley** are kidnapped and tortured by **Lucas Jackson**

Henry. Summers is rescued by the FBI at the **Blue Devil Brewery.** ["Beyond the Sea"]

SUN, LINDA: A Memphis murder victim of the vampiric Trinity. The fact that her name is Sun (a soundalike for "son") helps to link her murder to the Trinity killers. ["3"]

SURNOW, RONALD: Aeronautical scientist who works at the **Mahan Propulsion Laboratory.** For four years he's been working on a project to crack Mach 15. He is killed when **Roland Fuller** locks him in a wind tunnel and turns on the jet engine inside it, the second scientist on the project to die within six months. ["Roland"]

SWAIM, JEFFREY: The real name of **Dr. Blockhead.** ["Humbug"]

SWASTIKA: An ancient symbol of great power used by many cultures, including China and India, before it became associated with the Nazis in this century. **Golda** and the **Calusari** use a reverse swastika with four dots between its arms as a protective talisman when dealing with the possession of **Charlie Holvey.** ["The Calusari"]

SWENSON, KAREN: A victim of the mysterious killings in **Bellefleur, Oregon,** which have targeted certain members

of the high school class of '89. [Pilot]

[T]

TABER, GARY: A forty-two-year-old real estate agent who is inside an elevator when he believes that its digital display is telling him there is no air. Finally the digital display says, "KILL 'EM ALL," so he kills four people who are in the elevator with him, and then a security guard kills him. Mulder finds a greenish-yellow residue under Taber's fingernail. ["Blood"]

TABERNACLE OF TERROR: **Hepcat Helm**'s description of the funhouse he operates. ["Humbug"]

TACOMA, WASHINGTON: Mulder takes a commercial flight there en route to **Deadhorse, Alaska.** ["End Game"]

TAKEO, KAZUO: Supposedly a high-ranking Japanese diplomat whom Mulder catches at the scene of a murder. He is assassinated in Washington, D.C., along Embassy Row by a red-haired man (see **Malcolm Gerlach**). Takeo's body is found floating in the C&O Canal (see also **"Rat-Tail Productions"**). ["Nisei"]

TALAPUS: A ship photographed by a satellite. The picture is found by Mulder in the

leather satchel taken from a Japanese man who attempts to flee a murder scene. The *Talapus* is a salvage ship from San Diego that had been searching for a sunken World War II Japanese submarine. The sub was supposedly carrying a cargo of gold bullion. The satellite photos track the ship through the Panama Canal to the naval shipyard at Newport News, Virginia, where the name has been obliterated and it has been hidden in plain sight at dockside. Mulder sneaks aboard, only to see cars with black-suited soldiers arrive outside; they begin to board the ship. Mulder has to leap off the ship before he has a chance to search it. But in a nearby warehouse he discovers what appears to be a crashed UFO, which is what he thinks the *Talapus* recovered. ["Nisei"]

TALBOT, DET.: He brings **Eugene Tooms** to the emergency room after finding him beaten up and unconscious out on the street somewhere. Tooms tells Talbot that Mulder was his assailant. ["Tooms"]

TANAKA, PETER: Systems analyst on the **Cascade Volcano Research Team.** He is infected with a subterranean organism, which manifests as a six-inch spike bursting from his throat, followed by sand spilling from the wound. ["Firewalker"]

TAPIA, DONALD "DEKE": The U.S. marshal in charge of the pursuit of the two prisoners who have escaped from the **Cumberland State Correctional Facility.** He grudgingly accepts Mulder's assistance in the case, but suspects him when mysterious decontamination-suited men carry away a key witness. ["F. Emasculata"]

TAROT DEALER: A male professional psychic murdered by the **Puppet.** In his rush to meet **Clyde Bruckman,** the killer neglects to remove this victim's eyes (although he does leave a salad fork in his left eye). ["Clyde Bruckman's Final Repose"]

TASHMOO FEDERAL CORRECTIONAL FACILITY: In Pennsylvania. **John Barnett** was a prisoner here, as is **Joe Crandall; Dr. Joe Ridley** served as a prison physician there until 1989, when he vanished to continue his research in Mexico and Belize. ["Young at Heart"]

TASSEOGRAPHY: The art of divining the future by reading tea leaves. Practiced by the **Doll Collector.** ["Clyde Bruckman's Final Repose"]

TAYLOR, CORP. BRYCE: The officer stationed at the U.S. Space Surveillance Center who alerts **Col. Henderson** to a UFO sighting. He orders **Karen Koretz** to file a report but is countermanded by Henderson. ["Fallen Angel"]

TAYLOR RECITAL HALL: In Washington, D.C., where a friend of Scully's has a cello recital. **John Barnett** finds out about it from Scully's answering machine and disguises himself as a piano tuner in order to kill Scully there, unaware that the FBI knows he is there. ["Young at Heart"]

TEAGUE, STEVEN: A "monkey wrencher," a radical environmentalist who drives spikes into trees and sabotages logging equipment. He is an early victim of the ancient wood mites that are released by loggers who illegally cut down an old-growth tree. ["Darkness Falls"]

TED'S BAIT & TACKLE: Mulder and Scully stop here upon arrival at **Heuvelmans Lake,** where Mulder suspects that **Big Blue,** the Southern Serpent, may be responsible for some human disappearances. The owner of this shop, **Ted Bertram,** is a huge Big Blue fan, although he's never actually seen it. ["Quagmire"]

TEE-TOTALLERS: A golf driving range with a too-cute name, where **Robert Modell** leads Mulder and Scully. When Agent **Collins** apprehends him there, Modell wills the agent to douse himself with gasoline and light it. ["Pusher"]

TEGRETOL: A prescription drug that prevents seizures caused by epilepsy. Scully finds a bottle in **Robert Modell**'s medicine cabinet. ["Pusher"]

TELLER, JOHN: An officer of the Johnston County, Oklahoma, sheriff's office. He insists that nothing unusual is happening in **Connerville.** Mulder's suggestion that **Darin Peter Oswald** has murdered people by creating lightning is the craziest thing Teller has ever heard in his life. This skepticism does nothing to protect him from being killed by Darin's wrath, although his death is ruled accidental. ["D.P.O."]

TEPES, VLAD: Also known as Vlad the Impaler of fifteenth-century Romania. This historical figure inspired Bram Stoker to create the character he called Dracula. The **Club Tepes** in Los Angeles is named after Vlad. Most of the people who frequent the after-sunset club are pale-skinned and wear black. ["3"]

TERLE, CATHERINE ANN: Her body is desecrated by **Donnie Pfaster** at the Montifiore Cemetery in Minneapolis. ["Irresistible"]

TERREL, LISA: A member of the Girl Scout troop that witnessed and photographed a UFO near Lake **Okobogee** in 1967. ["Conduit"]

THIBODEAUX, RUBY: She was raped by **Harry Cokely** in 1945 in Terrence, Nebraska (a one-hour drive from Aubrey, Missouri). He carved the word "sister" on her chest, but she survived and he was sent to prison. As a result of the rape, she bore a child she gave up for adoption. He grew up to become the father of **B. J. Morrow.** Thibodeaux now lives in Edmond, Nebraska. She has a scar on her face from where Cokely slashed her. ["Aubrey"]

THE THINKER: A new member of the **Lone Gunmen.** He's not seen because he's agoraphobic and will only communicate with people via computer. ["One Breath"] A radical anarchist and hacker, he has set up a random access code program to break in to Defense Department files, little suspecting he would ever succeed. Fearing for his life, he arranges to pass a tape of the **MJ documents** on to Mulder, and is later captured by a black ops unit. His real name may have been Kenneth Soona. ["Anasazi"]

THOMAS: An FBI agent, first name unknown, present when **Liz Hawley** identifies **Lucas Henry**'s photograph. ["Beyond the Sea"]

THOMAS, GERD: The peeping Tom. He formerly ran a day care center. He knew about **Dr. Larson**'s tests and believed that Larson had turned the children into monsters. Larson was also using Thomas to inoculate cattle with alien DNA. ["Red Museum"]

THOMPSON, MIKE: The detective in charge of investigating the Atlantic City murders of several homeless men. He resents the FBI's intrusion, but with good reason: he knows what's behind the murders, and is out to cover it up in order to protect local tourism. ["The Jersey Devil"]

TIERNAN, MERV: An orderly at the **Excelsis Dei Convalescent Home.** He is lured up to the roof and when he leans out a window is pushed and falls to his death. Traces of ibotenic acid, a powerful hallucinogen, are found in his body. ["Excelsis Dei"]

TILDESKAN: A port town in Norway; Mulder and Scully meet **Capt. Henry Trondheim** in a bar there and convince him to take them to find the USS **Argent.** ["Dod Kalm"]

TILESTON, VIRGINIA: Scully takes the four remaining **Gregors** to the federal stockade here for protection, but they are killed by the **Pilot** posing as a federal marshal. ["Colony"]

TILLMAN, LT. BRIAN: Of the Aubrey, Missouri, police. He is having an affair with Det. **B. J. Morrow.** ["Aubrey"]

TIPPY, MR.: The pet dog whose bones are found in an old medical bag buried in a back yard. There is nothing sinister about this, as it turns out (see **Dr. Richard Godfrey**). ["Syzygy"]

TOEWS, JACKSON: **Donnie Pfaster**'s supervisor at the **Janelli-Heller Funeral Home.** ["Irresistible"]

TOOMS, EUGENE VICTOR: Although he appears to be in his early thirties, he is some sort of genetic mutant who has lived a great deal longer; the first known record of him is in the 1903 census. He lives at 66 **Exeter Street,** and records show a Eugene Tooms has lived at that address since 1903. A serial killer who has committed five homicides in Baltimore every thirty years beginning in 1903, Tooms cuts out the liver from his victim and consumes it. He also takes a small trophy from each victim. He can elongate and contort his body into inhuman proportions in order to crawl through seemingly impossibly small spaces. Eleven-inch-long fingerprints were found at seven of the nineteen crime scenes. In modern times he has worked for the Baltimore County Animal Shelter. After making his fifth present-day kill, he builds a nest for his thirty-year hibernation underneath the escalator at the new mall built at 66 Exeter. Mulder finds the nest and Tooms attacks and tries to kill him, but Mulder escapes and turns on the escalator, which catches Tooms and pulls him into its gears, crushing him to death. ["Squeeze"; "Tooms"] While investigating the locked-room disappearance of businessman **Patrick Newirth,** Mulder checks a heat vent, obviously thinking of Tooms or someone like him as a possible suspect. ["Soft Light"]

TORONTO, CANADA: The ultimate destination of the escaped convict **Paul.** He never gets there. ["F. Emasculata"]

TORRENCE, BOBBY: A prisoner at the **Cumberland State Correctional Facility** in Virginia who receives a package originally addressed to **Dr. Robert Torrence.** It contains a pig's leg, wrapped in a Spanish-language newspaper, that is infected with larvae of the *F. Emasculata* insect. Bobby Torrence is infected as a result, and dies some time thereafter; his body is incinerated. ["F. Emasculata"]

TORRENCE, DR. ROBERT: A scientist involved in the **Biodiversity Project** who, while in the field, succumbs to the parasite that lives in the insect *Faciphaga Emasculata.* ["F. Emasculata"]

TOWNSEND, WISCONSIN: A small town whose twelve thousand inhabitants are evacuated when an alien spacecraft crashes into the woods nearby. The government explains this action with a fictional toxic train spill, even though there is no railway nearby. When Scully uses her clearance to get to the truth, she discovers that a Libyan jet with a nuclear warhead is the real cause for the crisis — but this is just another level of misinformation. The military is unable to capture the invisible alien pilot, whose own mission is centered on **Max Fenig.** ["Fallen Angel"]

TOWNSEND YMCA: The federal government commandeers this building to use as a relief center for evacuees during **Operation Falcon.** ["Fallen Angel"]

TOW-TRUCK DRIVER: He is looking for Gary Mosier when he stops to talk to **Carl Wade,** whose car has broken down by the side of the road. But Wade becomes irate and warns the driver to leave him alone. ["Oubliette"]

TRAIN CAR: The site of a mysterious experiment. In an operating theater inside it, a body is operated on by four Japanese doctors, who draw a green fluid out of it. In the middle of the procedure, black-garbed soldiers burst in and shoot the doctors. Then they put the gray alien corpse into a body bag (see also **Knoxville, Tennessee**). ["Nisei"]

TRAVEL TIME TRAVEL AGENCY: In Richmond, Virginia. Because he could not remember where he was abducted, **Duane Barry** stops here with his hostage, **Dr. Hakkie,** in order to get directions, only to take three employees hostage as well. ["Duane Barry"]

TREGO INDIAN RESERVATION: In Browning, Montana. They are having a property line fight with rancher **Jim**

Parker, plus a nagging problem with werewolves. ["Shapes"]

TREPKOS, DANIEL: Volcanologist who invented the robot named **Firewalker.** His intent was to find out how the Earth was created by exploring the fire where it all began. ["Firewalker"]

TRIMBLE, SGT. LEONARD "RAPPO": A quadruple amputee at the **Fort Evanston** military hospital, wounded by friendly fire during the Gulf War. A bitter young man who blames his fellow soldiers and their commanding officers for his condition, he uses his powers of astral projection to take vengeance on them. He is smothered to death by **Lt. Col. Victor Stans** while his spirit is out of his body. ["The Walk"]

TRINITY KILLERS: X-File number X256933VW. A trio of vampiric killers who call themselves the **Father,** the **Son,** and the **Unholy Spirit.** They have committed murders across the United States. ["3"]

TROITSKY, DR. KIP: Astronomer who works at the U.S. Naval Observatory in Washington, D.C. ["Little Green Men"]

TRONDHEIM, HENRY: American sea captain who relocated to Norway, presumably his ancestral home, to pursue a fishing career. He tells Mulder and Scully of the ancient Norse legends about a stone from the sky falling into the sea. Trapped on the USS *Argent* when his boat, the *Zeal,* is stolen, Trondheim becomes so desperate to survive that he is willing to sacrifice the lives of Scully and Mulder. He drowns when the *Argent*'s outer hull is breached and flooded with freezing sea water. ["Dod Kalm"]

TRUITT, JOHN: County coroner in **Bellefleur, Oregon**. [Pilot]

TRUMAN, MATT: FBI photo analysis specialist. ["Roland"]

TRUSTNO1: The secret password Mulder uses on the files in his personal computer at home. ["Little Green Men"]

THE TRUTH ABOUT ALIENS: Title of a manuscript written by **Roky Crikenson** in screenplay format. ["Jose Chung's *From Outer Space*"]

TSKANY, CHARLEY: The sheriff in Browning, Montana. He supports the Indians and their beliefs, since he is the Native American tribal law for the **Trego Indian reservation.** He calls Mulder "Running Fox" and "Sneaky Fox." ["Shapes"]

TURBELLARIA: A flatworm, or fluke. During an autopsy Scully removes a twelve-inch fluke from the body of a man found in a sewer in Newark, New Jersey. It had attached itself to the bile duct and was feeding off the liver. It attaches itself with a scolex, a suckerlike mouth with four hooking spikes. A carnivorous scavenger, some species depend on using more than one host to complete their life cycle. ["The Host"]

TWENTY-FIRST CENTURY RECYCLING PLANT: In Jerusalem, Ohio. **Simon Gates** takes **Kevin Kryder** here to kill him. ["Revelations"]

2400 MOTEL: In **Braddock Heights, Maryland.** Mulder and Scully stay here when investigating a series of inexplicable murders committed by ordinary people. ["Wetwired"]

TWO GREY HILLS, NEW MEXICO: Home of **Albert** and **Eric Hosteen,** on the Navajo reservation in New Mexico. Eric finds an alien corpse nearby after an earthquake reveals its hiding place. ["Anasazi"]

TWO MEDICINE RANCH: **Jim Parker**'s ranch in Browning, Montana. ["Shapes"]

2SHY: The on-line alias **Virgil Incanto** uses to lure lonely women into his murderous trap. ["2Shy"]

TYNES, MRS.: **Kevin Kryder**'s fifth-grade teacher at Ridgeway Elementary School in Loveland, Ohio. ["Revelations"]

TYSON: **Sheriff Daniels**'s deputy. He comes to arrest Daniels for being involved in the death of **Samuel Hartley.** ["Miracle Man"]

TYVEK: A company that manufactures decontamination suits. ["F. Emasculata"]

[U]

ULLRICH, DR. JIM: The Florida state medical examiner who conducts an autopsy on the prison guard **Fornier** and finds Fornier's lungs filled with the larvae of the green bottle fly. ["The List"]

UNHOLY SPIRIT: One of the vampiric trio of killers. She is impaled on a large nail on a garage wall. Her body is destroyed when the house and garage are burned down. ["3"]

UNIT 53: A firefighter unit that suffers casualties when it encounters the alien crash near **Townsend, Wisconsin.** ["Fallen Angel"]

UNIVERSITY OF MARYLAND: Where Scully earned her medical degree, prior to her FBI training at Quantico. ["The Jersey Devil"] She and Mulder discuss near-death experiences with Dr. Raymond Varnes of UM's biology department. ["Lazarus"]

UNIVERSITY OF WASHINGTON MEDICAL CENTER: The Seattle hospital where **Lucy Householder** is taken when she suffers a spontaneous nosebleed. Mulder arrives there at 10.31 the morning after the kidnapping of **Amy Jacobs.** ["Oubliette"]

UPSHAW, DON: An orderly at the **Excelsis Dei Convalescent Home.** He disappears and his body is found in the basement, buried in a mushroom patch. ["Excelsis Dei"]

URANUS UNLIMITED: An investment firm that based its marketing plans on astrological forecasts. Owned by **Claude Dukenfield,** a victim of the **Puppet.** ["Clyde Bruckman's Final Repose"]

U.S. COAST GUARD HEADQUARTERS: Mulder goes there to inquire about the salvage ship *Talapus.* The Coast Guard had gone out to search it but were called back by the DEA. ["Nisei"]

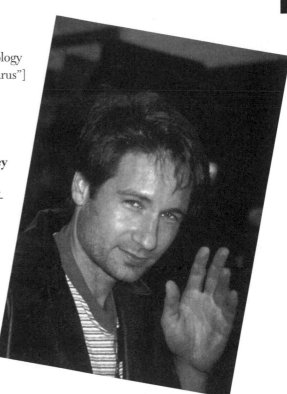

USHER, GEORGE: A Baltimore businessman found murdered in his locked office. **Tooms**'s third victim in 1993 and the one that leads Mulder and Scully to the trail of the flexible killer. ["Squeeze"]

U.S. MEDICAL RESEARCH INSTITUTE OF INFECTIOUS DISEASES: When the pathologists who conduct the original autopsy on FBI agent **Barrett Weiss** become ill, the body is brought here for further examination in a secure, sterile environment. ["End Game"]

U.S. SPACE SURVEILLANCE CENTER: A top-secret military installation at Cheyenne Mountain, Colorado. Its monitors detected a possible alien craft entering Earth's atmosphere off the Connecticut coast and tracked it to the area of **Townsend, Wisconsin.** ["Fallen Angel"]

[V]

VACATION VILLAGE MOTORLODGE: Motel in Germantown, Maryland, where Scully hides out when she realizes that CIA agent **Chapel** is a threat. Chapel, a.k.a. the **Pilot,** follows her there disguised as Mulder and takes her hostage. ["Colony"]

VALADEO, DANNY: He tracks down the son of **Ruby Thibodeaux** for Scully and reveals that the child's adopted name was Raymond Morrow. ["Aubrey"]

VALLEE, MAJ. ROBERT: Phony Gray Alien #1. He is planning to abduct and interrogate **Harold Lamb** and **Chrissy Giorgio** when all of them are abducted by real space aliens. Vallee is later found and he dies from an abdominal wound. ["Jose Chung's *From Outer Space*"]

VALLEY WOODS HIGH SCHOOL: Where fifteen-year-old **Amy Jacobs** is a student in Seattle. ["Oubliette"]

VANCE, LEONARD: The man **Samuel Hartley** raised from the dead in 1983. He then went to work for the **Rev. Hartley's Miracle Ministry.** He hates how deformed he is and so to get revenge he starts killing people who come to be healed by Samuel. After Samuel is beaten to death in his jail cell, he appears to Vance and confronts him about the crimes. He forgives Vance, who then commits suicide by taking poison. ["Miracle Man"]

VANKIN: Co-author, with Whelan, of *50 Greatest Conspiracies of All Time,* a book read by the **Thinker.** ["Anasazi"]

VARNES, DR. RAYMOND: Chairman of the biology department at the **University of Maryland;** Mulder and Scully consult him about near-death experiences. ["Lazarus"]

VENABLE PLAZA HOTEL: In Boston. A party is being held there in honor of Lord and Lady **Marsden** when fire breaks out on the fourteenth floor where their children are sleeping. Their caretaker **Bob (Cecil L'ively)** rescues them. ["Fire"]

VENANGO COUNTY: The location of **Franklin, Pennsylvania,** the site of several unexplained homicides. ["Blood"]

VIBUTI: A Sanskrit term meaning "holy ash," a mysterious substance that contains neither organic or inorganic material. According to **Chuck Burk,** it is produced when spirit beings are present, or when a person's psychic energy is transported from one place to another. It is found on several occasions at the **Holvey** home, always after an inexplicable occurrence or **Calusari** ritual. ["The Calusari"]

VIRTUA FIGHTER 2: The arcade game favored by **Darin Peter Oswald.** ["D.P.O."]

VITARIS, PAUL: Thirty-five-year-old black member of a witches' coven. He is killed by **Calgagni** while under the control of the demon. ["Die Hand Die Verletzt"]

VOSBERG: Member of the **Cascade Volcano Research Team** working at the California Institute of Technology in Pasadena. ["Firewalker"]

VOYAGER: The two spacecraft launched August 20 and September 5, 1977. The satellites contained messages which it was hoped could be interpreted by any extraterrestrial intelligence that might encounter them. These messages included recordings, the first of which is the *Brandenburg Concerto No. 2 in F* by Bach. ["Little Green Men"]

[W]

WADE, CARL: The assistant to the school photographer for Valley Woods High in Seattle. He is fired the day after the photo shoot. When he sees fifteen-year-old **Amy Jacobs** he is immediately attracted to her, in an unhealthy way. He has a darkroom in the small, windowless basement of his cabin near Easton, Washington. He creates a photo montage of himself and Amy, then he goes out and kidnaps the girl. He previously kidnapped an eight-year-old girl named **Lucy Householder** and kept her prisoner in his basement dungeon, or oubliette, for five years, until she escaped. He was never captured for that crime, but did later spend fifteen years in a mental institution due to a bipolar condition. He was released not long before he kidnapped Amy. By the time the FBI tracks him to his home, he has already fled with Amy. He is hunted down and shot to death by Mulder. ["Oubliette"]

WALDHEIM, KURT: UN Secretary General whose recorded voice was carried aboard the Voyager spacecraft. ["Little Green Men"]

WALK-INS: People who believe that other spirits can temporarily take possession of their bodies. ["Red Museum"]

WALLACE, CAROL: An ailing woman who dies minutes after **Samuel Hartley** tries to heal her with a laying on of hands. ["Miracle Man"]

WALLACE, FATHER THOMAS: A priest and a murder victim of the vampiric **Trinity.** The fact that he is a "father" helps to link him as a victim of the Trinity murders. ["3"]

WALLENBERG, STEVE: The FBI agent killed during the apprehension of **John Barnett** in 1989, he left behind a wife and two children. Mulder blamed himself for his death. ["Young at Heart"]

WALSH, CLAYTON: The fourth **Dudley, Arkansas,** resident to contract **Creutzfeldt-Jakob disease,** after **George Kearns, Paula Gray,** and an unknown truck driver. ["Our Town"]

WALTOS, DET.: He is investigating the murder of a nude woman found in **Walter Skinner**'s Washington, D.C., hotel room. He considers Skinner a suspect. ["Avatar"]

W.A.O.: The Wild Again Organization, an animal rights group opposed to keeping animals locked up in zoos. ["Fearful Symmetry"]

WASHINGTON COUNTY REGIONAL AIRPORT: A small-craft airport near **Lula Philips**'s hideout. Background noise of an airplane on her ransom phone call helps the FBI locate her general vicinity. ["Lazarus"]

WASHINGTON INSTITUTE OF TECHNOLOGY: Where the **Mahan Propulsion Laboratory** is located. ["Roland"]

WATERGATE HOTEL & OFFICE COMPLEX: Scully and Mulder meet secretly in the underground parking lot of this famous Washington, D.C., building. ["Little Green Men"]

WATERS, BERNADETTE: A woman listed in Mulder's files, who bore a small diamond-shaped scar behind her left ear, as did **Max Fenig.** Mulder believes her claim to be an abductee. ["Fallen Angel"]

WATKINS, DONNA: While jogging with her husband, Ted, this Greenwich, Connecticut, resident discovers **Teena Simmons** and the corpse of her father **Joel Simmons.** ["Eve"]

WATKINS, GINA: A clerk at the county hospital in **Townsend, Wisconsin.** She is unable to find any record that deputy sheriff **Jason Wright** had ever been a patient there. ["Fallen Angel"]

WATKINS, RICHARD: Part of the first X-file case in 1946. In the Pacific Northwest and in Browning, Montana, people were killed and ripped apart. When the killer was trapped and shot in Glacier National Park, the body of Watkins was found instead of the body of the animal they had cornered. It was believed that this wave of crimes had ended, but the mysterious murders erupted again in 1959, '64, '78, and '94. ["Shapes"]

WATKINS, TED: With his wife, Donna, finds the body of his neighbor **Joel Simmons,** sitting in a swing, drained of blood, with its lips cut off. ["Eve"]

WAYNESBURG, PENNSYLVANIA: Location of First Church of the Redemption, where the **Rev. Patrick Finley** is murdered by the Millennium Man (**Simon Gates**). ["Revelations"]

WEBSTER: CIA agent teamed up with CIA agent **Saunders** to investigate **HTG Industrial Technologies.** ["Shadows"]

WEISS, BARRETT: FBI special agent stationed in Syracuse, New York, who checks out **Dr. Aaron Baker** for Mulder but

is killed by the **Pilot,** his body locked in the trunk of his car. The Pilot impersonates him when Mulder and Scully arrive on the scene. No cause of death could be found; when Scully reads Weiss's autopsy report, however, she learns that his blood was unnaturally clotted. ["Colony"] Further examinations at the **U.S. Medical Research Institute of Infectious Diseases** reveal an alien virus in his blood. ["End Game"]

WELL-MANICURED MAN: An older, high-ranking member of the **Elders,** who is suspicious of the **Cigarette-Smoking Man**'s claims that the **MJ** files DAT has been recovered. Calm, serene, and utterly Machiavellian, he makes CSM look like a street punk. He approaches Scully at **William Mulder**'s funeral, admits his involvement in events surrounding the DAT, and advises her that her life is in danger. His motives are not benevolent: he merely feels that her death would draw attention to him and his associates. He and a younger **Deep Throat,** CSM, and William Mulder can be seen in an old picture, circa 1973, found by Fox Mulder. ["The Blessing Way"] He calls CSM on the carpet after **Krycek** kills **Melissa Scully.**

Fox Mulder meets him for the first time at the late **Victor Klemper**'s greenhouse, where he offers hints about William Mulder's activities as a member of the intelligence community and suggests that Nazi scientists were involved in creating human–alien hybrids using physical materials recovered from the Roswell UFO crash in 1947. ["Paper Clip"] He meets with Mulder in Central Park after Mulder finds his secret phone number, and confirms that a UFO was downed by American pilots during the final days of World War II. ["Apocrypha"]

WELLS, MS.: An employee of the Fairfield County Social Services Hostel in Greenwich, Connecticut who takes care of **Teena Simmons** after her father's death. ["Eve"]

WERBER, DR. HEITZ: At the Oregon State Psychiatric Hospital, he examines **Billy Miles,** who confesses to having been abducted and controlled by a mysterious light. [Pilot] He conducted hypnotic regression therapy sessions with Mulder in 1989, heard by Scully on tapes in the X-File on the disappearance of **Samantha Mulder.** ["Conduit"]

WERNER: **Eugene Tooms**'s fourth victim in 1993, eviscerated and killed (in that order) in his suburban Baltimore home. ["Squeeze"]

WEST TISBURY, MASSACHU-SETTS: A town on Martha's Vineyard, where Mulder's father lives. ["Colony"]

WESTIN: FBI agent who takes part in the raid on **Lula Philips**'s hideout, disguised as a phone worker for cover. ["Lazarus"]

WHARTON, COL. JACOB: The Marine in command at the **Folkstone INS Processing Center,** in charge of supervising 12,000 refugees. He's killed by **Pierce Bauvais** but awakens in his coffin — buried alive. ["Fresh Bones"]

WHELAN: Co-author, with Vankin, of *50 Greatest Conspiracies of All Time,* a book read by the **Thinker.** ["Anasazi"]

WHITE, DET. ANGELA: She is investigating the strange deaths in Comity and tells Mulder and Scully what she knows. It is believed that the deaths are connected to a Satanic cult, but there is no hard evidence of this. ["Syzygy"]

WHITE, KATE: One of the four teens who use an occult book that summons a demon. ["Die Hand Die Verletzt"]

WHITE "SAMANTHA": An alien clone in a white lab coat

whom Mulder meets at the **Women's Health Services Center** in Rockville, Maryland. This clone introduces Mulder to the **original "Samantha"** alien from whom she and the others were cloned; they trick Mulder into helping them in the hope he would protect the original. White "Samantha" is killed by the **Pilot,** along with the rest of the "Samantha" clones. ["End Game"]

WHITING INSTITUTE: A highly secure medical facility that houses **Eve Six. Teena Simmons** and **Cindy Reardon** are taken there after Mulder apprehends them for the murders of their "fathers" and **Dr. Sally Kendrick.** ["Eve"]

WICCA: The religion of modern witches. They are occult, but they do not practice black magic. ["Die Hand Die Verletzt"]

WICHITA, KANSAS: Scully traces the package that infected **Bobby Torrence** to the address of **Pinck Pharmaceuticals** in this city. ["F. Emasculata"]

WILCZEK, BRAD: Visionary founder of the Eurisko Corporation. A computer genius in the Steve Wozniak rather than the Bill Gates vein. Forced out by CEO **Benjamin**

Drake (with a hefty payoff of about $400 million). Idealistic, precocious, and manipulative, he was opposed to any use of Eurisko's software in military or governmental applications. He falsely confesses to murdering Drake and FBI agent **Jerry Lamana** in order to protect the artificial intelligence of the COS (central operating system) in the **Eurisko Building.** Later helps Mulder destroy the system, but is "disappeared" by the government. According to **Deep Throat,** Wilczek is being "persuaded" to yield his AI knowledge to the military. ["Ghost in the Machine"]

WILKINS: An intensive care nurse for Scully at the Northeast Georgetown Medical Center. ["One Breath"]

WILLIG, HENRY: One of the experimental subjects of **Dr. Saul Grissom**'s Vietnam-era experiments in sleep deprivation. He was in the Marines in 1970 and was assigned to Special Force and Recon Squad J-7. Of the thirteen original squad members, he is one of only two survivors. He is killed by one of **Augustus Cole**'s unusual hallucinations, but Willig welcomes death after twenty-four years without sleep. ["Sleepless"]

WILLIS, JACK: An older, diabetic FBI agent, born in 1955, who was one of Scully's instructors at the FBI academy and shares her birthday, February 23. Willis and Scully dated for about a year, but she broke it off because he was too intense about his work. Assigned to a series of bank robberies by the violent-crimes section, Willis becomes almost obsessed with his subjects and he is furious at the relationship between **Warren Dupre** and **Lula Philips,** even expressing jealousy at their fatalistically romantic relationship. After Dupre shoots him during the **Maryland Marine Bank** robbery, Willis is technically dead for thirteen minutes before being revived. After this he begins to display erratic behavior that includes chopping three fingers off Dupre's corpse, becoming left-handed, kidnapping Scully, declaring his love for Lula Philips, and forgetting such details as his own birthday and the fact that he is diabetic. One explanation is that the shock of his experience, combined with his obsession with Dupre and Philips, caused him to believe Dupre's spirit is now living in his body. (Mulder is inclined to believe that this is not a delusion.) Willis dies of apparent hyperglycemia (too much blood sugar) after killing Philips. ["Lazarus"]

WILMER, LT. TERRY: The sole survivor of a U.S. Navy submarine (presumably the USS *Allegiance*) stranded in Arctic ice. He claims to have hidden from the **Pilot** by concealing himself under the body of a dead chief petty officer. After Mulder handcuffs Wilmer to himself, Wilmer reveals that he is really the **Pilot** in disguise. ["End Game"]

WILMORE, CRAIG: A student at Grover Cleveland Alexander High School in Comity. He's mentioned in passing by **Terri Roberts.** ["Syzygy"]

WINDLESHAM, ENGLAND: Site of Sir Arthur Conan Doyle's tomb. Mulder had a tryst with **Phoebe Green** there, apparently on the tomb itself, when they were students at Oxford. ["Fire"]

WINN, MS.: **Robert Dorland**'s assistant. When she gives **Lauren Kyte** a hard time, a mysterious force causes her hot coffee to spill into her lap. ["Shadows"]

WINSTON: The guard at the **Cumberland State Correctional Facility** in Virginia who delivers **Bobby Torrence**'s last package to him. ["F. Emasculata"]

WINSTON, BONNIE: A member of the Girl Scout troop that witnessed and photographed a UFO near **Lake Okobogee** in 1967. ["Conduit"]

WINTER, LARRY: The supervisor for Venango County, Pennsylvania. ["Blood"]

WINTERS, DR.: The veterinarian who performs the autopsy on **Mona Wustner**'s dog. He determines that the dog has died of poisoning by eating a rat that had eaten strychnine. ["Teso dos Bichos"]

WITCH HUNT: A HISTORY OF THE OCCULT IN AMERICA: The book checked out by **Dave Duran.** Reading from it at a Black Mass altar in Milford Haven, New Hampshire, summons a demon. ["Die Hand Die Verletzt"]

WITCH'S PEGS: Three-pronged stakes driven into the ground to ward off evil spirits in the Ozarks, dismissed by **Sheriff Tom Arens** as a leftover superstition. ["Our Town"]

WITHERS, JACK: Deputy sheriff of Sioux City, Iowa, who favors a mundane explanation for **Ruby Morris**'s disappearance, and considers her mother to be a flake. Investigates the murder of **Greg Randall.** ["Conduit"]

WOLF INDUSTRIES: A company that supplies the CIA with surveillance equipment. **Max Fenig** owns a Wolf's Ear 2000, a sort of souped-up police scanner that can pick up over a hundred channels per second. ["Fallen Angel"]

WOMEN'S CARE FAMILY SERVICES AND CLINIC: The abortion clinic where **Dr. Landon Prince** was killed. The authorities initially suspected right-wing religious extremists in the case, not realizing it was the work of an extraterrestrial assassin. ["Colony"]

WOMEN'S HEALTH SERVICES CENTER: The abortion clinic in Rockville, Maryland, where Mulder encounters more "Samantha" clones and discovers that he has been used. Later burned to the ground by the **Pilot.** ["End Game"]

WONG, CHERYL: A woman listed in Mulder's files, who bore a small diamond-shaped scar behind her left ear, as did **Max Fenig.** Mulder believes her claim to be an abductee. ["Fallen Angel"]

WOOSLEY, SCOTT: A Boy Scout leader who disappeared at **Heuvelmans Lake** in Georgia. All that's ever found of him is his lower torso, which still has his wallet in the back

pocket. Did **Big Blue** chow down on a man whose motto was "Be prepared?" ["Quagmire"]

WORKMAN, JENNIFER: **Lauren Mackalvey**'s roommate. She reveals that Lauren met her final date over the Internet, and gives Mulder copies of **2Shy**'s letters. Quotations from rare sixteenth-century Italian poetry in the letters help locate the killer, who must be a scholar with access to exclusive academic libraries. ["2Shy"]

WORMHOLES: Theoretical portals where matter's interaction with time is radically sped up or slowed down. Mulder believes they were used in the **Philadelphia Experiment** in 1944, and erroneously thinks they might explain the disappearance of the USS **Argent** and the accelerated aging of **Lt. Richard Harper.** ["Dod Kalm"]

"WOW" SIGNAL: In August 1977, astronomer **Jerry Ehman** found a transmission of apparent extraterrestrial origin on a printout and called it a "wow" signal. This was a signal thirty times stronger than galactic background noise. It came through on a frequency not used by terrestrial satellites. ["Little Green Men"]

WRIGHT, JASON: A young sheriff's deputy in **Townsend, Wisconsin,** who is severely burned by a bright light while investigating what appeared to be a forest fire near the town. He dies of his injuries. ["Fallen Angel"]

WRIGHT, BELINDA: The widow of Jason Wright. The government refuses to release his body to her and threatens to cut off his pension if she protests. She has a three-year-old son. ["Fallen Angel"]

WUSTNER, MONA: A graduate student working with Ecuadoran artifacts at the Boston Museum of Natural History whose death is part of a series of unsolved murders revolving around the **Amaru** Urn. ["Teso dos Bichos"]

WYATT, MRS.: She is working at the blood drive table at a Franklin, Pennsylvania, department store. ["Blood"]

WYSNECKI, MARGARET: A sixty-six-year-old widow, retired from the **Laramie Tobacco** company, who disappears in Richmond, Virginia, presumably a victim of **Chester Ray Banton**'s shadow. ["Soft Light"]

[X]

X, MR.: A middle-aged black man, he first appears in "The

Host" as Mulder's new inside contact at the FBI, his new **Deep Throat.** He is a shadowy character who is working for the **Cigarette-Smoking Man** but is trying to undermine his activities. ["Wetwired"] Warns Mulder that he could not find out what he needed to know about the **Duane Barry** case. Mulder suspects that X knows Scully's whereabouts. ["Ascension"] Reveals that a U.S. Navy attack fleet is en route to destroy the **Pilot** and his spacecraft. Angered when Scully signals him at Mulder's apartment, he plays dumb and refuses to tell Scully where Mulder was going but reluctantly gives Assistant Director **Skinner** this information after a less than friendly discussion. ["End Game"] Denies all knowledge of **Chester Ray Banton** when Mulder turns to him for help, only to orchestrate an attempted abduction of Banton that leaves two of X's subordinates reduced to burn marks on the floor of Banton's hospital room. X later kills **Dr. Christopher Davey** at the **Polarity Magnetics** lab and delivers Banton to an unknown government agency for study. ["Soft Light"] X apparently did not respond to Mulder's signal — a taped X in his window lit

from within — during the events surrounding the theft of the **MJ documents.** ["Anasazi"]

[Y]

YAJE: Pronounced "YAH-hay." A vine used to prepare hallucinogenic potions by shamans in Ecuador. **Dr. Alonso Bilac** was taking large doses during a series of murders at the Boston Museum of Natural History, perhaps to open himself up to possession by a jaguar spirit. ["Teso dos Bichos"]

YALOFF PSYCHIATRIC HOSPITAL: In Piedmont, Virginia. Mulder and Scully take **Chester Ray Banton** there for safekeeping. Mulder is unwise enough to mention Banton's location to **X,** resulting in an ill-fated abduction attempt. ["Soft Light"]

YAMAGUCHI, DR.: The pathologist who does the autopsy on **Charlie Morris.** He notes that Morris was drowned in sea water. ["Born Again"]

YANI: The Greek janitor in **George Usher**'s office building. He doesn't clean Usher's office the night Usher is killed. ["Squeeze"]

YAPPI, THE STUPENDOUS: A publicity-hungry psychic whose abilities are dubious. He accuses Mulder of being a skeptic

who is sending out "negative energy" and insists that Mulder leave the scene of the **Doll Collector**'s murder. His predictions are very vague (the killer "is aged seventeen to thirty-four and may or may not have a beard"), but he does seem able to read a rude thought in Mulder's mind. Yappi's predictions are published in the **Midnight Inquisitor.** Those convinced of his abilities can make use of them, for a price, by calling 1-900-555-YAPP. ["Clyde Bruckman's Final Repose"] He is the narrator on part of the "alien autopsy" video. ["Jose Chung's *From Outer Space*"]

YUNG, DAVID: An acquaintance of **Kristen Kilar**'s. Mulder follows him but is knocked out and is thus unable to prevent him from being attacked and killed by the **Father** and the **Unholy Spirit.**

[Z]

ZAMA, DR. SHIRO: The name adopted by **Dr. Ishimaru.** He is traveling incognito on a train boarded by Mulder and is later killed in a restroom by the red-haired man (**Malcolm Gerlach).** Ishimaru was involved in experimenting on humans, and he is the one who put the monitoring chip implant in Scully's neck. Other people, who believed wrongly that they were abducted by aliens, have also been taken to train cars where Ishimaru conducted his experiments on them. ["731"]

ZEAL: **Henry Trondheim**'s boat, a fifty-ton trawler with double hulls. It is stolen by members of the pirate whaler **Olafssen**'s crew, leaving Mulder, Scully, Trondheim, and **Olafssen** stranded on the USS *Argent*. ["Dod Kalm"]

ZELMA, MADAME: A fake gypsy psychic and palm reader. The **Puppet** consults her, hoping to find out the reasons for his actions. Then he kills her, gouging her eyes out with the shards of her crystal ball. **Clyde Bruckman** finds her body in the Dumpster outside his apartment building. ["Clyde Bruckman's Final Repose"]

ZENZOLA, DR. JO: At the Middlesex County Hospital in Sayreville, New Jersey, she examines a sewer worker who was attacked and briefly pulled underwater by some unseen creature that left a vicious wound on his back. The worker claims he has a bad taste in his mouth. Later the man is in

his shower when a large fluke exits his body through his mouth. ["The Host"]

ZEUS FABER: A U.S. Navy submarine, active at the end of World War II. Mulder discovers its name written on a chart on the *Piper Maru*, prompting Scully to visit a former crewman of the *Zeus*. At the end of the war, the *Zeus* was assigned to locate a downed bomber carrying a third A-bomb headed for Japan. This was a cover story; the real mission was to protect a downed UFO. ["Piper Maru"] An alien entity from the UFO possessed the captain, **Kyle Sanford**, but abandoned him when the sub was attacked by a Japanese destroyer. It survived beneath the sea for fifty years before using **Alex Krycek** to return to its craft, now hidden by the U.S. government. ["Apocrypha"]

ZEUS STORAGE: Located at 1616 Pandora Street in Maryland. It contains a secret lab that has five bodies suspended in huge liquid-filled cylinders. Experiments with extraterrestrial viruses are being conducted on humans. ["The Erlenmeyer Flask"]

ZINNZSER, STEVEN: A Mutual UFO Network (MUFON) member living in the **Allentown** area. He was murdered by **Kazuo Takeo** because Zinnzser intercepted a satellite transmission of an alien autopsy and had been selling the videotape of it through magazine ads. He operated under the name **Rat-Tail Productions.** ["Nisei"]

ZIRINKA: An astrologer in the city of **Comity.** The sign on her business reads ASTROLOGY, NUMEROLOGY, RUNES, READINGS. She reveals that the Earth is entering a planetary alignment with Mars, Mercury, and Uranus and states that she believes this is behind the strange things going on in Comity. Mars, Mercury, and Uranus come into conjunction once every eighty-four years, but this time Uranus is in the House of Aquarius. ["Syzygy"]

ZOE: A teenage girl who sneaks onto **Ellens Air Force Base** to watch mysterious lights in the sky; she and her boyfriend Emil help Mulder infiltrate the base. ["Deep Throat"]

the X-Files

Series One

Episode 1.1
"The X-Files" (pilot)
Original UK airdates:
Sky One: January 19, 1994
BBC 2: September 19, 1994

Episode 1.2
"Deep Throat"
Original UK airdates:
Sky One: January 26, 1994
BBC 2: September 26, 1994

Episode 1.3
"Squeeze"
Original UK airdates:
Sky One: February 2, 1994
BBC 2: October 3, 1994

Episode 1.4
"Conduit"
Original UK airdates:
Sky One: February 9, 1994
BBC 2: October 10, 1994

Episode 1.5
"The Jersey Devil"
Original UK airdates:
Sky One: February 16, 1994
BBC 2: October 17, 1994

Episode 1.6
"Shadows"
Original UK airdates:
Sky One: February 23, 1994
BBC 2: October 24, 1994

Episode 1.7
"Ghost in the Machine"
Original UK airdates:
Sky One: March 2, 1994
BBC 2: November 3, 1994

Episode 1.8
"Ice"
Original UK airdates:
Sky One: March 9, 1994
BBC 2: November 10, 1994

Episode 1.9
"Space"
Original UK airdates:
Sky One: March 16, 1994
BBC 2: November 17, 1994

Episode 1.10
"Fallen Angel"
Original UK airdates:
Sky One: March 23, 1994
BBC 2: November 24, 1994

Episode 1.11
"Eve"
Original UK airdates:
Sky One: April 4, 1994
BBC 2: December 1, 1994

Episode 1.12
"Fire"
Original UK airdates:
Sky One: April 18, 1994
BBC 2: December 15, 1994

Episode 1.13
"Beyond the Sea"
Original UK airdates:
Sky One: April 25, 1994
BBC 2: December 17, 1994

Episode 1.14
"Genderbender"
Original UK airdates:
Sky One: May 2, 1994
BBC 2: December 22, 1994

Episode 1.15
"Lazarus"
Original UK airdates:
Sky One: May 9, 1994
BBC 2: January 5, 1995

Episode 1.16
"Young at Heart"
Original UK airdates:
Sky One: May 16, 1994
BBC 2: January 12, 1995

Episode 1.17
"E.B.E."
Original UK airdates:
Sky One: May 23, 1994
BBC 2: January 19, 1995

Episode 1.18
"Miracle Man"
Original UK airdates:
Sky One: May 30, 1994
BBC 2: January 26, 1995

Episode 1.19
"Shapes"
Original UK airdates:
Sky One: June 6, 1994
BBC 2: February 2, 1995

Episode 1.20
"Darkness Falls"
Original UK airdates:
Sky One: June 13, 1994
BBC 2: February 9, 1995

Episode 1.21
"Tooms"
Original UK airdates:
Sky One: June 20, 1994
BBC 2: February 16, 1995

Episode 1.22
"Born Again"
Original UK airdates:
Sky One: June 27, 1994
BBC 2: February 23, 1995

Episode 1.23
"Roland"
Original UK airdates:
Sky One: July 4, 1994
BBC 2: March 2, 1995

Episode 1.24
"The Erlenmeyer Flask"
Original UK airdates:
Sky One: July 11, 1994
BBC 2: March 16, 1995

Series Two

Episode 2.1
"Little Green Men"
Original UK airdates:
Sky One: February 21, 1995
BBC 2: August 28, 1995

Episode 2.2
"The Host"
Original UK airdates:
Sky One: February 28, 1995
BBC 2: September 4, 1995

Episode 2.3
"Blood"
Original UK airdates:
Sky One: March 7, 1995
BBC 2: September 11, 1995

Episode 2.4
"Sleepless"
Original UK airdates:
Sky One: March 14, 1995
BBC 2: September 18, 1995

Episode 2.5
"Duane Barry"
Original UK airdates:
Sky One: March 21, 1995
BBC 2: September 25, 1995

Episode 2.6
"Ascension"
Original UK airdates:
Sky One: March 28, 1995
BBC 2: October 2, 1995

Episode 2.7
"3"
Original UK airdates:
Sky One: April 4, 1995
BBC 2: October 9, 1995

Episode 2.8
"One Breath"
Original UK airdates:
Sky One: April 11, 1995
BBC 2: October 16, 1995

Episode 2.9
"Firewalker"
Original UK airdates:
Sky One: April 18, 1995
BBC 2: October 23, 1995

Episode 2.10
"Red Museum"
Original UK airdates:
Sky One: April 25, 1995
BBC 2: October 30, 1995

Episode 2.11
"Excelsis Dei"
Original UK airdates:
Sky One: May 2, 1995
BBC 2: November 6, 1995

Episode 2.12
"Aubrey"
Original UK airdates:
Sky One: May 9, 1995
BBC 2: November 13, 1995

Episode 2.13
"Irresistible"
Original UK airdates:
Sky One: May 16, 1995
BBC 2: November 20, 1995

Episode 2.14
"Die Hand Die Verletzt"
(The Hand That Wounds)
Original UK airdates:
Sky One: May 23, 1995
BBC 2: November 27, 1995

Episode 2.15
"Fresh Bones"
Original UK airdates:
Sky One: May 30, 1995
BBC 2: December 4, 1995

Episode 2.16
"Colony"
Original UK airdates:
Sky One: June 6, 1995
BBC 2: December 11, 1995

Episode 2.17
"End Game"
Original UK airdates:
Sky One: June 13, 1995
BBC 2: December 18, 1995

Episode 2.18
"Fearful Symmetry"
Original UK airdates:
Sky One: June 20, 1995
BBC 1: January 9, 1996

Episode 2.19
"Dod Kalm" (Dead Calm)
Original UK airdates:
Sky One: June 27, 1995
BBC 1: January 16, 1996

Episode 2.20
"Humbug"
Original UK airdates:
Sky One: July 4, 1995
BBC 1: January 23, 1996

Episode 2.21
"The Calusari"
Original UK airdates:
Sky One: July 11, 1995
BBC 1: January 30, 1996

Episode 2.22
"F. Emasculata"
Original UK airdates:
Sky One: July 18, 1995
BBC 1: February 6, 1996

Episode 2.23
"Soft Light"
Original UK airdates:
Sky One: July 25, 1995
BBC 1: February 13, 1996

Episode 2.24
"Our Town"
Original UK airdates:
Sky One: August 2, 1995
BBC 1: February 20, 1996

Episode 2.25
"Anasazi"
Original UK airdates:
Sky One: August 8, 1995
BBC 1: February 27, 1996

Series Three

Episode 3.1
"The Blessing Way"
Original UK airdates:
Sky One: March 5, 1996
BBC 1: September 12, 1996

Episode 3.2
"Paper Clip"
Original UK airdates:
Sky One: March 12, 1996
BBC 1: September 19, 1996

Episode 3.3
"D.P.O."
Original UK airdates:
Sky One: March 19, 1996
BBC 1: September 26, 1996

Episode 3.4
"Clyde Bruckman's Final
Repose"
Original UK airdates:
Sky One: March 26, 1996
BBC 1: October 3, 1996

Episode 3.5
"The List"
Original UK airdates:
Sky One: April 2, 1996
BBC 1: October 10, 1996

Episode 3.6
"2Shy"
Original UK airdates:
Sky One: April 9, 1996
BBC 1: October 17, 1996

Episode 3.7
"The Walk"
Original UK airdates:
Sky One: April 16, 1996
BBC 1: October 24, 1996

Episode 3.8
"Oubliette"
Original UK airdates:
Sky One: April 23, 1996
BBC 1: October 31, 1996

Episode 3.9
"Nisei"
Original UK airdates:
Sky One: April 30, 1996
BBC 1: November 7, 1996

Episode 3.10
"731"
Original UK airdates:
Sky One: May 7, 1996
BBC 1: November 14, 1996

Episode 3.11
"Revelations"
Original UK airdates:
Sky One: May 14, 1996
BBC 1: November 21, 1996

Episode 3.12
"War of the Coprophages"
Original UK airdates:
Sky One: May 21, 1996
BBC 1: November 28, 1996

Episode 3.13
"Syzygy"
Original UK airdates:
Sky One: May 28, 1996
BBC 1: December 5, 1996

Episode 3.14
"Grotesque"
Original UK airdates:
Sky One: June 4, 1996
BBC 1: December 12, 1996

Episode 3.15
"Piper Maru"
Original UK airdates:
Sky One: June 11, 1996
BBC 1: December 19, 1996

Episode 3.16
"Apocrypha"
Original UK airdates:
Sky One: June 18, 1996
BBC 1: to be scheduled

Episode 3.17
"Pusher"
Original UK airdates:
Sky One: June 25, 1996
BBC 1: to be scheduled

Episode 3.18
"Teso dos Bichos"
Original UK airdates:
Sky One: July 2, 1996
BBC 1: to be scheduled

Episode 3.19
"Hell Money"
Original UK airdates:
Sky One: July 9, 1996
BBC 1: to be scheduled

Episode 3.20
"Jose Chung's *From Outer Space*"
Original UK airdates:
Sky One: July 16, 1996
BBC 1: to be scheduled

Episode 3.21
"Avatar"
Original UK airdates:
Sky One: July 23, 1996
BBC 1: to be scheduled

Episode 3.22
"Quagmire"
Original UK airdates:
Sky One: July 30, 1996
BBC 1: to be scheduled

Episode 3.23
"Wetwired"
Original UK airdates:
Sky One: August 6, 1996
BBC 1: to be scheduled

Episode 3.24
"Talitha Cumi"
Original UK airdates:
Sky One: August 13, 1996
BBC 1: to be scheduled